DIET TRENDS MAY COME AND GO, BUT ONE FORMULA REMAINS THE SAME: EXTRA CALORIES = UNWANTED POUNDS

Today, many people believe that watching fat intake is all that matters. While that is important, we may overlook the fact that extra calories—even from low-fat and fat-free foods—put on pounds. Even in our fat-conscious age, many Americans are eating more calories than they require, and are putting their health and lives at risk.

This revised second edition of *THE CALORIE COUNTER* follows in the tradition of the entire bestselling Counter series from Annette Natow and Jo-Ann Heslin. Rely on this handy guide from the nutrition experts for counting calories safely and wisely. Look inside to determine an estimated daily calorie intake for your body and lifestyle—then turn to *THE CALORIE COUNTER* for up-to-date, comprehensive listings of thousands of foods, as well as tips on weight control and everyday healthy living.

Annette B. Natow, Ph.D., R.D., and Jo-Ann Heslin, M.A., R.D., are the authors of twenty-six books on nutrition. Both are former faculty members of Adelphi University and the State University of New York, Downstate Medical Center. They are editors of the *Journal of Nutrition for the Elderly*, and serve as editorial board members for the *Environmental Nutrition Newsletter*.

Books by Annette B. Natow and Jo-Ann Heslin

The Antioxidant Vitamin Counter
Calcium Counts
The Calorie Counter (Second Edition)
The Cholesterol Counter (Fifth Edition)
Count on a Healthy Pregnancy
The Diabetes Carbohydrate and Calorie Counter
Eating Out Food Counter
The Fat Attack Plan
The Fat Counter (Fourth Edition)
The Food Shopping Counter
Megadoses
The Most Complete Food Counter
No-Nonsense Nutrition for Kids
The Pocket Encyclopedia of Nutrition
The Pocket Fat Counter (Second Edition)
The Pocket Protein Counter
The Pregnancy Nutrition Counter
The Protein Counter
The Sodium Counter
Published by POCKET BOOKS

For information regarding special discounts for bulk purchases, please contact Simon & Schuster Special Sales at 1-800-456-6798 or business@simonandschuster.com

THE
CALORIE
COUNTER

SECOND EDITION
REVISED AND UPDATED

Annette B. Natow, Ph.D., R.D.
and **Jo-Ann Heslin, M.A., R.D.**

POCKET BOOKS
New York   London   Toronto   Sydney   Singapore

An *Original* Publication of POCKET BOOKS

POCKET BOOKS, a division of Simon & Schuster Inc.
1230 Avenue of the Americas, New York, NY 10020

Copyright © 2000 by Annette Natow and Jo-Ann Heslin

All rights reserved, including the right to reproduce
this book or portions thereof in any form whatsoever.
For information address Pocket Books, 1230 Avenue
of the Americas, New York, NY 10020

ISBN: 0-671-02564-3

First Pocket Books printing April 2000

10   9   8   7

POCKET and colophon are registered trademarks of
Simon & Schuster Inc.

Cover photo by Thomas Francisco/FoodPix

Printed in the U.S.A.

_____

To our families who support us through every project: Harry, Allen, Irene, Sarah, Meryl, Laura, Marty, George, Emily, Steven, Joe, Kristen, Brian and Karen

ACKNOWLEDGMENTS

Without the tireless cooperation of Steven Natow, M.D., and Stephen Llano, *The Calorie Counter* would never have been completed. Our thanks to all the food manufacturers and processors who shared product information. A special thanks to our insightful and supportive agent, Nancy Trichter, and our wonderfully perceptive editor, Jane Cavolina.

"Man is to be compared to a clock, going all the time, rather than to an automobile engine, working only at intervals. . . . In order to have energy to spend . . . we must first acquire it . . . protein, fat and carbohydrate . . . are the fuels which supply energy for the human machine."

MARY SWARTZ ROSE, PH.D.
Feeding the Family
The Macmillan Company, 1919

INTRODUCTION

Regardless of what you hear from experts or read in the newspaper CALORIES STILL COUNT.

The correct message is simple: EXCESS CALORIES PUT ON POUNDS. Every 3500 calories you eat that you don't use to keep your body going wind up being stored as one pound of fat. This message got muddied lately as a lot of emphasis was put on reducing fat. The implication was that if you were careful about how much fat you ate, you could forget about calories. That simply is not true. CALORIES COUNT. Over the last ten years fat consumption has been going down steadily and at the same time weight keeps going up. One third of Americans are overweight—8 percent more than a decade ago. A study from the National Institutes of Health shows that Americans aged 25 to 30 now weigh an average of 171 pounds, up from 161 pounds in 1986.

While reducing the fat you eat is good advice to keep you healthy, you cannot disregard the total number of calories you eat if you want to maintain or get to your best weight. Some lowfat foods and even some foods labeled reduced fat still contain lots of calories. Eating too much of them will sabotage your efforts to stay at your best weight. This is where *The Calorie Counter* will help. In it you'll find calorie counts for more than 20,000 foods, so that you can easily find out how many calories are in the foods you eat.

CALORIES—CAUTION: Americans are eating 230 calories more each day than they did in 1978. These calories add up!

Eating too many calories can make you fat and that can increase your risk for:

heart attack
stroke
high blood pressure
high blood cholesterol and triglyceride levels
diabetes
some cancers
gall bladder disease
gout
hiatus hernia
indigestion
osteoarthritis
foot problems
surgery complications
sleep apnea (short periods of not breathing while sleeping)

How many calories do you need? It depends on your best weight.

1. How to find your best weight

You can always look at one of those height/weight charts. But which one? There are several, and experts don't agree on which one is best to use. One simple approach is to use your weight in your early twenties as a benchmark. If your weight was normal then, that's a good weight to maintain for the rest of your life, if you can. Still another easy and reliable way to estimate your best weight is to use this simple formula.

Women: Give yourself 100 pounds for the first 5 feet of

WHAT IS A CALORIE?

The number of calories in a food is determined by burning the food. The amount of heat produced by the burning food is measured and converted into calories. The same thing happens when food is used or "burned" in your body—it gives off heat. By measuring the amount of heat given off, the calorie cost of keeping the body going can be measured. That's also how the number of calories used up in jogging, bicycling, cleaning house and other activities is measured. Americans, on average, consume 2,095 calories a day. Men eat more: 2,478 calories; women less: 1,732 calories.

your height and add 5 pounds for each additional inch over 5 feet (or subtract 5 pounds for each inch under 5 feet). For example, if you're 5 feet, 4 inches tall:

    100 pounds (for first 5 feet)
    <u>+ 20 pounds</u> (4 additional inches times 5 pounds each)
    120 pounds is your best weight

Men: Give yourself 106 pounds for the first 5 feet of your height and add 6 pounds for each additional inch over 5 feet (or subtract 6 pounds for each inch under 5 feet). For example, if you're 5 feet, 9 inches tall:

    106 pounds (for the first 5 feet)
    <u>+ 54 pounds</u> (9 additional inches times 6 pounds each)
    160 pounds is your best weight

2. How many calories do you need to maintain or to reach your best weight?

You can make a pretty good estimate of the number of calories you need every day once you have figured out your

CALORIES IN FOOD

Practically everything you eat and drink contains calories, except for water. The carbohydrate, protein and fat in foods supply the calories. Carbohydrate and protein each contain 4 calories in a gram (about ¼ of a teaspoon), while fat has more than double that amount—9 calories in a gram.

For example, a teaspoon of sugar, all carbohydrate, or unsweetened gelatin, all protein, has 16 calories, while a teaspoon of oil, all fat, has 40 calories.

It follows that foods that are high in fat contain more calories than foods that are high in carbohydrate or protein. On the other hand, foods that are high in water and indigestible fiber, like vegetables and fruits, have fewer calories.

It gets complicated because most foods and drinks are combinations of carbohydrate, protein, fat, water and, often, fiber, so the best way for you to find out how many calories are in a specific food is to look it up in *The Calorie Counter.*

best weight The more active you are, the more calories you need:

    13 calories a pound if you are not very active
    15 calories a pound if you are moderately active
    17 calories a pound if you are very active
    20 calories a pound if you are extremely active

For example, if you are moderately active and your best weight is 145 pounds, you need 2,175 calories a day to maintain your weight (145 × 15 calories = 2,175 calories).

BODY MASS INDEX (BMI)

BMI is often used to determine if a person is overweight. Weight and height are calculated together to estimate body fat.

To figure your BMI:

1. Multiply your weight in pounds by 700.
2. Divide that number by height in inches.
3. Then divide that result by height in inches again.

Desirable body fat levels increase as people age. An easy rule of thumb you can use as a guide is: a person is overweight with a BMI of 25 to 30. A BMI of more than 30 indicates obesity.

You can see that calories and activity go hand in hand. The more active you are, the more calories you use up. And you don't have to run in a marathon to make this work for you. New research points to the value of moderate activity in improving health and fitness besides using up calories. A paper published by a group of twenty health and fitness experts in the *Journal of the American Medical Association* recommends that every American adult accumulate thirty minutes or more of moderate intensity physical activity every day. This includes walking, climbing stairs, gardening or even cleaning house. And the thirty minutes do not have to be done all at once. Activity throughout the day adds up. In the words of former United States Surgeon General C. Everett Koop, "Just get off your seat and on your feet."

If you are very inactive, spending as little as 500 extra calories a week in added activity can provide some health benefits. Adding 1,000 calories worth of moderate activity a week gives you even more. Experts advise aiming for activities using up 2,000 calories or more each week. Two hours of tennis and three hours of walking use up about 2,000 calories. While five hours of housework will burn 1,000 calories. Use the table "Calories Used in 30 Minutes of Activity" to find out how many calories you are using up.

CALORIES USED IN 30 MINUTES OF ACTIVITY

Activity	130 Pounds	180 Pounds
Archery	139	193
Baseball, infield/outfield	122	168
Basketball	182	252
Bicycling, 5 miles per hour (level)	75	105
Bowling	105	147
Canoeing, 4 miles per hour	182	252
Dancing		
moderate	109	150
vigorous	148	204
Fencing	130	180
Football	129	130
Golf		
foursome	105	146
twosome	141	195
Handball	254	351
Hiking	177	246
Hockey		
field	237	336
ice	261	363
Horseback riding		
walk	85	117
trot	176	243
Ice skating	148	205
Judo	332	459
Karate	332	459

Activity	130 Pounds	180 Pounds
Motorcycling	95	131
Mountain climbing	261	362
Paddle ball	225	312
Playing cards	51	69
Pool	57	81
Roller blading	165	228
Rowing machine	356	498
Running		
5.5 miles per hour	280	387
7 miles per hour	348	482
Sculling	356	492
Skiing		
downhill	251	347
cross country	305	422
Soccer	233	322
Square dancing	177	246
Squash	135	187
Swimming		
backstroke	98	135
breaststroke	124	171
crawl	125	173
Tennis	181	250
Volleyball	148	205
Walking		
2 miles per hour	91	126
4.5 miles per hour	172	239
downstairs	173	239
upstairs	452	626
Water skiing	203	282
Weight training	204	282
Wrestling	332	459

KEEP MOVING—IT ADDS UP:

Take the stairs, instead of an elevator
Park your car at the far end of the parking lot
For short errands, walk instead of taking the car
When you have just a few dishes, wash them by hand
Use hand power instead of electric appliances when beating, mixing, slicing food or opening cans

USING YOUR CALORIE COUNTER

This book lists the calorie content of over 20,000 foods. Now you can compare the calorie values of your favorite foods and choose substitutes for them before you go out to shop or to eat. This will help you save time while making choices when you are deciding what to buy or eat.

The Calorie Counter lists foods alphabetically. For each category, you will find nonbranded (generic) foods listed first, in alphabetical order, followed by an alphabetical listing of brand-name foods. The nonbranded listing will help you determine calorie values for foods when you do not find your favorite brand listed. They also help you to evaluate generic and store brands. Large categories are divided into subcategories such as canned, dried, fresh and frozen to make it easier to find what you are looking for. The book is divided into two parts—Part One: Brand-Name, Nonbranded and Take-Out Foods, and Part Two: Restaurant Foods. Part Two will help you estimate the calories in restaurant foods.

Most foods are listed alphabetically. But, in some cases, foods are grouped by category. For example, a chicken stir fry and chicken salad are found under the category CHICKEN DISHES. Other group categories include:

DEFINITIONS

as prep (as prepared): refers to food that has been prepared according to package directions

home recipe: describes homemade dishes; those included can be used as a guide to the calorie values of similar products you may prepare or take-out food you buy ready to eat

lean and fat: describes meat with some fat on its edges that is not cut away before cooking or poultry prepared with skin and fat as purchased

lean only: lean portion, trimmed of all visible fat

shelf stable: refers to prepared products found on the supermarket shelf that are ready to eat or to be heated and do not require refrigeration

take-out: describes prepared dishes that you purchase ready to eat; those included serve as a guide to the calorie values of similar products you may purchase

ABBREVIATIONS:

avg	=	average
diam	=	diameter
fl	=	fluid
frzn	=	frozen
g	=	gram
in	=	inch
lb	=	pound
lg	=	large
med	=	medium
mg	=	milligram
oz	=	ounce
pkg	=	package
prep	=	prepared
pt	=	pint
qt	=	quart
reg	=	regular
sec	=	second
serv	=	serving
sm	=	small
sq	=	square
tbsp	=	tablespoon
tr	=	trace
tsp	=	teaspoon
w/	=	with
w/o	=	without
<	=	less than

EQUIVALENT MEASURES

3 teaspoons	=	1 tablespoon
4 tablespoons	=	¼ cup
8 tablespoons	=	½ cup
12 tablespoons	=	¾ cup
16 tablespoons	=	1 cup
1000 milligrams	=	1 gram
28 grams	=	1 ounce

LIQUID MEASUREMENTS

2 tablespoons	=	1 ounce
2 ounces	=	¼ cup
4 ounces	=	½ cup
6 ounces	=	¾ cup
8 ounces	=	1 cup
2 cups	=	1 pint
4 cups	=	1 quart

DRY MEASUREMENTS

4 ounces	=	¼ pound
8 ounces	=	½ pound
12 ounces	=	¾ pound
16 ounces	=	1 pound

NOTES

Discrepancies in figures are due to rounding, product reformulation and reevaluation. Labeling law allows rounding of values. Because most of the data is analysis data, obtained directly from manufacturers, not from labels, in some cases our values may not be exactly the same as label information because they have not been rounded.

PART ONE

BRAND NAME, NONBRANDED AND TAKE-OUT FOODS

FOOD	PORTION	CALS.
ABALONE		
fresh fried	3 oz	161
ACEROLA		
fresh	1	2
ACEROLA JUICE		
juice	1 cup	51
ADZUKI BEANS		
Eden		
Organic	½ cup (4.6 oz)	110
ALE		
(*see* BEER AND ALE, and MALT)		
ALFALFA		
sprouts	1 tbsp	1
ALLSPICE		
ground	1 tsp	5
ALMONDS		
almond butter honey & cinnamon	1 tbsp	96
almond butter w/ salt	1 tbsp	101
almond butter w/o salt	1 tbsp	101
almond paste	1 oz	127
jordan almonds	10 (1.4 oz)	190
Beer Nuts		
Almonds	1 pkg (1 oz)	180
Dole		
Blanched Slivered	1 oz	170
Blanched Whole	1 oz	170
Chopped Natural	1 oz	170
Sliced Natural	1 oz	170
Whole Natural	1 oz	170
Hain		
Almond Butter Natural Raw	2 tbsp	190
Almond Butter Toasted	2 tbsp	220
Nutella		
Spread	1 tbsp (0.5 oz)	85
Planters		
Almonds	1 oz	170
Gold Measure Slivered	1 pkg (2 oz)	340
Honey Roasted	1 oz	160
AMARANTH		
(*see also* CEREAL, COOKIES)		
uncooked	1 cup (6.8 oz)	729

FOOD	PORTION	CALS.
Arrowhead		
Seeds	¼ cup (1.6 oz)	170
ANASAZI BEANS		
Arrowhead		
Dried	¼ cup (1.5 oz)	150
Bean Cuisine		
Dried	½ cup	115
ANCHOVY		
CANNED		
in oil	5	42
in oil	1 can (1.6 oz)	95
FRESH		
fillets	3 (0.4 oz)	21
ANISE		
seed	1 tsp	7
ANTELOPE		
roasted	3 oz	127
APPLE		
DRIED		
rings	10	155
Del Monte		
Sliced	⅓ cup (1.4 oz)	80
Sonoma		
Pieces	10-12 pieces (1.4 oz)	110
FRESH		
apple	1	81
w/o skin sliced	1 cup	62
w/o skin sliced & cooked	1 cup	91
Cool Cut		
Apples & Caramel Dip	1 pkg (4.25 oz)	180
Dole		
Apple	1	80
Tastee		
Candy Apple	1 (3 oz)	160
Caramel Apple	1 (3 oz)	160
FROZEN		
Stouffer's		
Escalloped	1 cup (6 oz)	180
APPLE JUICE		
After The Fall		
Organic	1 bottle (10 oz)	110

FOOD	PORTION	CALS.
After The Fall (CONT.)		
Vermont Apple	1 bottle (10 oz)	110
Vermont Apple	1 bottle (8 oz)	90
Vermont Harvest Moon Sparkling Apple Cider	8 fl oz	110
Apple & Eve		
Cider	6 fl oz	80
Juice	6 fl oz	80
Nothin' But Juice	6 fl oz	78
Everfresh		
Apple Juice	1 can (8 oz)	110
Hi-C		
Jammin' Apple	8 fl oz	130
Hood		
Select Cider	1 cup (8 oz)	120
Minute Maid		
Box	8.45 fl oz	120
Juices To Go	1 can (11.5 fl oz)	160
Juices To Go	1 bottle (10 fl oz)	140
Juices To Go	1 bottle (16 fl oz)	110
Naturals	8 fl oz	110
Mott's		
From Concentrate as prep	8 fl oz	120
Fruit Basket Cocktail as prep	8 fl oz	120
Natural	8 fl oz	120
Ocean Spray		
100% Juice	8 fl oz	110
Odwalla		
Live Apple	8 fl oz	140
Red Cheek		
From Concentrate	8 fl oz	120
Natural	8 fl oz	120
Seneca		
Clarified frzn, as prep	8 fl oz	120
Granny Smith frzn as prep	8 fl oz	120
Natural frzn as prep	8 fl oz	120
Sippin' Pak		
100% Pure	8.45 fl oz	110
Snapple		
Apple Crisp	10 fl oz	140
Tree Of Life		
East Coast Apple	8 fl oz	120
Tropicana		
Season's Best	8 oz	110

FOOD	PORTION	CALS.
Veryfine		
100% Juice	1 bottle (10 oz)	150
Juice-Ups	8 fl oz	120

APPLESAUCE
Mott's

Chunky	5 oz	110
Cinnamon	5 oz	120
Fruit Snacks Apple Spice	4 oz	70
Fruit Snacks Cinnamon	4 oz	90
Fruit Snacks Sweetened	4 oz	90
Sweetened	5 oz	110
Seneca		
Cinnamon	½ cup	100
Golden Delicious	½ cup	100
McIntosh	½ cup	100
Natural	½ cup	60
Regular	½ cup	100
Tree Of Life		
Applesauce	½ cup (4.3 oz)	50
White House		
Chunky	4 oz	80

APRICOT JUICE

nectar	1 cup	141
Del Monte		
Nectar	8 fl oz	140
Kern's		
Nectar	6 fl oz	110
Libby		
Nectar	1 can (11.5 fl oz)	220

APRICOTS
CANNED

halves heavy syrup pack w/ skin	1 cup (9.1 oz)	214
halves water pack w/ skin	1 cup (8.5 oz)	65
halves water pack w/o skin	1 cup (8 oz)	51
puree from heavy syrup pack w/ skin	¾ cup (9.1 oz)	214
puree from light pack w/ skin	¾ cup (8.9 oz)	160
puree from water pack w/ skin	¾ cup (8.5 oz)	65
puree juice pack w/ skin	1 cup (8.7 oz)	119
Del Monte		
Halves Unpeeled In Heavy Syrup	½ cup (4.5 oz)	100
Halves Unpeeled Lite	½ cup (4.3 oz)	60
Libby		
Halves Unpeeled Lite	½ cup (4.4 oz)	60

FOOD	PORTION	CALS.
DRIED		
halves	10	83
Del Monte		
Sun Dried	⅓ cup (1.4 oz)	80
Sonoma		
Dried	10 pieces (1.4 oz)	120
FRESH		
apricots	3	51
ARROWHEAD		
fresh boiled	1 med (⅓ oz)	9
ARROWROOT		
flour	1 cup (4.5 oz)	457
ARTICHOKE		
CANNED		
Progresso		
Hearts	2 pieces (2.9 oz)	35
Hearts Marinated	⅓ cup (3 oz)	160
FRESH		
boiled	1 med (4 oz)	60
hearts cooked	½ cup	42
Dole		
Large Whole	1	23
ARUGULA		
raw	½ cup	2
ASIAN FOOD		
(*see also* DINNER, EGG ROLLS, PASTA, SUSHI)		
CANNED		
chow mein chicken	1 cup	95
FRESH		
wonton wrappers	1	23
FROZEN		
Banquet		
Chow Mein Chicken	1 pkg (9 oz)	400
Birds Eye		
Easy Recipe Meal Starter Oriental Stir Fry as prep	1 serv	280
Easy Recipe Meal Starter Spicy Asian	1 serv	280
Easy Recipe Meal Starter Teriyaki Stir Fry as prep	1 serv	280
Chun King		
Beef Pepper Steak	1 pkg (13 oz)	300

FOOD	PORTION	CALS.
Chun King (CONT.)		
Chow Mein Chicken	1 pkg (13 oz)	370
Imperial Chicken	1 pkg (13 oz)	460
Sweet & Sour Pork	1 pkg (13 oz)	450
Walnut Chicken	1 pkg (13 oz)	460
Green Giant		
Create A Meal LoMein Stir Fry as prep	1¼ cups (10 oz)	320
Create A Meal Sweet & Sour Stir Fry as prep	1¼ cups (10 oz)	290
Create A Meal Szechuan Stir Fry as prep	1¼ cups (10 oz)	340
Create A Meal Teriyaki Stir Fry as prep	1¼ cups (10 oz)	240
Lean Cuisine		
Chicken Chow Mein With Rice	1 pkg (9 oz)	220
Chicken Oriental w/ Vegetables & Vermicelli	1 pkg (9 oz)	250
Oriental Style Dumplings	1 pkg (9 oz)	300
Teriyaki Stir Fry	1 pkg (10 oz)	290
Luigino's		
Chicken & Almonds With Rice	1 pkg (8 oz)	250
Chop Suey Pork With Rice	1 pkg (8.5 oz)	210
Lo Mein Chicken	1 pkg (8 oz)	320
Lo Mein Shrimp	1 pkg (8 oz)	190
Oriental Beef & Peppers With Rice	1 pkg (8 oz)	230
Pasta Favorites		
Chicken Lo Mein	1 pkg (10.5 oz)	270
Rice Gourmet		
Chicken Teriyaki Rice Bowl	1 bowl (10.9 oz)	430
Stouffer's		
Chicken Chow Mein w/ Rice	1 pkg (10.6 oz)	260
Tyson		
Stir Fry Kit With Yoshida Oriental Sauce	10.6 oz	330
Sweet & Sour Kit With Sweet & Sour Sauce	14.85 oz	440
Weight Watchers		
Smart Ones Chicken Chow Mein	1 pkg (9 oz)	200
Smart Ones Hunan Style Rice & Vegetables	1 pkg (10.34 oz)	280
Smart Ones King Pao Noodles & Vegetables	1 pkg (10 oz)	250
Smart Ones Spicy Szechaun Style Vegetables & Chicken	1 pkg (9 oz)	220
READY-TO-EAT		
shrimp chips	1¼ cups (1 oz)	140

FOOD	PORTION	CALS.
TAKE-OUT		
Sesame Seed Paste Bun	1 (2.5 oz)	220
cha siu bao steamed buns w/ chicken filling	1 (2.3 oz)	160
chicken teriyaki w/ rice	1 serv (11 oz)	430
chop suey w/ beef & pork	1 cup	300
chow mein chicken	1 cup	255
chow mein vegetable	1 serv (8 oz)	90
shu mai chicken & vegetable dumplings	6 (3.6 oz)	160
spring roll	1 (3.5 oz)	112
sweet & sour pork	1 serv (8 oz)	250
sweet red bean bun	1 (2.5 oz)	130
szechuan chicken w/ lo mein	1 cup (5.3 oz)	190
ASPARAGUS		
CANNED		
Del Monte		
Salad Tips Tender Green	½ cup (4.4 oz)	20
Spears Cut Tender Green	½ cup (4.4 oz)	20
Spears Extra Long Tender Green	½ cup (4.4 oz)	20
Spears Tender Green	½ cup (4.4 oz)	20
Tips Tender Green	½ cup (4.4 oz)	20
Green Giant		
Cut Spears	½ cup (4.2 oz)	20
Cut Spears 50% Less Sodium	½ cup (4.2 oz)	20
Extra Long Spears	4.5 oz	20
Spears	4.5 oz	20
LeSueur		
Spears Extra Large	4.5 oz	20
Seneca		
Asparagus	½ cup	20
FRESH		
cooked	4 spears	14
Dole		
Spears	5	18
FROZEN		
Big Valley		
Spears	5-6 (3 oz)	20
Green Giant		
Harvest Fresh Cuts	⅔ cup (3 oz)	25
ATEMOYA		
fresh	½ cup	94
AVOCADO		
FRESH		
avocado	1	324
mashed	1 cup	370

FOOD	PORTION	CALS.

BACON
(*see also* BACON SUBSTITUTES)

FOOD	PORTION	CALS.
breakfast strips cooked	3 strips	156
pan fried	3 strips	109
Black Label		
Center Cut cooked	3 slices (0.5 oz)	70
Cooked	2 slices (0.5 oz)	80
Low Salt cooked	2 slices (0.5 oz)	80
Hillshire		
Bacon	1 slice	120
Hormel		
Bacon Bits	1 tbsp (7 g)	30
Bacon Pieces	1 tbsp (7 g)	25
Microwave cooked	2 slices (0.5 oz)	70
Old Smokehouse		
Cooked	2 slices (0.5 oz)	80
Oscar Mayer		
Bacon Bits	1 tbsp (0.2 oz)	25
Bacon Pieces	1 tbsp (0.2 oz)	25
Center Cut cooked	2 slices (0.4 oz)	70
Cooked	2 slices (0.5 oz)	70
Lower Sodium cooked	2 slices (0.5 oz)	70
Thick Cut cooked	1 slice (0.4 oz)	60
Range Brand		
Cooked	2 slices (0.7 oz)	100
Red Label		
Cooked	2 slices (0.5 oz)	80
Shannon		
Irish	1 oz	70

BACON SUBSTITUTES

FOOD	PORTION	CALS.
bacon substitute	1 strip	25
Bac-Os		
Chips or Bits	1½ tbsp (7 g)	30
Harvest Direct		
Bacon Bits	3.5 oz	320
Lightlife		
Fakin' Bacon	3 strips (2 oz)	79
Louis Rich		
Turkey Bacon	1 slice (0.5 oz)	35
McCormick		
Bac'n Pieces	2 tsp	20
Morningstar Farms		
Breakfast Strips	2 (0.5 oz)	60

FOOD	PORTION	CALS.
Mr. Turkey		
Slice	1	25
Worthington		
Stripples	2 strips (0.5 oz)	60
BAGEL		
FRESH		
cinnamon raisin	1 (3½ in)	194
cinnamon raisin toasted	1 (3½ in)	194
egg	1 (3½ in)	197
egg toasted	1 (3½ in)	197
oat bran	1 (3½ in)	181
oat bran toasted	1 (3½ in)	181
onion	1 (3½ in)	195
plain	1 (3½ in)	195
plain toasted	1 (3½ in)	195
poppy seed	1 (3½ in)	195
Alvarado St. Bakery		
Sprouted Wheat	1 (3.3 oz)	260
Sprouted Wheat Cinnamon/Raisin	1 (3.3 oz)	280
Sprouted Wheat Onion/Poppyseed	1 (3.3 oz)	320
Sprouted Wheat Sesame	1 (3.3 oz)	320
Uncle B's		
Plain	1 (2.8 oz)	210
Wonder		
Blueberry	1 (3 oz)	210
Cinnamon Raisin	1 (3 oz)	210
Onion	1 (3 oz)	210
Plain	1 (3 oz)	210
Rye	1 (3 oz)	220
Wheat	1 (3 oz)	210
FROZEN		
Amy's Organic		
Cinnamon Raisin	1 (3.5 oz)	240
Plain	1 (3.5 oz)	230
Poppy Seed	1 (3.5 oz)	230
Sesame	1 (3.5 oz)	240
Otis Spunkmeyer		
Barnstormin' Blueberry	1 (3.6 oz)	250
Barnstormin' Cinnamon Raisin	1 (3.6 oz)	230
Barnstormin' Onion	1 (3.6 oz)	230
Barnstormin' Plain	1 (3.6 oz)	240
Sara Lee		
Blueberry	1 (2.8 oz)	210

FOOD	PORTION	CALS.
Sara Lee (CONT.)		
Cinnamon Raisin	1 (2.8 oz)	220
Egg	1 (2.8 oz)	210
Oat Bran	1 (2.8 oz)	210
Onion	1 (2.8 oz)	210
Plain	1 (2.8 oz)	210
Poppy Seed	1 (2.8 oz)	210
Sesame Seed	1 (2.8 oz)	210
Tree Of Life		
Onion	1 (3 oz)	210
Plain	1 (3 oz)	210
Poppy	1 (3 oz)	210
Raisin	1 (3 oz)	210
Sesame	1 (3 oz)	210

BAKING POWDER

FOOD	PORTION	CALS.
baking powder	1 tsp	2
low sodium	1 tsp	5
Calumet		
Baking Powder	¼ tsp (1 g)	0
Clabber Girl		
Baking Powder	1 tsp	0
Davis		
Baking Powder	1 tsp	6
Watkins		
Baking Powder	¼ tsp (1 g)	0

BAKING SODA

FOOD	PORTION	CALS.
baking soda	1 tsp	0
Arm & Hammer		
Baking Soda	1 tsp	0

BALSAM PEAR

FOOD	PORTION	CALS.
leafy tips cooked	½ cup	10
pods cooked	½ cup	12

BANANA

FOOD	PORTION	CALS.
banana chips	1 oz	147
fresh	1	105
powder	1 tbsp	21
Dole		
Fresh	1	120
Rainforest Farms		
Slices Dried	5 slices (1.3 oz)	60

FOOD	PORTION	CALS.
BANANA JUICE		
Libby		
Nectar	1 can (11.5 fl oz)	190
BARBECUE SAUCE		
(*see also* SAUCE)		
Hain		
Honey	1 tbsp	14
Healthy Choice		
Hickory	2 tbsp (1.1 oz)	26
Hot & Spicy	2 tbsp (1.1 oz)	25
Original	2 tbsp (1.1 oz)	25
House Of Tsang		
Hong Kong	1 tbsp (0.6 oz)	10
Hunt's		
Barbeque	¼ cup (2.2 oz)	57
Bold Hickory	2 tbsp (1.2 oz)	47
Bold Original	2 tbsp (1.2 oz)	46
Hickory	2 tbsp (1.2 oz)	38
Hickory & Brown Sugar	2 tbsp (1.3 oz)	75
Honey Hickory	2 tbsp (1.2 oz)	38
Honey Mustard	2 tbsp (1.2 oz)	48
Hot & Spicy	2 tbsp (1.2 oz)	48
Light	2 tbsp (1.2 oz)	23
Mesquite Barbecue	2 tbsp (1.2 oz)	40
Mild	2 tbsp (1.2 oz)	41
Mild Dijon	2 tbsp (1.2 oz)	39
Original	2 tbsp (1.2 oz)	39
Teriyaki	2 tbsp (1.2 oz)	46
Kraft		
Char-Grill	2 tbsp (1.3 oz)	60
Extra Rich Original	2 tbsp (1.2 oz)	50
Hickory Smoke	2 tbsp (1.2 oz)	40
Hickory Smoke Onion Bits	2 tbsp (1.2 oz)	45
Honey	2 tbsp (1.3 oz)	50
Honey Hickory	2 tbsp (1.3 oz)	60
Honey Mustard	2 tbsp (1.3 oz)	60
Hot	2 tbsp (1.2 oz)	40
Hot Hickory Smoke	2 tbsp (1.2 oz)	40
Kansas City Style	2 tbsp (1.2 oz)	50
Mesquite Smoke	2 tbsp (1.2 oz)	40
Molasses	2 tbsp (1.3 oz)	70
Onion Bits	2 tbsp (1.2 oz)	45
Original	2 tbsp (1.2 oz)	40

FOOD	PORTION	CALS.
Kraft (CONT.)		
Roasted Garlic	2 tbsp (1.2 oz)	50
Spicy Honey	2 tbsp (1.3 oz)	60
Teriyaki	2 tbsp (1.3 oz)	60
Thick 'N Spicy Brown Sugar	2 tbsp (1.2 oz)	60
Thick 'N Spicy Hickory Bacon	2 tbsp (1.2 oz)	60
Thick 'N Spicy Hickory Smoke	2 tbsp (1.2 oz)	50
Thick 'N Spicy Honey	2 tbsp (1.3 oz)	60
Thick 'N Spicy Honey Mustard	2 tbsp (1.3 oz)	60
Thick'N Spicy Hickory Smoke	2 tbsp (1.2 oz)	50
Thick'N Spicy Honey	2 tbsp (1.2 oz)	60
Thick'N Spicy Kansas City Style	2 tbsp (1.3 oz)	60
Thick'N Spicy Mesquite Smoke	2 tbsp (1.2 oz)	50
Thick'N Spicy Original	2 tbsp (1.2 oz)	50
Lawry's		
Dijon Honey	¼ cup	203
McIlhenny		
Sauce	2 tbsp (1.1 oz)	70
Red Wing		
"K" Sauce	2 tbsp (1.2 oz)	45
Watkins		
Bold	2 tsp (0.4 oz)	25
Honey	2 tsp (0.4 oz)	25
Mesquite	2 tsp (0.4 oz)	25
Original	2 tsp (0.4 oz)	25
Smokehouse	2 tsp (0.4 oz)	25
BARLEY		
flour	1 cup (5.2 oz)	511
malt flour	1 cup (5.7 oz)	585
pearled cooked	1 cup (5.5 oz)	193
pearled uncooked	1 cup (7 oz)	704
Arrowhead		
Barley	¼ cup (1.7 oz)	170
Hulless	¼ cup (1.6 oz)	140
BASIL		
fresh chopped	2 tbsp	1
leaves fresh	5	1
Watkins		
Liquid Spice	1 tbsp (0.5 oz)	120
BASS		
freshwater raw	3 oz	97
sea cooked	3 oz	105

FOOD	PORTION	CALS.
sea raw	3 oz	82
striped baked	3 oz	105

BAY LEAF

crumbled	1 tsp	2
Watkins		
Bay Leaves	¼ tsp (0.5 g)	0

BEANS

(*see also individual bean names*)

CANNED

Allen

Baked	½ cup (4.5 oz)	150
B&M		
99% Fat Free Baked Beans	½ cup (4.6 oz)	160
Baked With Honey	½ cup (4.7 oz)	170
Barbeque Baked Beans	½ cup (4.7 oz)	170
Brick Oven Baked	½ cup (4.6 oz)	180
Extra Hearty Baked	½ cup (4.6 oz)	190
Brown Beauty		
Mexican Beans With Jalapeno	½ cup (4.5 oz)	120
Bush's		
Baked	½ cup (4.6 oz)	150
Baked With Onions	½ cup (4.6 oz)	150
Homestyle Baked	½ cup (4.6 oz)	160
Vegetarian	½ cup (4.6 oz)	140
Chi-Chi's		
Refried	½ cup (4.2 oz)	100
Refried Beans Fat Free	½ cup (4.2 oz)	120
Refried Beans Vegetarian	½ cup (4.2 oz)	100
Crest Top		
Pork And Beans	½ cup (4.5 oz)	130
Eden		
Organic Baked w/ Sweet Sorghum & Orangic Mustard	½ cup (4.6 oz)	150
Friend's		
Maple Baked	8 oz	240
Original Baked	½ cup (4.6 oz)	170
Green Giant		
Pork And Beans w/ Tomato Sauce	½ cup (4.5 oz)	120
Spicy Chili	½ cup (4.5 oz)	110
Three Bean Salad	½ cup (4.2 oz)	90
Health Valley		
Honey Baked	½ cup	110

FOOD	PORTION	CALS.
Heartland		
Iron Kettle Baked	½ cup (4.6 oz)	150
Hormel		
Beans & Wieners	1 can (7.5 oz)	290
Hunt's		
Big John's Beans & Fixin's	½ cup (4.7 oz)	127
Pork & Beans	½ cup (4.5 oz)	130
Kid's Kitchen		
Microwave Meals Beans & Wieners	1 cup (7.5 oz)	310
Little Pancho		
Refried & Green Chili	½ cup	80
McIlhenny		
Spicy	1 oz	7
Old El Paso		
Mexe-Beans	½ cup (4.6 oz)	110
Refried	½ cup (4.2 oz)	110
Refried Fat Free	½ cup (4.4 oz)	110
Refried Spicy	½ cup (4.3 oz)	140
Refried Vegetarian	½ cup (4.1 oz)	100
Refried With Cheese	½ cup (4.2 oz)	130
Refried With Green Chilies	½ cup (4.3 oz)	110
Refried With Sausage	½ cup (4.1 oz)	200
S&W		
Barbecue Beans Ranch Recipe	½ cup (4.5 oz)	100
Taco Bell		
Home Originals Fat Free Refried Beans	½ cup (4.6 oz)	110
Home Originals Fat Free Refried Beans w/ Mild Chilies	½ cup (4.5 oz)	110
Home Originals Refried Beans	½ cup (4.7 oz)	140
Trappey		
Mexi-Beans With Jalapeno	½ cup (4.5 oz)	130
Pork And Beans	½ cup (4.5 oz)	110
Pork And Beans With Jalapeno	½ cup (4.5 oz)	130
Van Camp's		
Baked Beans Fat Free	½ cup (4.6 oz)	130
Baked Beans Premium	½ cup (4.6 oz)	140
Beanee Weenee	1 cup (9 oz)	320
Beanee Weenee Baked Flavor	1 cup (9 oz)	410
Beanee Weenee Barbeque	1 cup (9 oz)	340
Brown Sugar Beans	½ cup (4.6 oz)	170
Mexican Style Chili Beans	½ cup (4.6 oz)	110
Pork And Beans	½ cup (4.6 oz)	110
Vegetarian In Tomato Sauce	½ cup (4.6 oz)	110

FOOD	PORTION	CALS.
Wagon Master		
Pork And Beans	½ cup (4.5 oz)	110
FROZEN		
Natural Touch		
Nine Bean Loaf	1 in slice (3 oz)	160
MIX		
Bean Cuisine		
Florentine Beans With Bow Ties	½ cup	199
Pasta & Beans Country French With Gemelli	½ cup	214
Melting Pot		
Terrazza Napoli Mixed Beans	1 cup	200
TAKE-OUT		
baked beans	½ cup	190
barbecue beans	3.5 oz	120
four bean salad	3.5 oz	100

BEAR
simmered	3 oz	220

BEAVER
roasted	3 oz	140
simmered	3 oz	141

BEECHNUTS
dried	1 oz	164

BEEF
(*see also* BEEF DISHES, VEAL)

CANNED		
corned beef	3 oz	85
Hormel		
Corned Beef	2 oz	120
Cubed Beef	½ cup (4.9 oz)	130
Potted Meat	4 tbsp (2 oz)	100
Treet		
50% Less Fat	2 oz	120
Beef	2 oz	150
Underwood		
Roast Beef	2.08 oz	140
Roast Beef Mesquite Smoked	2.08 oz	126
Roast Beef Light	2.08 oz	90
DRIED		
Hormel		
Pillow Pack	10 slices (1 oz)	45

FOOD	PORTION	CALS.
Rough Cut		
Beef Steak Hot	1 pkg (1 oz)	70
Beef Steak Original	1 pkg (1 oz)	60
Beef Steak Peppered	1 pkg (1 oz)	60
FRESH		
bottom round lean & fat trim 0 in Choice roasted	3 oz	172
bottom round lean & fat trim 0 in Select braised	3 oz	171
bottom round lean & fat trim 0 in Select roasted	3 oz	150
bottom round lean & fat trim 0 in braised	3 oz	193
bottom round lean & fat trim ¼ in Choice braised	3 oz	241
bottom round lean & fat trim ¼ in Choice roasted	3 oz	221
bottom round lean & fat trim ¼ in Select braised	3 oz	220
bottom round lean & fat trim ¼ in Select roasted	3 oz	199
brisket flat half lean & fat trim 0 in braised	3 oz	183
brisket flat half lean & fat trim ¼ in braised	3 oz	309
brisket point half lean & fat trim 0 in braised	3 oz	304
brisket point half lean & fat trim ¼ in braised	3 oz	343
brisket whole lean & fat trim 0 in braised	3 oz	247
brisket whole lean & fat trim ¼ in braised	3 oz	327
chuck arm pot roast lean & fat trim 0 in braised	3 oz	238
chuck arm pot roast lean & fat trim ¼ in braised	3 oz	282
chuck blade roast lean & fat trim 0 in braised	3 oz	284
chuck blade roast lean & fat trim ¼ in braised	3 oz	293
corned beef brisket cooked	3 oz	213
eye of round lean & fat trim 0 in Choice roasted	3 oz	153
eye of round lean & fat trim 0 in Select roasted	3 oz	137
eye of round lean & fat trim ¼ in Choice roasted	3 oz	205
eye of round lean & fat trim ¼ in Select roasted	3 oz	184
flank lean & fat trim 0 in braised	3 oz	224
flank lean & fat trim 0 in broiled	3 oz	192

FOOD	PORTION	CALS.
ground extra lean broiled medium	3 oz	217
ground extra lean broiled well done	3 oz	225
ground extra lean fried medium	3 oz	216
ground extra lean fried well done	3 oz	224
ground extra lean raw	4 oz	265
ground lean broiled medium	3 oz	231
ground lean broiled well done	3 oz	238
ground regular broiled medium	3 oz	246
ground regular broiled well done	3 oz	248
porterhouse steak lean & fat trim ¼ in Choice broiled	3 oz	260
porterhouse steak lean only trim ¼ in Prime broiled	3 oz	185
rib eye small end lean & fat trim 0 in Choice broiled	3 oz	261
rib large end lean & fat trim 0 in roasted	3 oz	300
rib large end lean & fat trim ¼ in broiled	3 oz	295
rib large end lean & fat trim ¼ in roasted	3 oz	310
rib small end lean & fat trim 0 in broiled	3 oz	252
rib small end lean & fat trim ¼ in broiled	3 oz	285
rib small end lean & fat trim ¼ in roasted	3 oz	295
rib whole lean & fat trim ¼ in Choice broiled	3 oz	306
rib whole lean & fat trim ¼ in Choice roasted	3 oz	320
rib whole lean & fat trim ¼ in Prime roasted	3 oz	348
rib whole lean & fat trim ¼ in Select broiled	3 oz	274
rib whole lean & fat trim ¼ in Select roasted	3 oz	286
shank crosscut lean & fat trim ¼ in Choice simmered	3 oz	224
short loin top loin lean & fat trim 0 in Choice broiled	3 oz	193
short loin top loin lean & fat trim 0 in Choice broiled	1 steak (5.4 oz)	353
short loin top loin lean & fat trim 0 in Select broiled	1 steak (5.4 oz)	309
short loin top loin lean & fat trim ¼ in Choice braised	3 oz	253
short loin top loin lean & fat trim ¼ in Choice broiled	1 steak (6.3 oz)	536
short loin top loin lean & fat trim ¼ in Prime broiled	1 steak (6.3 oz)	582
short loin top loin lean & fat trim ¼ in Select broiled	1 steak (6.3 oz)	473
short loin top loin lean only trim 0 in Choice broiled	1 steak (5.2 oz)	311

FOOD	PORTION	CALS.
short loin top loin lean only trim ¼ in Choice broiled	1 steak (5.2 oz)	314
shortribs lean & fat Choice braised	3 oz	400
t-bone steak lean & fat trim ¼ in Choice broiled	3 oz	253
t-bone steak lean only trim ¼ in Choice broiled	3 oz	182
tenderloin lean & fat trim 0 in Select broiled	3 oz	194
tenderloin lean & fat trim ¼ in Choice broiled	3 oz	259
tenderloin lean & fat trim ¼ in Choice roasted	3 oz	288
tenderloin lean & fat trim ¼ in Choice broiled	3 oz	208
tenderloin lean & fat trim ¼ in Prime broiled	3 oz	270
tenderloin lean & fat trim ¼ in Select roasted	3 oz	275
tenderloin lean only trim 0 in Select broiled	3 oz	170
tenderloin lean only trim ¼ in Choice broiled	3 oz	188
tenderloin lean only trim ¼ in Select broiled	3 oz	169
tip round lean & fat trim 0 in Choice roasted	3 oz	170
tip round lean & fat trim 0 in Select roasted	3 oz	158
tip round lean & fat trim ¼ in Choice roasted	3 oz	210
tip round lean & fat trim ¼ in Prime roasted	3 oz	233
tip round lean & fat trim ¼ in Select roasted	3 oz	191
top round lean & fat trim 0 in Choice braised	3 oz	184
top round lean & fat trim 0 in Select braised	3 oz	170
top round lean & fat trim ¼ in Choice braised	3 oz	221
top round lean & fat trim ¼ in Choice broiled	3 oz	190
top round lean & fat trim ¼ in Choice fried	3 oz	235
top round lean & fat trim ¼ in Prime broiled	3 oz	195
top round lean & fat trim ¼ in Select braised	3 oz	175
top round lean & fat trim ¼ in Select braised	3 oz	199
top sirloin lean & fat trim 0 in Choice broiled	3 oz	194
top sirloin lean & fat trim 0 in Select broiled	3 oz	166
top sirloin lean & fat trim ¼ in Choice broiled	3 oz	228
top sirloin lean & fat trim ¼ in Choice fried	3 oz	277
top sirloin lean & fat trim ¼ in Select broiled	3 oz	208
tripe raw	4 oz	111
Healthy Choice		
Ground Extra Lean	4 oz	130
Laura's Lean		
Eye Of Round	4 oz	150
Flank Steak	4 oz	160
Ground	4 oz	180
Ground Round	4 oz	160
Ribeye Steak	4 oz	150

FOOD	PORTION	CALS.
Laura's Lean (CONT.)		
Sirloin Tip Round	4 oz	140
Sirloin Top Butt	4 oz	140
Strip Steak	4 oz	150
Tenderloins	4 oz	150
Top Round	4 oz	140
Maverick Ranch		
Ground Round Extra Lean	4 oz	130
READY-TO-EAT		
Boar's Head		
Corned Beef Brisket	2 oz	80
Eye Round Pepper Seasoned	2 oz	90
Roast Beef Cajun	2 oz	80
Top Round Deluxe	2 oz	90
Top Round Oven Roasted No Salt Added	2 oz	90
Healthy Choice		
Deli-Thin Roast Beef	6 slices (2 oz)	60
Fresh-Trak Roast Beef	1 slice (1 oz)	30
Jordan's		
Healthy Trim 97% Fat Free Roast Beef Medium	1 slice (1 oz)	30
Healthy Trim 97% Fat Free Roast Beef Rare	1 slice (1 oz)	30
TAKE-OUT		
roast beef medium	2 oz	70
roast beef rare	2 oz	70

BEEF DISHES
CANNED

corned beef hash	3 oz	155
Dinty Moore		
Meatball Stew	1 cup (8.4 oz)	250
Sliced Potatoes & Beef	1 can (7.5 oz)	230
Stew	1 cup (8.3 oz)	230
Stew	1 cup (8.2 oz)	230
Hormel		
Beef Goulash	1 can (7.5 oz)	230
Roast Beef With Gravy	2 oz	60
Mary Kitchen		
Corned Beef Hash	1 cup (8.3 oz)	410
Corned Beef Hash 50% Reduced Fat	1 cup (8.3 oz)	280
Roast Beef Hash	1 cup (8.3 oz)	390
Roast Turkey Hash	1 can (14.9 oz)	420

FOOD	PORTION	CALS.
Mary Kitchen (CONT.)		
Sausage Hash	1 cup (8.3 oz)	410
FROZEN		
Hot Pocket		
Stuffed Sandwich Barbecue	1 (4.5 oz)	340
Stuffed Sandwich Beef & Cheddar	1 (4.5 oz)	360
Stuffed Sandwich Beef Fajita	1 (4.5 oz)	360
Lean Pockets		
Stuffed Sandwich Beef & Broccoli	1 (4.5 oz)	250
Luigino's		
Creamed Sauce Shaved Cured Beef With Croutons	1 pkg (8 oz)	360
Egg Noodles Rich Gravy Swedish Meatballs	1 cup (7.5 oz)	280
Egg Noodles Rich Gravy Swedish Meatballs	1 pkg (9 oz)	340
Tyson		
Microwave BBQ Sandwich	1 sandwich	200
MIX		
Casbah		
Gyro as prep	1 patty (2 oz)	145
Hamburger Helper		
BBQ Beef as prep	1 cup	320
Beef Pasta as prep	1 cup	270
Beef Romanoff as prep	1 cup	280
Beef Stew as prep	1 cup	260
Beef Taco as prep	1 cup	280
Beef Teriyaki as prep	1 cup	290
Cheddar & Broccoli as prep	1 cup	350
Cheddar Melt as prep	1 cup	310
Cheddar'n Bacon as prep	1 cup	330
Cheeseburger Macaroni as prep	1 cup	360
Cheesy Hashbrowns as prep	1 cup	400
Cheesy Italian as prep	1 cup	320
Cheesy Shells as prep	1 cup	330
Chili Macaroni as prep	1 cup	290
Fettuccine Alfredo as prep	1 cup	300
Four Cheese Lasagne as prep	1 cup	330
Italian Parmesan w/ Rigatoni as prep	1 cup	300
Lasagne as prep	1 cup	270
Meat Loaf as prep	1/6 loaf	270
Meaty Spaghetti & Cheese as prep	1 cup	290
Mushroom & Wild Rice as prep	1 cup	310
Nacho Cheese as prep	1 cup	320

FOOD	PORTION	CALS.
Hamburger Helper (CONT.)		
Pizza Pasta w/ Cheese Topping as prep	1 cup	280
Pizzabake as prep	⅙ pie	270
Potatoes Au Gratin as prep	1 cup	280
Potatoes Stroganoff as prep	1 cup	250
Reduced Sodium Cheddar Spirals as prep	1 cup	300
Reduced Sodium Italian Herby as prep	1 cup	270
Reduced Sodium Southwestern Beef as prep	1 cup	300
Rice Oriental as prep	1 cup	280
Salisbury as prep	1 cup	270
Spaghetti as prep	1 cup	270
Stroganoff as prep	1 cup	320
Swedish Meatballs as prep	1 cup	290
Three Cheeses as prep	1 cup	340
Zesty Italian as prep	1 cup	300
Zesty Mexican as prep	1 cup	280
SHELF-STABLE		
Dinty Moore		
Microwave Cup Corned Beef Hash	1 pkg (7.5 oz)	350
Microwave Cup Hearty Burger Stew	1 pkg (7.5 oz)	240
Microwave Cup Stew	1 pkg (7.5 oz)	190
Hormel		
Microcup Meals Stew	1 cup (7.5 oz)	190
Lunch Bucket		
Beef Stew	1 pkg (7.5 oz)	180
TAKE-OUT		
beef bourguignon	1 serv (7 oz)	254
bulgoghi korean grilled beef	1 serv (5.2 oz)	256
irish stew	1 cup (7 oz)	280
shepherds pie	1 serv (7 oz)	282
stew w/ vegetables	1 cup	220
BEEFALO		
roasted	3 oz	160
BEER AND ALE		
alcohol free beer	7 fl oz	50
beer light	12 oz can	100
beer regular	12 oz can	146
pilsener lager beer	7 fl oz	85
Amstel		
Light	12 oz	95
Anheuser Busch		
Natural Light	12 oz	110

FOOD	PORTION	CALS.
Bud		
Light	12 oz	108
Coors		
Beer	12 oz	132
Extra Gold	12 oz	147
Light	12 oz	101
Guiness		
Kaliber nonalcoholic	12 oz	43
Killian's		
Beer	12 oz	212
Kingsbury		
Nonalcoholic	12 fl oz	60
Michelob		
Light	12 oz	134
Miller		
Lite	12 oz	96
Molson		
Light	12 oz	109
Piels		
Light	12 oz	136
Schmidts		
Light	12 oz	96
Winterfest		
Beer	12 oz	167

BEETS
CANNED

FOOD	PORTION	CALS.
harvard	½ cup	89
pickled	½ cup	75
Del Monte		
Pickled Crinkle Style Sliced	½ cup (4.5 oz)	80
Sliced	½ cup (4.3 oz)	35
Whole	½ cup (4.3 oz)	35
Whole Tiny	½ cup (4.3 oz)	35
Green Giant		
Harvard	⅓ cup (3.1 oz)	60
Sliced	½ cup (4.2 oz)	35
Sliced No Salt Added	½ cup (4.2 oz)	35
Whole	½ cup (4.2 oz)	35
LeSueur		
Baby Whole	½ cup (4.3 oz)	35
Seneca		
Cut	½ cup	35
Diced	½ cup	35

FOOD	PORTION	CALS.
Seneca (CONT.)		
Harvard	½ cup	90
Pickled	2 tbsp	20
Pickled With Onions	2 tbsp	20
Sliced	½ cup	35
Whole	½ cup	35
FRESH		
greens cooked	½ cup	20
greens raw	½ cup	4
raw sliced	½ cup (2.4 oz)	29
sliced cooked	½ cup (3 oz)	38
whole cooked	2 (3.5 oz)	44
whole raw	2 (5.7 oz)	70

BEVERAGES

(*see* BEER AND ALE, CHAMPAGNE, COFFEE, DRINK MIXERS, FRUIT DRINKS, ICED TEA, LIQUOR/LIQUEUR, MALT, MILKSHAKE, SODA, SPORTS DRINKS, TEA/ HERBAL TEA, WATER, WINE, WINE COOLER)

BISCUIT

FOOD	PORTION	CALS.
FROZEN		
Jimmy Dean		
Chicken Twin	2 (3.2 oz)	280
Sausage Twin	2 (3.4 oz)	330
Steak Twin	2 (3.2 oz)	270
Rudy's Farm		
Ham Twin	2 (3 oz)	160
Sausage & Cheese Twin	2 (3 oz)	290
Sausage Twin	2 (2.7 oz)	296
HOME RECIPE		
buttermilk	1 (2 oz)	212
plain	1 (2 oz)	212
MIX		
buttermilk	1 (2 oz)	191
plain	1 (2 oz)	191
Arrowhead		
Biscuit Mix	¼ cup (1.2 oz)	120
Bisquick		
Mix	⅓ cup (1.4 oz)	170
Reduced Fat	⅓ cup (1.4 oz)	150
Sweet	¼ cup (1.4 oz)	170
Gold Medal		
Biscuits	2	180
Jiffy		
As prep	1	150

FOOD	PORTION	CALS.
Jiffy (CONT.)		
Biscuit	¼ cup (1.1 oz)	130
Buttermilk as prep	1	170
READY-TO-EAT		
Arnold		
Old Fashioned	1	60
REFRIGERATED		
buttermilk	1 (1 oz)	98
plain	1 (1 oz)	98
1869 Brand		
Buttermilk	1 (1.1 oz)	100
Hungry Jack		
Butter Tastin' Flaky	1 (1.2 oz)	100
Cinnamon & Sugar	1 (1.2 oz)	110
Flaky	1 (1.2 oz)	100
Flaky Buttermilk	1 (1.2 oz)	100
Pillsbury		
Big Country Butter Tastin'	1 (1.2 oz)	100
Big Country Buttermilk	1 (1.2 oz)	100
Big Country Southern Style	1 (1.2 oz)	100
Buttermilk	1 (2.2 oz)	150
Country	1 (2.2 oz)	150
Grands Blueberry	1 (2.1 oz)	210
Grands Butter Tastin'	1 (2.1 oz)	200
Grands Buttermilk	1 (2.1 oz)	200
Grands Buttermilk Reduced Fat	1 (2.1 oz)	190
Grands Extra Rich	1 (2.1 oz)	220
Grands Flaky	1 (2.1 oz)	200
Grands Golden Corn	1 (1.2 oz)	210
Grands HomeStyle	1 (2.1 oz)	210
Grands Southern Style	1 (2.1 oz)	200
Southern Style Flakey	1 (1.2 oz)	100
Tender Layer Buttermilk	1 (2.2 oz)	160
Roman Meal		
Biscuit	2 (2.4 oz)	180
Honey Nut Oat Bran	1 (1.5 oz)	131
TAKE-OUT		
buttermilk	1	127
plain	1 (35 g)	276
tea biscuit	1 (3 oz)	210
w/ egg	1 (4.8 oz)	316
w/ egg & bacon	1 (5.2 oz)	458
w/ egg & ham	1 (6.7 oz)	442
w/ egg & sausage	1 (6.3 oz)	581

FOOD	PORTION	CALS.
w/ egg & steak	1 (5.2 oz)	410
w/ egg cheese & bacon	1 (5.1 oz)	477
w/ ham	1 (4 oz)	386
w/ sausage	1 (4.4 oz)	485
w/ steak	1 (4.9 oz)	455

BISON
roasted	3 oz	122

BLACK BEANS
CANNED
Allen
Seasoned	½ cup (4.5 oz)	120

Eden
Organic	½ cup (4.6 oz)	100
Organic w/ Ginger & Lemon	½ cup (4.6 oz)	120

Green Giant
Black Beans	½ cup (4.5 oz)	50

Old El Paso
Black Beans	½ cup (4.6 oz)	100
Refried	½ cup (4.2 oz)	120

Progresso
Black Beans	½ cup (4.6 oz)	100

Trappey
Seasoned	½ cup (4.5 oz)	120

MIX
Bean Cuisine
Black Turtle	½ cup	115
Pasta & Beans Black Beans With Fusilli	½ cup	174

Mahatma
Black Beans & Rice	1 cup	200

BLACKBERRIES
canned in heavy syrup	½ cup	118
fresh	½ cup	37

Allen-Wolco
Canned	½ cup (5.3 oz)	60

Big Valley
Frozen	⅔ cup (4.9 oz)	70

BLACKBERRY JUICE
Kool-Aid
Scary Blackberry Ghoul-Aid Drink as prep w/ sugar	1 serv (8 oz)	100

BLACKEYE PEAS
CANNED
Allen
Blackeye Peas	½ cup (4.5 oz)	110

FOOD	PORTION	CALS.
Allen (CONT.)		
Fresh Shell	½ cup (4.4 oz)	120
With Bacon	½ cup (4.5 oz)	105
With Snaps	½ cup (4.4 oz)	120
Dorman		
Fresh Shell	½ cup (4.4 oz)	120
East Texas Fair		
Blackeye Peas	½ cup (4.5 oz)	110
Fresh Shell	½ cup (4.4 oz)	120
With Snaps	½ cup (4.4 oz)	120
Green Giant		
Blackeye Peas	½ cup (4.4 oz)	90
Homefolks		
Fresh Shell	½ cup (4.4 oz)	120
With Jalapeno	½ cup (4.4 oz)	120
With Snaps	½ cup (4.4 oz)	120
Sunshine		
With Bacon	½ cup (4.5 oz)	105
Trappey		
With Bacon	½ cup (4.5 oz)	120
With Bacon & Jalapeno	½ cup (4.4 oz)	110
DRIED		
cooked	1 cup	198
Hurst		
HamBeens California w/ Ham	1 serv	120
FROZEN		
Birds Eye		
Blackeye Peas	½ cup (2.8 oz)	110
Fresh Like	3.5 oz	138

BLINTZE

Empire		
Apple	2 (4.4 oz)	220
Blueberry	2 (4.4 oz)	190
Cheese	2 (4.4 oz)	200
Cherry	2 (4.4 oz)	200
Potato	2 (4.4 oz)	190
Golden		
Apple Raisin	1 (2.25 oz)	80
Blueberry	1 (2.25 oz)	90
Cheese	1 (2.25 oz)	80
Cherry	1 (2.25 oz)	95
Potato	1 (2.25 oz)	90
TAKE-OUT		
cheese	1 (2.7 oz)	160

FOOD	PORTION	CALS.
BLUEBERRIES		
canned in heavy syrup	1 cup	225
fresh	1 cup	82
Big Valley		
Frozen	¾ cup (4.9 oz)	70
Sonoma		
Dried	¼ cup (1.3 oz)	140
BLUEBERRY JUICE		
After The Fall		
Maine Coast	1 cup (8 oz)	90
BLUEFISH		
fresh baked	3 oz	135
BOAR		
wild roasted	3 oz	136
BOK CHOY		
Dole		
Shredded	½ cup	5
BONIATO		
fresh	½ cup	90
BORAGE		
fresh chopped cooked	3.5 oz	25
raw chopped	½ cup	9
BOTTLED WATER		
(*see* WATER)		
BOYSENBERRIES		
in heavy sirup	1 cup	226
BRAINS		
beef pan-fried	3 oz	167
beef simmered	3 oz	136
lamb braised	3 oz	124
lamb fried	3 oz	232
pork braised	3 oz	117
veal braised	3 oz	115
veal fried	3 oz	181
BRAN		
corn	1 cup (2.7 oz)	170
oat	½ cup (1.6 oz)	116
oat cooked	½ cup (3.8 oz)	44
rice	½ cup (2.1 oz)	187
wheat	½ cup (2 oz)	63

FOOD	PORTION	CALS.
Arrowhead		
Oat Bran	⅓ cup (1.4 oz)	150
Wheat Bran	¼ cup (0,6 oz)	30
Good Shepherd		
Wheat Bran	1 oz	80
Hodgson Mill		
Oat	¼ cup (1.3 oz)	120
Wheat	¼ cup (0.5 oz)	30
Mother's		
Oat Bran	½ cup	150
Quaker		
Oat Bran	½ cup (1.4 oz)	150
Roman Meal		
Oat	1 oz	94
Stone-Buhr		
Oat	⅓ cup (1 oz)	90

BRAZIL NUTS
dried unblanched	1 oz	186

BREAD
(*see also* BAGEL, BISCUIT, BREADSTICK, CROISSANT, ENGLISH MUFFIN, MUFFIN, ROLL, SCONE)

CANNED

boston brown	1 slice (1.6 oz)	88
B&M		
Brown Bread	½ in slice (2 oz)	130
Brown Bread Raisins	½ in slice (2 oz)	130

FROZEN

Kineret		
Challah	⅛ loaf (2 oz)	150
New York		
Garlic	1 slice (2 oz)	190
Garlic Reduced Fat	1 slice (2 oz)	160
Texas Garlic Toast	1 in slice (1.4 oz)	160
Pepperidge Farm		
Garlic	1 slice (1.8 oz)	170
Garlic Sourdough 30% Reduced Fat	1 slice (1.8 oz)	170
Monterey Jack Jalapeno Cheese	1 slice (2 oz)	145
Mozzeralla Garlic Cheese	1 slice (2 oz)	201

HOME RECIPE

banana	1 slice (2 oz)	195
cornbread as prep w/ 2% milk	1 piece (2.3 oz)	173
cornbread as prep w/ whole milk	1 piece (2.3 oz)	176
datenut	½ in slice	92

FOOD	PORTION	CALS.
irish soda bread	1 slice (2 oz)	174
pumpkin	1 slice (1 oz)	94
white as prep w/ nonfat dry milk	1 slice	78
white as prep w/ 2% milk	1 slice	81
white as prep w/ whole milk	1 slice	82
whole wheat	1 slice	79
MIX		
cornbread	1 piece (2 oz)	189
Aunt Jemima		
Corn Bread Easy Mix	⅓ cup (1.3 oz)	150
Natural Ovens		
Cracked Wheat	2 slices (2.4 oz)	140
English Muffin Bread	2 slices (2.4 oz)	140
Executive Fitness Sunny Millet	2 slices (2.6 oz)	160
Garden Bread	1 oz	50
Glorious Cinnamon & Raisin Fat Free	2 slices (2.1 oz)	110
Honey 'N Flax	2 slices (2.5 oz)	140
Hunger Filler Bread	2 slices (2.1 oz)	110
Light Wheat	2 slices (2.2 oz)	84
Nutty Natural Wheat Bread	2 slices (2.5 oz)	140
Seven Grain Herb	2 slices (2.5 oz)	140
Soft Hearth Whole Wheat	2 slices (2 oz)	100
Soft Sandwich Very Low Fat	2 slices (2.3 oz)	110
Stay Slim	2 slices (2 oz)	100
READY-TO-EAT		
baguette whole wheat	2 oz	140
cracked wheat	1 slice	65
egg	1 slice (1.4 oz)	115
french	1 slice (1 oz)	78
french	1 loaf (1 lb)	1270
gluten	1 slice	47
italian	1 loaf (1 lb)	1255
italian	1 slice (1 oz)	81
navajo fry	1 (10.5 in diam)	527
navajo fry	1 (5 in diam)	296
oat bran	1 slice	71
oat bran reduced calorie	1 slice	46
oatmeal	1 slice	73
oatmeal reduced calorie	1 slice	48
pita	1 reg (2 oz)	165
pita	1 sm (1 oz)	78
pita whole wheat	1 sm (1 oz)	76
pita whole wheat	1 reg (2 oz)	170
protein	1 slice	47

FOOD	PORTION	CALS.
pumpernickel	1 slice	80
raisin	1 slice	71
rice bran	1 slice	66
rye	1 slice	83
rye reduced calorie	1 slice	47
seven grain	1 slice	65
sourdough	1 slice (1 oz)	78
vienna	1 slice (1 oz)	78
wheat reduced calorie	1 slice	46
wheat berry	1 slice	65
wheat bran	1 slice	89
wheat germ	1 slice	74
white	1 slice	67
white reduced calorie	1 slice	48
white toasted	1 slice	67
white cubed	1 cup	80
whole wheat	1 slice	70
Alvarado St. Bakery		
Barley	1 slice (1.2 oz)	70
California Style	1 slice (1.2 oz)	60
French	1 slice (1.2 oz)	80
Multi-Grain	1 slice (1.2 oz)	60
Multi-Grain No-Salt	1 slice (1.2 oz)	60
Oat Berry	1 slice (1.2 oz)	70
Raisin	1 slice (1.1 oz)	80
Rye Seed	1 slice (1.2 oz)	60
Sourdough	1 slice (1.2 oz)	80
Wheat	1 slice (1.3 oz)	90
Arnold		
12 Grain Natural	1 slice (0.8 oz)	60
Augusto Pan De Aqua	1 oz	80
Bran'nola Country Oat	1 slice (1.3 oz)	90
Bran'nola Dark Wheat	1 slice (1.3 oz)	90
Bran'nola Hearty Wheat	1 slice (1.3 oz)	100
Bran'nola Nutty Grains	1 slice (1.3 oz)	90
Bran'nola Original	1 slice (1.3 oz)	90
Cinnamon Chip	1 slice	80
Cinnamon Raisin	1 slice (0.9 oz)	70
Country Bran Bakery Light	1 slice (0.8 oz)	40
Cranberry	1 slice (0.9 oz)	70
French Twin Loaves Francisco	2 slices (2 oz)	150
French Stick Francisco	1 slice (1 oz)	70
French Stick Savoni	1 oz	80
Italian Bakery Light	1 slice (0.7 oz)	40

FOOD	PORTION	CALS.
Arnold (CONT.)		
Italian Francisco	1 slice (1 oz)	70
Italian Stick Francisco	1 oz	90
Oatmeal Bakery	1 slice	60
Oatmeal Bakery Light	1 slice	40
Oatmeal Raisin	1 slice (0.9 oz)	60
Pita Wheat	½ pocket (1 oz)	71
Pita White	½ pocket (0.5 oz)	71
Pumpernickel	l slice (1.1 oz)	70
Rye Bakery Soft Light	1 slice (1.1 oz)	40
Rye Bakery Soft Seeded	1 slice (1.1 oz)	70
Rye Bakery Soft Unseeded	1 slice (1.1 oz)	70
Rye Dill	1 slice (1.1 oz)	60
Rye Real Jewish Dijon	1 slice	70
Rye Real Jewish Melba Thin	1 slice (0.7 oz)	40
Rye Real Jewish Unseeded	1 slice	80
Rye Real Jewish With Caraway	1 slice	70
Rye Real Jewish Without Seeds	1 slice (1.1 oz)	70
Sourdough Francisco	1 slice	90
Wheat Brick Oven	1 slice (0.8 oz)	60
Wheat Golden Light	1 slice (0.8 oz)	40
Wheat Natural	1 slice (1.3 oz)	80
Wheat Berry Honey	1 slice (1.1 oz)	80
White Brick Oven	1 slice (0.8 oz)	60
White Country	1 slice (1.3 oz)	100
White Extra Fiber Brick Oven	1 slice (0.9 oz)	50
White Light Brick Oven	1 slice (0.8 oz)	40
White Premium Light	1 slice	40
White Thin Sliced Brick Oven	1 slice	40
Whole Wheat 100% Light Brick Oven	1 slice (0.8 oz)	40
Whole Wheat 100% Stoneground	1 slice (0.8 oz)	50
August Bros.		
Pumpernickel	1 slice	80
Rye Onion	1 slice	80
Rye Thin Unseeded	1 slice	40
Rye With Seeds	1 slice (1 lb loaf)	80
Rye Without Seeds	1 slice	80
Rye N' Pump	1 slice	90
Beefsteak		
Pumpernickel	1 slice (1 oz)	70
Rye Hearty	1 slice (1 oz)	70
Rye Light	2 slices (1.6 oz)	70
Rye Mild	2 slices (1.4 oz)	90
Rye Soft	1 slice (1 oz)	70

FOOD	PORTION	CALS.
Beefsteak (CONT.)		
Wheat Hearty	1 slice (1 oz)	70
Wheat Soft	1 slice (1 oz)	70
White Robust	1 slice (1 oz)	70
Bread Du Jour		
French	3 in slice (2 oz)	140
Cedar's		
Mountain Bread Six Grain	1 piece (2.4 oz)	200
Damascus		
Wraps Tomato	1, 12-inch (4 oz)	240
Dicarlo's		
Foccaccia	⅛ bread (2 oz)	130
French Parisian	2 slices (1 oz)	70
Freihofer's		
Country Potato	1 slice (1.3 oz)	100
Country White	1 slice (1.3 oz)	100
Wheat Light	1 slice (1.6 oz)	80
White Light	2 slices (1.6 oz)	80
Whole Wheat 100%	1 slice (1.3 oz)	90
Home Pride		
Hearty Buttermilk & Biscuit White	1 slice (1.3 oz)	100
Hearty Deli Rye	1 slice (2 oz)	140
Hearty Golden Honey Wheat	1 slice (1.3 oz)	90
Hearty Honey Oats & Cracked Wheat	1 slice (1.4 oz)	100
Hearty Seven Grain Multi Grain	1 slice (1.3 oz)	100
Honey Wheat	1 slice (1 oz)	70
Seven Grain	1 slice (0.9 oz)	60
Wheat	1 slice (0.9 oz)	70
Wheat Light	3 slices (2.1 oz)	110
White	1 slice (0.9 oz)	70
White Grain	1 slice (1 oz)	60
White Light	3 slices (0.9 oz)	110
Whole Wheat Hearty 100% Stoneground	1 slice (1.4 oz)	90
Mediterranean Magic		
Focaccia	⅕ loaf (1.8 oz)	140
Parisian		
French Stick Extra Sour	2 oz	150
French Stick Sweet	2 oz	154
Pepperidge Farm		
Sandwich Pocket Wheat	1 (2 oz)	160
Sandwich Pocket White	1 (2 oz)	150
Roman Meal		
Brown & Serve Mini Loaf	½ loaf (2 oz)	136
Cracked Wheat	1 slice (1.4 oz)	92

FOOD	PORTION	CALS.
Roman Meal (CONT.)		
Hearty Wheat Light	1 slice (0.8 oz)	42
Honey Nut Oat Bran	1 slice (1 oz)	72
Honey Oat Bran	1 slice (1 oz)	70
Oat	1 slice (1 oz)	69
Oat Bran	1 slice (1 oz)	68
Oat Bran Light	1 slice (0.8 oz)	42
Round Top	1 slice (1 oz)	67
Sandwich	1 slice (0.8 oz)	55
Seven Grain	1 slice (1 oz)	67
Seven Grain Light	1 slice (0.8 oz)	42
Sourdough Light	1 slice (0.8 oz)	41
Sourdough Whole Grain Light	1 slice (0.8 oz)	40
Sun Grain	1 slice (1 oz)	70
Twelve Grain	1 slice (1 oz)	70
Twelve Grain Light	1 slice (0.8 oz)	42
Wheat Light	1 slice (0.8 oz)	41
Wheatberry Honey	1 slice (1 oz)	67
Wheatberry Light	1 slice (0.8 oz)	42
White Light	1 slice (0.8 oz)	41
Whole Grain 100%	1 slice (1.4 oz)	91
Whole Grain Sourdough	1 slice (1 oz)	66
Whole Wheat 100%	1 slice (1 oz)	64
Whole Wheat 100% Light	1 slice (0.8 oz)	42
Sunmaid		
Raisin	1 slice	70
Tree Of Life		
100% Spelt	1 slice (1.8 oz)	130
Millet	1 slice (1.8 oz)	130
Rye Sour Dough	1 slice (1.8 oz)	110
Sprouted Seven Grain	1 slice (1.8 oz)	110
Valley Lahvosh		
Valley Wraps	1 (1 oz)	100
ZA		
Pit-Za Hearty Multi-Grain	⅑ bread (2 oz)	130
Pit-Za Salt-Free Garlic Whole Wheat	⅑ bread (2 oz)	150
REFRIGERATED		
Pillsbury		
Crusty French Loaf	⅕ loaf (2.2 oz)	150
Grands Wheat	1 (2.1 oz)	200
Roman Meal		
Loaf	1 slice (1 oz)	85
Stefano's		
Stuffed Bread Broccoli & Cheese	½ bread (6 oz)	450

FOOD	PORTION	CALS.
TAKE-OUT		
chapatis as prep w/ fat	1 bread (1.6 oz)	95
focaccia onion	1 piece (4.6 oz)	282
focaccia rosemary	1 piece (3.5 oz)	251
focaccia tomato olive	1 piece (4.7 oz)	270
garlic bread	2 slices (2 oz)	190
naan	1 bread (3.5 oz)	286
paratha	1 bread (2.1 oz)	201

BREAD COATING

FOOD	PORTION	CALS.
Don's Chuck Wagon		
All Purpose Mix	¼ cup (1 oz)	100
Fish & Chips Mix	¼ cup (1 oz)	100
Fish Mix	¼ cup (1 oz)	95
Frying Mix Chicken	¼ cup (1 oz)	95
Frying Mix Seafood Seasoned	¼ cup (1 oz)	95
Mushroom Mix	¼ cup (1 oz)	95
Onion Ring Mix	¼ cup (1 oz)	100
Little Crow		
Fryin' Magic	0.5 oz	43
Mrs. Dash		
Crispy Coating	2 tbsp (0.6 oz)	65
Oven Fry		
Extra Crispy For Chicken	⅛ pkg (0.5 oz)	60
Extra Crispy For Pork	⅛ pkg (0.5 oz)	60
Shake 'N Bake		
Buffalo Wings	⅒ pkg (0.4 oz)	40
Classic Italian Chicken or Pork	⅛ pkg (0.4 oz)	40
Country Mild Recipe	⅛ pkg (0.3 oz)	35
Glazes Barbecue Chicken Or Pork	⅛ pkg (0.4 oz)	45
Glazes Honey Mustard Chicken Or Pork	⅛ pkg (0.4 oz)	45
Glazes Tangy Honey Chicken Or Pork	⅛ pkg (0.4 oz)	45
Home Style Flour Recipe For Chicken	⅛ pkg (0.4 oz)	40
Hot & Spicy Chicken Or Pork	⅛ pkg (0.4 oz)	40
Original For Chicken	⅛ pkg (0.4 oz)	40
Original For Fish	¼ pkg (0.7 oz)	80
Original For Pork	⅛ pkg (0.4 oz)	45

BREAD MACHINE MIX

FOOD	PORTION	CALS.
Sassafras		
Apricot Oatmeal	1 slice (1.4 oz)	140
Wanda's		
Dried Tomato Cheddar	¼ cup mix per serv (1.2 oz)	140

FOOD	PORTION	CALS.
Wanda's (CONT.)		
European White	¼ cup mix per serv (1.2 oz)	130
Oatmeal	¼ cup mix per serv (1.2 oz)	120
Oatmeal Cinnamon	¼ cup mix per serv (1.2 oz)	120
Old World Rye	¼ cup mix per serv (1.9 oz)	90
Onion	⅓ cup mix per serv (1.2 oz)	120
Orange Cinnamon	¼ cup mix per serv (1.3 oz)	130
Oregano Garlic	¼ cup mix per serv (1.2 oz)	130
Rosemary Basil	¼ cup mix per serv (1.2 oz)	130
Rye	¼ cup mix per serv (1.2 oz)	120
Rye Caraway	¼ cup mix per serv (1.2 oz)	120
Sourdough	¼ cup mix per serv (1.2 oz)	120
Sunflower Sesame Poppyseed	¼ cup mix per serv (1.2 oz)	120
Ten Grain	¼ cup mix per serv (1.4 oz)	140
Wheat	¼ cup mix per serv (1.2 oz)	130
White	¼ cup mix per serv (1.2 oz)	130
Whole Wheat	¼ cup mix per serv (1.3 oz)	130

BREADCRUMBS

FOOD	PORTION	CALS.
dry	1 cup	426
dry seasoned	1 cup (4 oz)	441
fresh	⅔ cup	76
Arnold		
Italian	½ oz	50
Plain	½ oz	50
Contadina		
Plain	⅓ cup	100
Progresso		
Italian Style	¼ cup (1 oz)	110

FOOD	PORTION	CALS.
Progresso (CONT.)		
Lemon Herb	¼ cup (0.9 oz)	100
Plain	¼ cup (1 oz)	100
Tomato Basil	¼ cup (1.1 oz)	120
BREADFRUIT		
fresh	¼ small	99
seeds cooked	1 oz	48
seeds raw	1 oz	54
seeds roasted	1 oz	59
BREADNUTTREE SEEDS		
dried	1 oz	104
BREADSTICKS		
plain	1 sm	25
plain	1	41
Angonoa		
Cheese	5 (1 oz)	120
Cheese Mini	16 (1 oz)	120
Garlic	6 (1 oz)	120
Italian Style Plain	5 (1 oz)	120
Low Sodium With Sesame Seed	6 (1 oz)	130
Onion	6 (1 oz)	120
Pizza Mini	26 (1 oz)	120
Sesame Mini	16 (1 oz)	130
Sesame Royale	6 (1 oz)	130
Whole Wheat Mini	14 (1 oz)	130
Bread Du Jour		
Original	1 (1.9 oz)	130
Sourdough	1 (1.9 oz)	130
J.J. Cassone		
Garlic	1 (1.6 oz)	150
New York		
Garlic Soft	1 (1.5 oz)	140
Pillsbury		
Soft	1 (1.4 oz)	110
Soft Garlic & Herb	1 (2.1 oz)	180
Roman Meal		
Brown & Serve Soft	1 (2.7 oz)	181
Refrigerated	1 (1.4 oz)	117
Stella D'Oro		
Deli Garlic Fat Free	5	60
Deli Original Fat Free	5	60
Garlic		35

FOOD	PORTION	CALS.
Stella D'Oro (CONT.)		
Grissini Garlic Fat Free	3	60
Grissini Original Fat Free	3	60
Onion	1	40
Regular	1	40
Regular Sodium Free	2	80
Sesame Low Fat	2	70
Sesame Sodium Free	1	50
Traditional Garlic Fat Free	2	70
Traditional Original Fat Free	2	70
Wheat	1	40

BREAKFAST BARS

(*see also* BREAKFAST DRINKS, CEREAL BARS, NUTRITION SUPPLEMENTS)

FOOD	PORTION	CALS.
Carnation		
Chewy Chocolate Chip	1 (1.26 oz)	150
Chewy Peanut Butter Chocolate Chip	1 (1.26 oz)	140
Health Valley		
Breakfast Bakes Apple Cinnamon	1 bar	110
Breakfast Bakes California Strawberry	1 bar	110
Breakfast Bakes Mountain Blueberry	1 bar	110
Breakfast Bakes Red Raspberry	1 bar	110
Weight Watchers		
Apple Cinnamon	1 (1 oz)	100
Blueberry	1 (1 oz)	100
Raspberry	1 (1 oz)	100

BREAKFAST DRINKS

(*see also* NUTRITION SUPPLEMENTS)

FOOD	PORTION	CALS.
Carnation		
Instant Breakfast Cafe Mocha	1 pkg	130
Instant Breakfast Cafe Mocha	1 pkg + skim milk (9 fl oz)	220
Instant Breakfast Cafe Mocha	1 can (10 fl oz)	220
Instant Breakfast Classic Chocolate Malt	1 pkg + skim milk (9 fl oz)	220
Instant Breakfast Classic Chocolate Malt	1 pkg	130
Instant Breakfast Creamy Milk Chocolate	1 pkg	130
Instant Breakfast Creamy Milk Chocolate	1 pkg + skim milk (9 fl oz)	220
Instant Breakfast Creamy Milk Chocolate	8 fl oz	220
Instant Breakfast Creamy Milk Chocolate	1 can (10 fl oz)	220
Instant Breakfast French Vanilla	1 pkg + skim milk	220
Instant Breakfast French Vanilla	1 pkg	130
Instant Breakfast No Sugar Added Classic Chocolate	1 pkg + skim milk (9 fl oz)	160

FOOD	PORTION	CALS.
Carnation (CONT.)		
Instant Breakfast No Sugar Added Classic Chocolate	1 pkg	70
Instant Breakfast No Sugar Added Creamy Milk Chocolate	1 pkg + skim milk (9 fl oz)	160
Instant Breakfast No Sugar Added Creamy Milk Chocolate	1 pkg	70
Instant Breakfast No Sugar Added French Vanilla	1 pkg + skim milk (9 fl oz)	150
Instant Breakfast No Sugar Added French Vanilla	1 pkg	70
Instant Breakfast No Sugar Added Strawberry Creme	1 pkg + skim milk (9 fl oz)	150
Instant Breakfast No Sugar Added Strawberry Creme	1 pkg	70
Instant Breakfast Strawberry Creme	1 pkg	130
Instant Breakfast Strawberry Creme	1 pkg + skim milk	220

BROCCOFLOWER

FOOD	PORTION	CALS.
fresh raw	½ cup (1.8 oz)	16
Dole		
Fresh	⅕ head	35

BROCCOLI
FRESH

FOOD	PORTION	CALS.
chinese broccoli (gai lan) cooked	1 cup (3.1 oz)	19
chopped cooked	½ cup	22
raw chopped	½ cup	12
Dole		
Spear	1 med	40
Fresh Alternatives		
BroccoSprouts	½ cup (1 oz)	10

FROZEN

FOOD	PORTION	CALS.
Amy's Organic		
Pocket Sandwich Broccoli & Cheese	1 (4.5 oz)	270
Big Valley		
Chopped	¾ cup (3 oz)	25
Cuts	¾ cup (3 oz)	25
Birds Eye		
Baby Broccoli Blend	1 cup (3.4 oz)	70
Baby Florets	1 cup (3 oz)	25
In Cheese Sauce	½ cup (3.9 oz)	110
Fresh Like		
Spear	3.5 oz	26

FOOD	PORTION	CALS.
Green Giant		
Butter Sauce	4 oz	50
Cheese Sauce	⅔ cup (3.9 oz)	70
Chopped	¾ cup (2.8 oz)	25
Cuts	1 cup (2.9 oz)	25
Harvest Fresh Cut	⅔ cup (3.2 oz)	25
Harvest Fresh Spears	3.5 oz	25
Select Florets	1⅓ cups (2.9 oz)	25
Select Spears	3 oz	25
Stouffer's		
Au Gratin	1 serv (4 oz)	100
Tree Of Life		
Broccoli	1 cup (3.1 oz)	25

BROWNIE
FROZEN
Greenfield

FOOD	PORTION	CALS.
Fat Free Homestyle	1 (1.3 oz)	110
Otis Spunkmeyer		
Blue Yonder w/ Walnuts	1 (2 oz)	230
Weight Watchers		
Brownie A La Mode	1 (3.14 oz)	190
Double Fudge Brownie Parfait	1 (5.3 oz)	190
HOME RECIPE		
plain	1 (0.8 oz)	112
MIX		
plain	1 (1.2 oz)	139
plain low calorie	1 (0.8 oz)	84
Estee		
Brownie Mix as prep	2	100
Jiffy		
Fudge as prep	1	160
Sweet Rewards		
Reduced Fat Fudge	1	140
Reduced Fat Fudge No Cholesterol Recipe	1	140
READY-TO-EAT		
plain	1 lg (2 oz)	227
plain	1 sm (1 oz)	115
Dolly Madison		
Fudge	1 (3 oz)	330
Health Valley		
Bar w/ Fudge Filling	1 bar	110
Hostess		
Brownie Bites	3 (1.3 oz)	170

FOOD	PORTION	CALS.
Hostess (CONT.)		
Fudge	1 (3 oz)	330
Light	1 (1.4 oz)	140
Little Debbie		
Fudge	1 pkg (2.1 oz)	270
Fudge	1 pkg (3.6 oz)	450
Fudge	1 pkg (2.9 oz)	360
Fudge	1 pkg (2.5 oz)	310
Tastykake		
Fudge Walnut	1 (3 oz)	370
TAKE-OUT		
plain	1, 2 in sq (2.1 oz)	243

BRUSSELS SPROUTS
FRESH

cooked	½ cup	30
cooked	1 sprout	8
raw	½ cup	19
raw	1 sprout	8
Dole		
Sprouts	½ cup	19
FROZEN		
Big Valley		
Whole	5-8 pieces (3 oz)	35
Birds Eye		
Brussels Sprouts	6 (3 oz)	35
Fresh Like		
Sprouts	3.5 oz	37
Green Giant		
Butter Sauce	⅔ cup (3.6 oz)	60

BUCKWHEAT

groats roasted cooked	1 cup (5.9 oz)	647
groats roasted uncooked	1 cup (5.7 oz)	567
Wolff's		
Brown Groats Roasted	1 cup (8 oz)	900
Flour	1 cup (8 oz)	860
Kasha Coarse cooked	¼ cup (1.6 oz)	170
Kasha Fine cooked	¼ cup (1.6 oz)	170
Kasha Medium cooked	¼ cup (1.6 oz)	170
Kasha Whole cooked	¼ cup (1.6 oz)	170
White Grits	1 cup (8 oz)	840

BUFFALO

water buffalo roasted	3 oz	111

FOOD	PORTION	CALS.
BULGUR		
cooked	1 cup (6.3 oz)	151
Casbah		
Pilaf Mix as prep	1 cup	200
Salad Mix as prep	⅔ cup	90
Good Shepherd		
Bulgur	¼ cup (43 g)	150
Hodgson Mill		
Bulgur	¼ cup (1.4 oz)	120
BURBOT (FISH)		
fresh baked	3 oz	98
BURDOCK ROOT		
cooked	1 cup	110
BUTTER		
(*see also* BUTTER BLENDS, BUTTER SUBSTITUTES, MARGARINE)		
clarified butter	3½ oz	876
stick	1 pat (5 g)	36
stick	1 stick (4 oz)	813
whipped	1 pat (4 g)	27
Crystal		
Salted Stick	1 tbsp (0.5 oz)	102
Unsalted Stick	1 tbsp (0.5 oz)	102
Hotel Bar		
Stick	1 tsp	35
Keller's		
Stick	1 tsp	35
Land O'Lakes		
Light Stick	1 tbsp	50
Light Unsalted Stick	1 tbsp	50
Stick	1 tbsp (0.5 oz)	100
Unsalted Stick	1 tbsp (0.5 oz)	100
Unsalted Tub	1 tbsp	60
Whipped	1 tbsp (0.3 oz)	70
BUTTER BEANS		
CANNED		
Allen		
Baby	½ cup (4.5 oz)	120
Large	½ cup (4.5 oz)	120
Green Giant		
Butter Beans	½ cup (4.5 oz)	90
Sunshine		
Butter Beans	½ cup (4.5 oz)	120

FOOD	PORTION	CALS.
Trappey		
Baby White With Bacon	½ cup (4.5 oz)	130
Large White With Bacon	½ cup (4.5 oz)	110
Van Camp's		
Butter Beans	½ cup	110
FROZEN		
Birds Eye		
Butter Beans	½ cup (2.7 oz)	100
Speckled	½ cup (2.7 oz)	100

BUTTER BLENDS

(*see also* BUTTER, BUTTER SUBSTITUTES, MARGARINE)

stick	1 stick	811
Brummel & Brown		
Spread Make With Yogurt	1 tbsp (0.5 oz)	50
Country Morning		
Blend Light Stick	1 tbsp (0.5 oz)	50
Blend Light Tub	1 tbsp (0.5 oz)	50
Blend Stick	1 tbsp	100
Blend Tub	1 tbsp	100
Blend Unsalted Stick	1 tbsp	100

BUTTER SUBSTITUTES

(*see also* BUTTER BLENDS, MARGARINE)

Butter Buds		
Mix	1 tsp (2 g)	5
Sprinkles	1 tsp (2 g)	5
Molly McButter		
Cheese	1 tsp	5
Light Sodium	1 tsp	5
Natural Butter	1 tsp	5
Roasted Garlic	1 tsp	5
Morningstar Farms		
Roasted Soy Butter	2 tbsp (1.1 oz)	170
Mrs. Bateman's		
Butterlike Baking Butter	1 tbsp (0.5 oz)	36
Butterlike Saute Butter	1 tbsp (0.5 oz)	40
Natural Touch		
Roasted Soy Butter	2 tbsp (1.1 oz)	170
Watkins		
Butter Sprinkles	1 tsp (2 g)	5
Imitation Butter Flavored Mist	1 tbsp (0.5 oz)	120

BUTTERFISH

baked	3 oz	159

FOOD	PORTION	CALS.

BUTTERNUTS
dried	1 oz	174

BUTTERSCOTCH
(see also CANDY)
Nestle
Morsels Butterscotch	1 tbsp	80

CABBAGE
(see also COLESLAW)
FRESH
chinese pak-choi raw shredded	½ cup	5
chinese pak-choi shredded cooked	½ cup	10
chinese pe-tsai raw shredded	1 cup	12
chinese pe-tsai shredded cooked	1 cup	16
danish raw	1 head (2 lbs)	228
danish raw shredded	½ cup (1.2 oz)	9
danish shredded cooked	½ cup (2.6 oz)	17
green raw	1 head (2 lbs)	228
green raw shredded	½ cup (1.2 oz)	9
green shredded cooked	½ cup (2.6 oz)	17
napa cooked	1 cup (3.8 oz)	13
red raw shredded	½ cup	10
red shredded cooked	½ cup	16
savoy raw shredded	½ cup	10
savoy shredded cooked	½ cup	18

Dole
Cabbage	1/12 med head	18
Napa shredded	½ cup	6

CAKE
(see also BROWNIE, CAKE MIX, COOKIES, DANISH PASTRY, DOUGHNUT, PIE)
angelfood	1 cake (11.9 oz)	876
angelfood home recipe	1/12 cake (1.9 oz)	142
apple crisp home recipe	1 recipe 6 serv (29.6 oz)	1377
boston cream pie frzn	⅙ cake (3.2 oz)	232
carrot w/ cream cheese icing home recipe	1 cake, 10 in diam	6175
cheesecake	⅙ cake (2.8 oz)	256
cheesecake	1 cake, 9 in diam	3350
cheesecake home recipe	1/12 cake (4.5 oz)	456
cherry fudge w/ chocolate frosting	⅛ cake (2.5 oz)	187
chocolate cupcake creme filled w/ frosting home recipe	1 (1.8 oz)	188
chocolate w/o frosting home recipe	1/12 cake (3.3 oz)	340
chocolate w/o frosting home recipe	2 layers (39.9 oz)	4067

FOOD	PORTION	CALS.
coffeecake creme-filled chocolate frosting home recipe	1/6 cake (3.2 oz)	298
coffeecake crumb topped cinnamon home recipe	1/12 cake (2.1 oz)	240
coffeecake fruit	1/8 cake (1.8 oz)	156
cream puff shell home recipe	1 (2.3 oz)	239
devil's food cupcake w/ chocolate frosting	1	120
devil's food w/ creme filling	1 (1 oz)	105
eclair home recipe	1 (3 oz)	262
fruitcake	1 piece (1.5 oz)	139
fruitcake dark home recipe	1 cake, 7½ in x 2¼ in	5185
pound	1 cake, 8½ x 3½ x 3 in	1935
pound	1/10 cake (1 oz)	117
pound fat free	1 cake (12 oz)	961
sheet cake w/ white frosting home recipe	1 cake, 9 in sq	4020
sheet cake w/o frosting home recipe	1/9 cake	315
sheet cake w/o frosting home recipe	1 cake, 9 in sq	2830
sour cream pound	1/10 cake (1 oz)	117
sponge	1/12 cake (1.3 oz)	110
sponge home recipe	1/12 cake (2.2 oz)	140
sponge w/ creme filling	1 (1.5 oz)	155
tiramisu	1 cake (4.4 lbs)	5732
toaster pastry apple	1 (1¾ oz)	204
toaster pastry blueberry	1 (1¾ oz)	204
toaster pastry brown sugar cinnamon	1 (1¾ oz)	206
toaster pastry cherry	1 (1¾ oz)	204
toaster pastry strawberry	1 (1¾ oz)	204
white w/ coconut frosting home recipe	1/12 cake (3.9 oz)	399
white w/o frosting home recipe	1/12 cake (2.6 oz)	264
white w/ white frosting	1/16 cake	260
white w/ white frosting	1 cake, 9 in diam	4170
yellow w/ chocolate frosting	1/8 cake (2.2 oz)	242
yellow w/ chocolate frosting	1 cake, 9 in diam	3895
yellow w/o frosting home recipe	1/12 cake (2.4 oz)	245
yellow w/o frosting home recipe	2 layers (28.7 oz)	2947
Baby Watson		
Cheesecake	1 slice (3.8 oz)	390
Cheesecake Light	1/16 cake (3.9 oz)	280
Baker Maid		
Creole Royal Pineapple Apricot	3 slices (5 oz)	270
Creole Royal Pineapple Apricot	1 slice (1.7 oz)	90
Carousel		
New York Cheese Cake	1 cake (3 oz)	250

FOOD	PORTION	CALS.
Dolly Madison		
Apple Crumb	1 (1.6 oz)	160
Banana Dream Flip	1 (3.5 oz)	390
Bear Claw	1 (2.75 oz)	270
Carrot	1 (4 oz)	360
Chocolate Snack Squares	1 (1.6 oz)	210
Cinnamon Buttercrumb	1 (1.6 oz)	170
Cinnamon Buttercrumb Low Fat	1 (1.5 oz)	140
Cinnamon Stix	1 (1.3 oz)	170
Creme Cakes	2 (1.9 oz)	210
Cupcakes Chocolate	1 (2 oz)	210
Cupcakes Spice	1 (2 oz)	230
Dunkin' Stix	1 (1.3 oz)	170
Frosty Angel	1 (3.5 oz)	330
Holiday Cupcakes	1 (1.9 oz)	180
Honey Bun	1 (3.7 oz)	440
Koo Koos	1 (1.8 oz)	200
Mini Coconut Loaf	1 (3.5 oz)	350
Mini Pound Cake	1 (3.2 oz)	310
Raspberry Square	1 (1.8 oz)	190
Sweet Roll Apple	1 (2.2 oz)	200
Sweet Roll Cherry	1 (2.2 oz)	210
Sweet Roll Cinnamon	1 (2.2 oz)	230
Texas Cinnamon Bun	1 (4.2 oz)	440
Zingers Devil's Food	2 (2.6 oz)	270
Zingers Yellow	2 (2.5 oz)	280
Dutch Mill		
Dessert Shells Chocolate Covered	1 (0.5 oz)	80
Entenmann's		
Apple Puffs	1 (3 oz)	280
Apple Strudel Old Fashioned	1 serv (1.5 oz)	120
Cheese Topped Buns	1 (2.3 oz)	240
Cinnamon Buns	1 (2.1 oz)	230
Cinnamon Filbert Ring	1 serv (1.5 oz)	190
Coffee Cake Cheese	1 serv (1.6 oz)	150
Coffee Cake Cheese Filled Crumb	1 serv (1.4 oz)	130
Coffee Cake Crumb	1 serv (1.3 oz)	160
Danish Ring	1 serv (1.5 oz)	180
Danish Ring Pecan	1 serv (1.5 oz)	190
Danish Ring Walnut	1 serv (1.5 oz)	190
Danish Twist Lemon	1 serv (1.2 oz)	140
Danish Twist Raspberry	1 serv (1.2 oz)	140
Devil's Food Cake Fudge Iced	1 serv (1.2 oz)	130
French Crumb Cake All Butter	1 serv (1.6 oz)	180

FOOD	PORTION	CALS.
Entenmann's (CONT.)		
Louisiana Crunch Cake	1 serv (1.7 oz)	180
Pound Loaf All Butter	1 serv (1 oz)	110
Pound Loaf Sour Cream	1 serv (1 oz)	120
Stollen Fruit	1/8 cake (2 oz)	210
Thick Fudge Golden Cake	1 serv (1.2 oz)	130
Freihofer's		
Angel Food	1/5 cake (2 oz)	150
Cinnamon Swirl Buns	1 (2.8 oz)	290
Coffee Cake Cinnamon Pecan	1/8 cake (2 oz)	220
Crumb	1/8 cake (2 oz)	240
Homestyle Golden Loaf	1/8 cake (1.8 oz)	200
Pound	1/5 cake (2.8 oz)	330
Greenfield		
Blondie Apple Spice	1 (1.4 oz)	120
Blondie Fat Free Chocolate Chip	1 (1.3 oz)	110
Hostess		
Angel Food	1/8 cake (2 oz)	160
Chocodiles	1 (1.6 oz)	240
Chocolicious	1 (1.6 oz)	190
Coffee Crumb	1 (1.1 oz)	130
Crumb Cake Light	1 (1 oz)	90
Cupcakes Chocolate	1 (1.8 oz)	180
Cupcakes Orange	1 (1.5 oz)	160
Cupcakes Light Chocolate	1 (1.6 oz)	140
Ding Dongs	2 (2.7 oz)	360
Ho Ho's	2 (2 oz)	250
Honey Bun Glazed	1 (2.7 oz)	320
Honey Bun Iced	1 (3.4 oz)	410
Shortcake Dessert Cups	1 (1 oz)	100
Sno Balls	1 (1.8 oz)	180
Suzy Q's	1 (2 oz)	230
Sweet Roll Cherry	1 (2.2 oz)	210
Sweet Roll Cinnamon	1 (2.2 oz)	230
Twinkies	1 (1.5 oz)	150
Twinkies Light	1 (1.5 oz)	130
Jell-O		
Cheesecake Snack Original	1 (3.3 oz)	160
Cheesecake Snack Strawberry	1 (3.3 oz)	150
Kellogg's		
Pop-Tarts Apple Cinnamon	1 (1.8 oz)	210
Pop-Tarts Blueberry	1 (1.8 oz)	210
Pop-Tarts Brown Sugar Cinnamon	1 (1.8 oz)	210
Pop-Tarts Cherry	1 (1.8 oz)	200

FOOD	PORTION	CALS.
Kellogg's (CONT.)		
Pop-Tarts Chocolate Graham	1 (1.8 oz)	210
Pop-Tarts Frosted Apple Cinnamon	1 (1.8 oz)	190
Pop-Tarts Frosted Blueberry	1 (1.8 oz)	200
Pop-Tarts Frosted Brown Sugar Cinnamon	1 (1.8 oz)	210
Pop-Tarts Frosted Cherry	1 (1.8 oz)	200
Pop-Tarts Frosted Chocolate Vanilla Creme	1 (1.8 oz)	200
Pop-Tarts Frosted Chocolate Fudge	1 (1.8 oz)	200
Pop-Tarts Frosted Grape	1 (1.8 oz)	200
Pop-Tarts Frosted Raspberry	1 (1.8 oz)	210
Pop-Tarts Frosted S'mores	1 (1.8 oz)	200
Pop-Tarts Frosted Strawberry	1 (1.8 oz)	200
Pop-Tarts Frosted Wild Berry	1 (2 oz)	210
Pop-Tarts Frosted Wild Watermelon	1 (2 oz)	210
Pop-Tarts Low Fat Blueberry	1 (1.8 oz)	190
Pop-Tarts Low Fat Cherry	1 (1.8 oz)	190
Pop-Tarts Low Fat Frosted Brown Sugar Cinnamon	1 (1.8 oz)	190
Pop-Tarts Low Fat Frosted Chocolate Fudge	1 (1.8 oz)	190
Pop-Tarts Low Fat Frosted Strawberry	1 (1.8 oz)	190
Pop-Tarts Low Fat Strawberry	1 (1.8 oz)	190
Pop-Tarts Strawberry	1 (1.8 oz)	200
Little Debbie		
Apple Delights	1 pkg (1.2 oz)	140
Apple-Roos	1 pkg (1.5 oz)	150
Banana Nut Muffin Loaves	1 pkg (1.9 oz)	210
Banana Twins	1 pkg (2.2 oz)	250
Be My Valentine	1 pkg (2.2 oz)	280
Cherry Cordials	1 pkg (1.3 oz)	160
Choc-o-Jel	1 pkg (1.2 oz)	150
Choco-Cakes	1 pkg (2.1 oz)	250
Choco-Cakes	1 pkg (2.2 oz)	240
Chocolate	1 pkg (3 oz)	360
Chocolate Chip	1 pkg (2.4 oz)	290
Chocolate Twins	1 pkg (2.4 oz)	240
Christmas Tree Cakes	1 pkg (1.5 oz)	190
Coconut	1 pkg (2.1 oz)	270
Coconut	1 pkg (2.4 oz)	300
Coconut Rounds	1 pkg (1.2 oz)	140
Coffee Cake Apple	1 pkg (1.9 oz)	220
Coffee Cake Apple Streusel	1 pkg (2 oz)	220
Devil Cremes	1 pkg (1.6 oz)	190
Devil Cremes	1 pkg (3.2 oz)	380

FOOD	PORTION	CALS.
Little Debbie (CONT.)		
Devil Squares	1 pkg (2.2 oz)	260
Easter Basket Cakes	1 pkg (2.5 oz)	310
Fancy Cakes	1 pkg (2.4 oz)	300
Fudge Crispy	1 pkg (1.1 oz)	170
Fudge Round	1 pkg (2.5 oz)	290
Fudge Round	1 pkg (3 oz)	350
Fudge Rounds	1 pkg (1.2 oz)	140
Golden Cremes	1 pkg (1.5 oz)	170
Golden Cremes	1 pkg (3 oz)	330
Holiday Cake Chocolate	1 pkg (2.4 oz)	290
Holiday Cake Vanilla	1 pkg (2.5 oz)	310
Honey Bun	1 pkg (4 oz)	510
Honey Bun	1 pkg (3 oz)	380
Jelly Rolls	1 pkg (2.1 oz)	230
Lemon Stix	1 pkg (1.5 oz)	210
Marshmallow Supremes	1 pkg (1.1 oz)	130
Mint Sprints	1 pkg (1.5 oz)	230
Nutty Bar	1 pkg (2 oz)	290
Pecan Twins	1 pkg (2 oz)	220
Pumpkin Delights	1 pkg (1.1 oz)	130
Smiley Faces Cherry	1 pkg (1.2 oz)	140
Smiley Faces Pumpkin	1 pkg (1 oz)	130
Snack Cake Chocolate	1 pkg (2.5 oz)	300
Snack Cake Vanilla	1 pkg (2.6 oz)	320
Spice	1 pkg (2.5 oz)	300
Star Crunch	1 pkg (1.1 oz)	140
Star Crunch	1 pkg (2.6 oz)	330
Swiss Rolls	1 pkg (2.1 oz)	250
Swiss Rolls	1 pkg (2.7 oz)	320
Swiss Rolls	1 pkg (3.2 oz)	380
Teddy Berries	1 pkg (1.2 oz)	130
Vanilla	1 pkg (3 oz)	370
Vanilla Cremes	1 pkg (1.4 oz)	170
Zebra Cakes	1 pkg (2.6 oz)	150
Nabisco		
Frosted Strawberry	1 (1.7 oz)	190
Nature's Choice		
Toaster Pastries Fat Free Apple Cinnamon	1 (1.9 oz)	180
Toaster Pastries Fat Free Blueberry	1 (1.9 oz)	180
Toaster Pastries Fat Free Raspberry	1 (1.9 oz)	180
Toaster Pastries Fat Free Strawberry	1 (1.9 oz)	180
Toaster Pastries Low Fat Cherry	1 (1.9 oz)	180
Toaster Pastries Low Fat Frosted Blueberry	1 (1.9 oz)	190

FOOD	PORTION	CALS.
Nature's Choice (CONT.)		
Toaster Pastries Low Fat Frosted Chocolate	1 (1.9 oz)	200
Toaster Pastries Low Fat Frosted Cinnamon	1 (1.9 oz)	190
Toaster Pastries Low Fat Frosted Strawberry	1 (1.9 oz)	190
Toaster Pastries Low Fat Peach Apricot	1 (1.9 oz)	180
Pepperidge Farm		
Apple Turnover	1 (3.1 oz)	330
Blueberry Turnovers	1 (3.1 oz)	340
Cherry Turnover	1 (3.1 oz)	320
Large Layer Chocolate Fudge	⅛ cake (2.4 oz)	260
Large Layer Coconut	⅛ cake (2.4 oz)	260
Large Layer Vanilla	⅛ cake (2.4 oz)	250
Mini Turnover Apple	1 (1.4 oz)	140
Mini Turnover Cherry	1 (1.4 oz)	140
Mini Turnover Strawberry	1 (1.4 oz)	140
Peach Turnover	1 (3.1 oz)	340
Raspberry Turnovers	1 (3.1 oz)	330
Perugina		
Pannettone Au Beurre	⅙ cake (2.9 oz)	310
Pet-Ritz		
Cobbler Apple	⅙ cake (4.33 oz)	290
Cobbler Blackberry	⅙ cake (4.33 oz)	250
Cobbler Blueberry	⅙ cake (4.33 oz)	270
Cobbler Cherry	⅙ cake (4.33 oz)	280
Cobbler Peach	⅙ cake (4.33 oz)	260
Cobbler Strawberry	⅙ cake (4.33 oz)	290
Pillsbury		
Apple Turnovers	1 (2 oz)	170
Cherry Turnovers	1 (2 oz)	180
Sara Lee		
Banana	⅙ cake (2.3 oz)	230
Banana Sundae	⅒ cake (2.8 oz)	270
Carrot	⅙ cake (3.2 oz)	320
Cheesecake Cherry	¼ cake (4.7 oz)	350
Cheesecake Chocolate Chip	¼ cake (4.2 oz)	410
Cheesecake Chocolate Mousse	⅕ cake	400
Cheesecake French	⅙ cake	350
Cheesecake Singles Fudge Brownie Crumble	1 slice (4 oz)	400
Cheesecake Singles Strawberry Drizzle	1 slice (4 oz)	380
Cheesecake Strawberry	¼ pie (4.7 oz)	330

FOOD	PORTION	CALS.
Sara Lee (CONT.)		
Cheesecake Strawberry French	⅙ cake	320
Cheesecake Bars Chocolate Dipped Original	1 bar (2.7 oz)	190
Cheesecake Bites Chocolate Praline Pecan	5 pieces (4 oz)	480
Cheesecake Bites Chocolate Praline Pecan	1 piece (0.8 oz)	100
Cheesecake Bites Chocolate Dipped Original	5 pieces (4 oz)	500
Cheesecake Bites Chocolate Dipped Original	1 piece (0.8 oz)	100
Cheesecake Bites Toasted Almond Crunch	5 pieces (4 oz)	470
Cheesecake Bits Toasted Almond Crunch	1 (0.8 oz)	90
Coffee Cake Butter Streusel	⅙ cake (1.9 oz)	220
Coffee Cake Cheese	⅙ cake (1.9 oz)	180
Coffee Cake Crumb	⅛ cake (2 oz)	220
Coffee Cake Pecan	⅙ cake (1.9 oz)	230
Coffee Cake Raspberry	⅙ cake (1.9 oz)	200
Harvest Pumpkin Spice	⅛ cake (2.9 oz)	270
Layer Cake Coconut	⅛ cake (2.8 oz)	280
Layer Cake Double Chocolate	⅛ cake (2.8 oz)	260
Layer Cake Fudge Golden	⅛ cake (2.8 oz)	270
Layer Cake German Chocolate	⅛ cake (2.9 oz)	280
Layer Cake Vanilla	⅛ cake (2.8 oz)	250
Original Cheesecake Reduced Fat	¼ cake (4.2 oz)	310
Pound Cake	¼ cake (2.7 oz)	320
Pound Cake Chocolate Swirl	1 slice (1 oz)	110
Pound Cake Family Size	⅙ cake (2.7 oz)	310
Pound Cake Free & Light	¼ cake (2.5 oz)	200
Pound Cake Golden	1 slice (1 oz)	120
Pound Cake Reduced Fat	1 slice (1 oz)	100
Pound Cake Strawberry	¼ cake (2.9 oz)	290
Red White & Blueberry	⅒ cake (3 oz)	210
Slice Chocolate	1 (3 oz)	320
Strawberry Shortcake	⅛ cake (2.5 oz)	180
Sinbad		
Baklava	1 piece (2 oz)	337
Tastykake		
Banana Creamie	1 (1.5 oz)	170
Bear Claw Appled	1 (3 oz)	280
Bear Claw Cinnamon	1 (3 oz)	300
Big Texas	1 (3 oz)	300
Breakfast Bun Chocolate Raisin	1 (3.2 oz)	330
Bunny Trail Treats	1 (1.3 oz)	150
Chocolate Creamie	1 (1.5 oz)	180

FOOD	PORTION	CALS.
Tastykake (CONT.)		
Chocolate Krimpies	2 (2.2 oz)	240
Coffee Roll Glazed	1 (3 oz)	300
Coffee Roll Vanilla	1 (3.2 oz)	320
Cupcakes Butter Cream Cream Filled Iced	2 (2.2 oz)	240
Cupcakes Chocolate Cream Filled Iced	2 (2.2 oz)	230
Cupcakes Cupcake	2 (2.1 oz)	200
Cupcakes Low Fat Chocolate Cream Filled	2 (2.2 oz)	200
Cupcakes Low Fat Vanilla Cream Filled	2 (2.2 oz)	190
Cupid Kake	1 (1.3 oz)	150
Honey Bun Glazed	1 (3.2 oz)	350
Honey Bun Iced	1 (3.2 oz)	350
Junior Chocolate	1 (3.3 oz)	330
Junior Coconut	1 (3.3 oz)	310
Junior Koffee Kake	1 (2.5 oz)	270
Junior Pound Kake	1 (3 oz)	320
Kandy Kakes Chocolate	3 (2 oz)	250
Kandy Kakes Coconut	2 (2.7 oz)	330
Kandy Kakes Peanut Butter	2 (1.3 oz)	190
Koffee Kake Cream Filled	2 (2 oz)	240
Koffee Kake Low Fat Apple	2 (2 oz)	170
Koffee Kake Low Fat Lemon	2 (2 oz)	180
Koffee Kake Low Fat Raspberry	2 (2 oz)	170
Kreepy Kakes	2 (2.2 oz)	240
Kreme Krimpies	2 (2 oz)	230
Krimpets Butterscotch Iced	2 (2 oz)	210
Krimpets Jelly Filled	2 (2 oz)	190
Krimpets Strawberry	2 (2 oz)	210
Kringle Kake	1 (1.3 oz)	150
Santa Snacks	2 (2.2 oz)	240
Sparkle Kake	1 (1.3 oz)	150
Tasty Tweets	2 (2.2 oz)	240
Tropical Delight Coconut	2 (2 oz)	190
Tropical Delight Guava	2 (2 oz)	190
Tropical Delight Papaya	2 (2 oz)	200
Tropical Delight Pineapple	2 (2 oz)	200
Vanilla Creamie	1 (1.5 oz)	190
Witchy Treat	1 (1.3 oz)	150
Toastettes		
Frosted Blueberry	1 (1.7 oz)	190
Frosted Brown Sugar Cinnamon	1 (1.7 oz)	190
Frosted Cherry	1 (1.7 oz)	190
Frosted Fudge	1 (1.7 oz)	190
Strawberry	1 (1.7 oz)	190

FOOD	PORTION	CALS.
Tortuga		
Cayman Island Rum Cake	1 piece (2 oz)	194
Weight Watchers		
Chocolate Raspberry Royale	1 (3.5 oz)	190
Chocolate Eclair	1 (2.1 oz)	150
Danish Coffee Cake Apple Cinnamon	1 piece (1.9 oz)	160
Danish Coffee Cake Cheese	1 piece (1.9 oz)	160
Danish Coffee Cake Raspberry	1 piece (1.9 oz)	160
Double Fudge	1 piece (2.75 oz)	190
French Style Cheesecake	1 piece (3.9 oz)	170
New York Style Cheesecake	1 piece (2.5 oz)	150
Strawberry Parfait Royale	1 (5.24 oz)	180
Triple Chocolate Eclair	1 (2.14 oz)	160
Well-Bred Loaf		
Banana Bread	1 slice (3.5 oz)	330
Banana Nut	1 slice (4.3 oz)	440
Blueberry	1 slice (4.3 oz)	440
Carrot	1 slice (4.3 oz)	480
Carrot Traditional	1 slice (4.3 oz)	440
Chocolate Chip	1 slice (4.3 oz)	490
Cinnamon Walnut	1 slice (4.3 oz)	480
Coconut Rum	1 slice (4.3 oz)	490
Cranberry	1 slice (4.3 oz)	460
Marble	1 slice (4.3 oz)	530
Pound All Butter	1 slice (4.3 oz)	470
Pound Mandarin Orange	1 slice (4 oz)	460
Raisin	1 slice (4.3 oz)	460
TAKE-OUT		
angelfood	1/12 cake (1 oz)	73
apple crisp	1/2 cup (5 oz)	230
boston cream pie	1/8 cake (3.3 oz)	293
carrot w/ cream cheese icing	1/12 cake (3.9 oz)	484
cheesecake w/ cherry topping	1/12 cake (5 oz)	359
chocolate w/ chocolate frosting	1/8 cake (2.2 oz)	235
coffeecake cheese	1/6 cake (2.7 oz)	258
coffeecake crumb topped cheese	1/6 cake (2.7 oz)	258
coffeecake crumb topped cinnamon	1/9 cake (2.2 oz)	263
cream puff w/ custard filling	1 (4.6 oz)	336
eclair w/ chocolate icing & custard filling	1	205
french apple tart	1 (3.5 oz)	302
fruitcake	1/36 cake (2.9 oz)	302
gingerbread	1/9 cake (2.6 oz)	264
panettone dal forno	1/9 cake (1.9 oz)	212
petit fours	2 (0.9 oz)	120

FOOD	PORTION	CALS.
pineapple upside down	⅑ cake (4 oz)	367
pound fat free	1 oz	80
pound cake	1 slice (1 oz)	120
sheet cake w/ white frosting	⅑ cake	445
strudel apple	1 piece (2½ oz)	195
tiramisu	1 piece (5.1 oz)	409
yellow w/ vanilla frosting	⅛ cake (2.2 oz)	239

CAKE ICING

FOOD	PORTION	CALS.
chocolate as prep w/ butter	1/12 box (1.5 oz)	161
chocolate as prep w/ butter	1 box (13.7 oz)	1908
chocolate as prep w/ butter home recipe	1/12 recipe (1.8 oz)	200
chocolate as prep w/ butter home recipe	1 recipe (21.1 oz)	2409
chocolate as prep w/ margarine	1 box (13.7 oz)	1909
chocolate as prep w/ margarine	1/12 box (1.5 oz)	161
chocolate as prep w/ margarine home recipe	1/12 recipe (1.8 oz)	200
chocolate as prep w/ margarine home recipe	1 recipe (21.1 oz)	2411
chocolate ready-to-use	1/12 pkg (1.3 oz)	151
chocolate ready-to-use	1 pkg (16 oz)	1834
coconut ready-to-use	1 pkg (16 oz)	1903
coconut ready-to-use	1/12 pkg (1.3 oz)	157
cream cheese ready-to-use	1 pkg (16 oz)	1906
cream cheese ready-to-use	1/12 pkg (1.3 oz)	157
glaze home recipe	1 recipe (11.5 oz)	1173
glaze home recipe	1/12 recipe (1 oz)	97
seven minute home recipe	1 recipe (13.6 oz)	1231
seven minute home recipe	1/12 recipe (1.1 oz)	102
sour cream ready-to-use	1/12 pkg (1.3 oz)	157
sour cream ready-to-use	1 pkg (16 oz)	1904
vanilla as prep w/ butter	1/12 pkg (1.5 oz)	182
vanilla as prep w/ butter	1 pkg (14.5 oz)	2188
vanilla as prep w/ butter home recipe	1/12 recipe (1.7 oz)	165
vanilla as prep w/ butter home recipe	1 recipe (20.1 oz)	1972
vanilla as prep w/ margarine	1 pkg (14.5 oz)	2190
vanilla as prep w/ margarine	1/12 pkg (1.5 oz)	182
vanilla as prep w/ margarine home recipe	1/12 recipe (1.7 oz)	195
vanilla as prep w/ margarine home recipe	1 recipe (20.1 oz)	2326
vanilla ready-to-use	1/12 pkg (1.3 oz)	159
vanilla ready-to-use	1 pkg (16 oz)	1936
white as prep w/ water	1 pkg (11.1 oz)	770
white as prep w/ water	1/12 pkg (0.9 oz)	64
Duncan Hines		
Chocolate Creamy Homestyle	2 tbsp	130
Milk Chocolate Creamy Homestyle	2 tbsp	130

FOOD	PORTION	CALS.
Duncan Hines (CONT.)		
Vanilla Creamy Homestyle	2 tbsp	140
Estee		
Frosting as prep	⅕ pkg	100
Jiffy		
Fudge	¼ cup (1.2 oz)	150
White	¼ cup (1.2 oz)	150
Sweet Rewards		
Ready-To-Spread Reduced Fat Chocolate	2 tbsp (1.2 oz)	120
Ready-To-Spread Reduced Fat Milk Chocolate	2 tbsp (1.2 oz)	120
Ready-To-Spread Reduced Fat Vanilla	2 tbsp (1.2 oz)	120

CAKE MIX
 (*see also* CAKE)

FOOD	PORTION	CALS.
angelfood	10 in cake (20.9 oz)	1535
angelfood	1/12 cake (1.8 oz)	129
carrot w/o frosting	2 layers (29.6 oz)	2886
carrot w/o frosting	1/12 cake (2.5 oz)	239
cheesecake no-bake	⅛ cake (3.5 oz)	271
chocolate pudding type w/o frosting	1/12 cake (2.7 oz)	270
chocolate pudding type w/o frosting	2 layers (32.4 oz)	3234
chocolate w/o frosting	2 layers (26.8 oz)	2393
chocolate w/o frosting	1/12 cake (2.3 oz)	198
chocolate w/o frosting low sodium	1/10 cake (1.3 oz)	116
coffeecake crumb topped cinnamon	⅛ cake (2 oz)	178
devil's food w/o frosting	1/12 cake (2.3 oz)	198
fudge w/o frosting	1/12 cake (2.3 oz)	198
german chocolate pudding type w/ coconut nut frosting	1/12 cake (3.9 oz)	404
gingerbread	⅑ cake (2.4 oz)	207
lemon w/o frosting no sugar low sodium	1/10 cake (1.3 oz)	118
marble pudding type w/o frosting	1/12 cake (2.6 oz)	253
marble pudding type w/o frosting	2 layers (30.6 oz)	3021
white pudding type w/o frosting	1/12 cake (2.4 oz)	244
white pudding type w/o frosting	2 layers (29 oz)	2915
white w/o frosting	1/12 cake (2.2 oz)	190
white w/o frosting	2 layer cake (26 oz)	2265
white w/o frosting no sugar low sodium	1/10 cake (1.3 oz)	118
yellow pudding-type w/o frosting	1/12 cake (2.6 oz)	257
yellow pudding-type w/o frosting	2 layers (31 oz)	3084
yellow w/o frosting	2 layers (26.5 oz)	2415
yellow w/o frosting	1/12 cake (2.2 oz)	202
yellow w/ chocolate frosting	1 cake, 9 in diam	3895

FOOD	PORTION	CALS.
Aunt Jemima		
Coffee Cake Easy Mix	⅓ cup (1.4 oz)	170
Bisquick		
Mix	⅓ cup (1.4 oz)	170
Reduced Fat	⅓ cup (1.4 oz)	150
Duncan Hines		
Angel Food as prep	1/12 pkg (1.3 oz)	140
Butter Recipe Golden as prep	1/12 cake	320
Cupcake Yellow as prep	1	180
Dark Chocolate Fudge as prep	1/12 cake	290
Devil's Food Moist Deluxe as prep	1/12 cake (1.5 oz)	290
French Vanilla	1/12 cake (1.5 oz)	250
Fudge Marble Moist Deluxe as prep	1/12 cake (1.5 oz)	250
Lemon Supreme Moist Deluxe	1/12 cake (1.5 oz)	250
White Moist Deluxe as prep	1/12 cake	190
Yellow Moist Deluxe as prep	1/12 cake (1.5 oz)	250
Yellow Moist Deluxe as prep	1/12 cake	250
Estee		
Chocolate as prep	⅕ cake	190
White as prep	⅕ cake	200
Hain		
Whole Wheat Baking Mix	1½ oz	150
Jell-O		
No Bake Cherry Cheesecake as prep	⅛ cake (4.8 oz)	340
No Bake Double Layer Chocolate as prep	⅛ cake (4.4 oz)	260
No Bake Double Layer Cookies And Creme as prep	⅛ cake (4.5 oz)	390
No Bake Double Layer Lemon as prep	⅛ cake (4.4 oz)	260
No Bake Homestyle Cheesecake as prep	⅙ cake (4.6 oz)	360
No Bake Peanut Butter Cup as prep	⅛ cake (3.8 oz)	380
No Bake Reduced Fat Strawberry Swirl Cheesecake as prep	⅛ cake (4 oz)	250
No Bake Strawberry Cheesecake as prep	⅛ cake (4.8 oz)	340
Real Cheesecake as prep	⅛ cake (4.6 oz)	360
Jiffy		
Devil's Food as prep	⅕ cake	220
Golden Yellow as prep	⅕ cake	220
White as prep	⅕ cake	210
Pillsbury		
Strawberry	1/12 cake	260
Royal		
Cheese Cake Lite No-Bake	⅛ pie	130
Cheese Cake Real No-Bake	⅛ pie	160

FOOD	PORTION	CALS.
Sweet Rewards		
Reduced Fat Devils Food	1/12 cake	200
Reduced Fat Devils Food No Cholesterol Recipe	1/12 cake	190
Reduced Fat White Whole Egg Recipe	1/12 cake	200
Reduced Fat Yellow	1/12 cake	200
Reduced Fat Yellow No Cholesterol Recipe	1/12 cake	190
Wanda's		
Double Chocolate	1/4 cup mix per serv (1.4 oz)	170

CALABAZA
fresh	1/2 cup	32

CALZONE
TAKE-OUT
cheese	1 (12 oz)	1020

CANADIAN BACON
grilled	1 pkg (6 oz)	257
Boar's Head		
Canadian Bacon	2 oz	70
Hormel		
Canadian Bacon	2 oz	70
Oscar Mayer		
Canadian Bacon	2 slices (1.6 oz)	50

CANDY
(*see also* MARSHMALLOW)

butterscotch	1 piece (6 g)	24
butterscotch	1 oz	112
candy corn	1 oz	105
caramels	1 pkg (2.5 oz)	271
caramels	1 piece (8 g)	31
caramels chocolate	1 piece (6 g)	22
caramels chocolate	1 bar (2.3 oz)	231
carob bar	1 (3.1 oz)	453
crisped rice bar almond	1 bar (1 oz)	130
crisped rice bar chocolate chip	1 bar (1 oz)	115
dark chocolate	1 oz	150
fondant chocolate coated	1 sm (0.4 oz)	40
fondant chocolate coated	1 lg (1.2 oz)	128
gumdrops	10 sm (0.4 oz)	135
gumdrops	10 lg (3.8 oz)	420
hard candy	1 oz	106
jelly beans	10 sm (0.4 oz)	40

FOOD	PORTION	CALS.
jelly beans	10 lg (1 oz)	104
lollipop	1 (6 g)	22
marzipan	1 oz	128
milk chocolate	1 bar (1.55 oz)	226
milk chocolate crisp	1 bar (1.45 oz)	203
milk chocolate w/ almonds	1 bar (1.45 oz)	215
peanut bar	1 (1.4 oz)	209
peanuts chocolate covered	10 (1.4 oz)	208
peanuts chocolate covered	1 cup (5.2 oz)	773
pretzels chocolate covered	1 oz	130
pretzels chocolate covered	1 (0.4 oz)	50
sesame crunch	1 oz	146
sesame crunch	20 pieces (1.2 oz)	181
sweet chocolate	1 bar (1.45 oz)	201
sweet chocolate	1 oz	143
100 Grand		
Bar	1 bar (1.5 oz)	200
3 Musketeers		
Bar	2 fun size (1.2 oz)	140
Bar	1 (2.1 oz)	260
Andes		
Chocolate Covered Mint Patties	1 (0.5 oz)	60
Baby Ruth		
Bar	1 (2.1 oz)	270
Fun Size	2 pieces	200
Barricini		
Dark Chocolate Raspberry Creme Shells	1 piece (0.3 oz)	47
Bits O Brickle		
Candy	1 tbsp (0.5 oz)	80
Bonus		
Bar	1 bar (2.1 oz)	290
Breath Savers		
Sugar Free Mint Cinnamon	1 piece (2 g)	10
Sugar Free Peppermint	1 piece (2 g)	10
Sugar Free Spearmint	1 piece (2 g)	10
Sugar Free Wintergreen	1 piece (2 g)	10
Brock		
Butterscotch Discs	3 pieces (0.6 oz)	70
Candy Corn	21 pieces (1.4 oz)	150
Candy Rolls	2 rolls (0.5 oz)	50
Caramel Dots	3 pieces (1.3 oz)	140
Cinnamon Discs	3 pieces (0.6 oz)	70
Circus Peanuts	11 pieces (2.5 oz)	260
Coconut Mountains	4 pieces (1.4 oz)	170

FOOD	PORTION	CALS.
Brock (cont.)		
Fruit Basket	3 pieces (0.6 oz)	60
Fruit Kisses	3 pieces (0.6 oz)	70
Glitters	2 pieces (0.5 oz)	50
Gummy Bears	5 pieces (1.4 oz)	130
Gummy Squirms	5 pieces (1.3 oz)	120
Jelly Beans	12 pieces (1.4 oz)	140
Lemon Drops	3 pieces (0.5 oz)	60
Orange Slices	4 pieces (1.5 oz)	140
Party Mints	9 pieces (0.5 oz)	60
Peanut Butter Crunch	3 pieces (0.6 oz)	80
Pops Assorted	2 (0.5 oz)	60
Sour Balls	3 pieces (0.6 oz)	70
Sour Sharks	23 pieces (2.5 oz)	30
Spearmint Starlights	3 pieces (0.6 oz)	60
Spice Drops	12 pieces (1.4 oz)	130
Starlight Mints	3 pieces (0.6 oz)	60
Toffee	6 pieces (1.5 oz)	170
Butterfinger		
BB's	1 pkg (1.7 oz)	230
Bar	1 (2.1 oz)	280
Fun Size	2 bars (1.6 oz)	200
Cellas		
Chocolate Covered Cherries Dark Chocolate	2 pieces (1 oz)	100
Chocolate Covered Cherries Milk Chocolate	2 pieces (1 oz)	110
Certs		
Breath Mints	1 piece (1.67 g)	6
Mini Sugar Free	1 piece (0.365 g)	1
Sugar Free	1 piece (1.67 g)	7
Charleston Chew		
Candy	1 pkg (1.9 oz)	230
Charms		
Blow Pop	1 (0.6 oz)	70
Lollipop Sour	1 (0.6 oz)	70
Lollipop Sweet	1 (0.6 oz)	70
Chuckles		
Candy	4 pieces (1.4 oz)	140
Chunky		
Bar	1 (1.4 oz)	200
Clorets		
Mints	1 piece (1.67 g)	6

FOOD	PORTION	CALS.
Crunch		
Fun Size	4 bars (1.5 oz)	200
Del Monte		
Radical Raizins Cinnamon	1 pkg (0.7 oz)	70
Radical Raizins Rainbow	1 pkg (0.7 oz)	70
Dove		
Dark Chocolate	¼ bar (1.5 oz)	230
Dark Chocolate	1 bar (1.3 oz)	200
Dark Chocolate Minatures	7 (1.5 oz)	220
Milk Chocolate	1 bar (1.3 oz)	200
Milk Chocolate	¼ bar (1.5 oz)	230
Milk Chocolate Miniatures	7 (1.5 oz)	230
Truffles	3 (1.2 oz)	200
Dream		
Caramel & Nougat In Milk Chocolate	1 bar (1 oz)	90
Estee		
Caramels Vanilla & Chocolate	5	115
Dark Chocolate	½ bar (1.4 oz)	200
Milk Chocolate	½ bar (1.4 oz)	230
Milk Chocolate w/ Almonds	½ bar (1.4 oz)	230
Milk Chocolate w/ Crisp Rice	½ bar (1.2 oz)	370
Milk Chocolate w/ Fruit & Nuts	½ bar (1.4 oz)	220
Mint Chocolate	½ bar (1.4 oz)	200
Peanut Brittle	⅓ box (1.3 oz)	160
Peanut Butter Cups	5	200
Sugar Free Assorted Fruit	5	30
Sugar Free Assorted Mint	5	30
Sugar Free Butterscotch	2	25
Sugar Free Fruit Gum Drops	23	80
Sugar Free Gourmet Jelly Beans	26	70
Sugar Free Gummy Apple Rings	5	70
Sugar Free Gummy Bears Assorted Fruit	17	100
Sugar Free Licorice Gum Drops	11	90
Sugar Free Peppermint Swirl	3	30
Sugar Free Sour Citrus Slices	9	60
Sugar Free Toffee	5	30
Sugar Free Tropical Fruit	5	30
Favorite Brands		
Candy Corn	24 pieces (1.4 oz)	150
Cinnamon Imperials	52 (0.5 oz)	80
Circus Peanuts	5 pieces (1.6 oz)	160
Gummallo Apple Ring	5 pieces (1.4 oz)	120
Gummallo Peach Ring	5 pieces (1.4 oz)	120
Gummi Bears	18 pieces (1.4 oz)	130

FOOD	PORTION	CALS.
Favorite Brands (CONT.)		
Gummi Dinos	7 pieces (1.3 oz)	120
Gummi Worms	4 pieces (1.4 oz)	130
Jelly Beans	13 (1.4 oz)	150
Marshmallow Eggs	3 (1.3 oz)	140
Neon Worms	4 pieces (1.4 oz)	120
Sour Gummi Bears	16 pieces (1.4 oz)	110
Sour Gummi Worms	4 pieces (1.6 oz)	130
Ferrero Rocher		
Candy	2 pieces (0.9 oz)	150
Franklin		
Crunch 'N Munch Candied	1.25 oz	170
Crunch 'N Munch Caramel	1.25 oz	160
Crunch 'N Munch Maple Walnut	1.25 oz	160
Crunch 'N Munch Toffee	1.25 oz	160
Godiva		
Almond Butter Dome	3 pieces (1.5 oz)	240
Bouchee Au Chocolat	1 piece (1.5 oz)	210
Bouchee Ivory Raspberry	1 pieces (1 oz)	160
Gold Ballotin	3 pieces (1.5 oz)	210
Truffle Amaretto Di Saronno	2 pieces (1.5 oz)	210
Truffle Deluxe Liqueur	2 pieces (1.5 oz)	210
Goldenberg's		
Peanut Chews	3 pieces (1.3 oz)	180
Goo Goo Supreme		
With Pecans	1 pkg (1.5 oz)	188
Goobers		
Peanuts	1 pkg (1.38 oz)	210
Good & Fruity		
Candy	1 box (1.8 oz)	140
Good & Plenty		
Snacksize	3 boxes (1.5 oz)	140
Haviland		
Chocolate Covered Thin Mints	6 (1.5 oz)	170
Heath		
Bar	1 (1.4 oz)	210
Hershey		
Amazin'Fruit Gummy Candy	2 snack pkg (1.4 oz)	130
Jolly Rancher		
Candies	3 pieces (0.6 oz)	60
Joyva		
Halvah	1.5 oz	240
Halvah Chocolate Covered	1 bar (2 oz)	380
Jells Raspberry	3 pieces (1.6 oz)	200

FOOD	PORTION	CALS.
Joyva (CONT.)		
Joys Raspberry	1 (1.6 oz)	200
Marshmallow Twists Chocolate Covered	2 (1.5 oz)	190
Rings Orange & Raspberry	3 pieces (1.5 oz)	190
Sesame Crunch	3 pieces (0.5)	80
Sticks Orange	3 pieces (1.6 oz)	200
Twists Vanilla & Cherry	2 pieces (1.5 oz)	190
Juicefuls		
Candy	3 pieces (0.5 oz)	60
Junior Mints		
Candies	1 pkg (1.6 oz)	190
Snack Size	1 pkg (0.7 oz)	75
Just Born		
Hot Tamales	1 pkg (2.1 oz)	220
Mike and Ike Berry Fruits	1 pkg (2.1 oz)	220
Mike and Ike Cherry & Bubble Gum	1 pkg (2.1 oz)	220
Mike and Ike Chewy Grape	1 pkg (2.1 oz)	220
Mike and Ike Lemon Watermelon	1 pkg (2.1 oz)	220
Mike and Ike Original	1 pkg (1.2 oz)	220
Mike and Ike Strawberry & Banana	1 pkg (2.1 oz)	220
Mike and Ike Tropical Fruits	1 pkg (2.1 oz)	220
Super Hot Tamales	1 pkg (2.1 oz)	220
Teenee Beanee Assorted Fruits	36 pieces (1.4 oz)	150
Teenee Beanee Berry Berry	36 pieces (1.4 oz)	150
Teenee Beanee Tropical Mix	36 pieces (1.4 oz)	150
Lifesavers		
Big Tablet Candy Cane	4 pieces (0.5 oz)	60
Cards 'N Candy	4 pieces (0.4 oz)	40
Christmas Tin	4 pieces (0.5 oz)	60
Egg-Sortment	1 roll (0.4 oz)	40
Fruit Juicers Lollipops	1	40
Gummi Bunnies	3 pkg (1.6 oz)	140
Gummi Savers Five Flavor	1 roll (1.5 oz)	130
Gummi Savers Five Flavor	1 pkg (1.8 oz)	160
Gummi Savers Mixed Berry	1 roll (1.5 oz)	130
Gummi Savers Mixed Berry	1 pkg (1.8 oz)	160
Gummi Savers Tangy Fruits	1 pkg (1.8 oz)	160
Gummi Savers Tangy Fruits	1 roll (1.5 oz)	130
Gummi Savers Variety	2 pkg (1.3 oz)	120
Gummi Savers Wacky Frootz	1 roll (1.5 oz)	130
Gummi Savers Wacky Frootz	1 pkg (1.8 oz)	160
Holes Five Flavor	20 pieces (5 g)	20
Holes Island Fruit	20 pieces (5 g)	20
Holes Sour 'N Sweet	16 pieces (5 g)	20

FOOD	PORTION	CALS.
Lifesavers (CONT.)		
Holes Sunshine Fruits	20 pieces (0.2 oz)	20
Holes Super Tart	20 pieces (5 g)	20
Holes Tangerine	1 candy	2
Holes Wild Fruits	20 pieces (5 g)	20
Lollipops Candy Cane	1 (0.4 oz)	40
Lollipops Christmas	1 (0.4 oz)	40
Lollipops Easter	1 (0.4 oz)	40
Lollipops Fruit Flavors	1 (0.4 oz)	45
Lollipops Swirled Flavors	1 (0.4 oz)	40
Lollipops Valentine	1 (0.4 oz)	40
Roll Butter Rum	2 pieces (5 g)	20
Roll Candy Cane	4 pieces (0.4 oz)	40
Roll Cryst-O-Mint	2 pieces (5 g)	20
Roll Five Flavor	2 pieces (5 g)	20
Roll Fruits On Fire	2 pieces (5 g)	20
Roll Pep-O-Mint	3 pieces (5 g)	20
Roll Spear-O-Mint	3 pieces (5 g)	20
Roll Sunshine Fruits	2 pieces (5 g)	20
Roll Tangy Fruit Swirl	2 pieces (5 g)	20
Roll Tangy Fruit Watermelon	1 pieces (5 g)	20
Roll Tangy Fruits	2 pieces (5 g)	20
Roll Tropical Fruits	2 pieces (5 g)	20
Roll Wild Cherry	1 pieces (5 g)	20
Roll Wild Flavors	2 pieces (5 g)	20
Roll Wild Sour Berries	2 pieces (5 g)	20
Roll Wint-O-Green	3 pieces (5 g)	20
Sack'it Butter Rum	4 pieces (0.5 oz)	60
Sack'it Five Flavor	4 pieces (0.5 oz)	60
Sack'it Holiday Tin	4 pieces (0.5 oz)	60
Sack'it Pep-O-Mint	4 pieces (0.5 oz)	60
Sack'it Tangy Fruits	4 pieces (0.5 oz)	60
Sack'it Wild Cherry	4 pieces (0.5 oz)	60
Sack'it Wint-O-Green	4 pieces (0.5 oz)	60
Sugar Free Iced Mint	1 pieces (2 g)	10
Sugar Free Vanilla Mint	1 pieces (2 g)	10
Valentine Book	2 pieces (5 g)	20
Lindt		
Truffles Milk Chocolate	3 pieces (1.3 oz)	210
M&M's		
Almond	1.5 oz	220
Almond	1 pkg (1.3 oz)	200
Mint	1 pkg (1.7 oz)	230
Mint	1.5 oz	200

FOOD	PORTION	CALS.
M&M's (CONT.)		
Peanut	½ bag king size (1.6 oz)	240
Peanut	1 fun size (0.7 oz)	110
Peanut	1 pkg (1.7 oz)	250
Peanut	1.5 oz	220
Peanut Butter	1 fun size (0.7 oz)	110
Peanut Butter	1.5 oz	220
Peanut Butter	1 pkg (1.6 oz)	240
Plain	1 pkg fun size (0.7 oz)	100
Plain	½ pkg king size (1.6 oz)	220
Plain	1 pkg (1.7 oz)	230
Plain	1.5 oz	200
Mars		
Almond Bar	2 fun size (1.3 oz)	190
Almond Bar	1 bar (1.8 oz)	240
Mayfair		
Mints	5 pieces (1.3 oz)	180
Milk Duds		
Pieces	1 box (1.8 oz)	230
Snack Size	4 boxes (1.3 oz)	160
Milkshake		
Bar	1 bar (1.8 oz)	220
Milky Way		
Bar	2 fun size (1.4 oz)	180
Bar	⅓ king size (1.2 oz)	160
Bar	1 (2.1 oz)	280
Dark	1 fun size (0.7 oz)	90
Dark	1 bar (1.8 oz)	220
Miniature	5 (1.5 oz)	190
NECCO		
Mint	1 piece	12
Nestle		
Areo Bar	1 bar (1.45 oz)	210
Buncha Crunch	1 pkg (1.4 oz)	90
Crunch	1 bar (1.55 oz)	230
Milk Chocolate	1 bar (1.45 oz)	220
Treasures Crunch	4 pieces (1.4 oz)	210
Turtles Bite Size	1 piece (0.4 oz)	50
Turtles Pecan Caramel Candy	2 pieces (1.2 oz)	160
Newman's Own		
Organics Espresso Sweet Dark Chocolate	1 bar (1.2 oz)	190
Nips		
Butter Rum	2 pieces (0.5 oz)	60
Caramel	2 pieces (0.5 oz)	60

FOOD	PORTION	CALS.
Nips (CONT.)		
Chocolate Mint	2 pieces (0.5 oz)	60
Chocolate Parfait	2 pieces (0.5 oz)	60
Peanut Butter Parfait	2 pieces (0.5 oz)	60
Ocean Spray		
Fruit Waves Assorted	3 pieces (0.3 oz)	35
Oh Henry!		
Bar	1 (1.8 oz)	230
Palmer		
Milk Chocolate Lollipop	1 (0.9 oz)	130
PayDay		
Bar	1 (1.85 oz)	240
Pearson's		
Licorice	2 pieces (0.5 oz)	60
Mint Patties	5 (1.3 oz)	150
Pez		
Candy	1 roll (0.3 oz)	30
Sugar Free	1 roll (0.3 oz)	30
Planters		
Original Peanut Bar	1 pkg (1.6 oz)	230
Pom Pom		
Candies	1 pkg (1.6 oz)	200
Raisinets		
Candy	1 pkg (1.58 oz)	200
Fun Size	3 pkg (1.7 oz)	210
Reese's		
Sticks	1 (0.7 oz)	120
Riesen		
Candy	5 pieces (1.4 oz)	180
Rokeach		
Cotton Candy	2 cups (1 oz)	110
Russell Stover		
Assorted Creams	3 pieces (1.4 oz)	180
Looney Tunes Peanut Butter Nougat w/ Peanuts in Milk Chocolate	1 snack size (0.7 oz)	90
Pecan Roll	1 (2 oz)	300
See's		
Lollypop Butterscotch	1	90
Lollypop Cafe Latte	1	90
Lollypop Chocolate	1	90
Lollypop Peanut Butter	1	90
Simply Lite		
Sugar Free Lil'l Bits Chocolately	36 pieces (1.4 oz)	130
Sugar Free Lil'l Bits Peanut Buttery	36 pieces (1.4 oz)	140

FOOD	PORTION	CALS.
Simply Lite (CONT.)		
Sugar Free Patteez	5 pieces (1.3 oz)	110
Skittles		
Original	2 pkg fun size (1.6 oz)	180
Original	1 pkg (2.8 oz)	250
Original	½ king size (1.3 oz)	150
Original	1.5 oz	170
Tropical	1 bag (2.2 oz)	250
Tropical	1.5 oz	170
Tropical	2 bags fun size (1.4 oz)	160
Wild Berry	2 bags fun size (1.4 oz)	160
Wild Berry	1 bag (2.2 oz)	250
Wild Berry	1.5 oz	170
Smucker's		
Fruit Fillers Strawberry	1 pkg (0.9 oz)	80
Jelly Beans	1 pkg (0.7 oz)	70
Snickers		
Bar	1 bar (2.1 oz)	280
Bar	2 bars fun size (1.4 oz)	190
Bar	⅓ king size (1.2 oz)	170
Miniatures	4 (1.3 oz)	170
Munch Bar	1 (1.4 oz)	230
Peanut Butter	1 bar (2 oz)	310
Sno-Caps		
Candies	1 pkg (2.3 oz)	300
Sour Punch		
Candy Straws Sour Apple	6 pieces (1.4 oz)	130
Spice Stix		
And Drops	14 pieces (1.6 oz)	140
Starburst		
California Fruits	8 pieces (1.4 oz)	160
California Fruits	1 stick (2.1 oz)	240
Original Fruits	⅓ king size (1.2 oz)	140
Original Fruits	8 pieces (1.4 oz)	160
Orignal Fruits	1 stick (2.1 oz)	240
Strawberry Fruits	8 pieces (1.4 oz)	160
Strawberry Fruits	1 stick (2.1 oz)	240
Tropical Fruits	1 stick (2.1 oz)	240
Tropical Fruits	8 pieces (1.4 oz)	160
Sugar Babies		
Candies	1 pkg (1.7 oz)	190
Sugar Daddy		
Candies	1 pkg (1.7 oz)	200

FOOD	PORTION	CALS.
Swedish Fish		
Original	19 pieces (1.4 oz)	160
Sweet Escapes		
Triple Chocolate Wafer Bars	1 (0.7 oz)	80
Sweet'N Low		
Sugar Free Butter Toffee	4 pieces (0.5 oz)	30
Sugar Free Butterscotch	1 piece	7
Sugar Free Cinnamon	1 piece	7
Sugar Free Fancy Fruit	1 piece	7
Sugar Free Fruit Flavors	1 piece	7
Sugar Free Hard Candy Coffee	4 pieces (0.5 oz)	30
Sugar Free Peppermint	1 piece	7
Sugar Free Soft Candy Fruitie Flavors	1 piece	11
Sugar Free Soft Candy Tropical Flavors	1 piece	11
Sugar Free Watermelon	1 piece	7
Sugar Free Wild Cherry	1 piece	7
Switzer		
Cherry Bites	12 pieces (1.6 oz)	50
Licorice Bites	12 pieces (1.6 oz)	46
Terry's		
Orange Milk Chocolate	5 pieces (1.5 oz)	240
Tootsie Roll		
Candy	1 (1 oz)	110
Dots	12 (1.5 oz)	160
Midgees	6 (1.4 oz)	160
Pop	1 (0.6 oz)	60
Twix		
Caramel	1 pkg (2 oz)	280
Caramel	1 (1 oz)	140
Caramel	1 fun size (0.5 oz)	80
Caramel	1 king size (0.8 oz)	120
Peanut Butter	1 (0.9 oz)	130
Twizzlers		
Candy	4 pieces (1.4 oz)	130
Pull-N-Peel Cherry	1 piece (1.1 oz)	110
Velamints		
Cocoamint	1 piece (1.7 g)	5
Peppermint	1 piece (1.7 g)	5
Spearmint	1 piece (1.7 g)	5
Wintergreen	1 piece (1.7 g)	5
Very Special		
Chocolate Bottles Liquor Filled	3 pieces (1 oz)	150
Whitman's		
Assorted	3 pieces (1.4 oz)	190

FOOD	PORTION	CALS.
Whitman's (CONT.)		
Dark Chocolate	3 pieces (1.4 oz)	200
Little Ambassadors	7 pieces (1.4 oz)	190
Pecan Delight	1 bar (2 oz)	310
Pecan Roll	1 bar (2 oz)	300
Sampler	3 pieces (1.4 oz)	200
Snoopy Treats Caramel Peanuts Milk Chocolate	1 snack size (1.4 oz)	80
Whoppers		
Candy	1 pkg (1.8 oz)	230
York		
Peppermint Patty	1 snack size (0.5 oz)	57
Zero		
Bar	2 pieces (1.4 oz)	170
HOME RECIPE		
divinity	1 recipe 48 pieces (19 oz)	1891
divinity	1 (11 g)	38
fondant	1 recipe 60 pieces (32.6 oz)	3327
fondant	1 piece (0.6 oz)	57
fudge brown sugar w/ nuts	1 piece (0.5 oz)	56
fudge brown sugar w/ nuts	1 recipe 60 pieces (30.7 oz)	3453
fudge chocolate	1 piece (0.6 oz)	65
fudge chocolate	1 recipe 48 pieces (29 oz)	3161
fudge chocolate marshmallow	1 recipe (43.1 oz)	5182
fudge chocolate marshmallow	1 piece (0.7 oz)	84
fudge chocolate marshmallow w/ nuts	1 piece (0.8 oz)	96
fudge chocolate marshmallow w/ nuts	1 recipe 60 pieces (43.1 oz)	5182
fudge chocolate marshmallow w/ nuts	1 recipe 60 pieces (46.1 oz)	5742
fudge chocolate w/ nuts	1 recipe 48 pieces (32.7 oz)	3967
fudge chocolate w/ nuts	1 piece (0.7 oz)	81
fudge peanut butter	1 piece (0.6 oz)	59
fudge peanut butter	1 recipe 36 pieces (20.4 oz)	2161
fudge vanilla	1 piece (0.6 oz)	59
fudge vanilla	1 recipe 48 pieces (27.5 oz)	2893
fudge vanilla w/ nuts	1 recipe 60 pieces (31 oz)	3666

FOOD	PORTION	CALS.
fudge vanilla w/ nuts	1 piece (0.5 oz)	62
peanut brittle	1 recipe (17.6 oz)	2288
peanut brittle	1 oz	128
praline	1 recipe 23 pieces (31.8 oz)	4116
praline	1 piece (1.4 oz)	177
taffy	1 piece (0.5 oz)	56
taffy	1 recipe 48 pieces (25 oz)	2677
toffee	1 piece (0.4 oz)	65
toffee	1 recipe 48 pieces (19.4 oz)	2997
truffles	1 piece (0.4 oz)	59
truffles	1 recipe 49 pieces (21.5 oz)	2985

CANTALOUPE

fresh cubed	1 cup	57
fresh half	½	94
Big Valley		
Balls frzn	¾ cup (4.9 oz)	40
Dole		
Fresh	¼	50

CAPERS

Progresso		
Capers	1 tsp (5 g)	0
Reese		
Capers	1 tsp (5 g)	0

CARAWAY

seed	1 tsp	7

CARDAMON

ground	1 tsp	6

CARDOON

fresh cooked	3.5 oz	22
raw shredded	½ cup	36

CARIBOU

roasted	3 oz	142

CARISSA

fresh	1	12

CAROB

carob mix	3 tsp	45

FOOD	PORTION	CALS.
CARP		
fresh cooked	3 oz	138
roe raw	3½ oz	130
CARROT JUICE		
canned	6 oz	73
Hain		
Juice	6 fl oz	80
Hollywood		
Juice	6 fl oz	80
Odwalla		
Juice	8 fl oz	70
CARROTS		
CANNED		
Allen		
Sliced	½ cup (4.5 oz)	35
Crest Top		
Sliced	½ cup (4.5 oz)	35
Del Monte		
Cut	½ cup (4.3 oz)	35
Sliced	½ cup (4.3 oz)	35
Green Giant		
Sliced	½ cup (4.2 oz)	25
LeSueur		
Baby Whole	½ cup (4.2 oz)	35
Seneca		
Diced	½ cup	30
Sliced	½ cup	30
FRESH		
baby raw	1 (0.5 oz)	6
raw	1 (2.5 oz)	31
raw shredded	½ cup	24
slices cooked	½ cup	35
Dole		
Medium	1	40
FROZEN		
Big Valley		
Carrots	½ cup (3 oz)	35
Birds Eye		
Baby Whole	⅔ cup (3 oz)	35
Fresh Like		
Carrots	3.5 oz	42
Green Giant		
Harvest Fresh Baby	⅔ cup (3 oz)	20

FOOD	PORTION	CALS.
Green Giant (CONT.)		
Select Baby Cut	¾ cup (2.8 oz)	30
CASABA		
cubed	1 cup	45
fresh	¹⁄₁₀	43
CASHEWS		
cashew butter w/o salt	1 tbsp	94
Beer Nuts		
Cashews	1 pkg (1 oz)	170
Fisher		
Honey Roasted Halves	1 oz	150
Honey Roasted Whole	1 oz	150
Oil Roasted Halves	1 oz	170
Oil Roasted Whole	1 oz	170
Frito Lay		
Salted	1 oz	180
Guy's		
Whole Salted	1 oz	170
Hain		
Cashew Butter Raw	2 tbsp	190
Cashew Butter Raw Unsalted	2 tbsp	210
Cashew Butter Toasted	2 tbsp	210
Planters		
Fancy Oil Roasted	1 oz	170
Fancy Oil Roasted	1 pkg (2 oz)	340
Halves Lightly Salted Oil Roasted	1 oz	160
Halves Oil Roasted	1 oz	170
Honey Roasted	1 oz	150
Honey Roasted	1 pkg (2 oz)	310
Munch'N Go Honey Roasted	1 pkg (2 oz)	310
Munch'N Go Singles Oil Roasted	1 pkg (2 oz)	330
Oil Roasted	1 pkg (1 oz)	160
Oil Roasted	1 pkg (1.5 oz)	250
CASSAVA		
raw	3.5 oz	120
CATFISH		
channel breaded & fried	3 oz	194
CATSUP		
(*see* KETCHUP)		
CAULIFLOWER		
FRESH		
cooked	½ cup (2.2 oz)	14

FOOD	PORTION	CALS.
flowerets cooked	3 (2 oz)	12
flowerets raw	3 (2 oz)	14
green cooked	1½ cup (3.2 oz)	29
green raw	1 head 7 in diam (18 oz)	158
green raw	1 cup (2.2 oz)	20
green raw floweret	1 (0.9 oz)	8
raw	½ cup (1.8 oz)	13
Dole		
Cauliflower	⅙ med head	18
FROZEN		
Big Valley		
Florets	¾ cup (3 oz)	25
Birds Eye		
Frzn	⅔ cup	25
In Cheese Sauce	½ cup (4.1 oz)	80
Fresh Like		
Cauliflower	3.5 oz	26
Green Giant		
Cheese Sauce	½ cup (3.5 oz)	60
Florets	1 cup (2.8 oz)	25
JARRED		
Vlasic		
Hot & Spicy	1 oz	4
Sweet	1 oz	35

CAVIAR
black	1 tbsp	40
red	1 tbsp	40

CELERIAC
fresh cooked	3.5 oz	25
raw	½ cup	31

CELERY
DRIED
seed	1 tsp	8

FRESH
raw	1 stalk (1.3 oz)	6
raw diced	½ cup	10
Dole		
Stalks	2 med	20

FROZEN
Fresh Like
Celery	3.5 oz	14

CELTUCE
raw	3.5 oz	22

FOOD	PORTION	CALS.
CEREAL		
corn flakes low sodium	1 cup (0.9 oz)	100
corn grits white regular & quick as prep w/ water & salt	¾ cup (6.4 oz)	109
corn grits white regular or quick as prep	¾ cup (6.4 oz)	109
corn grits yellow regular & quick as prep w/ water & salt	¾ cup (6.4 oz)	109
corn grits yellow regular & quick not prep	1 cup (5.5 oz)	579
crispy rice	1 cup (1 oz)	111
crispy rice low sodium	1 cup (0.9 oz)	105
farina as prep w/ water	¾ cup (6.1 oz)	88
farina not prep	1 tbsp (0.4 oz)	40
oatmeal instant w/ cinnamon & spice as prep w/ water	1 pkg (5.6 oz)	177
oatmeal instant w/ raisins & spice as prep w/ water	1 cup (5.5 oz)	161
oatmeal instant w/ bran & raisins as prep w/ water	1 pkg (6.8 oz)	158
oatmeal instant as prep w/ water	1 cup (8.2 oz)	138
oatmeal regular & quick as prep w/ water	¾ cup (6.1 oz)	149
oatmeal regular & quick not prep	⅓ cup (0.9 oz)	104
puffed rice	1 cup (0.5 oz)	56
puffed wheat	1 cup (0.4 oz)	44
shredded mini wheats	1 cup (1.1 oz)	107
shredded wheat rectangular	1 biscuit (0.8 oz)	85
shredded wheat round	2 biscuits (1.3 oz)	136
whole wheat hot natural as prep w/ water	¾ cup (6.4 oz)	113
Albers		
Hominy Quick Grits uncooked	¼ cup	140
Arrowhead		
4 Grain + Flax	¼ cup (1.6 oz)	150
7 Grain	⅓ cup (1.4 oz)	140
Amaranth Flakes	1 cup (1.2 oz)	130
Apple Corns	1 cup (1.5 oz)	150
Bear Mush	¼ cup (1.6 oz)	160
Bran Flakes	1 cup (1 oz)	100
Kamut Flakes	1 cup (1.1 oz)	120
Maple Corns	1 cup (1.9 oz)	190
Multi Grain Flakes	1 cup (1.2 oz)	140
Nature O's	1 cup (1.1 oz)	130
Oat Bran Flakes	1 cup (1.2 oz)	110
Oat Flakes Rolled	⅓ cup (1.2 oz)	130
Oat Groats	¼ cup (1.5 oz)	160

FOOD	PORTION	CALS.
Arrowhead (CONT.)		
Oatmeal Instant Original	1 oz	100
Puffed Corn	1 cup (0.8 oz)	80
Puffed Kamut	1 cup (0.6 oz)	50
Puffed Millet	1 cup (0.9 oz)	90
Puffed Rice	1 cup (0.8 oz)	90
Puffed Wheat	1 cup (0.9)	90
Rice & Shine	¼ cup (1.5 oz)	150
Spelt Flakes	1 cup (1.1 oz)	100
Wheat Flakes Rolled	⅓ cup (1.2 oz)	110
Barbara's		
Apple Cinnamon Toasted O's	¾ cup	110
Bite Size Shredded Oats	1¼ cups (2 oz)	220
Breakfast O's	1 cup (1 oz)	120
Brown Rice Crisps	1 cup (1 oz)	120
Cocoa Crunch Stars	1 cup (1 oz)	110
Corn Flakes	1 cup (1 oz)	110
Frosted Corn Flakes	1 cup (1 oz)	110
Honey Crunch Stars	1 cup (1 oz)	110
Honey Nut Toasted O's	¾ cup	120
Organic Ultra Minis Frosted	¾ cup (1.9 oz)	190
Organic Ultra Minis Original	¾ cup (1.9 oz)	190
Organic Fruity Punch	1 cup (1 oz)	110
Puffins	¾ cup (0.9 oz)	90
Shredded Spoonfuls	¾ cup (1.1 oz)	120
Shredded Wheat	2 biscuits (1.4 oz)	140
General Mills		
Apple Cinnamon Cheerios	¾ cup (1 oz)	120
Basic 4	1 cup (1.9 oz)	200
Berry Berry Kix	¾ cup (1 oz)	120
Body Buddies Natural Fruit	1 cup (1 oz)	120
Boo Berry	1 cup (1 oz)	120
Cheerios	1 cup (1 oz)	110
Cinnamon Grahams	¾ cup (1 oz)	120
Cinnamon Toast Crunch	¾ cup (1 oz)	130
Cocoa Puffs	1 cup (1 oz)	120
Cookie Crisp	1 cup (1 oz)	120
Corn Chex	1 cup (1 oz)	110
Count Chocula	1 cup (1 oz)	120
Country Corn Flakes	1 cup (1 oz)	120
Crispy Wheaties 'n Raisins	1 cup (1.9 oz)	190
Fiber One	½ cup (1 oz)	60
Frankenberry	1 cup (1 oz)	120
French Toast Crunch	¾ cup (1 oz)	120

FOOD	PORTION	CALS.
General Mills (CONT.)		
Frosted Cheerios	1 cup (1 oz)	120
Golden Grahams	¾ cup (1 oz)	120
Grand Slams Major League	1 cup (1 oz)	120
Honey Frosted Wheaties	¾ cup (1 oz)	110
Honey Nut Cheerios	1 cup (1 oz)	120
Honey Nut Clusters	1 cup (1.9 oz)	210
Honey Nut Chex	¾ cup (1 oz)	120
Jurassic Park Crunch	1 cup (1 oz)	120
Kaboom	1¼ cup (1 oz)	120
Kix	1⅓ cup (1 oz)	120
Lucky Charms	1 cup (1 oz)	120
Multi-Bran Chex	1 cup (2 oz)	200
Multi-Grain Cheerios Plus	1 cup (1 oz)	110
Oatmeal Crisp Almond	1 cup (1.9 oz)	220
Oatmeal Crisp Apple Cinnamon	1 cup (1.9 oz)	210
Oatmeal Crisp Raisin	1 cup (1.9 oz)	210
Raisin Nut Bran	¾ cup (1.9 oz)	200
Reese's Peanut Butter Puffs	¾ cup (1 oz)	130
Rice Chex	1¼ cup (1.1 oz)	120
Team Cheerios	1 cup (1 oz)	120
Total Corn Flakes	1⅓ cup (1 oz)	110
Total Raisin Bran	1 cup (1.9 oz)	180
Total Whole Grain	¾ cup (1 oz)	110
Trix	1 cup (1 oz)	120
USA Olympic Crunch	1 cup (1 oz)	120
Wheat Chex	1 cup (1.9 oz)	180
Wheat Hearts	¼ cup (1.3 oz)	130
Wheaties	1 cup (1 oz)	110
Good Shepherd		
Millet Rice Flakes Wheat Free	1 oz	95
Spelt	1 oz	90
Spelt Flakes	1 oz	100
Grist Mill		
Apple Cinnamon Natural	½ cup (1.9 oz)	260
Bran	½ cup (1.9 oz)	250
Oat & Honey Natural	½ cup (1.9 oz)	270
Oat Honey & Raisin Natural	½ cup (1.9 oz)	260
Health Valley		
10 Bran O's Apple Cinnamon	¾ cup	100
Bran w/ Apples & Cinnamon	¾ cup	160
Golden Flax	½ cup	190
Healthy Crunches & Flakes Almond	¾ cup	130
Healthy Crunches & Flakes Apple Cinnamon	¾ cup	130

FOOD	PORTION	CALS.
Health Valley (CONT.)		
Healthy Crunches & Flakes Honey Crunch	¾ cup	130
Hot Cereal Cups Amazing Apple!	1 pkg	220
Hot Cereal Cups Banana Gone Nuts!	1 pkg	240
Hot Cereal Cups Maple Madness!	1 pkg	240
Hot Cereal Cups Terrific 10 Grain!	1 pkg	220
Oat Bran O'S	¾ cup	100
Organic Amaranth Flakes	¾ cup	100
Organic Blue Corn Bran Flakes	¾ cup	100
Organic Bran w/ Raisin	¾ cup	160
Organic Fiber 7 Flakes	¾ cup	100
Organic Healthy Fiber Flakes	¾ cup	100
Organic Oat Bran Flakes	¾ cup	100
Organic Oat Bran Flakes w/ Raisins	¾ cup	110
Puffed Honey Sweetened Corn	1 cup	110
Puffed Honey Sweetened Crisp Brown Rice	1 cup	110
Raisin Bran Flakes	1¼ cup	190
Real Oat Bran	½ cup	200
Healthy Choice		
Almond Crunch With Raisins	1 cup (2 oz)	210
Golden Multi- Grain Flakes	¾ cup (1.1 oz)	110
Toasted Brown Sugar Squares	1 cup (2 oz)	190
Heartland		
Coconut	1 oz	130
Plain	1 oz	130
Raisin	1 oz	130
Kashi		
Go Berry Tart	½ cup (4.9 oz)	260
Kellogg's		
All-Bran	½ cup (1.1 oz)	80
All-Bran Bran Buds	⅓ cup (1 oz)	80
All-Bran Extra Fiber	½ cup (0.9 oz)	50
Apple Jacks	1 cup (1.2 oz)	120
Cocoa Frosted Flakes	¾ cup (1.1 oz)	120
Cocoa Krispies	¾ cup (1.1 oz)	120
Complete Oat Bran Flakes	¾ cup (1 oz)	110
Complete Wheat Bran Flakes	¾ cup (1 oz)	90
Corn Flakes	1 cup (1 oz)	100
Corn Pops	1 cup (1.1 oz)	120
Cracklin' Oat Bran	¾ cup (1.7 oz)	190
Crispix	1 cup (1 oz)	110
Froot Loops	1 cup (1.1 oz)	120
Frosted Flakes	¾ cup (1.1 oz)	120

FOOD	PORTION	CALS.
Kellogg's (CONT.)		
Honey Crunch Corn Flakes	¾ cup (1.1 oz)	120
Just Right Crunchy Nuggets	1 cup (2 oz)	210
Just Right Fruit & Nut	1 cup (2.1 oz)	220
Mini-Wheats Apple Cinnamon Squares	¾ cup (1.9 oz)	180
Mini-Wheats Blueberry Squares	¾ cup (1.9 oz)	180
Mini-Wheats Frosted	1 cup (1.8 oz)	180
Mini-Wheats Frosted Bite Size	24 pieces (2.1 oz)	200
Mini-Wheats Raisin Squares	¾ cup (1.9 oz)	180
Mini-Wheats Strawberry Squares	¾ cup (1.8 oz)	170
Mueslix Apple & Almond Crunch	¾ cups (1.9 oz)	200
Mueslix Raisin & Almond	⅔ cup (1.9 oz)	200
Nutri-Grain Almond Raisin	1¼ cup (1.7 oz)	180
Nutri-Grain Golden Wheat	¾ cup (1 oz)	100
Product 19	1 cup (1 oz)	100
Raisin Bran	1 cup (2.1 oz)	200
Rice Krispies	1¼ cup (1.2 oz)	120
Rice Krispies Razzle Dazzle	¾ cup (1 oz)	110
Rice Krispies Treats	¾ cup (1 oz)	120
Smacks	¾ cup (1 oz)	100
Smart Start	1 cup (1.8 oz)	180
Special K	1 cup (1.1 oz)	110
Kolln		
Crispy Oats	1 cup (1.8 oz)	190
Oat Bran Crunch	⅔ cup (2.1 oz)	220
Oat Muesli Fruit	¾ cup (2 oz)	200
Kraft		
Morning Traditions Banana Nut Crunch	1 cup (2 oz)	250
Morning Traditions Blueberry Morning	1¼ cup (1.9 oz)	220
Morning Traditions Cranberry Almond Crunch	1 cup (1.9 oz)	220
Morning Traditions Great Grains Crunchy Pecan	⅔ cup (1.9 oz)	220
Morning Traditions Great Grains Raisins Dates & Pecans	⅔ cup (1.9 oz)	210
Little Crow		
Coco Wheat	3 tbsp (36 g)	130
Maltex		
Cereal	1 oz	105
Maypo		
30 Second	1 oz	100
Vermont Style	1 oz	105
With Oat Bran	1 oz	130

FOOD	PORTION	CALS.
McCann's		
Irish Oatmeal	1 oz	110
Mother's		
Oatmeal Instant	½ cup (1.4 oz)	150
Whole Wheat Natural	½ cup (1.4 oz)	130
Mueslix		
Crispy Blend	⅔ cup (1.9 oz)	200
Nabisco		
100% Bran	⅓ cup (1 oz)	80
Cream Of Rice	1 oz	100
Cream Of Wheat Instant as prep	1 cup	120
Cream Of Wheat Quick as prep	1 cup	120
Cream Of Wheat Regular as prep	1 cup	120
Frosted Shredded Wheat Bite Size	1 cup (1.8 oz)	190
Honey Nut Shredded Wheat Bite Size	1 cup (1.8 oz)	200
Mix'n Eat Cream Of Wheat Apple & Cinnamon	1 pkg (1¼ oz)	130
Mix'n Eat Cream Of Wheat Brown Sugar Cinnamon	1 pkg (1¼ oz)	130
Mix'n Eat Cream Of Wheat Maple Brown Sugar	1 pkg (1¼ oz)	130
Mix'n Eat Cream Of Wheat Our Original	1 pkg (1¼ oz)	100
Original Shredded Wheat	2 biscuits (1.6 oz)	160
Original Shredded Wheat 'N Bran	1¼ cup (2.1 oz)	200
Original Shredded Wheat Spoon Size	1 cup (1.7 oz)	170
Nutri-Grain		
Almond Raisin	1¼ cup (2 oz)	200
Golden Wheat	¾ cup (1.1 oz)	100
Post		
Alpha-Bits	1 cup (1 oz)	130
Bran Flakes	¾ cup (1 oz)	100
Cocoa Pebbles	¾ cup (1 oz)	120
Fruit & Fibre Dates Raisins & Walnuts	1 cup (1.9 oz)	210
Fruit & Fibre Peaches Raisins & Almonds	1 cup (1.9 oz)	210
Fruity Pebbles	¾ cup (1 oz)	110
Golden Crisp	¾ cup (1 oz)	110
Grape-Nuts	¾ cup (1 oz)	100
Honey Bunches Of Oats	¾ cup (1 oz)	120
Honey Bunches Of Oats With Almonds	¾ cup (1.1 oz)	130
Honeycomb	1⅓ cups (1 oz)	110
Post Toasties	1 cup (1 oz)	100
Raisin Bran	1 cup (2 oz)	190
Waffle Crisp	1 cup (1 oz)	130

FOOD	PORTION	CALS.
Pritikin		
Apple Raisin Spice	1 pkg (1.6 oz)	170
Multigrain	1 pkg	160
Quaker		
Instant Grits Original	1 pkg (1 oz)	100
Multigrain	½ cup (1.4 oz)	130
Oatmeal Instant	1 pkg (1 oz)	100
Oatmeal Instant Apples & Cinnamon	1 pkg (1.2 oz)	130
Oatmeal Instant Bananas & Cream	1 pkg (1.2 oz)	130
Oatmeal Instant Blueberries & Cream	1 pkg (1.2 oz)	130
Oatmeal Instant Cinnamon & Spice	1 pkg (1.6 oz)	170
Oatmeal Instant Kid's Choice Chocolate Chip Cookie	1 pkg (1.5 oz)	160
Oatmeal Instant Kid's Choice Cookie'n Cream	1 pkg (1.5 oz)	160
Oatmeal Instant Kid's Choice Fruity Marshmallow	1 pkg (1.4 oz)	150
Oatmeal Instant Kid's Choice Oatmeal Raisin Cookie	1 pkg (1.5 oz)	160
Oatmeal Instant Kid's Choice Radical Raspberry	1 pkg (1.4 oz)	150
Oatmeal Instant Kid's Choice S'mores	1 pkg (1.5 oz)	160
Oatmeal Instant Kid's Choice Strawberries'n Stuff	1 pkg (1.4 oz)	150
Oatmeal Instant Kid's Choice Twisted Strawberry Banana	1 pkg (1.4 oz)	150
Oatmeal Instant Maple & Brown Sugar	1 pkg (1.5 oz)	160
Oatmeal Instant Peaches & Cream	1 pkg (1.2 oz)	140
Oatmeal Instant Raisin & Spice	1 pkg (1.5 oz)	150
Oatmeal Instant Raisin Date & Walnut	1 pkg (1.3 oz)	140
Oatmeal Instant Strawberries & Cream	1 pkg (1.2 oz)	140
Oatmeal Quick'n Hearty Microwave	1 pkg (1 oz)	110
Oatmeal Quick'n Hearty Microwave Apple Spice	1 pkg (1.6 oz)	170
Oatmeal Quick'n Hearty Microwave Brown Sugar Cinnamon	1 pkg (1.5 oz)	150
Oatmeal Quick'n Hearty Microwave Cinnamon Double Raisin	1 pkg (1.6 oz)	170
Oatmeal Quick'n Hearty Microwave Honey Bran	1 pkg (1.4 oz)	150
Oats Old Fashion	½ cup (1.4 oz)	150
Oats Quick	½ cup (1.4 oz)	150
Oats Steel Cut	½ cup (1.4 oz)	150
Whole Wheat Hot Natural	½ cup (1.4 oz)	130

FOOD	PORTION	CALS.
Ralston		
Almond Delight	1 cup (1.8 oz)	210
Bran Flakes	¾ cup (1.1 oz)	110
Chex Multi-Bran	1¼ cup (2 oz)	220
Cocoa Crispy Rice	1 cup (1.8 oz)	200
Cocoa Crunchies	¾ cup (1.1 oz)	120
Cookie Crisp	1 cup (1 oz)	120
Corn Flakes	1¼ cup (1.1 oz)	120
Crisp Crunch	¾ cup (1.1 oz)	120
Crisp Rice	1¼ cup (1.2 oz)	130
Frosted Flakes	¾ cup (1.1 oz)	120
Fruit Rings	¾ cup (0.9 oz)	100
Magic Stair	¾ cup (1.1 oz)	120
Muesli Blueberry	1 cup (1.9 oz)	200
Muesli Cranberry	¾ cup (1.9 oz)	200
Muesli Peach	¾ cup (1.9 oz)	200
Muesli Raspberry	¾ cup (2 oz)	220
Muesli Strawberry	1 cup (1.9 oz)	210
Multi Vitamin Whole Grain Flakes	1 cup (1.1 oz)	120
Nutty Nuggets	½ cup (1.7 oz)	180
Raisin Bran	¾ cup (1.9 oz)	190
Tasteeos	1¼ cup (1.1 oz)	130
Tasteeos Apple Cinnamon	1 cup (1.2 oz)	130
Tasteeos Honey Nut	1 cup (1.2 oz)	130
Roman Meal		
Apple Cinnamon	1.2 oz	105
Cream Of Rye	1.3 oz	111
Oats Wheat Dates Raisins Almonds	1.3 oz	129
Oats Wheat Honey Coconuts Almonds	1.3 oz	155
Original	1 oz	83
Original With Oats	1.2 oz	108
Stone-Buhr		
4 Grain	⅓ cup (1.6 oz)	140
7 Grain	⅓ cup (1.6 oz)	140
Bran Flakes	¼ cup (0.6 oz)	64
Cracked Wheat	¼ cup (2.4 oz)	210
Manna Golden	6 tsp (1.6 oz)	160
Rolled Oats Old Fashion	6 tsp (1.6 oz)	150
Scotch Oats	¼ cup (1.6 oz)	150
Sunbelt		
Muesli	1.9 oz	210
Uncle Roy's		
Muesli Swiss Style	½ cup (1.6 oz)	170

FOOD	PORTION	CALS.
Wheatena		
Cereal	⅓ cup (1.4 oz)	150

CEREAL BARS
(*see also* GRANOLA BARS, NUTRITION SUPPLEMENTS)

FOOD	PORTION	CALS.
Cap'n Crunch		
Bar	1 (0.8 oz)	90
Berries Bar	1 (0.8 oz)	90
Dolly Madison		
Apple	1 (1.3 oz)	120
Blueberry	1 (1.3 oz)	120
Raspberry	1 (1.3 oz)	120
Strawberry	1 (1.3 oz)	120
Estee		
Rice Crunchie Chocolate	1 (0.7 oz)	50
Rice Crunchie Chocolate Chip	1 (0.7 oz)	50
Rice Crunchie Peanut Butter	1 (0.7 oz)	60
Rice Crunchie Vanilla	1 (0.7 oz)	60
Glenny's		
Chocolate Crunch Creamy Low Fat	1 bar (1.75 oz)	190
Chocolate Crunch Toasted Almond	1 bar (1.75 oz)	200
Health Valley		
Crisp Rice Bars Apple Cinnamon	1	110
Crisp Rice Bars Orange Date	1	110
Crisp Rice Bars Tropical Fruit	1	110
Fiber 7 Flakes w/ Strawberry	1 bar	110
Oat Bran Flakes w/ Blueberry	1 bar	110
Raisin Bran Flakes w/ Apple Raisin	1 bar	110
Hostess		
Apple	1 (1.3 oz)	120
Banana Nut	1 (1.3 oz)	120
Blueberry	1 (1.3 oz)	120
Raspberry	1 (1.3 oz)	120
Strawberry	1 (1.3 oz)	120
Kellogg's		
Nutri-Grain Apple Cinnamon	1 (1.3 oz)	140
Nutri-Grain Blueberry	1 (1.3 oz)	140
Nutri-Grain Cherry	1 (1.3 oz)	140
Nutri-Grain Mixed Berry	1 (1.3 oz)	140
Nutri-Grain Peach	1 (1.3 oz)	140
Nutri-Grain Raspberry	1 (1.3 oz)	140
Nutri-Grain Strawberry	1 (1.3 oz)	140
Rice Krispies Treats	1 (0.8 oz)	90
Rice Krispies Treats Chocolate Chip Squares	1 (0.8 oz)	90

FOOD	PORTION	CALS.
Nature's Choice		
Fat Free Apple	1 bar (1.3 oz)	110
Fat Free Blueberry	1 bar (1.3 oz)	110
Fat Free Cranberry	1 bar (1.3 oz)	110
Fat Free Peach	1 bar (1.3 oz)	110
Fat Free Raspberry	1 bar (1.3 oz)	110
Fat Free Strawberry	1 bar (1.3 oz)	110
Low Fat Triple Berry	1 bar (1.3 oz)	130
Low Fat Very Cherry	1 bar (1.3 oz)	130

CHAMPAGNE

sekt german champagne	3.5 fl oz	84
Andre		
Blush	1 fl oz	22
Brut	1 fl oz	21
Cold Duck	1 fl oz	25
Extra Dry	1 fl oz	23
Ballatore		
Spumante	1 fl oz	23
Eden Roc		
Brut	1 fl oz	21
Brut Rosé	1 fl oz	22
Extra Dry	1 fl oz	21
Tott's		
Blanc de Noir	1 fl oz	22
Brut	1 fl oz	20
Extra Dry	1 fl oz	21

CHAYOTE

fresh cooked	1 cup	38
raw	1 (7 oz)	49
raw cut up	1 cup	32

CHEESE

(*see also* CHEESE DISHES, CHEESE SUBSTITUTES, COTTAGE CHEESE, CREAM CHEESE)

beaufort	1 oz	115
cacio di roma sheep's milk cheese	1 oz	130
cantal	1 oz	105
chabichou	1 oz	95
chaource	1 oz	83
cheddar low fat	1 oz	49
cheddar low sodium	1 oz	113
colby low fat	1 oz	49
colby low sodium	1 oz	113

FOOD	PORTION	CALS.
comte	1 oz	114
coulommiers	1 oz	88
crottin	1 oz	105
goat fresh	1 oz	23
goat hard	1 oz	128
goat semisoft	1 oz	103
goat soft	1 oz	76
gorgonzola	3.5 oz	376
limburger	1 oz	93
maroilles	1 oz	97
morbier	1 oz	99
picodon	1 oz	99
pont l'eveque	1 oz	86
pyrenees	1 oz	101
queso anego	1 oz	106
queso asadero	1 oz	101
queso chichuahua	1 oz	106
raclette	1 oz	102
reblochon	1 oz	88
rouy	1 oz	95
saint marcellin	1 oz	94
saint nectaire	1 oz	97
saint paulin	1 oz	85
sainte maure	1 oz	99
selles sur cher	1 oz	93
tome	1 oz	92
triple creme	1 oz	113
vacherin	1 oz	92
whey cheese	3.5 oz	440
yogurt cheese	1 oz	20
Alouette		
Brie Baby	1 oz	110
Brie Baby With Herbs	1 oz	110
French Onion	2 tbsp (0.8 oz)	70
Garlic	2 tbsp (0.8 oz)	70
Light Dill	2 tbsp (0.8 oz)	50
Light Garlic	2 tbsp (0.8 oz)	50
Light Herb	2 tbsp (0.8 oz)	50
Light Herbs & Garlic	2 tbsp (0.8 oz)	50
Light Spring Vegetable	2 tbsp (0.8 oz)	50
Salmon	2 tbsp (0.8 oz)	60
Scallions	2 tbsp (0.8 oz)	70
Spinach	2 tbsp (0.8 oz)	60

FOOD	PORTION	CALS.
Alpine Lace		
American	1 slice (0.66 oz)	50
American Fat Free	1 piece (1 oz)	45
American Hot Pepper Less Fat Less Sodium	1 piece (1 oz)	80
American Less Fat Less Sodium	1 piece (1 oz)	80
Cheddar Fat Free	1 piece (1 oz)	45
Cheddar Reduced Fat	1 piece (1 oz)	80
Colby Reduced Fat	1 piece (1 oz)	80
Fat Free For Parmesan Lovers	2 tsp (5 g)	10
Fat Free Mexican Macho	2 tbsp (1 oz)	30
Fat Free Singles	1 slice (0.66 oz)	25
Feta Reduced Fat	1 piece (1 oz)	60
Goat	1 oz	40
Mozzarella Fat Free	1 piece (1 oz)	45
Mozzarella Reduced Sodium Part Skim	1 piece (1 oz)	70
Muenster Reduced Sodium	1 piece (1 oz)	100
Provolone Smoked Reduced Fat	1 piece (1 oz)	70
Swiss Reduced Fat	1 piece (1 oz)	90
BabyBel		
Mini Light	1 (0.7 oz)	45
Boar's Head		
American	1 oz	100
Baby Swiss	1 oz	110
Canadian Cheddar	1 oz	110
Double Glouster White	1 oz	110
Double Glouster Yellow	1 oz	110
Havarti	1 oz	110
Havarti w/ Dill	1 oz	110
Havarti w/ Jalapeno	1 oz	110
Longhorn Colby	1 oz	110
Monerey Jack	1 oz	100
Monerey Jack w/ Jalapeno	1 oz	100
Mozzarella	1 oz	90
Muenster	1 oz	100
Muenster Low Sodium	1 oz	100
Provolone Picante Sharp	1 oz	100
Swiss	1 oz	110
Swiss No Salt Added	1 oz	110
Bongrain		
Chavrie	2 tbsp (0.8 oz)	40
Montrachet	1 oz	70
Montrachet Chive	1 oz	70
Montrachet Classic	1 oz	70

FOOD	PORTION	CALS.
Bongrain (CONT.)		
Montrachet Classic Herb	1 oz	70
Montrachet Herbs & Garlic	1 oz	70
Montrachet In Oil drained	1 oz	70
Montrachet With Ash	1 oz	70
Borden		
American Slices	1 oz	110
American Very Sharp	1 oz	110
Swiss Slices	1 oz	100
Breakstone's		
Ricotta	¼ cup (2.2 oz)	110
Bresse		
Brie	1 oz	110
Brie Light	1 oz	70
Brie With Herbs	1 oz	110
Creme De Brie	2 tbsp (1 oz)	90
Creme De Brie Herb	2 tbsp (1 oz)	90
Brier Run		
Cherve	1 oz	61
Quark	1 oz	34
Bristol Gold		
Cheddar Light	1 oz	70
French Onion Light	1 oz	70
Garlic & Herb Light	1 oz	70
Horseradish Light	1 oz	70
Smoke Light	1 oz	70
Wine Light	1 oz	70
Cheez Whiz		
Light	2 tbsp (1.2 oz)	80
Churney		
Feta	1 oz	80
Cracker Barrel		
Baby Swiss	1 oz	110
Cheddar Extra Sharp	1 oz	120
Cheddar Marbled Sharp	1 oz	110
Cheddar New York Aged	1 oz	120
Cheddar Sharp	1 oz	120
Cheddar Vermont Sharp	1 oz	110
Reduced Fat Cheddar Extra Sharp	1 oz	90
Reduced Fat Cheddar Sharp	1 oz	90
Reduced Fat Cheddar Vermont Sharp	1 oz	90
Whipped Spreadable Cream Cheese & Extra Sharp Cheddar	2 tbsp (0.9 oz)	80
Whipped Spreadable Cream Cheese & Sharp Cheddar	2 tbsp (0.9 oz)	80

FOOD	PORTION	CALS.
Cracker Barrel (CONT.)		
Whipped Spreadable Cream Cheese & Sharp Cheddar w/ Herbs	2 tbsp (0.9 oz)	80
Delice De France		
Cheese	1 oz	110
With Herbs	1 oz	110
Delico		
Alouette Cajun	2 tbsp (0.8 oz)	70
Alouette French Onion	2 tbsp (0.8 oz)	70
Alouette Garden Vegetable	2 tbsp (0.8 oz)	60
Alouette Garlic	2 tbsp (0.8 oz)	70
Alouette Horseradish & Chive	2 tbsp (0.8 oz)	60
Alouette Spinach	2 tbsp (0.8 oz)	60
Di Giorno		
Parmesan Grated	2 tsp (5 g)	25
Parmesan Shredded	2 tsp (5 g)	20
Parmesan Shredded	2 tsp (5 g)	20
Romano Grated	2 tsp (5 g)	25
Romano Shredded	2 tsp (5 g)	20
Easy Cheese		
Spread American	2 tbsp (1.2 oz)	100
Spread Cheddar	2 tbsp (1.2 oz)	100
Spread Cheddar'n Bacon	2 tbsp (1.2 oz)	100
Spread Nacho	2 tbsp (1.2 oz)	100
Spread Sharp Cheddar	2 tbsp (1.2 oz)	100
Father Time		
Cheddar Extra-Sharp Premium	1 oz	110
Formagg		
Formaggio D'Oro	1 oz	70
Friendship		
Farmer	2 tbsp (1 oz)	50
Farmer No Salt Added	2 tbsp (1 oz)	50
Hoop	2 tbsp (1 oz)	20
Frigo		
Asiago	1 oz	110
Blue	1 oz	100
Cheddar	1 oz	110
Cheddar Lite	1 oz	80
Feta	1 oz	100
Impastata	1 oz	60
Mozzarella Part Skim Low Moisture	1 oz	80
Mozzarella Whole Milk Low Moisture	1 oz	90
Mozzarella Lite Whole Milk Low Moisture	1 oz	60
Parmazest	1 oz	120

FOOD	PORTION	CALS.
Frigo (CONT.)		
Parmesan & Romano Dry Grated	1 oz	130
Parmesan & Romano Grated	1 oz	110
Parmesan Dry Grated	1 oz	130
Parmesan Grated	1 oz	110
Parmesan Whole	1 oz	110
Pizza Shredded	1 oz	65
Provolone	1 oz	100
Provolone Lite	1 oz	70
Ricotta Low Fat Low Salt	1 oz	30
Ricotta Part Skim	1 oz	40
Ricotta Whole Milk	1 oz	60
Romano Dry Grated	1 oz	130
Romano Grated	1 oz	110
Romano Whole	1 oz	110
String	1 oz	80
String Lite	1 oz	60
Swiss	1 oz	110
Taco Shredded	1 oz	110
Gerard		
Brie	1 oz	90
Handi-Snacks		
Cheez'n Breadsticks	1 pkg (1.1 oz)	120
Cheez'n Crackers	1 pkg (1.1 oz)	110
Cheez'n Pretzels	1 pkg (1 oz)	100
Mozzarella String Cheese	1 piece (1 oz)	80
Nacho Stix'n Cheez	1 pkg (1.1 oz)	110
Healthy Choice		
American Singles White	1 slice (0.7 oz)	30
American Singles Yellow	1 slice (0.7 oz)	30
Cheddar Fancy Shreds	¼ cup (1 oz)	45
Cheddar Shreds	¼ cup (1 oz)	45
Loaf	1 in cube (1 oz)	35
Mexican Shreds	¼ cup (1 oz)	45
Mozzarella	1 oz	45
Mozzarella Fancy Shreds	¼ cup (1 oz)	45
Mozzarella Shreds	¼ cup (1 oz)	45
Mozzarella String Cheese	1 stick (1 oz)	45
Pizza Fancy Shreds	¼ cup (1 oz)	45
Pizza String	1 stick (1 oz)	45
Heluva Good Cheese		
American	1 slice (0.7)	45
Cheddar Curds Snack	1 oz	113
Cheddar Extra-Sharp	1 oz	110

FOOD	PORTION	CALS.
Heluva Good Cheese (CONT.)		
Cheddar Mild	1 oz	110
Cheddar Mild Reduced Fat	1 oz	80
Cheddar Mild White	1 oz	110
Cheddar Sharp	1 oz	110
Cheddar Sharp White	1 oz	110
Cheddar Shredded	¼ cup (1 oz)	110
Cheddar Very Low Sodium	1 oz	110
Cheddar White Extra-Sharp	1 oz	110
Cheddar White Very Low Sodium	1 oz	110
Cheddar White Shredded	¼ cup (1 oz)	110
Colby	1 oz	117
Colby-Jack	1 oz	110
Cold Pack Cheddar Sharp	2 tbsp (1 oz)	90
Cold Pack Cheddar Sharp With Bacon	2 tbsp (1 oz)	90
Cold Pack Cheddar Sharp With Horseradish	2 tbsp (1 oz)	90
Cold Pack Cheddar Sharp With Jalapenos	2 tbsp (1 oz)	90
Cold Pack Cheddar Sharp With Port Wine	2 tbsp (1 oz)	90
Monterey Jack	1 oz	100
Monterey Jack Shredded	¼ cup (1 oz)	100
Monterey Jack With Jalapenos	1 oz	100
Mozzarella Part Skim Low Moisture Shredded	¼ cup (1 oz)	80
Mozzarella Whole Milk	1 oz	80
Muenster	1 oz	100
Swiss	1 oz	112
Washed Curd Cheese	1 oz	110
Hoffman		
American Yellow	1 oz	110
Hot Pepper	1 oz	90
Super Sharp	1 oz	110
Keller's		
Chub	2 tbsp (1 oz)	100
Kraft		
Cheddar Extra Sharp	1 oz	120
Cheddar Medium	1 oz	110
Cheddar Mild	1 oz	110
Cheddar Sharp	1 oz	120
Cheddary Melts Medium Cheddar	1 oz	110
Cheddary Melts Mild Cheddar	1 oz	110
Cheddary Melts Shreds Medium Cheddar	¼ cup (1.1 oz)	120
Cheddary Melts Shreds Mild Cheddar	¼ cup (1.1 oz)	120
Cheese Food w/ Garlic	1 oz	90

FOOD	PORTION	CALS.
Kraft (CONT.)		
Cheese Food w/ Jalapeno Peppers	1 oz	90
Colby	1 oz	110
Colby Monterey Jack	1 oz	110
Deluxe American	1 oz	100
Deluxe American White	1 oz	100
Deluxe Singles American	1 (1 oz)	110
Deluxe Singles American	1 (0.7 oz)	70
Deluxe Singles Pimento	1 (1 oz)	100
Deluxe Singles Swiss	1 (1 oz)	90
Deluxe Singles Swiss	1 slice (0.7 oz)	70
Free Grated	2 tsp (5 g)	15
Free Shredded Cheddar	¼ cup (0.9 oz)	40
Free Shredded Mozzarella	¼ cup (1 oz)	45
Grated Parm Plus! Garlic Herb	2 tsp (5 g)	15
Grated Parm Plus! Zesty Red Pepper	2 tsp (5 g)	15
Grated Parmesan	2 tsp (5 g)	20
Grated Romano	2 tsp (5 g)	20
Marbled Cheddar Mild	1 oz	110
Marbled Cheddar & Monterey Jack	1 oz	110
Marbled Cheddar & Whole Milk Mozzarella	1 oz	100
Marbled Colby Monterey Jack	1 oz	110
Monterey Jack	1 oz	110
Monterey Jack w/ Jalapeno Peppers	1 oz	110
Mozzarella Part Skim Low Moisture	1 oz	80
Mozzarella String Cheese Low Moisture Part Skim	1 piece (1 oz)	80
Pizza Shredded Four Cheese	¼ cup (0.9 oz)	90
Pizza Shredded Mozzarella & Cheddar	⅓ cup (1.1 oz)	120
Pizza Shredded Mozzarella & Provolone w/ Smoke Flavor	¼ cup (0.9 oz)	90
Reduced Fat Cheddar Mild	1 oz	90
Reduced Fat Cheddar Sharp	1 oz	90
Reduced Fat Colby	1 oz	80
Reduced Fat Monterey Jack	1 oz	80
Shredded Cheddar Medium	¼ cup (0.9 oz)	100
Shredded Cheddar Mild	¼ cup (0.9 oz)	100
Shredded Cheddar Sharp	1 oz (0.9 oz)	110
Shredded Cheddar & Monterey Jack	¼ cup (0.9 oz)	100
Shredded Colby & Monterey Jack	¼ cup (0.9 oz)	100
Shredded Hearty Italian	⅓ cup (1.1 oz)	100
Shredded Italian Style Classic Garlic	⅓ cup (1.1 oz)	100
Shredded Italian Style Mozzarelle & Parmesan	⅓ cup (1.1 oz)	100

FOOD	PORTION	CALS.
Kraft (CONT.)		
Shredded Lower Fat Cheddar Mild	¼ cup (0.9 oz)	80
Shredded Lower Fat Cheddar Sharp	¼ cup (0.9 oz)	80
Shredded Lower Fat Colby & Monterey Jack	¼ cup (0.9 oz)	80
Shredded Lower Fat Mozzarella	⅓ cup (1.1 oz)	80
Shredded Lower Fat Pizza Cheese	⅓ cup (1.1 oz)	90
Shredded Mexican Style Cheddar & Monterey Jack	⅓ cup (1.1 oz)	120
Shredded Mexican Style Cheddar & Monterey Jack w/ Jalapeno Peppers	⅓ cup (1.1 oz)	120
Shredded Mexican Style Four Cheese	⅓ cup (1.1 oz)	120
Shredded Mexican Style Taco Cheese	⅓ cup (1.1 oz)	120
Shredded Monterey Jack	¼ cup (0.9 oz)	100
Shredded Parmesan	2 tsp (5 g)	20
Shredded Part Skim Mozzarella	¼ cup (1.1 oz)	90
Shredded Swiss	¼ cup (0.9 oz)	100
Shredded Whole Milk Mozzarella	¼ cup (1.1 oz)	100
Shredded Finely Cheddar Mild	¼ cup (1.1 oz)	120
Shredded Finely Cheddar Sharp	¼ cup (1.1 oz)	120
Shredded Finely Colby & Monterey Jack	¼ cup (1 oz)	110
Shredded Finely Lower Fat Cheddar Milk	⅓ cup (1.1 oz)	100
Shredded Finely Lower Fat Cheddar Sharp	⅓ cup (1.1 oz)	100
Shredded Finely Part Skim Mozzarella	¼ cup (1.1 oz)	90
Shredded Finely Swiss	¼ cup (0.9 oz)	110
Singles American	1 (1.2 oz)	110
Singles American	1 (0.7 oz)	60
Singles American	1 (0.6 oz)	60
Singles Mild Mexican	1 (0.7 oz)	70
Singles Monterey	1 slice (0.7 oz)	70
Singles Pimento	1 (0.7 oz)	60
Singles Reduced Fat American	1 (0.7 oz)	50
Singles Reduced Fat American White	1 (0.7 oz)	50
Singles Sharp	1 slice (0.7 oz)	70
Singles Swiss	1 slice (0.7 oz)	70
Singles Nonfat American	1 (0.7 oz)	30
Singles Nonfat American White	1 (0.7 oz)	30
Singles Nonfat Sharp Cheddar	1 (0.7 oz)	35
Singles Nonfat Swiss	1 slice (0.7 oz)	30
Slices Cheddar Mild	1 (1 oz)	110
Slices Colby	1 (1.6 oz)	180
Slices Part Skim Mozzarella	1 (1.6 oz)	130
Slices Part Skim Mozzarella	1 (1.5 oz)	120
Slices Provolone Smoke Flavor	1 (1.5 oz)	150

FOOD	PORTION	CALS.
Kraft (CONT.)		
Slices Swiss	1 (1.3 oz)	150
Slices Swiss	1 (0.8 oz)	90
Slices Swiss	1 (1.5 oz)	170
Slices Swiss	1 (1.6 oz)	180
Slices Swiss Aged	1 (1.5 oz)	170
Slices Deli-Thin Part Skim Mozzarella	1 (1 oz)	80
Slices Deli-Thin Swiss	1 (0.8 oz)	90
Slices Deli-Thin Swiss Aged	1 (0.8 oz)	90
Slices Reduced Fat Swiss	1 (1.3 oz)	130
Spread Bacon	2 tbsp (1.1 oz)	90
Spread Olive & Pimento	2 tbsp (1.1 oz)	70
Spread Pimento	2 tbsp (1.1 oz)	80
Spread Pineapple	2 tbsp (1.1 oz)	70
Spread Pineapple	2 tbsp (1.1 oz)	70
Spread Roka Brand Blue	2 tbsp (1.1 oz)	90
Swiss	1 oz	110
Lactaid		
American	3.5 oz	328
Land O'Lakes		
American	1 slice (0.75 oz)	80
American	2 slices (1 oz)	100
American	1 oz	110
American Less Salt	1 oz	110
American Light	1 oz	70
American Sharp	1 oz	110
American & Swiss	1 oz	100
Baby Swiss	1 oz	110
Brick	1 oz	100
Chedarella	1 oz	100
Cheddar Light	1 oz	70
Gouda	1 oz	110
Jalapeno Light	1 oz	70
Monterey Jack	1 oz	110
Mozzarella	1 oz	80
Muenster	1 oz	100
Provolone	1 oz	100
Swiss	1 oz	110
Swiss Light	1 oz	80
Laughing Cow		
Assorted Wedge	1 (1 oz)	70
Babybel	1 oz	90
Babybel Mini	1 (0.7 oz)	70
Bonbel	1 oz	100

FOOD	PORTION	CALS.
Laughing Cow (CONT.)		
Bonbel Mini	1 (0.7 oz)	70
Cheesebits	6 pieces (1 oz)	70
Gouda Mini	1 (0.7 oz)	80
Original Wedge	1 (1 oz)	70
Wedge Light	1 (1 oz)	50
Lifetime		
Cheddar Fat Free	1 oz	40
Cheddar Fat Free Lactose Free	1 oz	40
Garden Vegetable Fat Free	1 oz	40
Jalapeno Jack Fat Free	1 oz	40
Jalapeno Jack Fat Free Lactose Free	1 oz	40
Mild Mexican Fat Free	1 oz	40
Monterey Jack Fat Free	1 oz	40
Mozzarella Fat Free	1 oz	40
Mozzarella Fat Free Lactose Free	1 oz	40
Onions & Chives Fat Free	1 oz	40
Sharp Cheddar Fat Free	1 oz	40
Smoked Cheddar Fat Free	1 oz	40
Swiss Fat Free	1 oz	40
Light N'Lively		
Singles American	1 (0.7 oz)	45
MayBud		
Edam	1 oz	100
Gouda	1 oz	100
Gouda Round	1 oz	100
New Holland		
Cheese	1 oz	90
Garlic	1 oz	90
Havarti Lower Fat Garden Vegetable	1 oz	80
Jalapeno	1 oz	80
Natural Vegetable	1 oz	80
Old English		
American Sharp	1 slice (1 oz)	100
Polly-O		
Mozzarella Free	1 oz	35
Mozzarella Lite	1 oz	60
Mozzarella Part Skim	1 oz	70
Mozzarella Part Skim Shredded	¼ cup	80
Mozzarella Shredded Free	¼ cup	45
Mozzarella Shredded Lite	¼ cup	60
Mozzarella Whole Milk	1 oz	80
Mozzarella Whole Milk Shredded	¼ cup	90
Ricotta Free	¼ cup	50

FOOD	PORTION	CALS.
Polly-O (CONT.)		
Ricotta Lite	¼ cup	70
Ricotta Part Skim	¼ cup	90
Ricotta Whole Milk	¼ cup	110
String	1 oz	80
String Lite	1 piece (1 oz)	60
President		
Feta Fat Free	1 oz	30
Price's		
Cheese & Bacon Spread	2 tbsp (1.1 oz)	90
Jalapeno Nacho Dip Hot	2 tbsp (1.1 oz)	80
Jalapeno Nacho Dip Mild	2 tbsp (1.1 oz)	80
Pimento Cheese Spread	2 tbsp (1.1 oz)	80
Pimento Cheese Spread Light	2 tbsp (1.1 oz)	60
Vegetable Garden	2 tbsp (1.1 oz)	70
Quaker		
Chub	2 tbsp (1 oz)	100
Rondele		
Light Soft Spreadable Garlic & Herb	2 tbsp (0.9 oz)	60
Soft Spreadable Garlic & Herbs	2 tbsp (1 oz)	100
Sargento		
4 Cheese Mexican Recipe Blend Shredded	¼ cup (1 oz)	110
6 Cheese Italian Recipe Blend Shredded	¼ cup (1 oz)	90
Blue Crumbled	¼ cup (1 oz)	100
Cheddar	1 slice (1 oz)	110
Cheddar Mild Shredded Classic Supreme	¼ cup (1 oz)	110
Cheddar Mild Shredded Fancy Supreme	¼ cup (1 oz)	110
Cheddar Mild Shredded Preferred Light	¼ cup (1 oz)	70
Cheddar Mild White Shredded Classic Supreme	¼ cup (1 oz)	110
Cheddar New York Sharp Shredded Classic Supreme	¼ cup (1 oz)	110
Cheddar Sharp Shredded Classic Supreme	¼ cup (1 oz)	110
Cheddar Sharp Shredded Fancy Supreme	¼ cup (1 oz)	110
Cheese For Nachos & Tacos Shredded	¼ cup (1 oz)	110
Cheese For Pizza Shredded	¼ cup (1 oz)	90
Cheese For Tacos Shredded	¼ cup (1 oz)	110
Cheese For Tacos Shredded Preferred Light	¼ cup (1 oz)	70
Colby	1 slice (1 oz)	110
Colby-Jack Shredded Fancy Supreme	¼ cup (1 oz)	110
Gourmet Parm	1 tbsp	20
Jarlsberg	1 slice (1.2 oz)	120
Monterey Jack	1 slice (1 oz)	100

FOOD	PORTION	CALS.
Sargento (CONT.)		
MooTown Snackers Cheddar	1 piece (0.8 oz)	100
MooTown Snackers Cheddar Mild Light	1 piece (0.8 oz)	60
MooTown Snackers Cheese & Pretzels	1 pkg (1 oz)	90
MooTown Snackers Cheese & Sticks	1 pkg (1 oz)	100
MooTown Snackers Colby-Jack	1 piece (0.8 oz)	90
MooTown Snackers Pizza Cheese & Sticks	1 pkg (1 oz)	100
MooTown Snackers String	1 piece (0.8 oz)	70
MooTown Snackers String Light	1 piece (0.8 oz)	60
Mozzarella	1 slice (1.5 oz)	130
Mozzarella Preferred Light	1 slice (1.5 oz)	100
Mozzarella Shredded Classic Supreme	¼ cup (1 oz)	80
Mozzarella Shredded Fancy Supreme	¼ cup (1 oz)	80
Mozzarella Shredded Preferred Light	¼ cup (1 oz)	70
Muenster	1 slice (1 oz)	100
Parmesan Fresh	1 oz	111
Parmesan Shredded	¼ cup (1 oz)	110
Parmesan & Romano Shredded	¼ cup (1 oz)	110
Pizza Double Cheese Shredded	¼ cup (1 oz)	90
Provolone	1 slice (1 oz)	100
Ricotta Light	¼ cup (2.2 oz)	60
Ricotta Old Fashioned	¼ cup (2.2 oz)	90
Ricotta Part Skim	¼ cup (2.2 oz)	80
Swiss	1 slice (0.7 oz)	80
Swiss Preferred Light	1 slice (1 oz)	80
Swiss Shredded Fancy Supreme	¼ cup (1 oz)	110
Swiss Wafer Thin	2 slices (1 oz)	110
Smart Beat		
American Fat Free	1 slice (0.6 oz)	25
Lactose Free Fat Free	1 slice (0.6 oz)	25
Mellow Cheddar Fat Free	1 slice (0.6 oz)	25
Sharp Cheddar Fat Free	1 slice (0.6 oz)	25
Treasure Cave		
Blue Crumbled	1 oz	110
Feta Crumbled	1 oz	80
Tree Of Life		
Cheddar 33% Reduced Fat Organic Milk	1 oz	90
Cheddar Low Sodium Raw Milk	1 oz	110
Cheddar Mild Organic Milk	1 oz	110
Cheddar Mild Raw Milk	1 oz	110
Cheddar Razor Sharp Raw Milk	1 oz	110
Cheddar Sharp Organic Milk	1 oz	110
Cheddar Sharp Raw Milk	1 oz	110
Colby Organic Milk	1 oz	120

FOOD	PORTION	CALS.
Tree Of Life (CONT.)		
Colby Raw Milk	1 oz	110
Farmer Part-Skim Organic Milk	1 oz	90
Jalapeno Jack Organic Milk	1 oz	110
Jalapeno Jack Semi-Soft Organic Milk	1 oz	110
Monterey Jack 35% Reduced Fat Organic Milk	1 oz	80
Monterey Jack Organic Milk	1 oz	100
Monterey Jack Semi-Soft Raw Milk	1 oz	110
Mozzarella Low Moisture Part Skim	1 oz	80
Mozzarella Low Moisture Part Skim Organic Milk	1 oz	80
Muenster Organic Milk	1 oz	100
Muenster Semi-Soft Raw Milk	1 oz	100
Provolone	1 oz	100
Swiss Raw Milk	1 oz	110
Velveeta		
Light	1 oz	60
Shredded	¼ cup (1.3 oz)	130
Shredded Mild Mexican w/ Jalapeno Pepper	¼ cup (1.3 oz)	120
Spread	1 oz	90
Spread Hot Mexican	1 oz	90
Spread Mild Mexican	1 oz	90
Weight Watchers		
Cheddar Mild Yellow	1 oz	80
Cheddar Sharp Yellow	1 oz	80
Fat Free Grated Italian Topping	1 tbsp	20
Fat Free Reduced Sodium Yellow	2 slices (0.75 oz)	30
Fat Free Sharp Cheddar	2 slices (0.75 oz)	30
Fat Free Swiss	2 slices (0.75 oz)	30
Fat Free White	2 slices (0.75 oz)	30
Fat Free Yellow	2 slices (0.75 oz)	30
WisPride		
Chunk	1 oz	110
Garlic & Herb Cup	2 tbsp (1.1 oz)	100
Hickory Smoked Cup	2 tbsp (1.1 oz)	100
Port Wine Ball	2 tbsp (1.1 oz)	100
Port Wine Cup	2 tbsp (1.1 oz)	100
Port Wine Light Cup	2 tbsp (1.1 oz)	80
Sharp Ball	2 tbsp (1.1 oz)	100
Sharp Cheddar Ball	2 tbsp (1.1 oz)	100
Sharp Cup	2 tbsp (1.1 oz)	100
Sharp Light Cup	2 tbsp (1.1 oz)	80

FOOD	PORTION	CALS.
WisPride (CONT.)		
Swiss Ball	2 tbsp (1.1 oz)	110

CHEESE DISHES
FROZEN
Stouffer's

Welsh Rarebit	½ cup (2.5 oz)	120

TAKE-OUT

fondue	½ cup (3.8 oz)	247
souffle	1 serv (7 oz)	504

CHEESE SUBSTITUTES

mozzarella	1 oz	70
Borden		
Cheese Two	1 oz	90
Taco-Mate	1 oz	100
Formagg		
American White	1 slice (0.66 oz)	60
American Yellow	1 slice (0.66 oz)	60
Caesar's Italian Garden American	1 oz	60
Cheddar	1 slice (0.66 oz)	60
Cheddar Shredded	1 oz	60
Classic American	1 oz	60
Macaroni And Cheese Sauce	⅔ cup (5 oz)	190
Mozzarella Shredded	1 oz	60
Old World Mozzarella	1 oz	60
Parmesan Grated	2 tsp (5 g)	15
Swiss	1 oz	60
Swiss White	1 slice (0.66 oz)	60
Vintage Provolone	1 oz	60
Zesty Jalapeno American	1 oz	60
Frigo		
Imitation Cheddar	1 oz	90
Imitation Mozzarella	1 oz	90
Georgio's		
Imitation Cheddar Shredded	¼ cup (1 oz)	90
Imitation Mozzarella Shredded	¼ cup (1 oz)	90
Sargento		
Classic Supreme Cheddar Shredded	¼ cup (1 oz)	90
Classic Supreme Mozzarella Shredded	¼ cup (1 oz)	80
Fancy Supreme Cheddar Shredded	¼ cup (1 oz)	90
White Wave		
Soy A Melt Cheddar	1 oz	80
Soy A Melt Fat Free Cheddar	1 oz	40
Soy A Melt Fat Free Mozzarella	1 oz	40

FOOD	PORTION	CALS.
White Wave (CONT.)		
Soy A Melt Garlic Herb	1 oz	80
Soy A Melt Jalapeno Jack	1 oz	80
Soy A Melt Monterey Jack	1 oz	80
Soy A Melt Mozzarella	1 oz	80
Soy A Melt Singles American	1 slice (0.75 oz)	60
Soy A Melt Singles Mozzarella	1 slice (0.75 oz)	60

CHERIMOYA
fresh	1	515

CHERRIES
CANNED
sour in heavy syrup	½ cup	232
sour in light syrup	½ cup	189
sour water packed	1 cup	87
sweet in heavy sirup	½ cup	107
sweet in light syrup	½ cup	85
sweet juice pack	½ cup	68
sweet water pack	½ cup	57
Del Monte		
Dark Pitted In Heavy Syrup	½ cup (4.2 oz)	120
Sweet Dark Whole Unpitted In Heavy Syrup	½ cup (4.2 oz)	120

DRIED
Sonoma		
Pitted	¼ cup (1.4 oz)	140

FRESH
sour	1 cup	51
sweet	10	49
Dole		
Cherries	1 cup	90

FROZEN
Big Valley		
Dark Sweet	¾ cup (4.9 oz)	90

CHERRY JUICE
After The Fall		
Black Cherry	1 can (12 oz)	170
Capri Sun		
Wild Cherry Drink	1 pkg (7 oz)	100
Hi-C		
Box	8.45 fl oz	140
Drink	8 fl oz	130
Juicy Juice		
Drink	1 bottle (6 fl oz)	90

FOOD	PORTION	CALS.
Juicy Juice (CONT.)		
Drink	1 box (8.45 fl oz)	130
Kool-Aid		
Black Cherry Drink as prep w/ sugar	1 serv (8 oz)	100
Bursts Cherry Drink	1 (7 oz)	100
Splash Drink	1 serv (8 oz)	110
Sugar Free Drink Mix as prep	1 serv (8 oz)	5
Tree Of Life		
Concentrate	8 tsp (1.4 oz)	110
Veryfine		
Juice-Ups	8 fl oz	130

CHERVIL
seed	1 tsp	1

CHESTNUTS
chinese cooked	1 oz	44
chinese dried	1 oz	103
chinese raw	1 oz	64
chinese roasted	1 oz	68
cooked	1 oz	37
creme de marrons	1 oz	73
dried peeled	1 oz	105
japanese cooked	1 oz	16
japanese dried	1 oz	102
japanese raw	1 oz	44
japanese roasted	1 oz	57
roasted	2 to 3 (1 oz)	70
roasted	1 cup	350

CHEWING GUM
bubble gum	1 block (8 g)	27
stick	1 (3 g)	10
Bazooka		
Fruit Chunk	1 piece (6 g)	25
Fruit Soft	1 piece (6 g)	25
Gum	1 piece (4 g)	15
Gum	1 piece (6 g)	25
Beech-Nut		
Peppermint	1 stick (3 g)	10
Spearmint	1 stick (3 g)	10
Brock		
Bubble Gum	1 piece (0.2 oz)	20
Bubble Yum		
Bananaberry Split	1 piece (0.3 oz)	25

FOOD	PORTION	CALS.
Bubble Yum (CONT.)		
Cotton Candy	1 piece (0.3 oz)	25
Grape	1 piece (0.3 oz)	25
Luscious Lime	1 piece (0.3 oz)	25
Regular	1 piece (0.3 oz)	25
Sour Apple	1 piece (0.3 oz)	25
Sour Cherry	1 piece (0.3 oz)	25
Sugarless	1 piece (0.2 oz)	15
Sugarless Grape	1 piece (0.2 oz)	15
Sugarless Peppermint	1 piece (0.2 oz)	15
Sugarless Strawberry	1 piece (0.2 oz)	15
Sugarless Variety	1 piece (0.2 oz)	15
Variety Pack	1 piece (0.3 oz)	25
Watermelon	1 piece (0.3 oz)	25
Wild Strawberry	1 piece (0.3 oz)	25
Bubblicious		
Gum	1 piece (7.9 g)	25
Care*Free		
Sugarless Bubble Gum	1 stick (3 g)	10
Sugarless Cinnamon	1 piece (3 g)	5
Sugarless Peppermint	1 piece (3 g)	5
Sugarless Spearmint	1 piece (3 g)	5
Sugarless Wild Cherry	1 stick (3 g)	10
Chiclets		
Original	1 piece (1.59 g)	6
Tiny Size	8 pieces (0.13 g)	tr
Clorets	1 piece (1.59 g)	6
Dentyne		
Cinn-A-Burst	1 piece (3.2 g)	9
Gum	1 piece (1.88 g)	6
Sugar Free	1 piece (1.88 g)	5
Doublemint		
Chewing Gum	1 piece	10
Extra Sugar Free		
Cinnamon	1 piece	8
Spearmint & Peppermint	1 stick	8
Winter Fresh	1 piece	8
Freedent		
Spearmint Peppermint & Cinnamon	1 stick	10
Freshen-Up		
Gum	1 piece (4.2 g)	13
Fruit Stripe		
Bubble Gum Jumbo Pack	1 stick (3 g)	10
Variety Pack Chewing & Bubble Gum	1 stick (3 g)	10

FOOD	PORTION	CALS.
Hubba Bubba		
Bubble Gum Cola	1 piece	23
Bubble Gum Sugarfree Grape	1 piece	13
Bubble Gum Sugarfree Original	1 piece	14
Original	1 piece	23
Strawberry Grape Raspberry	1 piece	23
Juicy Fruit		
Stick	1	10
Rain-Blo		
Bubble Gum Balls	1 piece (2 g)	5
Stick*Free		
Sugarless Peppermint	1 stick (3 g)	10
Sugarless Spearmint	1 stick (3 g)	10
Swell		
Bubble Gum	1 piece (3 g)	10
Trident		
Gum	1 piece (1.88 g)	5
Soft Bubble Gum	1 piece (3.3 g)	9
Winterfresh		
Stick	1 stick (3 g)	10
Wrigley's		
Spearmint	1 stick	10
CHIA SEEDS		
dried	1 oz	134

CHICKEN

(*see also* CHICKEN DISHES, CHICKEN SUBSTITUTES, DINNER, HOT DOGS)

CANNED

FOOD	PORTION	CALS.
Swanson		
Chunk Style Mixin' Chicken	2.5 oz	130
White	2.5 oz	100
White & Dark	2.5 oz	100
Underwood		
Chunky	2.08 oz	150
Chunky Light	2.08 oz	80
Smoky	2.08 oz	150
FRESH		
broiler/fryer back w/ skin batter dipped & fried	½ back (2.5 oz)	238
broiler/fryer back w/ skin floured & fried	1.5 oz	146
broiler/fryer back w/ skin roasted	1 oz	96
broiler/fryer back w/ skin stewed	½ back (2.1 oz)	158
broiler/fryer back w/o skin fried	½ back (2 oz)	167
broiler/fryer breast w/ skin batter dipped & fried	½ breast (4.9 oz)	364

FOOD	PORTION	CALS.
broiler/fryer breast w/ skin batter dipped & fried	2.9 oz	218
broiler/fryer breast w/ skin roasted	2 oz	115
broiler/fryer breast w/ skin roasted	½ breast (3.4 oz)	193
broiler/fryer breast w/ skin stewed	½ breast (3.9 oz)	202
broiler/fryer breast w/o skin fried	½ breast (3 oz)	161
broiler/fryer breast w/o skin roasted	½ breast (3 oz)	142
broiler/fryer breast w/o skin stewed	2 oz	86
broiler/fryer dark meat w/ skin batter dipped & fried	5.9 oz	497
broiler/fryer dark meat w/ skin floured & fried	3.9 oz	313
broiler/fryer dark meat w/ skin roasted	3.5 oz	256
broiler/fryer dark meat w/ skin stewed	3.9 oz	256
broiler/fryer dark meat w/o skin fried	1 cup (5 oz)	334
broiler/fryer dark meat w/o skin roasted	1 cup (5 oz)	286
broiler/fryer dark meat w/o skin stewed	1 cup (5 oz)	269
broiler/fryer dark meat w/o skin stewed	3 oz	165
broiler/fryer drumstick w/ skin batter dipped & fried	1 (2.6 oz)	193
broiler/fryer drumstick w/ skin floured & fried	1 (1.7 oz)	120
broiler/fryer drumstick w/ skin roasted	1 (1.8 oz)	112
broiler/fryer drumstick w/ skin stewed	1 (2 oz)	116
broiler/fryer drumstick w/o skin fried	1 (1.5 oz)	82
broiler/fryer drumstick w/o skin roasted	1 (1.5 oz)	76
broiler/fryer drumstick w/o skin stewed	1 (1.6 oz)	78
broiler/fryer leg w/ skin batter dipped & fried	1 (5.5 oz)	431
broiler/fryer leg w/ skin floured & fried	1 (3.9 oz)	285
broiler/fryer leg w/ skin roasted	1 (4 oz)	265
broiler/fryer leg w/ skin stewed	1 (4.4 oz)	275
broiler/fryer leg w/o skin fried	1 (3.3 oz)	195
broiler/fryer leg w/o skin roasted	1 (3.3 oz)	182
broiler/fryer leg w/o skin stewed	1 (3.5 oz)	187
broiler/fryer light meat w/ skin batter dipped & fried	4 oz	312
broiler/fryer light meat w/ skin floured & fried	2.7 oz	192
broiler/fryer light meat w/ skin roasted	2.8 oz	175
broiler/fryer light meat w/ skin stewed	3.2 oz	181
broiler/fryer light meat w/o skin fried	1 cup (5 oz)	268
broiler/fryer light meat w/o skin roasted	1 cup (5 oz)	242
broiler/fryer light meat w/o skin stewed	1 cup (5 oz)	223
broiler/fryer neck w/ skin stewed	1 (1.3 oz)	94
broiler/fryer neck w/o skin stewed	1 (.6 oz)	32
broiler/fryer skin batter dipped & fried	from ½ chicken (6.7 oz)	749

FOOD	PORTION	CALS.
broiler/fryer skin batter dipped & fried	4 oz	449
broiler/fryer skin floured & fried	from ½ chicken (2 oz)	281
broiler/fryer skin floured & fried	1 oz	166
broiler/fryer skin roasted	from ½ chicken (2 oz)	254
broiler/fryer skin stewed	from ½ chicken (2.5 oz)	261
broiler/fryer thigh w/ skin batter dipped & fried	1 (3 oz)	238
broiler/fryer thigh w/ skin floured & fried	1 (2.2 oz)	162
broiler/fryer thigh w/ skin roasted	1 (2.2 oz)	153
broiler/fryer thigh w/ skin stewed	1 (2.4 oz)	158
broiler/fryer thigh w/o skin fried	1 (1.8 oz)	113
broiler/fryer thigh w/o skin roasted	1 (1.8 oz)	109
broiler/fryer thigh w/o skin stewed	1 (1.9 oz)	107
broiler/fryer w/ skin floured & fried	½ chicken (11 oz)	844
broiler/fryer w/ skin floured & fried	½ breast (3.4 oz)	218
broiler/fryer w/ skin fried	½ chicken (16.4 oz)	1347
broiler/fryer w/ skin roasted	½ chicken (10.5 oz)	715
broiler/fryer w/ skin stewed	½ chicken (11.7 oz)	730
broiler/fryer w/ skin neck & giblets batter dipped & fried	1 chicken (2.3 lbs)	2987
broiler/fryer w/ skin neck & giblets roasted	1 chicken (1.5 lbs)	1598
broiler/fryer w/ skin neck & giblets stewed	1 chicken (1.6 lbs)	1625
broiler/fryer w/o skin fried	1 cup	307
broiler/fryer w/o skin roasted	1 cup (5 oz)	266
broiler/fryer w/o skin stewed	1 oz	54
broiler/fryer w/o skin stewed	1 cup (5 oz)	248
broiler/fryer wing w/ skin batter dipped & fried	1 (1.7 oz)	159
broiler/fryer wing w/ skin floured & fried	1 (1.1 oz)	103
broiler/fryer wing w/ skin roasted	1 (1.2 oz)	99
broiler/fryer wing w/ skin stewed	1 (1.4 oz)	100
capon w/ skin neck & giblets roasted	1 chicken (3.1 lbs)	3211
cornish hen w/ skin roasted	1 hen (8 oz)	595
cornish hen w/o skin & bone roasted	1 hen (3.8 oz)	144
cornish hen w/o skin & bone roasted	½ hen (2 oz)	72
cornish hen w/skin roasted	½ hen (4 oz)	296
roaster dark meat w/o skin roasted	1 cup (5 oz)	250
roaster light meat w/o skin roasted	1 cup (5 oz)	214
roaster w/ skin neck & giblets roasted	1 chicken (2.4 lbs)	2363
roaster w/ skin roasted	½ chicken (1.1 lbs)	1071
roaster w/o skin roasted	1 cup (5 oz)	469
stewing dark meat w/o skin stewed	1 cup (5 oz)	361
stewing w/ skin neck & giblets stewed	1 chicken (1.3 lbs)	1636
stewing w/ skin stewed	½ chicken (9.2 oz)	744

FOOD	PORTION	CALS.
stewing w/ skin stewed	6.2 oz	507
Perdue		
Boneless Breasts Cooked	3 oz	120
Boneless Breast Tenderloins Cooked	3 oz	100
Boneless Thighs Roasted	2 (3.5 oz)	200
Breast Quarters Cooked	3 oz	180
Burger Cooked	1 (3 oz)	170
Chicken Breast Seasoned Barbecue Cooked	3 oz	110
Chicken Breast Seasoned Italian Cooked	3 oz	100
Chicken Breast Seasoned Lemon Pepper Cooked	3 oz	90
Chicken Breast Seasoned Oriental Cooked	3 oz	100
Cornish Hen Split Dark Meat Roasted	1 half (6.5 oz)	210
Cornish Hen White Meat Cooked	3 oz	170
Drumsticks Roasted	1 (2 oz)	110
Drumsticks Skinless Roasted	2 (3.5 oz)	150
Ground Cooked	3 oz	180
Jumbo Drumsticks Roasted	1 (2 oz)	110
Jumbo Split Breast Roasted	1 (7 oz)	370
Jumbo Thighs Roasted	1 (3 oz)	240
Jumbo Whole Leg Roasted	2 (5.5 oz)	360
Jumbo Wings Roasted	2 (3 oz)	210
Leg Quarters Cooked	3 oz	210
Oven Stuffer Boneless Breast Cooked	3 oz	120
Oven Stuffer Boneless Breast Thin Sliced Cooked	1 slice (2 oz)	80
Oven Stuffer Boneless Thighs Roasted	1 (3.5 oz)	170
Oven Stuffer Dark Meat Roasted	3 oz	200
Oven Stuffer Drumstick Roasted	1 (3.5 oz)	190
Oven Stuffer White Meat Roasted	3 oz	160
Oven Stuffer Whole Breast Cooked	3 oz	150
Oven Stuffer Wing Drummettes Roasted	2 (2.5 oz)	170
Split Breast Skinless Roasted	1 (6 oz)	250
Split Breasts Roasted	1 (7 oz)	370
Thighs Roasted	1 (3 oz)	240
Thighs Skinless Roasted	1 (2.5 oz)	160
Whole White Meat Cooked	3 oz	160
Whole Leg Roasted	1 (5.5 oz)	360
Wingettes Roasted	3 (3 oz)	200
Wings Roasted	2 (3 oz)	210
Tyson		
Breast	3 oz	116
Cornish Hen	3.5 oz	250

FOOD	PORTION	CALS.
Tyson (CONT.)		
Drumstick	3 oz	131
Thigh	3 oz	152
Whole	3 oz	134
Wing	3 oz	147
Wampler Longacre		
Ground raw	1 oz	50
FROZEN		
Banquet		
Country Fried	1 serv (3 oz)	270
Drum Snackers	2.25 oz	190
Fried Breast	1 piece (4.45 oz)	240
Fried Hot & Spicy	1 serv (3 oz)	260
Fried Original	1 serv (3 oz)	270
Fried Thigh & Drumsticks	1 serv (3 oz)	260
Hot & Spicy Nuggets	2.5 oz	230
Hot Popcorn Chicken	1 pkg (3 oz)	290
Nuggets	3 oz	240
Nuggets Chicken & Cheddar	2.7 oz	280
Nuggets Chicken & Mozzarella	6 (2.8 oz)	210
Nuggets Southern Fried	6 (4.5 oz)	340
Nuggets Sweet & Sour	6 (4.5 oz)	320
Patties	1 (2.5 oz)	180
Patties Southern Fried	1 (2.5 oz)	190
Skinless Fried	1 serv (3 oz)	210
Skinless Fried Honey BBQ	1 serv (3 oz)	210
Southern Fried	1 serv (3 oz)	270
Tenders	3 pieces (3 oz)	260
Tenders Southern Fried	3 pieces (3 oz)	260
Wings Hot & Spicy	4 pieces (5 oz)	230
Country Skillet		
Chicken Chunks	5 (3.1 oz)	270
Chicken Nuggets	10 (3.3 oz)	280
Chicken Patties	2.5 oz	190
Southern Fried Chicken Chunks	5 (3.1 oz)	250
Southern Fried Chicken Patties	1 (2.5 oz)	190
Empire		
Nuggets	5 (3 oz)	180
Stix	4 (3.1 oz)	180
Ozark Valley		
Nuggets	4 (2.9 oz)	210
Patties	1 (3 oz)	210
Sensible Chef		
Fried Breast	1 (3 oz)	200

FOOD	PORTION	CALS.
Swanson		
Chicken Nibbles	3.25 oz	300
Chicken Nuggets	3 oz	230
Fried Chicken Breast Portion	4.5 oz	360
Pre-Fried Chicken Parts	3.25 oz	270
Thighs & Drumsticks	3.25 oz	290
Tyson		
BBQ Breast Fillets	3 oz	110
Boneless Breasts	3.5 oz	210
Boneless Skinless Breast	3.5 oz	130
Boneless Skinless Thighs	3.5 oz	200
Breaded Patties	3 oz	300
Breast Chunks	3 oz	240
Breast Fillets	3 oz	190
Breast Patties	2.6 oz	220
Breast Tenders	3 oz	220
Chick'n Cheddar	2.6 oz	220
Chick'n Chunks	2.6 oz	220
Cordon Blue Mini	1	90
Diced	3 oz	130
Drums & Thighs	3.5 oz	270
Grilled Sandwich	3.5 oz	200
Hors D'Oeuvres Mesquite Chunks	3.5 oz	100
Hot BBQ Breast Tenders	2.75 oz	110
Mesquite Breast Fillets	2.75 oz	100
Mesquite Breast Strips	2.75 oz	100
Mesquite Breast Tenders	2.75 oz	110
Microwave Chunks	3.5 oz	220
Microwave Chunks BBQ Sandwich	4 oz	230
Microwave Tenders	3.5 oz	230
Roasted Breast Fillets	1 oz	50
Roasted Breasts	1 oz	50
Roasted Drumsticks	1 oz	50
Roasted Half Chicken	1 oz	60
Roasted Thighs	1 oz	70
Roasted Whole Chicken	1 oz	60
Skinless Breast Tenders	3.5 oz	120
Southern Fried Breast Fillets	3 oz	220
Southern Fried Breast Patties	2.6 oz	220
Southern Fried Chick'n Chunks	2.6 oz	220
Thick & Crispy Patties	2.6 oz	220
Weaver		
Batter Dipped Breast	4.4 oz	310
Batter Dipped Drums & Thighs	3 oz	210

FOOD	PORTION	CALS.
Weaver (CONT.)		
Batter Dipped Wings	4 oz	400
Breast Fillets	4.5 oz	270
Breast Fillets Strips	3.3 oz	200
Breast Patties	3 oz	205
Chicken Nuggets	2.6 oz	190
Crispy Dutch Frye Assorted	3.6 oz	290
Crispy Dutch Frye Breasts	4.5 oz	350
Crispy Dutch Frye Drums & Thighs	3.5 oz	290
Crispy Dutch Frye Wings	4 oz	400
Crispy Light Skinless	2.9 oz	170
Croquettes	2 pieces	280
Croquettes With Gravy	2 pieces + ½ cup gravy	282
Honey Batter Tenders	3 oz	220
Hot Wings	2.7 oz	170
Mini Drums Crispy	3 oz	210
Mini Drums Herbs & Spice	3 oz	200
Premium Tenders	3 oz	170
Rondelets Cheese	1 (2.6 oz)	190
Rondelets Italian	1 (2.6 oz)	190
Rondelets Original	1 (3 oz)	190
READY-TO-EAT		
Banquet		
Breast Tenders Fat Free	3 (3.2 oz)	130
Boar's Head		
Breast Hickory Smoked	2 oz	60
Breast Oven Roasted	2 oz	50
Carl Buddig		
Chicken	1 oz	50
Chicken By George		
Cajun	1 breast (4 oz)	130
Caribbean Grill	1 breast (4 oz)	150
Garlic & Herb	1 breast (4 oz)	120
Italian Bleu Cheese	1 breast (4 oz)	130
Lemon Herb	1 breast (4 oz)	120
Lemon Oregano	1 breast (4 oz)	130
Mesquite Barbecue	1 breast (4 oz)	130
Mustard Dill	1 breast (4 oz)	140
Roasted	1 breast (4 oz)	110
Teriyaki	1 breast (4 oz)	130
Tomato Herb With Basil	1 breast (4 oz)	140
Empire		
Barbarcue Whole	5 oz	280
Battered & Breaded Cutlets	1 (3.3 oz)	200

FOOD	PORTION	CALS.
Empire (CONT.)		
Battered & Breaded Fried Breasts	3 oz	170
Battered & Breaded Nuggets	5 (3 oz)	200
Bologna	3 slices (1.8 oz)	200
Fried Drum & Thigh	3 oz	240
Falls		
BBQ	3 oz	150
Healthy Choice		
Deli-Thin Oven Roasted Breast	6 slices (2 oz)	45
Deli-Thin Smoked Breast	6 slices (2 oz)	60
Fresh-Trak Oven Roasted Breast	1 slice (1 oz)	30
Oven Roasted Breast	1 slice (1 oz)	25
Smoked Breast	1 slice (1 oz)	35
Hebrew National		
Deli Thin Oven Roasted	1.8 oz	45
Hillshire		
Deli Select Oven Roasted Breast	1 slice	10
Deli Select Smoked Breast	1 slice	10
Flavor Pack 90-99% Fat Free Smoked Breast	1 slice (0.75 oz)	20
Lunch 'N Munch Smoked Chicken/ Monterey Jack	1 pkg (4.5 oz)	350
Lunch 'N Munch Smoked Chicken/ Monterey/ Snickers	1 pkg (4.25 oz)	400
Louis Rich		
Carving Board Classic Baked	2 slices (1.6 oz)	45
Carving Board Grilled	2 slices (1.6 oz)	45
Deli-Thin Oven Roasted Breast	4 slices (1.8 oz)	50
Oven Roasted Deluxe Breast	1 slice (1 oz)	30
Mr. Turkey		
Deli Cuts Hardwood Smoked	3 slices	30
Deli Cuts Oven Roasted	3 slices	25
Oscar Mayer		
Free Oven Roasted Breast	4 slices (1.8 oz)	45
Lunchables Chicken/Monterey Jack	1 pkg (4.5 oz)	350
Lunchables Deluxe Chicken/Turkey	1 pkg (5.1 oz)	380
Lunchables Dessert Chocolate Pudding/ Chicken/ Jack	1 pkg (6.2 oz)	370
Perdue		
Cafe Meal Kit Stir Fry	1 serv (8.2 oz)	360
Cornish Hen Dark Meat Cooked	3 oz	200
Cornish Hen Split White Meat Roasted	½ hen (6.5 oz)	200
Nuggets Chicken & Cheese	5 (3 oz)	220
Nuggets Chik-Tac-Toe Cooked	5 (3 oz)	200

FOOD	PORTION	CALS.
Perdue (CONT.)		
Nuggets Football Basketball Baseball	4 (3 oz)	230
Nuggets Original	5 (3 oz)	200
Nuggets Star & Drumstick	4 (3 oz)	200
Original Tenderloins Cooked	3 oz	160
Original Cutlets Cooked	1 (3.5 oz)	230
Oven Roasted Breast	1 (5 oz)	190
Oven Roasted Drumsticks	2 (2.5 oz)	100
Oven Roasted Half Dark Meat	3 oz	170
Oven Roasted Half White Meat	3 oz	140
Oven Roasted Thighs	1 (3 oz)	170
Oven Roasted Whole Chicken Dark Meat	3 oz	170
Oven Roasted Whole Chicken White Meat	3 oz	140
Seasoned Whole Chicken Dark Meat	3 oz	190
Seasoned Whole Chicken White Meat	3 oz	160
Short Cuts Italian	3 oz	110
Short Cuts Lemon Pepper	½ cup (2.5 oz)	90
Short Cuts Mesquite	3 oz	110
Short Cuts Oven Roasted	3 oz	110
Wings Barbecued	3 oz	200
Wings Hot & Spicy	3 oz	190
Shady Brook		
Slow Roasted Breast	2 oz	60
Tyson		
Bologna	1 slice	44
Hickory Smoked Breast	1 slice	25
Honey Flavored Breast	1 slice	25
Oven Roasted Breast	1 slice	25
Oven Roasted Mesquite Breast	1 slice	25
Roasted Drumsticks w/ Skin	2 (3.8 oz)	220
Roll	1 slice	26
Wings Barbecue	6-7 (3.5 oz)	218
Wings Hot & Spicy	6-7 (3.5 oz)	218
Wings Roasted	6-7 (3.5 oz)	218
Wings Teriyaki	6-7 (3.5 oz)	218
Wampler Longacre		
Breast	1 oz	35
Chef's Select Breast	1 oz	35
Premium Oven Roasted Breast	1 oz	50
Roll	1 oz	65
Roll Sliced	1 slice (0.8 oz)	50
Weaver		
Roasted Wings	1 oz	70

FOOD	PORTION	CALS.
TAKE-OUT		
oven roasted breast of chicken	2 oz	60
CHICKEN DISHES		
(*see also* CHICKEN SUBSTITUTES, DINNER)		
CANNED		
Dinty Moore		
Noodles & Chicken	1 can (7.5 oz)	180
Stew	1 cup (8.5 oz)	220
Swanson		
Chicken & Dumplings	7.5 oz	220
Chicken Ala King	5.25 oz	190
Chicken Stew	7.6 oz	160
FROZEN		
Croissant Pocket		
Stuffed Sandwich Chicken Broccoli & Cheddar	1 piece (4.5 oz)	300
Hot Pocket		
Stuffed Sandwich Chicken & Cheddar With Broccoli	1 (4.5 oz)	300
Jimmy Dean		
Grilled Breast Sandwich	1 (5.5 oz)	330
Lean Pockets		
Stuffed Sandwich Chicken Fajita	1 (4.5 oz)	260
Stuffed Sandwich Chicken Parmesan	1 (4.5 oz)	260
Stuffed Sandwich Glazed Chicken Supreme	1 (4.5 oz)	240
Mrs. Paterson's		
Aussie Pie Chicken Low Fat	1 (5.5 oz)	380
Tyson		
Microwave Breast Sandwich	4.25 oz	328
White Castle		
Grilled Chicken Sandwich	2 (4 oz)	250
Grilled Chicken Sandwich w/ Sauce	2 (4.8 oz)	290
MIX		
Chicken Skillet Helper		
Stir-Fried Chicken as prep	1 cup	270
Hamburger Helper		
Reduced Sodium Cheddar Spirals Chicken Recipe as prep	1 cup	240
Reduced Sodium Italian Herb Chicken Recipe as prep	1 cup	200
Reduced Sodium Southwestern Beef Chicken Recipe as prep	1 cup	220
READY-TO-EAT		
Shady Brook		
Chicken Breast w/ Rice Pilaf	1 serv (12 oz)	350

FOOD	PORTION	CALS.
Shady Brook (CONT.)		
Teriyaki Breast	1 serv (12 oz)	490
Wampler Longacre		
Cacciatore	1 serv (4 oz)	118
Salad	1 oz	70
Salad Lite	1 oz	45
Smokey Barbecue	1 serv (4 oz)	175
Sweet N Sour	1 serv (4 oz)	106
Szechwan With Peanuts	1 serv (4 oz)	112
SHELF-STABLE		
Dinty Moore		
Microwave Cup Chicken & Dumpling	1 pkg (7.5 oz)	200
Microwave Cup Stew	1 pkg (7.5 oz)	180
Lunch Bucket		
Dumplings'n Chicken	1 pkg (7.5 oz)	140
Light'n Healthy Chicken Fiesta	1 pkg (7.5 oz)	170
TAKE-OUT		
boneless breaded & fried w/ barbecue sauce	6 pieces (4.6 oz)	330
boneless breaded & fried w/ honey	6 pieces (4 oz)	339
boneless breaded & fried w/ mustard sauce	6 pieces (4.6 oz)	323
boneless breaded & fried w/ sweet & sour sauce	6 pieces (4.6 oz)	346
breast & wing breaded & fried	2 pieces (5.7 oz)	494
chicken & noodles	1 cup	365
chicken a la king	1 cup	470
chicken paprikash	1½ cups	296
drumstick breaded & fried	2 pieces (5.2 oz)	430
thigh breaded & fried	2 pieces (5.2 oz)	430

CHICKEN SUBSTITUTES

FOOD	PORTION	CALS.
Harvest Direct		
TVP Poultry Chunks	3.5 oz	280
TVP Poultry Ground	3.5 oz	280
Knox Mountain Farm		
Chick'N Wheat Mix	1 serv (⅛ pkg)	110
Loma Linda		
Chicken Supreme Mix not prep	⅓ cup (0.9 oz)	90
Chik Nuggets	5 pieces (3 oz)	240
Fried Chik'n w/ Gravy	2 pieces (2.8 oz)	210
Morningstar Farms		
Chik Nuggets	4 pieces (3 oz)	160
Chik Patties	1 (2.5 oz)	150
Soy Is Us		
Chicken Not!	½ cup (1.75 oz)	140
White Wave		
Meatless Sandwich Slices	2 slices (1.6 oz)	80

FOOD	PORTION	CALS.
Worthington		
Chic-Ketts	2 slices (1.9 oz)	120
Chicken Sliced	2 slices (2 oz)	80
ChikStiks	1 (1.6 oz)	110
CrispyChik Patties	1 (2.5 oz)	170
Cutlets	1 slice (2.1 oz)	70
Diced Chik	¼ cup (1.9 oz)	40
FriChik	2 pieces (3.2 oz)	120
FriChik Low Fat	2 pieces (3 oz)	80
Golden Croquettes	4 pieces (3 oz)	210
Sliced Chik	3 slices (3.2 oz)	70

CHICKPEAS
CANNED
Allen		
Garbanzo	½ cup (4.4 oz)	120
East Texas Fair		
Garbanzo	½ cup (4.4 oz)	120
Eden		
Organic	½ cup (4.6 oz)	120
Goya		
Spanish Style	7.5 oz	150
Green Giant		
Garbanzo	½ cup (4.4 oz)	110
Old El Paso		
Garbanzo	½ cup (4.6 oz)	120
Progresso		
Chick Peas	½ cup (4.6 oz)	120

DRIED
Bean Cuisine		
Garbanzo	½ cup	115

CHICORY
greens raw chopped	½ cup	21
root raw	1 (2.1 oz)	44
witloof head raw	1 (1.9 oz)	9
witloof raw	½ cup (1.6 oz)	8

CHILI
Allen		
Mexican w/ Beans	½ cup (4.5 oz)	120
Amy's Organic		
Whole Meals Chili & Cornbread	1 pkg (10.5 oz)	320
Brown Beauty		
Mexican Chili Beans	½ cup (4.5 oz)	120

FOOD	PORTION	CALS.
Chili Man		
Seasoning Mix	1 tbsp (7 g)	25
Del Monte		
Sauce	1 tbsp (0.6 oz)	20
Eden		
Organic Chili Beans w/ Jalapeno & Red Peppers	½ cup (4.6 oz)	130
Hain		
Hot	¼ pkg	30
Medium	¼ pkg	30
Mild	¼ pkg	30
Spicy Tempeh	7.5 oz	160
Spicy Vegetarian	7.5 oz	160
Spicy Vegetarian Reduced Sodium	7.5 oz	170
Spicy With Chicken	7.5 oz	130
Health Valley		
Burrito	1 cup	160
Enchilada	1 cup	160
Fajita	1 cup	80
In A Cup Black Bean Mild	¾ cup	120
In A Cup Texas Style Spicy	¾ cup	120
Vegetarian Lentil Mild	1 cup	160
Vegetarian Lentil No Salt	1 cup	80
Vegetarian Mild	1 cup	160
Vegetarian Mild No Salt	1 cup	160
Vegetarian Spicy	1 cup	160
Vegetarian Spicy No Salt	1 cup	160
Vegetarian w/ 3 Beans Mild	1 cup	160
Vegetarian w/ Black Beans Mild	1 cup	160
Vegetarian w/ Black Beans Spicy	1 cup	160
Hormel		
Chunky w/ Beans	1 cup (8.7 oz)	270
Hot No Beans	1 cup (8.3 oz)	210
Hot With Beans	1 cup (8.7 oz)	270
Microcup Meals Chili Mac	1 cup (7.5 oz)	200
Microcup Meals Hot With Beans	1 cup (7.3 oz)	220
Microcup Meals No Beans	1 cup (7.3 oz)	190
Microcup Meals With Beans	1 cup (7.3 oz)	220
No Beans	1 cup (8.3 oz)	210
Turkey No Beans	1 cup (8.3 oz)	190
Turkey w/ Beans	1 cup (8.7 oz)	210
Vegetarian	1 cup (8.7 oz)	200
With Beans	1 cup (8.7 oz)	270
With Beans	1 cup (8.7 oz)	270

FOOD	PORTION	CALS.
Hunt's		
Chili Beans	½ cup (4.5 oz)	87
Hurst		
HamBeens Chili Beans	1 serv	130
Just Rite		
Hot With Beans	4 oz	195
With Beans	4 oz	200
Without Beans	4 oz	180
Lean Cuisine		
Three Bean w/ Rice	1 pkg (10 oz)	250
Lightlife		
Chili	4.3 oz	110
Luigino's		
Chili-Mac	1 pkg (8 oz)	230
Lunch Bucket		
Chili With Beans	1 pkg (7.5 oz)	300
Natural Touch		
Vegetarian	1 cup (8.1 oz)	170
Nile Spice		
Chili'n Beans Original	1 pkg	150
Chili'n Beans Spicy	1 pkg	150
Old El Paso		
Chili Seasoning Mix	1 tbsp (0.3 oz)	25
Chili With Beans	1 cup (8 oz)	200
Stouffer's		
With Beans	1 pkg (8.75 oz)	270
Swanson		
Homestyle Chili Con Carne	8¼ oz	270
Tabatchnick		
Vegetarian	7.5 oz	210
Tyson		
Chicken	3.5 oz	105
Van Camp's		
Chilee Beanee Weenee	1 can (8 oz)	240
Chili With Beans	1 cup (8.9 oz)	350
Wampler Longacre		
Turkey	1 serv (4 oz)	118
Watkins		
Powder	¼ tsp (0.5 g)	0
Seasoning	1¼ tsp (4 g)	15
Worthington		
Chili	1 cup (8.1 oz)	290
Low Fat	1 cup (8.1 oz)	170

FOOD	PORTION	CALS.
TAKE-OUT		
con carne w/ beans	8.9 oz	254
CHINESE CABBAGE		
(see CABBAGE)		
CHINESE FOOD		
(see ASIAN FOOD)		
CHINESE PRESERVING MELON		
cooked	½ cup	11
CHIPS		
(see also POPCORN, PRETZELS, SNACKS)		
CORN		
barbecue	1 bag (7 oz)	1036
barbecue	1 oz	148
cones nacho	1 oz	152
cones plain	1 oz	145
onion	1 oz	142
plain	1 bag (7 oz)	1067
plain	1 oz	153
puffs cheese	1 oz	157
puffs cheese	1 bag (8 oz)	1256
twists cheese	1 bag (8 oz)	1256
twists cheese	1 oz	157
Energy Food Factory		
Corn Pops Fat Free	0.5 oz	50
Corn Pops Nacho	0.5 oz	50
Corn Pops Original	0.5 oz	50
Fritos		
BBQ	29 (1 oz)	150
Chili Cheese	31 (1 oz)	160
King Size	12 (1 oz)	150
Original	32 (1 oz)	160
Sabrositas Flamin' Hot	30 (1 oz)	150
Sabrositas Lime'N Chile	28 (1 oz)	150
Scoops	11 (1 oz)	160
Texas Grill Honey BBQ	15 (1 oz)	150
Wild N'Mild Ranch	28 (1 oz)	160
Planters		
Corn Chips	34 chips (1 oz)	170
King Size	17 chips (1 oz)	160
Snacks To Go	1 pkg (1.5 oz)	240
Snyder's		
BBQ	1 oz	160

FOOD	PORTION	CALS.
Snyder's (CONT.)		
Chips	1 oz	160
Utz		
Barbeque	24 (1 oz)	160
Corn	24 (1 oz)	160
Wise		
Corn Crunchies	1 oz	160
Crispy Corn	1 oz	160
Crispy Corn Nacho Cheese	1 oz	160
Dipsy Doodles	1 pkg (1.5 oz)	240
MULTIGRAIN		
Barbara's		
Pinta Chips	13 (1 oz)	130
Pinta Chips Salsa	12 (1 oz)	130
Sunchips		
French Onion	13 (1 oz)	140
Harvest Cheddar	13 (1 oz)	140
Original	14 (1 oz)	140
POTATO		
barbecue	1 oz	139
barbecue	1 bag (7 oz)	971
cheese	1 oz	140
cheese	1 bag (6 oz)	842
light	1 oz	134
light	1 bag (6 oz)	801
potato	1 oz	152
potato	1 bag (8 oz)	1217
sour cream & onion	1 bag (7 oz)	1051
sour cream & onion	1 oz	150
sticks	1 oz	148
sticks	½ cup (0.6 oz)	94
sticks	1 pkg (1 oz)	148
Barbara's		
No Salt Added	1¼ cups (1 oz)	150
Regular	1¼ cups (1 oz)	150
Ripple	1¼ cups (1 oz)	150
Yogurt & Green Onion	1¼ cups (1 oz)	150
Barrel O' Fun		
Barbeque	1 oz	145
Chips	1 oz	150
Sour Cream & Onion	1 oz	150
Butterfield		
Sticks	1 pkg (1.7 oz)	250
Sticks	⅔ cup (1 oz)	150

FOOD	PORTION	CALS.
Cape Cod		
Chips	19 chips (1 oz)	150
Chester's		
Flamin'Hot	1 oz	140
Salsa	1 oz	140
Cottage Fries		
No Salt Added	1 oz	160
Energy Food Factory		
Potato Pops Au Gratin	0.5 oz	60
Potato Pops Fat Free	0.5 oz	50
Potato Pops Herb & Garlic	0.5 oz	50
Potato Pops Mesquite	0.5 oz	50
Potato Pops Original	0.5 oz	50
Potato Pops Salt N' Vinegar	0.5 oz	50
Herr's		
Potato	1 oz	140
Lay's		
Adobadas	16 (1 oz)	170
Baked KC Masterpiece BBQ	11 (1 oz)	120
Baked Original	11 (1 oz)	110
Baked Roasted Herb	12 (1 oz)	130
Baked Sour Cream & Onion	12 (1 oz)	120
Classic	20 (1 oz)	150
Deli Style Hot N'Tangy BBQ	18 (1 oz)	150
Deli Style Jalapeno	17 (1 oz)	150
Deli Style Original	17 (1 oz)	140
Deli Style Salt & Vinegar	16 (1 oz)	90
Flamin' Hot	17 pieces (1 oz)	150
KC Masterpiece BBQ	15 (1 oz)	150
Onion & Garlic	19 (1 oz)	150
Salt & Vinegar	17 pieces (1 oz)	150
Sour Cream & Onion	17 pieces (1 oz)	160
Toasted Onion & Cheese	17 pieces (1 oz)	160
Wavy Au Gratin	13 (1 oz)	150
Wavy Original	11 pieces (1 oz)	160
Wavy Ranch	11 (1 oz)	160
Wow Mesquite BBQ	20 (1 oz)	75
Wow Mesquite BBQ	20 (1 oz)	75
Wow Original	20 (1 oz)	75
Wow Original	1 pkg (0.75 oz)	55
Wow Sour Cream & Chive	19 (1 oz)	80
Wow Sour Cream & Chive	19 (1 oz)	80
Louise's		
"1g" Mesquite BBQ	1 oz	110

FOOD	PORTION	CALS.
Louise's (CONT.)		
"1g" Original	1 oz	110
70% Less Fat Mesquite BBQ	1 oz	110
70% Less Fat Original	1 oz	110
Fat-Free Maui Onion	1 oz	110
Fat-Free Mesquite BBQ	1 oz	110
Fat-Free No Salt	1 oz	110
Fat-Free Original	1 oz	110
Fat-Free Vinegar & Salt	1 oz	110
Mr. Phipps		
Tater Crisps Bar-B-Que	21 (1 oz)	130
Tater Crisps Original	23 (1 oz)	120
Tater Crisps Sour Cream 'n Onion	22 (1 oz)	130
New York Deli		
Chips	1 oz	160
Pringles		
BBQ	14 chips (1 oz)	150
Cheez-ums	14 chips (1 oz)	150
Fat Free	15 chips (1 oz)	75
Original	14 chips (1 oz)	160
Ranch	14 chips (1 oz)	150
Ridges Cheddar & Sour Cream	12 chips (1 oz)	150
Ridges Mesquite BBQ	12 chips (1 oz)	150
Ridges Original	12 chips (1 oz)	150
Right BBQ	16 chips (1 oz)	140
Right Original	16 chips (1 oz)	140
Right Ranch	16 chips (1 oz)	140
Right Sour Cream 'N Onion	16 chips (1 oz)	140
Rippled Original	10 chips (1 oz)	160
Sour Cream N'Onion	14 chips (1 oz)	160
Ruffles		
Baked	10 (1 oz)	110
Baked Cheddar & Sour Cream	9 (1 oz)	120
Buffalo Style	11 chips (1 oz)	160
Cheddar & Sour Cream	11 chips (1 oz)	160
French Onion	11 (1 oz)	150
MC Masterpiece Mesquite BBQ	11 (1 oz)	150
Original	12 chips (1 oz)	150
Ranch	13 (1 oz)	150
Reduced Fat	16 (1 oz)	130
The Works	12 (1 oz)	160
Wow Cheddar & Sour Cream	15 (1 oz)	75
Wow Cheddar & Sour Cream	15 (1 oz)	75
Wow Original	17 (1 oz)	5

FOOD	PORTION	CALS.
Ruffles (CONT.)		
Wow Original	17 (1 oz)	75
Snyder's		
BBQ	1 oz	150
Cheddar Bacon	1 oz	150
Chips	1 oz	150
Coney Island	1 oz	150
Grilled Steak & Onion	1 oz	150
Hot Buffalo Wings	1 oz	150
Kosher Dill	1 oz	150
No Salt	1 oz	150
Salt & Vinegar	1 oz	150
Sausage Pizza	1 oz	150
Sour Cream & Onion	1 oz	150
Sour Cream & Onion Unsalted	1 oz	150
State Line		
Chips	1 pkg (0.5 oz)	80
Utz		
Baked Crisps	12 (1 oz)	110
Carolina Barbeque	20 (1 oz)	150
Cheddar & Sour Cream	20 (1 oz)	160
Grandma	20 (1 oz)	140
Grandma BBQ	20 (1 oz)	140
Home Style Kettle	20 (1 oz)	140
Home Style Kettle BBQ	20 (1 oz)	140
Kettle Classics Crunchy	20 (1 oz)	150
Kettle Classics Crunchy Mesquite BBQ	20 (1 oz)	150
No Salt Added	20 (1 oz)	150
Onion & Garlic	20 (1 oz)	150
Reduced Fat BBQ	22 (1 oz)	140
Reduced Fat Ripple	24 (1 oz)	140
Regular	20 (1 oz)	150
Ripple	20 (1 oz)	150
Ripple Sour Cream & Onion	20 (1 oz)	160
Ripple Barbeque	20 (1 oz)	150
Salt'N Vinegar	20 (1 oz)	150
The Crab Chip	20 (1 oz)	150
Wavy	20 chips (1 oz)	150
Yes! Fat Free	20 (1 oz)	75
Yes! Fat Free Barbeque	20 (1 oz)	75
Yes! Fat Free Ripple	20 (1 oz)	75
Wise		
Natural	1 oz	160
Ridgies Barbecue	1 oz	150

FOOD	PORTION	CALS.
TORTILLA		
nacho	1 oz	141
nacho	1 bag (8 oz)	1131
nacho light	1 oz	126
nacho light	1 bag (6 oz)	757
plain	1 bag (7.5 oz)	1067
plain	1 oz	142
ranch	1 oz	139
ranch	1 bag (7 oz)	969
taco	1 bag (8 oz)	1089
taco	1 oz	136
Barbara's		
Blue Corn	15 (1 oz)	140
Blue Corn No Salt Added	15 (1 oz)	140
Barrel O' Fun		
Nacho	1 oz	140
Tostada Yellow	1 oz	140
White	1 oz	140
Doritos		
3D's Cooler Ranch	27 (1 oz)	140
3D's Nacho Cheesier	27 (1 oz)	140
Cooler Ranch	12 (1 oz)	140
Flamin' Hot	11 (1 oz)	140
Nacho Cheesier	11 (1 oz)	140
Salsa Verde	12 (1 oz)	150
Smokey Red	12 (1 oz)	150
Spicy Nacho	12 (1 oz)	140
Toasted Corn	13 (1 oz)	140
Wow Nacho Cheesier	1 pkg (0.75 oz)	70
Guiltless Gourmet		
Baked	22-26 chips (1 oz)	110
Hain		
Sesame	1 oz	140
Sesame Cheese	1 oz	160
Sesame No Salt Added	1 oz	140
Taco Style	1 oz	160
Herr's		
Restaurant Style White Corn	10 chips (1 oz)	140
La FAMOUS		
No Salt Added	1 oz	140
Tortilla	1 oz	140
Louise's		
95% Fat-Free	1 oz	120

FOOD	PORTION	CALS.
Mr. Phipps		
Nacho	28 (1 oz)	130
Original	28 (1 oz)	130
Old El Paso		
NACHIPS	9 chips (1 oz)	150
White Corn	11 chips (1 oz)	140
Santitas		
100% White Corn	6 (1 oz)	130
Restaurant Style Chips	7 (1 oz)	130
Restaurant Style Strips	10 (1 oz)	130
Snyder's		
Chips	1 oz	140
Enchilada	1 oz	140
Nacho Cheese	1 oz	140
No Salt	1 oz	140
Ranch	1 oz	140
Tostitos		
Baked Bite Size	20 (1 oz)	110
Baked Bite Size Salsa & Cream Cheese	16 (1 oz)	120
Baked Original	13 (1 oz)	110
Bite Size	15 (1 oz)	140
Crispy Rounds	13 (1 oz)	150
Nacho Style	6 (1 oz)	140
Restaurant Style	7 (1 oz)	140
Restaurant Style Hint Of Lime	6 (1 oz)	140
Santa Fe Gold	7 (1 oz)	140
Wow Original	6 (1 oz)	90
Wow Original	6 (1 oz)	90
Tyson		
Nacho Cheese	1 oz	140
Ranch Flavor	1 oz	140
Traditional	1 oz	140
Unsalted	1 oz	140
Utz		
Black Bean & Salsa	13 (1 oz)	150
Low Fat Baked	10 (1 oz)	120
Nacho	13 (1 oz)	150
Restaurant Style	6 (1 oz)	140
Spicy Nacho	13 (1 oz)	150
White Corn	12 (1 oz)	140
Wise		
Bravos	1 oz	150
VEGETABLE		
taro	10 (0.8 oz)	115
taro	1 oz	141

FOOD	PORTION	CALS.
Eden		
Vegetable Chips	50 (1 oz)	130
Wasabi Chip Hot & Spicy	50 (1 oz)	130
Hain		
Carrot Chips	1 oz	150
Carrot Chips Barbecue	1 oz	140
Carrot Chips No Salt Added	1 oz	150
Robert's American Gourmet		
Spirulina Spirals	1 oz	120
Soya King		
Soy	1 pkg (0.75 oz)	110
Terra Chips		
Sweet Potato	1 oz	140
Sweet Potato Spiced	1 oz	140
Taro Spiced	1 oz	130
Vegetable	1 oz	140
Top Banana		
Plantain Chips	1 oz	150

CHITTERLINGS

pork cooked	3 oz	258

CHIVES

freeze-dried	1 tbsp	1
fresh chopped	1 tbsp	1

CHOCOLATE

(*see also* CANDY, CAROB, COCOA, ICE CREAM TOPPINGS, MILK DRINKS)

BAKING

baking	1 oz	145
grated unsweetened	1 cup (4.6 oz)	690
liquid unsweetened	1 oz	134
squares unsweetened	1 square (1 oz)	148
Baker's		
Bittersweet	½ square (0.5 oz)	70
German's Sweet	2 squares (0.5 oz)	60
Semi-Sweet	½ square (0.5 oz)	70
Unsweetened	½ square (0.5 oz)	70
White	½ square (0.5 oz)	80
Nestle		
Choco Bake	0.5 oz	80
Premier White	0.5 oz	80
Semi-Sweet	0.5 oz	70
Unsweetened	0.5 oz	80

CHIPS

milk chocolate	1 cup (6 oz)	862

FOOD	PORTION	CALS.
semisweet	1 cup (6 oz)	804
semisweet	60 pieces (1 oz)	136
Baker's		
Chips	1 oz	143
Real Milk Chocolate	0.5 oz	70
Real Semi-Sweet	0.5 oz	60
Semi-Sweet	0.5 oz	70
M&M's		
Baking Bits Milk Chocolate	0.5 oz	70
Baking Bits Semi-Sweet	0.5 oz	70
Nestle		
Morsels Milk Chocolate	1 tbsp	70
Morsels Mint Chocolate	1 tbsp	70
Morsels Rainbow	1 tbsp	70
Morsels Mini Semi-Sweet	1 tbsp	70
Semi-Sweet Morsels	1 tbsp	40
MIX		
Quik		
Chocolate Powder	2 tbsp (0.8 oz)	90
Chocolate Powder No Sugar Added	2 tbsp (0.4 oz)	40

CHOCOLATE MILK
(*see* CHOCOLATE, COCOA, MILK DRINKS, MILKSHAKE)

CHOCOLATE SYRUP

chocolate fudge	1 tbsp (0.7 oz)	73
chocolate fudge	1 cup (11.9 oz)	1176
Estee		
Chocolate	2 tbsp	15
Marzetti		
Syrup	2 tbsp	40
Quik		
Chocolate	2 tbsp (1.3 oz)	100
Red Wing		
Syrup	2 tbsp (1.4 oz)	110

CHUTNEY

coconut	¼ cup	74
Sonoma		
Dried Tomato	1 tbsp (0.7 g)	35

CILANTRO

fresh	1 tsp (2 g)	tr
fresh	1 cup (1.6 oz)	11
Watkins		
Dried	¼ tsp (0.5 oz)	0

FOOD	PORTION	CALS.
CINNAMON		
ground	1 tsp	6
sticks	0.5 oz	39
Watkins		
Ground	¼ tsp (0.5 g)	0
CISCO		
raw	3 oz	84
smoked	3 oz	151
CLAM JUICE		
Doxsee		
Canned	3 fl oz	4
CLAMS		
CANNED		
liquid only	3 oz	2
liquid only	1 cup	6
meat only	3 oz	126
meat only	1 cup	236
Doxsee		
Chopped	6.5 oz	90
Gorton's		
Minced & Chopped	½ can	70
Progresso		
Creamy Clam	½ cup (4.2 oz)	100
Minced	¼ cup (2 oz)	25
Red Clam	½ cup (4.4 oz)	80
White Clam Sauce	½ cup (4.4 oz)	120
Snow's		
Minced	6.5 oz	90
FRESH		
cooked	20 sm	133
raw	20 sm (180 g)	133
raw	9 lg (180 g)	133
FROZEN		
Gorton's		
Microwave Crunchy Clam Strips	3.5 oz	330
TAKE-OUT		
breaded & fried	20 sm	379
CLOVES		
ground	1 tsp	7
COCOA		
(*see also* CHOCOLATE)		
hot cocoa	1 cup	218

FOOD	PORTION	CALS.
powder unsweetened	1 tbsp (5 g)	11
powder unsweetened	1 cup (3 oz)	197
Nestle		
Cocoa	1 tbsp	15
Swiss Miss		
Cocoa Diet	6 oz	20
Hot Cocoa Bavarian Chocolate	6 oz	110
Hot Cocoa Double Rich	6 oz	110
Hot Cocoa Milk Chocolate	6 oz	110
Hot Cocoa Milk Chocolate	1 serv	110
Hot Cocoa Mini-Marshmallow	1 serv	109
Hot Cocoa Rich Chocolate	1 serv	110
Hot Cocoa Sugar Free	1 serv	67
Hot Cocoa Sugar Free Milk Chocolate	1 serv	49
Hot Cocoa Sugar Free Mini-Marshmallow	1 serv	51
Hot Cocoa White Chocolate	1 serv	109
Hot Cocoa With Mini Marshmallows	6 oz	110
Hot Cocoa Lite	1 serv	74
Lite as prep	6 oz	70
Sugar Free With Sugar Free Marshmallows as prep	6 oz	50
Sugar Free as prep	6 oz	60
Ultra Slim-Fast		
Hot Cocoa as prep w/ water	8 oz	190
Weight Watchers		
Hot Cocoa Mix as prep	1 pkg	70

COCONUT

FOOD	PORTION	CALS.
coconut water	1 cup	46
coconut water	1 tbsp	3
cream canned	1 tbsp	36
cream canned	1 cup	568
dried sweetened flaked	1 cup	351
dried sweetened flaked	7 oz pkg	944
dried sweetened flaked canned	1 cup	341
dried sweetened shredded	1 cup	466
dried sweetened shredded	7 oz pkg	997
dried toasted	1 oz	168
fresh	1 piece (1.5 oz)	159
fresh shredded	1 cup	283
milk canned	1 tbsp	30
milk canned	1 cup	445
Baker's		
Angel Flake	1 tbsp (0.5 oz)	70

FOOD	PORTION	CALS.
Baker's (CONT.)		
Angel Flake (canned)	2 tbsp (0.5 oz)	70
Premium Shred	2 tbsp (0.5 oz)	70
Coco Lopez		
Cream Of Coconut	2 tbsp	120

COD
CANNED
atlantic	3 oz	89
roe	3.5 oz	118

DRIED
atlantic	3 oz	246

FRESH
atlantic cooked	3 oz	89
pacific baked	3 oz	95
roe baked w/ butter & lemon juice	3.5 oz	126
roe raw	3.5 oz	130
tarama	3.5 oz	547

FROZEN
Gorton's		
Fishmarket Fresh	5 oz	110
Van De Kamp's		
Lightly Breaded Fillets	1 (4 oz)	220

COFFEE
(*see also* COFFEE BEVERAGES, COFFEE SUBSTITUTES)

INSTANT
decaffeinated	1 rounded tsp (1.8 g)	4
decaffeinated as prep	6 oz	4
regular	1 rounded tsp	4
regular as prep	6 oz	4
regular w/ chicory	1 rounded tsp	6
regular w/ chicory as prep	6 oz	6

REGULAR
brewed	6 oz	4
Folgers		
Colombian Supreme	1 tbsp	16
Custom Roast	1 tbsp	16
Decaffeinated	1 tbsp	17
French Roast	1 tbsp	16
Gourmet Supreme	1 tbsp	16
Instant	1 tsp	8
Instant Decaffeinated	1 tsp	8
Singles	1 bag	21
Singles Decaffeinated	1 bag	21

FOOD	PORTION	CALS.
Folgers (CONT.)		
Special Roast	1 tbsp	16
Vacuum Pack	1 tbsp	16
Maryland Club		
Ground	1 tbsp	16
TAKE-OUT		
cafe au lait	1 cup (8 fl oz)	77
cafe brulot	1 cup (4.8 fl oz)	48
cappuccino	1 cup (8 fl oz)	77
coffee con leche	1 cup (8 fl oz)	77
espresso	1 cup (3 fl oz)	2
irish coffee	1 serv (9 fl oz)	107
latte w/ skim milk	13 oz	88
latte w/ whole milk	13 oz	152
mocha	1 mug (9.6 fl oz)	202

COFFEE BEVERAGES
(*see also* COFFEE SUBSTITUTES)

FOOD	PORTION	CALS.
General Foods		
Cappuccino Coolers French Vanilla as prep w/ 2% milk	1 serv	180
International Coffee Sugar Free Cafe Vienna as prep	1 serv (8 oz)	30
International Coffee Sugar Free Fat Free Suisse Mocha as prep	1 serv (8 oz)	25
International Coffees Cafe Francais as prep	1 serv (8 oz)	60
International Coffees Cafe Vienna as prep	1 serv (8 oz)	70
International Coffees Decaffeinated French Vanilla Cafe as prep	1 serv (8 oz)	60
International Coffees Decaffeinated Suisse Mocha as prep	1 serv (8 oz)	60
International Coffees French Vanilla Cafe as prep	1 serv (8 oz)	60
International Coffees Hazelnut Belgain Cafe as prep	1 serv (8 oz)	70
International Coffees Irish Creme Cafe as prep	1 serv (8 oz)	60
International Coffees Italian Cappuccino as prep	1 serv (8 oz)	60
International Coffees Kahlua Cafe as prep	1 serv (8 oz)	60
International Coffees Orange Cappuccino as prep	1 serv (8 oz)	70
International Coffees Suisse Mocha as prep	1 serv (8 oz)	60

FOOD	PORTION	CALS.
General Foods (CONT.)		
International Coffees Viennese Chocolate Cafe as prep	1 serv (8 oz)	50
International Coffees Sugar Free Fat Free Decaffeinated French Vanilla	1 serv (8 oz)	25
International Coffees Sugar Free Fat Free Decaffeinated Suisse Mocha	1 serv (8 oz)	25
International Coffees Sugar Free Fat Free French Vanilla Cafe as prep	1 serv (8 oz)	25
Maxwell House		
Cafe Cappuccino Amaretto as prep	1 serv (8 oz)	90
Cafe Cappuccino Decaffeinated Mocha as prep	1 serv (8 oz)	100
Cafe Cappuccino Decaffeinated Vanilla as prep	1 serv (8 oz)	90
Cafe Cappuccino Irish Cream as prep	1 serv (8 oz)	90
Cafe Cappuccino Mocha as prep	1 serv (8 oz)	100
Cafe Cappuccino Sugar Free Mocha as prep	1 serv (8 oz)	60
Cafe Cappuccino Sugar Free Vanilla as prep	1 serv (8 oz)	60
Cafe Cappuccino Vanilla as prep	1 serv (8 oz)	90
Iced Cappuccino as prep w/ 2% milk	1 serv (8 oz)	180
Starbucks		
Frappuccino	1 bottle (9.5 fl oz)	190

COFFEE SUBSTITUTES

Kava		
Instant	1 tsp	2
Natural Touch		
Kaffree Roma	1 tsp (2 g)	10
Roma Cappuccino	3 tbsp (0.4 oz)	50
Pero		
Instant Grain Beverage	1 tsp (1.5 g)	5
Postum		
Instant Coffee Flavor as prep	1 serv (8 oz)	10
Instant as prep	1 serv (8 oz)	10

COFFEE WHITENERS
(*see also* MILK SUBSTITUTES)

Coffee-Mate		
Liquid	1 tbsp (0.5 fl oz)	16
Powder	1 tsp (2 g)	10
Cremora		
Whitener	1 tsp	12

FOOD	PORTION	CALS.
Hood		
Non Dairy	1 tbsp (0.5 oz)	20
International Delight		
Amaretto	1 tbsp (0.6 fl oz)	45
Cinnamon Hazelnut	1 tbsp (0.6 fl oz)	45
Irish Creme	1 tbsp (0.6 fl oz)	45
No Fat Amaretto	1 tbsp (0.5 fl oz)	30
No Fat French Vanilla Royale	1 tbsp (0.5 fl oz)	30
No Fat Hawaiian Macadamia	1 tbsp (0.5 fl oz)	30
No Fat Irish Creme	1 tbsp (0.5 fl oz)	30
Suisse Chocolate Mocha	1 tbsp (0.6 fl oz)	45
Mocha Mix		
Fat-Free	1 tbsp (0.5 fl oz)	10
Lite	1 tbsp (0.5 fl oz)	10
Lite	4 fl oz	80
Original	1 tbsp (0.5 fl oz)	20
Signature Flavors French Vanilla	1 tbsp (0.5 fl oz)	35
Signature Flavors Irish Creme	1 tbsp (0.5 fl oz)	35
Signature Flavors Kahlua	1 tbsp (0.5 fl oz)	35
Signature Flavors Mauna Loa Macadamia Nut	1 tbsp (0.5 fl oz)	35
N-Rich Creamer		
Whitener	1 tsp	10

COLESLAW
Fresh Express

Cole Slaw	1½ cups (3 oz)	25

TAKE-OUT

coleslaw w/ dressing	½ cup	42
vinegar & oil coleslaw	3.5 oz	150

COLLARDS
CANNED
Allen

Collards	½ cup (4.1 oz)	30

Sunshine

Collards	½ cup (4.1 oz)	30

FRESH

cooked	½ cup	17
raw chopped	½ cup	6

FROZEN

chopped cooked	½ cup	31

COOKIES
(*see also* BROWNIE, CAKE, DOUGHNUT, PIE)

HOME RECIPE

chocolate chip as prep w/ butter	1 (0.42 oz)	78

FOOD	PORTION	CALS.
chocolate chip as prep w/ margarine	1 (0.56 oz)	78
oatmeal	1 (0.5 oz)	67
oatmeal w/ raisins	1 (0.52 oz)	65
peanut butter	1 (0.7 oz)	95
shortbread as prep w/ butter	1 (0.38 oz)	60
shortbread as prep w/ margarine	1 (0.38 oz)	60
sugar as prep w/ butter	1 (0.49 oz)	66
sugar as prep w/ margarine	1 (0.49 oz)	66
MIX		
chocolate chip	1 (0.56 oz)	79
oatmeal	1 (0.6 oz)	74
oatmeal raisin	1 (0.6 oz)	74
GoldnBrown		
Fat Free	1 (1.1 oz)	120
READY-TO-EAT		
animal	11 crackers (1 oz)	126
animal crackers	1 (2.5 g)	11
australian anzac biscuit	1	98
butter	1 (5 g)	23
chocolate chip	1 (0.4 oz)	48
chocolate chip low fat	1 (0.25 oz)	45
chocolate chip low sugar low sodium	1 (0.24 oz)	31
chocolate chip soft-type	1 (0.5 oz)	69
chocolate w/ creme filling	1 (0.35 oz)	47
chocolate w/ creme filling chocolate coated	1 (0.60 oz)	82
chocolate w/ creme filling sugar free low sodium	1 (0.35 oz)	46
chocolate w/ extra creme filling	1 (0.46 oz)	65
chocolate wafer	1 (0.2 oz)	26
chocolate wafer cookie crumbs	½ cup (5.9 oz)	728
fig bars	1 (0.56 oz)	56
fortune	1 (0.28 oz)	30
fudge	1 (0.73 oz)	73
gingersnaps	1 (0.24 oz)	29
graham	1 squares (0.24 oz)	30
graham chocolate covered	1 (0.49 oz)	68
graham honey	1 (0.24 oz)	30
ladyfingers	1 (0.38 oz)	40
macaroons	1 (0.8 oz)	97
marshmallow chocolate coated	1 (0.46 oz)	55
marshmallow pie chocolate coated	1 (1.4 oz)	165
meringue	1 (0.3 oz)	20
molasses	1 (0.5 oz)	65
neapolitan tri-color cookie	1 (0.6 oz)	79

FOOD	PORTION	CALS.
oatmeal	1 (0.6 oz)	81
oatmeal	1 (0.52 oz)	71
oatmeal soft-type	1 (0.5 oz)	61
oatmeal raisin	1 (0.6 oz)	81
oatmeal raisin low sugar no sodium	1 (0.24 oz)	31
oatmeal raisin soft-type	1 (0.5 oz)	61
peanut butter sandwich	1 (0.5 oz)	67
peanut butter sandwich sugar free low sodium	1 (0.35 oz)	54
peanut butter soft-type	1 (0.5 oz)	69
raisin soft-type	1 (0.5 oz)	60
shortbread	1 (0.28 oz)	40
shortbread pecan	1 (0.49 oz)	79
sugar	1 (0.52 oz)	72
sugar low sugar sodium free	1 (0.24 oz)	30
sugar wafers w/ creme filling	1 (0.12 oz)	18
sugar wafers w/ creme filling sugar free sodium free	1 (0.14 oz)	20
vanilla sandwich	1 (0.35 oz)	48
vanilla wafers	1 (0.21 oz)	28
Alternative Baking		
Vegan Chocolate Chip	1 serv (2.5 oz)	280
Vegan Expresso Chocolate Chip	1 serv (2 oz)	230
Vegan Lemon	1 serv (2.25 oz)	250
Vegan Oatmeal	1 serv (2.25 oz)	250
Vegan Peanut Butter	1 serv (2.25 oz)	270
Vegan Pumpkin	1 serv (2 oz)	200
Vegan Wheat Free Choco Cherry Chunk	1 serv (1.75 oz)	190
Vegan Wheat Free Hula Nut	1 serv (1.75 oz)	190
Vegan Wheat Free P-nut Fudge Fusion	1 serv (1.75 oz)	190
Vegan Wheat Free Snickerdoodle	1 serv (1.75 oz)	170
Amay's		
Chinese Style Almond	1 (0.5 oz)	80
Archway		
Almond Crescents	2 (0.8 oz)	100
Apple N'Raisin	1 (1.1 oz)	130
Apricot Filled	1 (1 oz)	110
Bells And Stars	3 (1 oz)	150
Blueberry Filled	1 (1 oz)	110
Carrot Cake	1 (1 oz)	120
Cherry Filled	1 (1 oz)	110
Cherry Nougat	3 (1 oz)	150
Chocolate Chip	1 (1 oz)	130
Chocolate Chip & Toffee	1 (1 oz)	140

FOOD	PORTION	CALS.
Archway (CONT.)		
Chocolate Chip Bag	3 (0.9 oz)	130
Chocolate Chip Drop	1 (1 oz)	140
Chocolate Chip Ice Box	1 (1 oz)	140
Chocolate Chip Mini	12 (1.1 oz)	150
Cinnamon Snaps	12 (1.1 oz)	150
Coconut Macaroon	1 (0.8 oz)	90
Cookie Jar Hermits	1 (1 oz)	110
Dark Chocolate	1 (1 oz)	110
Dutch Chocolate	1 (1 oz)	120
Fig Bars Low Fat	2 (1.1 oz)	100
Frosty Lemon	1 (1 oz)	120
Frosty Orange	1 (1 oz)	120
Fruit And Honey Bar	1 (1 oz)	110
Fruit Bar No Fat	1 (1 oz)	90
Fruit Cake	1 (1.1 oz)	140
Fudge Nut Bar	1 (1 oz)	110
Fun Chip Mini	12 (1.1 oz)	140
Gingersnaps	5 (1.1 oz)	130
Granola No Fat	1 (0.5 oz)	50
Holiday Pak	3 (1.1 oz)	150
Iced Gingerbread	3 (1.1 oz)	140
Iced Molasses	1 (1 oz)	110
Iced Oatmeal	1 (1 oz)	120
Lemon Snaps	12 (1.1 oz)	150
New Orleans Cake	1 (1 oz)	110
Nutty Nougat	3 (1.1 oz)	160
Oatmeal	1 (0.9 oz)	110
Oatmeal Apple Filled	1 (1 oz)	110
Oatmeal Date Filled	1 (1 oz)	110
Oatmeal Mini	12 (1.1 oz)	150
Oatmeal Pecan	1 (1 oz)	120
Oatmeal Raisin	1 (1 oz)	110
Oatmeal Raisin Bran	1 (1 oz)	110
Old Fashioned Molasses	1 (1 oz)	120
Old Fashioned Windmill	1 (0.7 oz)	100
Party Treats	3 (1.1 oz)	140
Peanut Butter	1 (1 oz)	140
Peanut Butter & Chip	3 (0.9 oz)	130
Peanut Butter N' Chips	1 (1 oz)	140
Peanut Butter Nougat	3 (1.1 oz)	160
Pecan Crunch	6 (1.1 oz)	150
Pecan Ice Box	1 (1 oz)	140
Pecan Malted Nougat	3 (1.1 oz)	160

FOOD	PORTION	CALS.
Archway (CONT.)		
Pfeffernusse	2 (1.3 oz)	140
Pineapple Filled	1 (0.9 oz)	100
Raisin Oatmeal	1 (1 oz)	130
Raisin Oatmeal Bag	3 (1 oz)	130
Raspberry Filled	1 (1 oz)	110
Rocky Road	1 (1 oz)	130
Ruth's Golden Oatmeal	1 (1 oz)	120
Select Assortment	3 (0.9 oz)	130
Soft Molasses Drop	1 (1 oz)	110
Soft Sugar	1 (1 oz)	110
Strawberry Filled	1 (1 oz)	110
Sugar	1 (1 oz)	120
Vanilla Wafer	5 (1.1 oz)	130
Wedding Cakes	3 (1.1 oz)	160
Bahlsen		
Afrika	8 (1.1 oz)	170
Butter Leaves	7 (1 oz)	140
Choco Leibniz	2 (1 oz)	140
Choco Star Dark Chocolate	3 (1.1 oz)	170
Choco Star Milk Chocolate	3 (1.1 oz)	180
Chocolate Hearts	4 (1 oz)	160
Delice	6 (1 oz)	140
Deloba	4 (0.9 oz)	130
Hit Chocolate Vanilla Filled	2 (1 oz)	140
Hit Vanilla Chocolate Filled	2 (1 oz)	140
Leibniz	6 (1 oz)	130
Nuss Dessert	3 (1.1 oz)	180
Probiers	6 (1.1 oz)	150
Twingo	6 (1.1 oz)	170
Waffeletten	4 (1 oz)	160
Waffelin	5 (1 oz)	160
Bakery Wagon		
Apple Walnut Raisin	1	100
Cobbler Apple Cranberry Fat Free	1	70
Cobbler Apple Fat Free	1	70
Cobbler Mixed Fruit Fat Free	1	70
Cobbler Raspberry Fat Free	1	70
Ginger Snaps	5	160
Honey Fruit Bars	1	100
Iced Molasses	1	100
Iced Molasses Mini	3	130
Oatmeal Apple Filled	1	90
Oatmeal Chocolate Chunk	1	100

FOOD	PORTION	CALS.
Bakery Wagon (CONT.)		
Oatmeal Date Filled	1	90
Oatmeal Raspberry Filled	1	100
Oatmeal Soft	1	100
Oatmeal Walnut Raisin	1	100
Vanilla Wafers Cholesterol Free	6	130
Barbara's		
Animal Cookies Vanilla	8 (1 oz)	130
Chocolate Chip	1 (0.6 oz)	80
Double Dutch Chocolate	1 (0.6 oz)	80
Fat Free Homestyle Chewy Chocolate	2 (0.9 oz)	80
Fat Free Homestyle Chocolate Mint	2 (0.9 oz)	80
Fat Free Homestyle Nutt'n Crispies	2 (0.9 oz)	80
Fat Free Homestyle Oatmeal Raisin	2 (0.9 oz)	80
Fat Free Mini Carmel Apple	6 (1 oz)	110
Fat Free Mini Cocoa Mocha	6 (1 oz)	100
Fat Free Mini Double Chocolate	6 (1 oz)	100
Fat Free Mini Oatmeal Raisin	6 (1 oz)	110
Fig Bars Fat Free	1 (0.7 oz)	60
Fig Bars Fat Free Raspberry	1 (0.7 oz)	60
Fig Bars Fat Free Whole Wheat	1 (0.7 oz)	60
Fig Bars Fat Free Whole Wheat Apple Cinnamon	1 (0.7 oz)	60
Fig Bars Low Fat	1 (0.7 oz)	60
Fig Bars Low Fat Blueberry	1 (0.7 oz)	60
Old Fashioned Oatmeal	1 (0.6 oz)	70
Snackimals Chocolate Chip	8 (1 oz)	120
Snackimals Oatmeal Wheat Free	8 (1 oz)	120
Snackimals Vanilla	8 (1 oz)	120
Traditional Shortbread	1 (0.6 oz)	80
Barnum's		
Animal Crackers	12 (1.1 oz)	140
Animal Crackers Chocolate	10 (1 oz)	130
Biscos		
Sugar Wafers	8 (1 oz)	140
Waffle Cremes	4 (1.2 oz)	180
Breaktime		
Chocolate Chip	1 (0.3 oz)	37
Coconut	1 (0.3 oz)	35
Ginger	1 (0.3 oz)	34
Oatmeal	1 (0.3 oz)	35
Sprinkles	1 (0.3 oz)	36
Bud's Best		
Caco Creme	7 (1 oz)	140

FOOD	PORTION	CALS.
Bud's Best (CONT.)		
Chocolate Chip	6 (1 oz)	140
French Vanilla	7 (1 oz)	150
Oatmeal	6 (1 oz)	130
Cadbury		
Fingers	3	85
Cafe		
Cinnamony Twists Chocolate Chip	1 (0.5 oz)	40
Sugar Free California Almond	4 (1 oz)	110
Twists Cinnamony	1 (0.3 oz)	40
Carriage Trade		
Finnish Ginger Snaps	3	60
Chip-A-Roos		
Cookies	3 (1.3 oz)	190
Chips Ahoy!		
Bit Size Chocolate Chip	14 (1.1 oz)	170
Chewy Chocolate Chip	3 (1.3 oz)	170
Chunky Chocolate Chip	1 (0.5 oz)	80
Real Chocolate Chip	3 (1.1 oz)	160
Reduced Fat	3 (1.1 oz)	150
Sprinkled Real Chocolate Chip	3 (1.3 oz)	170
Striped Chocolate Chip	1 (0.5 oz)	80
Chortles		
Cookies	½ pkg. (1 oz)	125
Cookie Lover's		
Blue Ribbon Brownies	1 (0.8 oz)	90
Classic Shortbread	1 (0.8 oz)	110
Dutch Chocolate Chip	1 (0.8 oz)	90
Fancy Peanut Butter	1 (0.8 oz)	100
Grahams Cinnamon Honey	2 (1 oz)	110
Grahams Honey	2 (1 oz)	100
Old-Time Raisin	1 (0.8 oz)	90
Dare		
Blueberry Cheesecake	1 (0.6 oz)	90
Butter Shortbread	1 (0.5 oz)	63
Butter Creme	1 (0.6 oz)	85
Carrot Cake	1 (0.6 oz)	92
Chocolate Chip	1 (0.5 oz)	77
Chocolate Fudge	1 (0.7 oz)	97
Cinnamon Danish	1 (0.4 oz)	47
Coconut Creme	1 (0.7 oz)	99
French Creme	1 (0.5 oz)	80
Harvest From The Rain Forest	1 (0.5 oz)	70
Key Lime Creme	1 (0.6 oz)	86

FOOD	PORTION	CALS.
Dare (CONT.)		
Lemon Creme	1 (0.7 oz)	95
Maple Leaf Creme	1 (0.6 oz)	83
Maple Walnut Fudge	1 (0.7 oz)	99
Milk Chocolate Fudge	1 (0.7 oz)	99
Oatmeal Raisin	1 (0.4 oz)	59
Social Tea	1 (0.2 oz)	26
Sun Maid Raisin Oatmeal	1 (0.5 oz)	52
Delacre		
Cookie Assortment	4 (1.1 oz)	130
Dunkaroos		
Chocolate Chip w/ Chocolate Frosting	1 pkg (1 oz)	120
Cinnamon Graham w/ Vanilla Frosting	1 pkg (1 oz)	130
Cookies'n Creme	1 pkg (1 oz)	120
Dutch Mill		
Chocolate Chip	3 (1.1 oz)	160
Coconut Macaroons	3 (1 oz)	120
Oatmeal Raisin	3 (1 oz)	130
Entenmann's		
Chocolate Chip	3 (0.9 oz)	140
Estee		
Chocolate Chip	4	150
Coconut	4	140
Fig Bars	2	100
Fudge	4	150
Lemon Thins	4	140
Oatmeal Raisin	4	130
Sandwich Chocolate	3	160
Sandwich Original	3	160
Sandwich Peanut Butter	3	160
Sandwich Vanilla	3	160
Shortbread	4	130
Sugar Free Chocolate Chip	3	110
Sugar Free Chocolate Walnut	3	110
Sugar Free Coconut	3	110
Sugar Free Grahams Chocolate	2	110
Sugar Free Grahams Cinnamon	2	90
Sugar Free Grahams Old Fashion	2	90
Sugar Free Lemon	3	110
Sugar Free Wafer Banana Split	5	155
Sugar Free Wafer Chocolate	5	150
Sugar Free Wafer Chocolate Peanut Butter Caramel	5	150
Sugar Free Wafer Lemon Creme	5	150

FOOD	PORTION	CALS.
Estee (CONT.)		
Sugar Free Wafer Peanut Butter Creme	5	150
Sugar Free Wafer Vanilla	5	150
Sugar Free Wafer Vanilla Strawberry	5	150
Vanilla Thins	4	140
Famous Amos		
Chocolate Chip	3 (1 oz)	140
Chocolate Chip Pecan	3 (1 oz)	150
Oatmeal Raisin	3 (1 oz)	134
Freihofer's		
Chocolate Chip	2 (0.9 oz)	120
Frookie		
Animal Frackers	14 (1 oz)	130
Chocolate Chip Wheat & Gluten Free	3 (1.1 oz)	140
Double Chocolate Wheat & Gluten Free	3 (1.1 oz)	130
Dream Creams Strawberry	4 (1 oz)	140
Dream Creams Vanilla	4 (1 oz)	140
Funky Monkeys Chocolate	16 (1 oz)	120
Funky Monkeys Vanilla	16 (1 oz)	120
Graham Cinnamon	2 (1 oz)	100
Graham Honey	2 (1 oz)	110
Lemon Wafers	8 (1 oz)	110
Old Fashioned Ginger Snaps	8 (1 oz)	120
Organic Chocolate Chip	3 (1.1 oz)	150
Organic Double Chocolate Chip	3 (1.1 oz)	140
Organic Iced Lemon	3 (1.3 oz)	165
Organic Oatmeal Raisin	3 (1.1 oz)	140
Peanut Butter Chunk Wheat & Gluten Free	3 (1.1 oz)	140
Sandwich Chocolate	2 (0.7 oz)	100
Sandwich Lemon	2 (0.7 oz)	100
Sandwich Peanut Butter	2 (0.7 oz)	100
Sandwich Vanilla	2 (0.7 oz)	100
Shortbread	5 (1 oz)	130
Vanilla Wafers	8 (1 oz)	110
Girl Scout		
Apple Cinnamon Reduced Fat	3 (1 oz)	120
Do-si-dos	3 (1.2 oz)	170
Lemon Drops	3 (1.2 oz)	160
Samoas	2 (1 oz)	160
Striped Chocolate Chip	3 (1.2 oz)	180
Tagalongs	2 (0.9 oz)	150
Thin Mints	4 (1 oz)	140
Trefoils	5 (1.1 oz)	160

FOOD	PORTION	CALS.
Golden Fruit		
Apple	1 (0.7 oz)	80
Cranberry	1 (0.7 oz)	70
Cranberry Low Fat	1 (0.7 oz)	70
Raisin	1 (0.7 oz)	80
Golden Grahams Treats		
Chocolate Chunk	1 bar (0.8 oz)	90
Honey Graham	1 bar (0.8 oz)	90
King Size Chocolate Chunk	1 bar (1.6 oz)	190
King Size Honey Graham	1 bar (1.6 oz)	180
Grandma's		
Chocolate Chip	1 (1.4 oz)	190
Fudge Chocolate Chip	1 (1.4 oz)	170
Fudge Sandwich	3	180
Fudge Vanilla Sandwich	3	120
Mini Fudge	9	150
Mini Peanut Butter	9	150
Mini Vanilla	9	150
Oatmeal Raisin	1 (1.4 oz)	160
Old Time Molasses	1 (1.4 oz)	160
Peanut Butter	1 (1.4 oz)	190
Peanut Butter Chocolate Chip	1 (1.4 oz)	190
Peanut Butter Sandwich	5	210
Rich N'Chewy	1 pkg	270
Vanilla Sandwich	3	180
Vanilla Sandwich	5	210
Handi-Snack		
Cookie Jammers Cookies & Fruit Spread	1 pkg (1.3 oz)	130
Health Valley		
Apple Spice	3	100
Apricot Delight	3	100
Biscotti Amaretto	2	120
Biscotti Chocolate	2	120
Biscotti Fruit & Nut	2	120
Cheesecake Bars Blueberry	1 bar	160
Cheesecake Bars Raspberry	1 bar	160
Cheesecake Bars Strawberry	1 bar	160
Chips Double Chocolate	3	100
Chips Old Fashioned	3	100
Chips Original	3	100
Chocolate Fudge Center	2	70
Chocolate Sandwich Bar Bavarian Creme	1 bar	150
Chocolate Sandwich Bars Caramel Creme	1 bar	150
Chocolate Sandwich Bars Vanilla Creme	1 bar	150

FOOD	PORTION	CALS.
Health Valley (CONT.)		
Date Delight Date Delight	3	100
Graham Amaranth	8	100
Graham Oat Bran	8	100
Graham Original Amaranth	6	120
Hawaiian Fruit	3	100
Jumbo Apple Raisin	1	80
Jumbo Raisin Raisin	1	80
Jumbo Raspberry	1	80
Marshmallow Bars Chocolate Chip	1	90
Marshmallow Bars Old Fashioned	1	90
Marshmallow Bars Tropical Fruit	1	90
Oat Bran Fruit Bars Raisin Cinnamon	1 bar	160
Raisin Oatmeal	3	100
Raspberry Fruit Center	1	70
Tarts Baked Apple Cinnamon	1	150
Tarts California Strawberry	1	150
Tarts Chocolate Fudge	1	150
Tarts Cranberry Apple	1	150
Tarts Mountain Blueberry	1	150
Tarts Red Raspberry	1	150
Tarts Sweet Red Cherry	1	150
Heyday		
Caramel & Peanut	1 (0.8 oz)	110
Fudge	1 (0.8 oz)	110
Honey Maid		
Cinnamon Grahams	10 (1.1 oz)	140
Honey Grahams	8 (1 oz)	120
Hydrox		
Original	3	150
Reduced Fat	3 (1.1 oz)	130
Keebler		
Chips Deluxe	1 (0.5 oz)	80
Chips Deluxe 25% Reduced Fat	1 (0.6 oz)	70
Chips Deluxe Chewy	1 (0.6 oz)	80
Chips Deluxe Chocolate Lovers	1 (0.6 oz)	90
Chips Deluxe Rainbow	1 (0.6 oz)	80
Chips Deluxe w/ Peanut Butter Cups	1 (0.6 oz)	90
Chocolate Wafers 30% Reduced Fat	8 (1.1 oz)	130
Classic Collection Dutch Chocolate Fudge Sandwich	1 (0.6 oz)	80
Classic Collection French Vanllia Creme Sandwich	1 (0.6 oz)	80
Classic Collection Hearty Oatmeal	2 (1 oz)	150

FOOD	PORTION	CALS.
Keebler (CONT.)		
Classic Collection Peanut Butter	2 (1 oz)	150
Classic Collection Sparkling Sugar	2 (1 oz)	140
Danish Wedding	4 (1 oz)	120
E.L. Fudge Butter Sandwich w/ Fudge Creme	2 (0.9 oz)	120
E.L. Fudge Chocolate Sandwich w/ Vanilla Creme	2 (0.9 oz)	120
E.L. Fudge Fudge w/ Fudge Creme	2 (0.9 oz)	120
Elfin Crackers	23 (1 oz)	130
Golden Vanilla Wafers	8 (1.1 oz)	150
Graham Cinnamon Crisp	8 (1 oz)	140
Graham Cinnamon Crisp Low Fat	8 (1 oz)	110
Graham Honey	8 (1.1 oz)	150
Graham Honey Low Fat	8 (1.1 oz)	120
Graham Original	8 (1 oz)	130
Iced Animal	6 (1.1 oz)	150
Krisp Kreem	5 (1 oz)	140
Soft Batch Chocolate Chip	1 (0.6 oz)	80
Soft Batch Homestyle Chocolate Chunk	1 (0.9 oz)	130
Soft Batch Oatmeal Raisin	1 (0.6 oz)	70
Vanilla Wafer 30% Reduced Fat	8 (1.1 oz)	130
Knott's Berry Farm		
Fruit Filled All Flavors	4 (1 oz)	120
LU		
Le Bastogne	2 (0.8 oz)	120
Le Dore	4 (1 oz)	140
Le Fondant	4 (1.1 oz)	170
Le Palmier	4 (1.2 oz)	180
Le Petit Beurre	4 (1.2 oz)	150
Le Petit Ecolier Dark Chocolate	2 (0.9 oz)	130
Le Petit Ecolier Hazelnut Milk Chocolate	2 (0.9 oz)	130
Le Petit Ecolier Milk Chocolate	2 (0.9 oz)	130
Le Pim's Orange	2 (0.9 oz)	90
Le Pim's Raspberry	2 (0.9 oz)	90
Le Raisin Dore	4 (1.2 oz)	160
Le Truffe Coconut	4 (1.2 oz)	190
Le Truffe Praline Chocolate	4 (1.2 oz)	170
Les Varietes	3 (0.9 oz)	140
Linden's		
Lemon	1 (1 oz)	120
Little Debbie		
Animal	1 pkg (1.5 oz)	190
Apple Flips	1 (1.2 oz)	150

FOOD	PORTION	CALS.
Little Debbie (cont.)		
Caramel Cookie Bars	1 pkg (1.2 oz)	160
Chocolate Chip Chewy	1 pkg (2 oz)	370
Chocolate Chip Crisp	1 pkg (1.5 oz)	210
Cookie Wreaths	1 pkg (0.6 oz)	90
Creme Filled Chocolate	1 pkg (1.2 oz)	180
Creme Filled Chocolate	1 pkg (1.8 oz)	260
Easter Puffs	1 pkg (1.2 oz)	140
Figaroos	1 pkg (1.5 oz)	160
Figaroos	1 pkg (2 oz)	200
Fudge Macaroons	1 pkg (1 oz)	140
Ginger	1 pkg (0.7 oz)	90
Oatmeal Crisp	1 pkg (1.5 oz)	210
Oatmeal Lights	1 pkg (1.3 oz)	140
Oatmeal Raisin	1 pkg (2.7 oz)	320
Peanut Butter	1 pkg (1.5 oz)	210
Peanut Butter & Jelly Sandwich	1 pkg (1.1 oz)	130
Peanut Butter Bars	1 pkg (1.9 oz)	270
Peanut Clusters	1 pkg (1.4 oz)	190
Pecan Spinwheels	1 pkg (1 oz)	110
Pecan Shortbread	1 pkg (1.5 oz)	220
Lorna Doone		
Cookies	4 (1 oz)	140
Mallopuffs		
Cookies	1 (0.6 oz)	70
Manischewitz		
Macaroons Chocolate	2 (0.9 oz)	90
Mother's		
Almond Shortbread	3	180
Butter	5	140
Checkerboard Wafers	8	150
Chocolate Chip	2	160
Chocolate Chip Angel	3	180
Chocolate Chip Bag	4	140
Chocolate Chip Parade	4	130
Circus Animals	6	140
Cocadas	5	150
Cookie Parade	4	140
Dinosaur Grrrahams	2	130
Double Fudge	3	170
Duplex Creme	3	170
English Tea	2	180
Fig Bar	2	130
Fig Bar Fat Free	1	70

FOOD	PORTION	CALS.
Mother's (CONT.)		
Fig Bar Whole Wheat	2	130
Fig Bar Whole Wheat Fat Free	1	70
Flaky Flix Fudge	2	140
Flaky Flix Vanilla	2	140
Frosted Holiday	4	130
Fudge Bowl Crowns	2	140
Fudge Bowl Nuggets	2	140
Gaucho Peanut Butter	2	190
Gingerbread Man	6	140
Iced Oatmeal	2	120
Iced Oatmeal Bag	4	120
Iced Raisin	2	180
MLB Double Header Duplex	3	170
Macaroon	2	150
Marias	3	170
North Poles	2	140
Oatmeal	2	110
Oatmeal Chocolate Chip	2	120
Oatmeal Raisin	5	150
Oatmeal Walnut Chocolate Chip	2	130
Pecan Goldens	2	170
Rainbow Wafers	8	150
Striped Shortbread	3	170
Sugar	2	140
Taffy	2	180
Triplet Assortment	2	140
Vanilla Wafers	6	150
Walnut Fudge	2	130
Zoo Pals	14	140
Mystic Mint		
Cookies	1 (0.5 oz)	90
Nabisco		
Brown Edge Wafers	5 (1 oz)	140
Bugs Bunny Chocolate Graham	13 (1.1 oz)	140
Bugs Bunny Cinnamon Graham	13 (1.1 oz)	140
Bugs Bunny Graham	13 (1.1 oz)	140
Cameo	2 (1 oz)	130
Chocolate Grahams	3 (1.1 oz)	160
Chocolate Chip Snaps	7 (1.1 oz)	150
Chocolate Snaps	7 (1.1 oz)	140
Cookie Break	3 (1.1 oz)	160
Danish Imported	5 (1.1 oz)	170
Family Favorites Fudge Covered Grahams	3 (1 oz)	140

FOOD	PORTION	CALS.
Nabisco (CONT.)		
Family Favorites Fudge Striped Shortbread	3 (1.1 oz)	160
Family Favorites Oatmeal	1 (0.5 oz)	80
Family Favorites Vanilla Sandwich	3 (1.2 oz)	170
Famous Chocolate Wafers	5 (1.1 oz)	140
Ginger Snaps Old Fashioned	4 (1 oz)	120
Grahams	8 (1 oz)	120
Mallomars	2 (0.9 oz)	120
Marshmallow Puffs	1 (0.75 oz)	90
Marshmallow Twirls	1 (1 oz)	130
Nilla Wafers	8 (1.1 oz)	140
Pecan Passion	1 (0.5 oz)	90
Pinwheels	1 (1 oz)	130
National		
Arrowroot	1 (5 g)	20
Newman's Own		
Fig Newman's Organic	2 (1.3 oz)	120
Newtons		
Apple Fat Free	2 (1 oz)	100
Cranberry Fat Free	2 (1 oz)	100
Fig	2 (1.1 oz)	110
Fig Fat Free	1 (1 oz)	100
Raspberry Fat Free	2 (1 oz)	100
Strawberry Fat Free	2 (1 oz)	100
Nutra/Balance		
Chocolate Chip	1 (2 oz)	260
Oatmeal Raisin	1 (2 oz)	240
Nutter Butter		
Bites Peanut Butter Sandwich	10 (1.1 oz)	150
Peanut Butter Sandwich	2 (1 oz)	130
Peanut Creme Patties	5 (1.1 oz)	160
Oreo		
Cookies	3 (1.2 oz)	160
Double Stuf	2 (1 oz)	140
Fudge Covered	1 (0.75 oz)	110
Halloween Treats	2 (1 oz)	140
Reduced Fat	3 (1.2 oz)	140
White Fudge Covered	1 (0.75 oz)	110
Otis Spunkmeyer		
Butter Sugar	1 med (1.3 oz)	160
Butter Sugar	1 (2 oz)	250
Carnival	1 med (1.3 oz)	170
Chocolate Chip	1 med (1.3 oz)	170
Chocolate Chip	1 bite size (0.75 oz)	100

FOOD	PORTION	CALS.
Otis Spunkmeyer (CONT.)		
Chocolate Chip	1 (2 oz)	250
Chocolate Chip Pecan	1 med (1.3 oz)	170
Chocolate Chip Walnut	1 med (1.3 oz)	180
Chocolate Chip Walnut	1 bite size (0.75 oz)	100
Chocolate Chip Walnut	1 (2 oz)	270
Double Chocolate Chip	1 bite size (0.75 oz)	100
Double Chocolate Chip	1 med (1.3 oz)	180
Oatmeal Raisin	1 bite size (0.75 oz)	90
Oatmeal Raisin	1 med (1.3 oz)	160
Otis Express Chocolate Chunk	1 (2 oz)	280
Otis Express Double Chocolate Chip	1 (2 oz)	270
Otis Express Oatmeal Raisin	1 (2 oz)	240
Otis Express Peanut Butter	1 (2 oz)	270
Peanut Butter	1 med (1.3 oz)	180
Pinnacle Checkpoint Chocolate Almond Coconut	1 (2.4 oz)	320
Pinnacle Mach One Mocha Chocolate Chunk	1 (2.4 oz)	300
Pinnacle Passport Peanut Butter Chocolate Chunk	1 (2.4 oz)	300
Pinnacle Ripcord Rocky Road	1 (2.4 oz)	310
Pinnacle Takeoff Triple Chocolate	1 (2.4 oz)	300
Pinnacle Transatlantic Turtle	1 (2.4 oz)	310
Travel Lite Low Fat Apple Cinnamon	1 (1.3 oz)	130
Travel Lite Low Fat Chocolate Chip	1 (1.3 oz)	130
Travel Lite Low Fat Ginger Spice	1 (1.3 oz)	130
Travel Lite Low Fat Oatmeal Rum Raisin	1 (1.3 oz)	130
White Chocolate Macadamia Nut	1 med (1.3 oz)	180
White Chocolate Macadamia Nut	1 (2 oz)	280
Pally		
Butter	4 (0.88 oz)	100
Peek Freans		
Petit Beret Creme Caramel	2 (0.8 oz)	110
Petit Beret Fudge Truffle	2 (0.8 oz)	110
Traditional Oatmeal	1 (0.7 oz)	90
Pepperidge Farm		
Biscotti Almond	1 (0.7 oz)	90
Biscotti Chocolate Hazelnut	1 (0.7 oz)	90
Biscotti Cranberry Pistachio	1 (0.7 oz)	90
Bordeaux	4	130
Brussels	3	150
Chessman	3	120
Chocolate Chip	3	140

FOOD	PORTION	CALS.
Pepperidge Farm (CONT.)		
Chocolate Chunk Soft Baked	1	130
Chocolate Chunk Soft Baked Milk Chocolate Macademia	1	130
Chocolate Chunk Soft Baked Reduced Fat	1	110
Chocolate Chunk Soft Baked White Chocolate Pecan	1	120
Fruitful Apricot- Raspberry Cut	3	140
Fruitful Strawberry Cut	3	140
Geneva	3	160
Lemon Nut Crunch	3	170
Lido	1	90
Milano	3	180
Milano Endless Chocolate	3	180
Milano Milk Chocolate	3	170
Mint Milano	2	130
Nantucket	1 (0.9 oz)	130
Nantucket Chocolate Chunk	1	140
Oatmeal Raisin	1	100
Orange Milano	2	130
Pecan Shortbread	1	70
Pirouettes Traditional	5 (1.2 oz)	170
Shortbread	2	140
Sugar	3	140
Ritz		
Chocolate Covered	3 (1 oz)	150
Royal		
Apple Bars	1 (1.1 oz)	100
Apple Cake	1 (1.1 oz)	110
Brownie Rounds	1 (1.1 oz)	130
Chocolate Chip	1 (1.1 oz)	140
Devilfood	1 (1 oz)	110
Oatmeal	1 (1.1 oz)	130
Raisin	1 (1 oz)	110
Strawberry Bars	1 (1.1 oz)	100
Sargento		
MooTown Snackers Cookies & Creme Honey Graham Sticks & Vanilla Creme w/Sprinkle	1 pkg (1.1 oz)	140
MooTown Snackers Cookies & Creme Vanilla Sticks & Chocolate Fudge Creme	1 pkg (1.1 oz)	140
Scotto's		
Biscotti Fat Free French Vanilla	4 (1 oz)	80

FOOD	PORTION	CALS.
Season		
Hamantashen Poppy	1 (1 oz)	150
Hamantasken Apricot	1 (1 oz)	150
Simple Pleasures		
Almond	1 (0.3 oz)	37
Cinnamon Snaps	1 (0.2 oz)	31
Digestive	1 (0.3 oz)	46
Encore Tea Cookie	1 (0.2 oz)	29
Lemon Social Tea	1 (0.2 oz)	29
Oatmeal	1 (0.5 oz)	74
Spice Snaps	1 (0.3 oz)	34
Sugar	1 (0.4 oz)	45
SnackWell's		
Fat Free Double Fudge	1 (0.5 oz)	50
Golden Devil's Food	1 (0.5 oz)	50
Reduced Fat Chocolate Chip	13 (1 oz)	130
Reduced Fat Chocolate Sandwich	2 (0.8 oz)	100
Reduced Fat Oatmeal Raisin	2 (1 oz)	110
Reduced Fat Vanilla Sandwich	2 (0.9 oz)	110
Social Tea		
Cookies	6 (1 oz)	120
Stella D'Oro		
Almond Toast Mandel	1	60
Angel Bars	1	80
Angel Wings	1	70
Angelica Goodies	1	110
Anginetti	1	30
Anisette Sponge	1	50
Anisette Toast	1	50
Anisette Toast Jumbo	1	110
Apple Pastry Low Sodium	1	80
Biscottini Cashews	1	110
Breakfast Treats	1	100
Castelets Chocolate	1	60
Chinese Dessert Cookies	1	170
Como Delight	1	150
Deep Night Fudge	1	65
Dutch Apple Bars	1	110
Egg Biscuits Low Sodium	3	120
Egg Biscuits Sugared	1	80
Egg Jumbo	1	50
Fruit Delight Apple Cinnamon Fat Free	1	70
Fruit Delight Peach Apricot Fat Free	1	70
Fruit Delight Raspberry Fat Free	1	70

FOOD	PORTION	CALS.

Stella D'Oro (CONT.)

FOOD	PORTION	CALS.
Fruit Slices	1	60
Fruit Slices Fat Free	1	50
Golden Bars	1	110
Holiday Rings & Stars	1	47
Holiday Trinkets	1	40
Hostess Assortment	1	40
Indulgente Cashew Biscottini	1 (1.1 oz)	150
Kichel Low Sodium	21	150
Lady Stella Assortment	1	40
Margherite Chocolate	1	70
Margherite Vanilla	1	70
Peach Apricot Pastry Sodium Free	1	80
Pfeffernusse Spice Drops	1	40
Prune Pastry Dietetic	1	90
Roman Egg Biscuits	1	140
Royal Nuggets	1	2
Sesame Regina	1	50
Swiss Fudge	1	70

Sunshine

FOOD	PORTION	CALS.
Almond Crescents	4 (1.1 oz)	150
Animal Crackers	1 box (2 oz)	260
Animal Crackers	14 (1.1 oz)	140
Classics Chocolate Chip With Pecans	1 (0.7 oz)	110
Classics Chocolate Chip With Walnuts	1 (0.7 oz)	100
Classics Premier Chocolate Chip	1 (0.7 oz)	100
Dixie Vanilla	2 (0.9 oz)	120
Fig Bars	2 (1 oz)	110
Fudge Family Bears Vanilla	2 (1 oz)	140
Fudge Mint Patties	2 (0.8 oz)	130
Fudge Striped Shortbread	3 (1.1 oz)	160
Ginger Snaps	7 (1 oz)	130
Grahams Cinnamon	2 (1.1 oz)	140
Grahams Fudge Dipped	4 (1.2 oz)	170
Grahams Honey	2 (1 oz)	120
Grahamy Bears	1 pkg (2 oz)	260
Grahamy Bears	10 (1.1 oz)	140
Iced Gingerbread	5 (1 oz)	130
Iced Oatmeal	2 (0.9 oz)	120
Jingles	6 (1.1 oz)	150
Lemon Coolers	5 (1 oz)	140
Mini Chocolate Chip Cookies	5 (1.1 oz)	160
Mini Fudge Royals	15 (1.1 oz)	160
Oatmeal Chocolate Chip	3 (1.3 oz)	170

FOOD	PORTION	CALS.
Sunshine (CONT.)		
Oatmeal Country Style	3 (1.2 oz)	170
School House Cookies	20 (1.1 oz)	140
Sugar Wafers Chocolate	3 (0.9 oz)	130
Sugar Wafers Peanut Butter	4 (1.1 oz)	170
Sugar Wafers Vanilla	3 (0.9 oz)	130
Tru Blu Chocolate	1 (0.6 oz)	80
Tru Blu Lemon	1 (0.6 oz)	80
Tru Blu Vanilla	1 (0.5 oz)	80
Vanilla Wafers	7 (1.1 oz)	150
Vienna Fingers	2 (1 oz)	140
Sweet Rewards		
Fat Free Blueberry w/ Drizzle	1 bar (1.3 oz)	120
Fat Free Double Fudge Supreme	1 bar (1.3 oz)	100
Fat Free Raspberry	1 bar (1.3 oz)	120
Fat Free Strawberry w/ Drizzle	1 bar (1.3 oz)	120
Low Fat Chocolate Chip	1 bar (1.1 oz)	110
Tastykake		
Chocolate Chip	1 (1.4 oz)	180
Chocolate Chip Bar	1 (2 oz)	270
Chocolate Fudge Iced	1 (1.4 oz)	170
Fudge Bar	1 (2 oz)	250
Lemon Bar	1 (2 oz)	260
Oatmeal Raisin Bar	1 (2 oz)	260
Oatmeal Raisin Boxed	3 (0.4 oz)	130
Oatmeal Raisin Iced	1 (1.4 oz)	170
Sugar Boxed	3 (0.4 oz)	120
Teddy Grahams		
Chocolate	24 (1 oz)	140
Cinnamon	24 (1 oz)	140
Honey	24 (1 oz)	140
The Source		
Barry's Raspberry Palmiers	1 (0.7 oz)	80
Tree Of Life		
Creme Supremes	2 (0.9 oz)	120
Creme Supremes Mint	2 (0.9 oz)	120
Fat Free Classic Carrot Cake	1 (0.8 oz)	60
Fat Free Devil's Food Chocolate	1 (0.8 oz)	70
Fat Free Golden Oatmeal Raisin	1 (0.8 oz)	70
Fat Free Harvest Fruit & Nut	1 (0.8 oz)	70
Fat Free Toasted Almond Butter	1 (0.8 oz)	70
Fruit Bars Apple Spice	2 (1.3 oz)	120
Fruit Bars Fat Free Fig	1 (0.8 oz)	70
Fruit Bars Fat Free Peach Apricot	1 (0.8 oz)	70

FOOD	PORTION	CALS.
Tree Of Life (CONT.)		
Fruit Bars Fat Free Wildberry	1 (0.8 oz)	70
Fruit Bars Fig	2 (1.3 oz)	120
Fruit Bars Peach Apricot	2 (1.3 oz)	120
Honey-Sweet Colossal Carrot Cake	1 (0.8 oz)	110
Honey-Sweet Lemon Burst	1 (0.8 oz)	110
Honey-Sweet Oh-So-Oatmeal	1 (0.8 oz)	110
Honey-Sweet Pecans-A-Plenty	1 (0.8 oz)	125
Monster Fat Free Carrot Cake	¼ cookie (0.9 oz)	60
Monster Fat Free Devil's Food Chocolate	¼ cookie (0.9 oz)	80
Monster Fat Free Gingerbread	¼ cookie (0.9 oz)	80
Monster Fat Free Maple Pecan	¼ cookie (0.9 oz)	90
Royal Vanilla	2 (0.9 oz)	120
Small World Animal Grahams	7 (1 oz)	120
Small World Chocolate Chip	7 (1 oz)	120
Soft-Bake Chocolate Chip	1 (0.8 oz)	125
Soft-Bake Double Fudge	1 (0.8 oz)	110
Soft-Bake Maui Macaroon	1 (0.8 oz)	135
Soft-Bake Oatmeal	1 (0.8 oz)	115
Soft-Bake Peanut Butter	1 (0.8 oz)	125
Wheat-Free American Oatmeal	1 (0.8 oz)	90
Wheat-Free California Carob	1 (0.8 oz)	105
Wheat-Free Georgia Peanut Butter	1 (0.8 oz)	95
Wheat-Free Mountain Maple Walnut	1 (0.8 oz)	100
Vienna Fingers		
Low Fat	2 (1 oz)	130
Walkers		
Shortbread Triangles	2 (0.7 oz)	100
Weight Watchers		
Apple Raisin Bar	1 (0.75 oz)	70
Chocolate Chip	2 (1.06 oz)	140
Chocolate Sandwich	2 (1.06)	140
Fruit Filled Fig	1 (0.7 oz)	70
Fruit Filled Raspberry	1 (0.7 oz)	70
Oatmeal Raisin	2 (1.06 oz)	120
Vanilla Sandwich	2 (1.06 oz)	140
White Eagle Bakery		
Chruscik	2 (1 oz)	140
Wortz		
Grahams Chocolate	2 (1 oz)	130
REFRIGERATED		
chocolate chip	1 (0.42 oz)	59
chocolate chip unbaked	1 oz	126
oatmeal	1 (0.4 oz)	56

FOOD	PORTION	CALS.
oatmeal raisin	1 (0.4 oz)	56
peanut butter	1 (0.4 oz)	60
peanut butter dough	1 oz	130
sugar	1 (0.42 oz)	58
sugar dough	1 oz	124
Pillsbury		
Bunny	2	130
Chocolate Chip	1 (1 oz)	130
Chocolate Chip Reduced Fat	1 (1 oz)	110
Chocolate Chip w/ Walnuts	1 (1 oz)	140
Chocolate Chunk	1 (1 oz)	130
Christmas Tree	2	130
Double Chocolate	1 (1 oz)	130
Flag	2	130
Frosty	2	130
M&M's	1 (1 oz)	130
Oatmeal Chocolate Chip	1 (1 oz)	120
One Step Pan Chocolate Chip	⅛ pan (1 oz)	130
One Step Pan M&M's	⅛ pan (1 oz)	130
Peanut Butter	1 (1 oz)	120
Pumpkin	2	130
Reeses	1 (1 oz)	130
Shamrock	2	130
Sugar	2	130
Sugar Holiday Red & Green	2	130
Valentine	2	130
White Chocolate Chunk	1 (1 oz)	130
TAKE-OUT		
biscotti with nuts chocolate dipped	1 (1.3 oz)	117
black & white	1 lg (3 oz)	302

CORIANDER

leaf dried	1 tsp	2
leaf fresh	¼ cup	1
seed	1 tsp	5

CORN

(*see also* BRAN, CEREAL, CORNMEAL)

CANNED

Del Monte

Cream Style Golden	½ cup (4.4 oz)	90
Cream Style Golden 50% Less Salt	½ cup (4.4 oz)	90
Cream Style Golden No Salt Added	½ cup (4.4 oz)	90
Cream Style Supersweet Golden	½ cup (4.4 oz)	60
Cream Style White	½ cup (4.4 oz)	100

FOOD	PORTION	CALS.
Del Monte (CONT.)		
Whole Kernel Golden	½ cup (4.4 oz)	90
Whole Kernel Golden Supersweet 50% Less Salt	½ cup (4.4 oz)	60
Whole Kernel Golden Supersweet No Salt Added	½ cup (4.4 oz)	60
Whole Kernel Golden Supersweet No Sugar	½ cup (4.4 oz)	60
Whole Kernel Golden Supersweet Vacuum Packed	½ cup (3.7 oz)	70
Whole Kernel Golden Supersweet Vacuum Packed No Salt Added	½ cup (3.7 oz)	70
Whole Kernel White Sweet	½ cup (4.4 oz)	80
Green Giant		
Cream Style	½ cup (4.5 oz)	100
Mexicorn	⅓ cup (2.7 oz)	60
Niblets	⅓ cup (2.7 oz)	70
Niblets 50% Less Sodium	⅓ cup (2.7 oz)	60
Niblets Extra Sweet	⅓ cup (2.6 oz)	50
Niblets No Added Sugar or Salt	⅓ cup (2.7 oz)	60
White Shoepeg	⅓ cup	80
Whole Sweet	½ cup (4.3 oz)	80
Whole Sweet 50% Less Sodium	½ cup (4.2 oz)	80
Seneca		
Cream Style	½ cup	80
Whole Kernel	½ cup	90
Whole Kernel Natural Pack	½ cup	80
DRIED		
Goya		
Giant White	⅓ cup (1.6 oz)	160
FRESH		
on-the-cob w/ butter cooked	1 ear	155
white cooked	½ cup	89
white raw	½ cup	66
yellow cooked	1 ear (2.7 oz)	83
yellow cooked	½ cup	89
yellow raw	1 ear (3 oz)	77
yellow raw	½ cup	66
FROZEN		
Birds Eye		
Baby Corn Blend	⅔ cup (2.9 oz)	60
Baby Gold & White	⅔ cup (3.3 oz)	80
In Butter Sauce	½ cup (4.6 oz)	110

FOOD	PORTION	CALS.
Fresh Like		
Cob Corn	1 ear (3 in)	96
Cob Corn	1 ear (5 in)	96
Cut	3.5 oz	85
Green Giant		
Butter Sauce Niblets	⅔ cup (4.3 oz)	130
Butter Sauce Shoepeg White	¾ cup (4 oz)	120
Cream Corn	½ cup (4.1 oz)	110
Extra Sweet Niblets	⅔ cup (3.1 oz)	70
Harvest Fresh Niblets	⅔ cup (3.4 oz)	80
Harvest Fresh Shoepeg White	½ cup (2.6 oz)	70
Niblets	⅔ cup (2.9 oz)	80
On The Cob Extra Sweet	1 ear (4.4 oz)	120
On The Cob Nibblers	1 ear (2.1 oz)	70
On The Cob Niblets	1 ear (5 oz)	160
Select Extra Sweet White	⅔ cup (2.9 oz)	50
Select Shoepeg White	¾ cup (3.2 oz)	100
Ore Ida		
Cob Corn	1 ear (6.1 oz)	180
Cob Corn Mini-Gold	1 ear (3.1 oz)	90
Stouffer's		
Souffle	½ cup (6 oz)	170
Tree Of Life		
Corn	⅔ cup (3.2 oz)	80

CORN CHIPS
(*see* CHIPS)

CORNISH HENS
(*see* CHICKEN)

CORNMEAL

FOOD	PORTION	CALS.
white	1 cup (4.8 oz)	505
whole grain	1 cup (4.3 oz)	442
yellow	1 cup (4.8 oz)	505
yellow self-rising	1 cup (4.3 oz)	407
Albers		
White	3 tbsp	110
Yellow	3 tbsp	110
Arrowhead		
Yellow	¼ cup (1.2 oz)	120
MIX		
Arrowhead		
Corn Bread	¼ cup (1.2 oz)	120
Hodgson Mill		
Yellow	¼ cup (1 oz)	100

FOOD	PORTION	CALS.
Hodgson Mill (CONT.)		
Yellow Self Rising	¼ cup (1 oz)	90
Kentucky Kernel		
White Corn Meal Mix	¼ cup (1 oz)	100
Miracle Maize		
Complete as prep	1 piece (1.5 oz)	193
Country Style as prep	1 piece 2 in x 2 in (1.8 oz)	230
Sweet as prep	1 piece 2 in x 2 in (1.8 oz)	236
Stone-Buhr		
Yellow Corn Meal	¼ cup (1 oz)	100
READY-TO-EAT		
Aurora		
Polenta	½ cup (5 oz)	110
TAKE-OUT		
hush puppies	1 (0.75 oz)	74
CORNSALAD		
raw	1 cup	12
CORNSTARCH		
cornstarch	1 cup (4.5 oz)	488
Hodgson Mill		
Cornstarch	2 tsp (0.4 oz)	35
COTTAGE CHEESE		
Axelrod		
Nonfat	½ cup (4.4 oz)	90
Borden		
4%	½ cup	120
Dry Curd 0.5%	½ cup	80
Unsalted 4%	½ cup	120
Breakstone's		
2% Fat Large Curd	½ cup (4.2 oz)	90
2% Fat Small Curd	½ cup (4.2 oz)	90
4% Fat Large Curd	½ cup (4.2 oz)	120
4% Fat Small Curd	½ cup (4.2 oz)	120
Cottage Doubles Peach	1 pkg (5.5 oz)	140
Dry Curd	¼ cup (1.9 oz)	45
Free	½ cup (4.4 oz)	80
Snack 2% Fat Small Curd	1 pkg (4 oz)	90
Snack 4% Fat Small Curd	1 pkg (4 oz)	110
Snack Free	1 pkg (4 oz)	70
Friendship		
California Style	½ cup (4 oz)	115

FOOD	PORTION	CALS.
Friendship (CONT.)		
Lowfat No Salt Added	½ cup (4 oz)	90
Lowfat Pineapple	½ cup (4 oz)	120
Lowfat 1%	½ cup (4 oz)	90
Nonfat	½ cup (4 oz)	80
Nonfat Plus Peach	½ cup (4 oz)	110
Pot Style	½ cup (4 oz)	90
With Pineapple	½ cup (4 oz)	140
Hood		
1% Fat	½ cup (4 oz)	90
1% Fat Chive & Onion	½ cup (4 oz)	90
1% Fat No Salt Added	½ cup (4 oz)	90
1% Fat Pepper & Herb	½ cup (4 oz)	90
1% Fat Pineapple Cherry	½ cup (4 oz)	110
4% Fat	½ cup (4 oz)	120
4% Fat Chive	½ cup (4 oz)	130
4% Fat Pineapple	½ cup (4 oz)	130
Nonfat	½ cup (4 oz)	80
Nonfat Pineapple	½ cup (4 oz)	110
Knudsen		
1.5% Fat Small Curd Pineapple	½ cup (4.6 oz)	120
2% Fat Small Curd	½ cup (4.2 oz)	100
4% Fat Large Curd	½ cup (4.5 oz)	130
4% Fat Small Curd	½ cup (4.3 oz)	120
Free	½ cup (4.2 oz)	80
On The Go! 1.5% Fat Peach	1 pkg (4 oz)	110
On The Go! 1.5% Fat Pineapple	1 pkg (4 oz)	110
On The Go! 1.5% Fat Strawberry	1 pkg (4 oz)	110
On The Go! 1.5% Fat Tropical Fruit	1 pkg (4 oz)	110
On The Go! 2% Fat	1 pkg (4 oz)	90
On The Go! Free	1 pkg (4 oz)	70
Lactaid		
1%	4 oz	72
Light N'Lively		
1% Fat	½ cup (4 oz)	80
1% Fat Garden Salad	½ cup (4.2 oz)	80
1% Fat Peach & Pineapple	½ cup (4.3 oz)	110
Fat Free	½ cup (4.4 oz)	80
Lite Line		
Lowfat 1½%	½ cup	90
Viva		
Nonfat	½ cup	70

COTTONSEED

kernels roasted	1 tbsp	51

FOOD	PORTION	CALS.
COUGH DROPS		
Halls		
Cough Drops	1 (3.8 g)	15
Plus	1 (4.7 g)	18
With Vitamin C	1 (3.8 g)	14
Lifesavers		
Menthol	2 (0.5 oz)	60
COUSCOUS		
cooked	1 cup (5.5 oz)	176
dry	1 cup (6.1 oz)	650
Casbah		
Almond Chicken Vegetarian	1 pkg (1.5 oz)	160
Asparagus Au Gratin Organic	1 pkg (1.5 oz)	150
Cheddar Broccoli	1 pkg (1.3 oz)	130
Hearty Harvest Zestful Organic as prep	1 pkg (10 fl oz)	180
Moroccan Stew	1 pkg (2 oz)	180
Pilaf as prep	1 cup	200
Tomato Parmesan	1 pkg (1.8 oz)	170
Kitchen Del Sol		
Aegean Citrus as prep	½ cup (1.1 oz)	110
Moroccan Ginger as prep	½ cup (1.1 oz)	120
Spicy Vegetable as prep	½ cup (1.1 oz)	120
Tomato & Olive	½ cup (1 oz)	120
Tomato & Olive	½ cup (1.1 oz)	120
Melting Pot		
Calypso Cranberry	1 cup	200
Lentil Curry	1 cup	170
Lucky Seven	1 cup	190
Mango Salsa	1 cup	190
Roasted Garlic	1 cup	170
Sesame Ginger	1 cup	180
Sun-Dried Tomatoes	1 cup	190
Wild Mushroom	1 cup	190
Near East		
As Prep	1¼ cup	260
COWPEAS		
frozen cooked	½ cup	112
leafy tips chopped cooked	1 cup	12
CRAB		
CANNED		
blue	1 cup	133
FRESH		
alaska king cooked	3 oz	82

FOOD	PORTION	CALS.
alaska king cooked	1 leg (4.7 oz)	129
blue cooked	1 cup	138
queen steamed	3 oz	98
TAKE-OUT		
baked	1 (3.8 oz)	160
cake	1 (2 oz)	160
soft-shell fried	1 (4.4 oz)	334

CRACKER CRUMBS

FOOD	PORTION	CALS.
cracker meal	1 cup (4 oz)	440
graham cracker crumbs	½ cup (4.4 oz)	540
Honey Maid		
Graham Cracker	0.5 oz	70
Kellogg's		
Corn Flake Crumbs	2 tbsp (0.4 oz)	40
Nabisco		
Nilla Cookie Crumbs	2 tbsp (0.5 oz)	70
Oreo		
Cookie Crumbs	2 tbsp (0.5 oz)	80
Premium		
Fat Free Cracker Crumbs	¼ cup (1 oz)	100
Ritz		
Cracker Crumbs	⅓ cup (1 oz)	140
Sunshine		
Graham	3 tbsp (0.6 oz)	80

CRACKERS

(*see also* CRACKER CRUMBS)

FOOD	PORTION	CALS.
cheese	14 (0.5 oz)	71
cheese	1 (1 in sq) (1 g)	5
cheese low sodium	1 (1 in sq) (1 g)	5
cheese low sodium	14 (0.5 oz)	71
cheese w/ peanut butter filling	1 (0.24 oz)	34
crispbread rye	1 (0.35 oz)	37
melba toast plain	1 (5 g)	19
melba toast pumpernickel	1 (5 g)	19
melba toast rye	1 (5 g)	19
melba toast wheat	1 (5 g)	19
milk	1 (0.42 oz)	55
oyster cracker	1 (1 g)	4
peanut butter sandwich	1 (7 g)	34
rusk toast	1 (0.35 oz)	41
rye w/ cheese filling	1 (0.24 oz)	34
rye wafers plain	1 (0.9 oz)	84
rye wafers seasoned	1 (0.8 oz)	84

FOOD	PORTION	CALS.
saltines	1 (3 g)	13
saltines fat free low sodium	6 (1 oz)	118
saltines fat free low sodium	3 (0.5 oz)	59
saltines low salt	1 (3 g)	13
snack cracker	1 (3 g)	15
snack cracker low salt	1 (3 g)	15
snack cracker w/ cheese filling	1 (7 g)	33
soup cracker	1 (1 g)	4
wheat w/ cheese filling	1 (0.24 oz)	35
wheat w/ peanut butter filling	1 (0.24 oz)	35
wheat thins	1 (2 g)	9
wheat thins	7 (0.5 oz)	67
wheat thins low salt	7 (0.5 oz)	67
whole wheat	1 (4 g)	18
whole wheat low salt	1 (4 g)	18
Adrienne's		
Gourmet Flatbread Caraway & Rye	2	20
Gourmet Flatbread Classic Island	2	20
Gourmet Flatbread Slightly Onion	2	20
Gourmet Flatbread Ten Grain	2	20
Ak-mak		
100% Whole Wheat	5 (1 oz)	116
Armenian Cracker Bread	1 sheet (1 oz)	100
Armenian Cracker Bread Whole Wheat	1 sheet (1 oz)	116
Round Cracker Bread No Seeds	1 (1 oz)	100
Round Cracker Bread Seeded	1 (1 oz)	100
Round Cracker Bread Whole Wheat	1 (1 oz)	116
American Heritage		
Sesame	9 (1.1 oz)	160
Wheat & Bran	9 (1 oz)	140
Barbara's		
Cheese Bites	26 (1 oz)	120
French Onion	3	60
Rite Lite Rounds	5 (0.5 oz)	55
Roasted Garlic & Herb	3	60
Sundried Tomato & Basil	3	60
Toasted Sesame	3	60
Wheatines All Flavors	1 lg sq (0.5 oz)	50
Better Cheddars		
Crackers	22 (1 oz)	70
Low Sodium	22 (1 oz)	150
Reduced Fat	24 (1 oz)	140
Burns & Ricker		
Bagel Crisps Garlic	5 (1 oz)	100

FOOD	PORTION	CALS.
Cheetos		
Bacon Cheddar	1 pkg	190
Cheddar Cheese	1 pkg	210
Golden Toast	1 pkg	240
Cheez-It		
Crackers	27 (1 oz)	160
Crackers	1 pkg (1.5 oz)	220
Crackers	1 pkg (2 oz)	290
Hot & Spicy	26 (1 oz)	160
Hot & Spicy	1 pkg (1.5 oz)	220
Low Sodium	27 (1 oz)	160
Party Mix	½ cup (1 oz)	140
Reduced Fat	30 (1 oz)	130
White Cheddar	1 pkg (1.5 oz)	220
White Cheddar	26 (1 oz)	160
Crown Pilot		
Crackers	1 (0.5 oz)	70
Doritos		
Jalapeno Cheese	1 pkg	230
Nacho Cheddar	1 pkg	240
Eden		
Brown Rice	5 (1 oz)	120
Escort		
Crackers	3 (0.5 oz)	70
Estee		
Sugar Free Cracked Pepper	18	120
Sugar Free Golden	10	130
Sugar Free Wheat	17	100
Frito Lay		
Cheddar Snacks	1 pkg	200
Frookie		
Cheddar	17 (1 oz)	140
Cracked Pepper	8 (0.7 oz)	70
Garden Vegetable	13 (1 oz)	130
Garlic & Herb	8 (0.7 oz)	70
Pizza	17 (1 oz)	130
Snack & Party	10 (1 oz)	140
Water Crackers	8 (0.7 oz)	70
Wheat & Onion	12 (1 oz)	120
Wheat & Rye	13 (1 oz)	120
Goya		
Butter Crackers	1	40
Crackers	1	30

FOOD	PORTION	CALS.
Hain		
Cheese	1 oz	130
Onion	1 oz	130
Onion No Salt Added	1 oz	130
Rich	1 oz	130
Rich No Salt Added	1 oz	130
Rye	1 oz	120
Rye No Salt Added	1 oz	120
Sesame	1 oz	140
Sesame No Salt Added	1 oz	140
Sour Cream & Chive	1 oz	130
Sour Cream & Chive No Salt Added	1 oz	130
Sourdough	0.5 oz	65
Sourdough Low Salt	1 oz	130
Vegetable	1 oz	130
Vegetable No Salt Added	1 oz	130
Harvest Crisps		
5 Grain	13 (1.1 oz)	130
Oat	13 (1.1 oz)	140
Health Valley		
Healthy Pizza Garlic & Herb	6	50
Healthy Pizza Italiano	6	50
Healthy Pizza Zesty Cheese	6	50
Low Fat Mild Jalapeno	6	60
Low Fat Mild Ranch	6	60
Low Fat Roasted Garlic	6	60
Original Oat Bran	6	120
Original Rice Bran	6	110
Whole Wheat	5	50
Whole Wheat Cheese	5	50
Whole Wheat Herb	5	50
Whole Wheat No Salt Vegetable	5	50
Whole Wheat Onion	5	50
Whole Wheat Vegetable	5	50
Healthy Choice		
Bread Crisps Garlic Herb	11 (1 oz)	110
Hi Ho		
Butter Flavored	9 (1.1 oz)	160
Cracked Pepper	9 (1.1 oz)	160
Crackers	9	160
Low Salt	9 (1.1 oz)	160
Multi Grain	9 (1.1 oz)	160
Reduced Fat	10 (1.1 oz)	140
Whole Wheat	9 (1.1 oz)	150

FOOD	PORTION	CALS.
J.J. Flats		
Breadflats Caraway	1	52
Breadflats Caraway And Salt	1	51
Breadflats Cinnamon	1	53
Breadflats Flavorall	1	52
Breadflats Garlic	1	52
Breadflats Oat Bran	1	49
Breadflats Onion	1	53
Breadflats Plain	1	53
Breadflats Poppy	1	53
Breadflats Sesame	1	55
Kavli		
Crackers	1 piece	40
Keebler		
Club 33% Reduced Fat	5 (0.6 oz)	70
Club 50% Reduced Sodium	4 (0.5 oz)	70
Club Original	4 (0.5 oz)	70
Munch'ems 55% Reduced Fat	35 (1 oz)	130
Munch'ems Cheddar	30 (1 oz)	130
Munch'ems Chili Cheese	28 (1.1 oz)	130
Munch'ems Ranch	33 (1 oz)	130
Munch'ems Salsa	28 (1.1 oz)	130
Munch'ems Seasoned Original	30 (1 oz)	130
Munch'ems Sour Cream & Onion 55% Reduced Fat	33 (1 oz)	130
Paks Cheese & Peanut Butter	1 pkg	190
Paks Club & Cheddar	1 pkg	190
Paks Toast & Peanut Butter	1 pkg	190
Paks Town House & Cheddar	1 pkg	200
Toasteds Buttercrisp	9 (1 oz)	140
Toasteds Onion	9 (1 oz)	140
Toasteds Sesame	9 (1 oz)	140
Toasteds Sesame Reduced Fat	10 (1 oz)	120
Toasteds Wheat	9 (1 oz)	140
Toasteds Wheat Reduced Fat	10 (1 oz)	120
Town House	5 (0.6 oz)	80
Town House 50% Reduced Sodium	5 (0.6 oz)	80
Town House Reduced Fat	6 (0.6 oz)	70
Town House Wheat	5 (0.6 oz)	80
Wheatables 50% Reduced Fat	29 (1 oz)	130
Wheatables Garden Vegetable	25 (1 oz)	140
Wheatables Original	26 (1 oz)	150
Wheatables Ranch	25 (1 oz)	150
Wheatables White Cheddar 30% Reduced Fat	27 (1 oz)	130

FOOD	PORTION	CALS.
Keebler (CONT.)		
Zesta Saltine 50% Reduced Sodium	5 (0.5 oz)	60
Zesta Saltine Fat Free	5 (0.5 oz)	50
Zesta Saltine Original	5 (0.5 oz)	60
Zesta Saltine Unsalted Top	5 (0.5 oz)	70
Zesta Soup & Oyster	42 (0.5 oz)	80
Krispy		
Cracked Pepper	5 (0.5 oz)	60
Fat Free	5 (0.5 oz)	60
Mild Cheddar	5 (0.5 oz)	60
Original	5 (0.5 oz)	60
Soup & Oyster Crackers	17 (0.5 oz)	60
Unsalted Tops	5 (0.5 oz)	60
Whole Wheat	5 (0.5 oz)	60
Lavash		
Bread Crisp Original	2 (0.5 oz)	60
Bread Crisp Sesame	2 (0.5 oz)	60
Little Debbie		
Cheese Crackers With Peanut Butter	1 pkg (0.9 oz)	140
Cheese Crackers With Peanut Butter	1 pkg (1.4 oz)	210
Toasty Crackers With Peanut Butter	1 pkg (0.9 oz)	140
Toasty Crackers With Peanut Butter	1 pkg (1.4 oz)	200
Wheat Crackers With Cheddar Cheese	1 pkg (0.9 oz)	140
NABS		
Cheese Peanut Butter Sandwich	6 (1.4 oz)	190
Peanut Butter Toast Sandwich	6 (1.4 oz)	190
Nabisco		
Bacon Flavored	15 (1.1 oz)	160
Chicken In A Biskit	14 (1 oz)	160
Garden Crisps	15 (1 oz)	130
Oat Thins	18 (1 oz)	140
Royal Lunch	1 (0.4 oz)	50
Swiss	15 (1 oz)	140
Tid-Bit Cheese	32 (1 oz)	150
Vegetable Thins	14 (1.1 oz)	160
Wheat Thins Original	16 (1 oz)	140
Wheat Thins Reduced Fat	18 (1 oz)	120
Zings!	1 pkg (1.8 oz)	240
Nips		
Cheese	29 (1 oz)	150
No-No		
Flatbreads Tortilla Corn Low Fat Sugar Free Everything	3 (1 oz)	95

FOOD	PORTION	CALS.
Old London		
Melba Toast Pumpernickel	0.5 oz	54
Melba Toast Rye	0.5 oz	52
Melba Toast Sesame	0.5 oz	55
Melba Toast Sesame Unsalted	0.5 oz	55
Melba Toast Wheat	0.5 oz	51
Melba Toast White	0.5 oz	51
Melba Toast White Unsalted	0.5 oz	51
Melba Toast Whole Grain	0.5 oz	52
Melba Toast Whole Grain Unsalted	0.5 oz	53
Rounds Bacon	0.5 oz	53
Rounds Garlic	0.5 oz	56
Rounds Onion	0.5 oz	52
Rounds Rye	0.5 oz	52
Rounds Sesame	0.5 oz	56
Rounds White	0.5 oz	48
Rounds Whole Grain	0.5 oz	54
Oysterettes		
Crackers	19 (0.5 oz)	60
Partners		
Walla Walla Sweet Onion Perservative Free	0.5 oz	65
Pepperidge Farm		
Butter Thins	4 (0.5 oz)	70
English Water Biscuits	4 (0.5 oz)	70
Goldfish Cheddar	55	140
Goldfish Cheese Trio	58	140
Goldfish Original	55	140
Goldfish Parmesan Cheese	60	140
Goldfish Pizza Flavored	55 (1 oz)	140
Goldfish Pretzel	43 (1 oz)	120
Goldfish Toasted Wheat	41	150
Hearty Wheat	3 (0.6 oz)	80
Sesame	3 (0.5 oz)	70
Snack Mix Fat Free Goldfish	⅔ cup (0.9 oz)	90
Peter Pan		
Cheese Peanut Butter	1 pkg	210
Toast Peanut Butter	1 pkg	210
Planters		
Cheese Peanut Butter Sandwiches	1 pkg (1.4 oz)	190
Toast Peanut Butter Sandwiches	1 pkg (1.4 oz)	190
Premium		
Saltine Bits	34 (1 oz)	150
Saltine Fat Free	5 (0.5 oz)	50
Saltine Low Sodium	5 (0.5 oz)	60

FOOD	PORTION	CALS.
Premium (CONT.)		
Saltine Original	5 (0.5 oz)	60
Saltine Unsalted Tops	5 (0.5 oz)	60
Soup & Oyster	23 (0.5 oz)	60
Ritz		
Bits	48 (1 oz)	160
Bits Sandwiches With Peanut Butter	13 (1 oz)	150
Bits Sandwiches With Real Cheese	14 (1.1 oz)	160
Crackers	5 (0.5 oz)	80
Low Sodium	5 (0.5 oz)	80
Sandwiches With Real Cheese	1 pkg (1.4 oz)	210
Savory Thins		
Toasted Onion & Garlic	15 (1 oz)	110
Sesmark		
Brown Rice	15 (1 oz)	120
Cheese Thins	15 (1 oz)	130
Rice Thins Original	15 (1 oz)	130
Rice Thins Teriyaki Flavored	13 (1 oz)	130
Savory Thins Original	15 (1 oz)	125
Sesame Thins Cheddar	9 (1 oz)	150
Sesame Thins Garlic	9 (1 oz)	150
Sesame Thins Original	9 (1 oz)	150
Sesame Thins Unsalted	11 (1 oz)	150
SnackWell's		
Cracked Pepper	7 (0.5 oz)	60
Fat Free Wheat	5 (0.5 oz)	60
Reduced Fat Cheese	38 (1 oz)	130
Reduced Fat Classic Golden	6 (0.5 oz)	60
Salsa Cheddar	32 (1 oz)	120
Snorkles		
Cheddar	56 (1 oz)	140
Sociables		
Crackers	7 (0.5 oz)	80
Sunshine		
Saltines Cracked Pepper	5 (0.5 oz)	60
Tree Of Life		
Bite Size Fat Free Corn & Salsa	12	60
Bite Size Fat Free Cracked Pepper	12	55
Bite Size Fat Free Garden Vegetable	12	55
Bite Size Fat Free Garlic & Herb	12	55
Bite Size Fat Free Soya Nut	12	60
Bite Size Fat Free Toasted Onion	12	60
Bite Size Fat Free Whole Wheat	12	60
Fat Free Oyster	40 (0.5 oz)	60

FOOD	PORTION	CALS.
Tree Of Life (CONT.)		
Saltine Cracked Pepper Fat Free	4 (0.5 oz)	60
Saltine Fat Free	4 (0.5 oz)	50
Triscuit		
Crackers	7 (1.1 oz)	140
Deli-Style Rye	7 (1.1 oz)	140
Garden Herb	6 (1 oz)	130
Low Sodium	7 (1.1 oz)	150
Reduced Fat	8 (1.1 oz)	130
Wheat 'n Bran	7 (1.1 oz)	140
Twigs		
Sesame & Cheese Sticks	15 (1 oz)	150
Uneeda Biscuit		
Unsalted Tops	2 (0.5 oz)	60
Venus		
Armenian Thin Bread	2 (0.9 oz)	100
Bran Wafers Salt Free	5 (0.5 oz)	60
Corn Crackers Salt Free	5 (0.5 oz)	60
Cracked Wheat Wafers Salt Free	5 (0.5 oz)	60
Cracker Bread	5 (0.5 oz)	60
Hors D'oeuvre	3 (0.5 oz)	60
Oat Bran Wafers	5 (0.5 oz)	60
Oat Bran Wafers Salt Free	5 (0.5 oz)	60
Old Brussels Cheddar Waferettes	5 (0.5 oz)	80
Old Brussels Jalapeno Waferettes	5 (0.5 oz)	80
Rye Wafers Low Salt	5 (0.5 oz)	60
Stoned Wheat Wafers Bite Size	7 (0.5 oz)	60
Water Crackers Fat Free	5 (0.5 oz)	55
Wheat Wafers Low Salt	5 (0.5 oz)	60
Wasa		
Crisp	3 (0.5 oz)	50
Crisp'N Light Sourdough Rye	3 (0.6 oz)	60
Crisp'N Light Wheat	2 (0.5 oz)	50
Crispbread Cinnamon Toast	1 (0.6 oz)	60
Crispbread Fiber Rye	1 (0.4 oz)	30
Crispbread Gluten & Wheat Free Corn	1 (0.4 oz)	40
Crispbread Hearty Rye	1 (0.5 oz)	45
Crispbread Light Rye	1 (0.3 oz)	25
Crispbread Multi Grain	1 (0.5 oz)	45
Crispbread Organic Rye	1 (0.3 oz)	25
Crispbread Sodium Free Rye	1 (0.3 oz)	30
Crispbread Sourdough Rye	1 (0.4 oz)	35
Crispbread Toasted Wheat	1 (0.5 oz)	50
Crispbread Whole Wheat	1 (0.5 oz)	50

FOOD	PORTION	CALS.
Waverly		
Crackers	5 (0.5 oz)	70
Wheat Thins		
Low Salt	16 (1 oz)	140
Multi-Grain	17 (1 oz)	130
Wheatworth		
Stone Ground	5 (0.5 oz)	80
Zwieback		
Crackers	1 (8 g)	35

CRANBERRIES
CANNED
Ocean Spray

CranOrange	¼ cup	120
Cranberry Sauce Jellied	¼ cup	110
Whole Berry Sauce	¼ cup	110

DRIED
Ocean Spray

Craisins	⅓ cup (1.4 oz)	130

FRESH

chopped	1 cup	54

CRANBERRY BEANS
Bean Cuisine

Dried	½ cup	115

CRANBERRY JUICE
After The Fall

Cape Cod Cranberry	1 bottle (10 oz)	130
Cranberry Ginger Ale	1 can (12 oz)	140
Apple & Eve		
Juice	6 fl oz	100
Crystal Light		
Cranberry Breeze Drink	1 serv (8 oz)	5
Cranberry Breeze Drink Mix as prep	1 serv (8 oz)	5
Everfresh		
Cranberry Cocktail	1 can (8 oz)	140
Ocean Spray		
Cocktail	8 fl oz	140
Lightstyle Low Calorie Cranberry Juice Cocktail	8 fl oz	40
Reduced Calorie Cocktail	8 fl oz	50
Seneca		
Cocktail frzn as prep	8 fl oz	140
Snapple		
Cranberry Royal	10 fl oz	150

FOOD	PORTION	CALS.
Tree Of Life		
Concentrate	8 tsp (1.4 oz)	110
Tropicana		
Twister Ruby Red	1 bottle (10 oz)	160
Veryfine		
Cocktail	1 bottle (10 oz)	180

CRAYFISH
(*see also* LOBSTER)

cooked	3 oz	97
raw	3 oz	76

CREAM
(*see also* SOUR CREAM, SOUR CREAM SUBSTITUTES, WHIPPED TOPPINGS)

LIQUID

Farmland		
Half & Half	2 tbsp	40
Light Cream	2 tbsp	30
Hood		
Half & Half	2 tbsp (1 oz)	40
Heavy	1 tbsp (0.5 oz)	50
Light	1 tbsp (0.5 oz)	30
Whipping Cream	1 tbsp (0.5 oz)	45
Parmalat		
Half & Half	2 tbsp (1 oz)	40

WHIPPED

heavy whipping	1 cup (4.1 oz)	411
light whipping	1 cup (4.2 oz)	345

CREAM CHEESE

Alpine Lace		
Fat Free Garden Vegetable	2 tbsp (1 oz)	30
Fat Free Garlic & Herbs	2 tbsp (1 oz)	30
Boar's Head		
Cream Cheese	2 tbsp (1 oz)	100
Breakstone's		
Temp-Tee Whipped	2 tbsp (0.8 oz)	80
Fleur De Lait		
Bermuda Onion & Chives	2 tbsp (0.9 oz)	90
Cinnamon Raisin	2 tbsp (0.9 oz)	90
Date Nut Rum	2 tbsp (0.9 oz)	90
Fresh Cut Garden Vegetable	2 tbsp (0.9 oz)	80
Garden Vegetable	2 tbsp (0.9 oz)	80
Garlic & Spice	2 tbsp (0.9 oz)	90
Herb & Spice	2 tbsp (0.9 oz)	90

FOOD	PORTION	CALS.
Fleur De Lait (CONT.)		
Irish Creme	2 tbsp (0.9 oz)	100
Lemon	2 tbsp (0.9 oz)	90
Lox	2 tbsp (0.9 oz)	90
Mandarin Orange	2 tbsp (0.9 oz)	90
Peach	2 tbsp (0.9 oz)	90
Pineapple	2 tbsp (0.9 oz)	90
Plain	2 tbsp (1 oz)	100
Strawberry	2 tbsp (0.9 oz)	90
Toasted Onion	2 tbsp (0.9 oz)	90
Wildberry	2 tbsp (0.9 oz)	90
Fresh Cut		
Bac'n & Horseradish	2 tbsp (0.9 oz)	90
Bermuda Onion & Chives	2 tbsp (0.9 oz)	90
Date Nut & Rum	2 tbsp (0.9 oz)	90
Garlic & Spice	2 tbsp (0.9 oz)	90
Herb & Spice	2 tbsp (0.9 oz)	90
Lox	2 tbsp (0.9 oz)	90
Peaches & Cream	2 tbsp (0.9 oz)	90
Strawberry	2 tbsp (0.9 oz)	90
Friendship		
NY Style Reduced Fat	2 tbsp (1 oz)	50
Healthy Choice		
Herbs & Garlic	2 tbsp (1 oz)	25
Plain	2 tbsp (1 oz)	25
Strawberry	2 tbsp (1 oz)	30
Heluva Good Cheese		
Cream Cheese	1 tbsp (1 oz)	100
Philadelphia		
Free	1 oz	30
Regular	1 oz	100
Soft	2 tbsp (1 oz)	100
Soft Apple Cinnamon	2 tbsp (1.1 oz)	100
Soft Cheesecake	2 tbsp (1 oz)	110
Soft Chives & Onions	2 tbsp (1.1 oz)	110
Soft Garden Vegetable	2 tbsp (1.1 oz)	110
Soft Honey Nut	2 tbsp (1.1 oz)	110
Soft Pineapple	2 tbsp (1.1 oz)	100
Soft Salmon	3 tbsp (1.1 oz)	100
Soft Strawberry	2 tbsp (1.1 oz)	100
Soft Free	2 tbsp (1.2 oz)	30
Soft Free Garden Vegetable	2 tbsp (1.2 oz)	30
Soft Free Strawberries	2 tbsp (1.2 oz)	45
Soft Light	2 tbsp (1.1 oz)	70

FOOD	PORTION	CALS.
Philadelphia (CONT.)		
Soft Light Jalapeno	2 tbsp (1.1 oz)	60
Soft Light Raspberry	2 tbsp (1.1 oz)	70
Soft Light Roasted Garlic	2 tbsp (1.1 oz)	70
Whipped	2 tbsp (0.7 oz)	70
Whipped Chives	2 tbsp (0.7 oz)	70
Whipped Smoked Salmon	2 tbsp (0.7 oz)	70
With Chives	1 oz	90
Ultra Delight		
Cheddar Cream Cheese	2 tbsp (0.9 oz)	60
Chive	2 tbsp (0.9 oz)	60
Garlic	2 tbsp (0.9 oz)	60
Mixed Berry	2 tbsp (0.9 oz)	70
Nacho	2 tbsp (0.9 oz)	60
Salsa	2 tbsp (0.9 oz)	60
Shrimp	2 tbsp (0.9 oz)	60
Strawberry	2 tbsp (0.9 oz)	60
Vegetable	2 tbsp (0.9 oz)	50

CREAM CHEESE SUBSTITUTES
Tofutti

Better Than Cream Cheese French Onion	1 oz	80
Better Than Cream Cheese Herb & Chive	1 oz	80
Better Than Cream Cheese Plain	1 oz	80

CREAM OF TARTAR
cream of tartar	1 tsp	8

CREPES
basic crepe unfilled	1	75

CRESS
(*see also* WATERCRESS)

garden cooked	½ cup	16
garden raw	½ cup	8

CROAKER
atlantic breaded & fried	3 oz	188

CROISSANT
apple	1 (2 oz)	145
cheese	1 (2 oz)	236
plain	1 (2 oz)	232
plain	1 mini (1 oz)	115
Rudy's Farm		
Ham & Swiss Sandwich	1 (3.4 oz)	310

FOOD	PORTION	CALS.
TAKE-OUT		
w/ egg & cheese	1 (4.5 oz)	368
w/ egg cheese & bacon	1 (4.5 oz)	413
w/ egg cheese & ham	1 (5.3 oz)	474
w/ egg cheese & sausage	1 (5.6 oz)	523
CROUTONS		
plain	1 cup (1 oz)	122
seasoned	1 cup (1.4 oz)	186
Arnold		
Crispy Cheddar Romano	0.5 oz	64
Crispy Cheese Garlic	0.5 oz	60
Crispy Fine Herbs	0.5 oz	50
Crispy Italian	0.5 oz	60
Crispy Onion & Garlic	0.5 oz	60
Crispy Seasoned	0.5 oz	60
Pepperidge Farm		
Garlic	6 (0.2 oz)	30
Homestyle	6 (0.2 oz)	30
Sourdough	6 (0.2 oz)	35
CUCUMBER		
FRESH		
raw	1 (11 oz)	38
raw sliced	½ cup (1.8 oz)	7
JARRED		
Rosoff's		
Salad	3 slices (1 oz)	12
Schorr's		
Cucumber Garden Salad	3 slices (1 oz)	12
TAKE-OUT		
cucumber salad	3.5 oz	50
kimchee	½ cup (1.8 oz)	36
tzatziki	½ cup (3.4 oz)	72
CUMIN		
seed	1 tsp	8
CURRANTS		
black fresh	½ cup	36
zante dried	½ cup	204
CUSK		
fillet baked	3 oz	106
CUSTARD		
HOME RECIPE		
baked	1 recipe 4 serv (19.8 oz)	549

FOOD	PORTION	CALS.
flan	1 recipe 10 serv (53.7 oz)	2206
MIX		
as prep w/ 2% milk	½ cup (4.7 oz)	148
as prep w/ 2% milk	1 recipe 4 serv (18.7 oz)	595
as prep w/ whole milk	½ cup (4.7 oz)	163
as prep w/ whole milk	1 recipe 4 serv (18.7 oz)	652
flan as prep w/ 2% milk	½ cup (4.7 oz)	135
flan as prep w/ 2% milk	1 recipe 4 serv (18.7 oz)	542
flan as prep w/ whole milk	½ cup (4.7 oz)	150
flan as prep w/ whole milk	1 recipe 4 serv (18.7 oz)	600
Jell-O		
Americana Custard Dessert as prep w/ 2% milk	½ cup (5 oz)	140
Flan as prep w/ 2% milk	½ cup (5.1 oz)	140
Royal		
Custard	mix for 1 serv	60
Flan Caramel Custard	mix for 1 serv	60
READY-TO-EAT		
Kozy Shack		
Flan	1 pkg (4 oz)	150
TAKE-OUT		
baked	½ cup (5 oz)	148
flan	½ cup (5.4 oz)	220
zabaione	½ cup (57.2 g)	135

CUTTLEFISH

steamed	3 oz	134

DANDELION GREENS

fresh cooked	½ cup	17
raw chopped	½ cup	13

DANISH PASTRY
FROZEN
Morton

Honey Buns	1 (2.28 oz)	250
Honey Buns Mini	1 (1.23 oz)	160
READY-TO-EAT		
Dolly Madison		
Danish Rollers	3 (2.8 oz)	290
Tastykake		
Cheese	1 (3 oz)	290
Lemon	1 (3 oz)	290
Raspberry	1 (3 oz)	290
TAKE-OUT		
almond	1 (4¼ in) 2.3 oz	280

FOOD	PORTION	CALS.
apple	1 (4¼ in) 2.5 oz	264
cheese	1 (3.2 oz)	353
cheese	1 (4¼ in) 2.5 oz	266
cinnamon	1 (3.1 oz)	349
cinnamon	1 (4¼ in) 2.3 oz	262
cinnimon nut	1 (4¼ in) 2.3 oz	280
fruit	1 (3.3 oz)	335
lemon	1 (4¼ in) 2.5 oz	264
raisin	1 (4¼ in) 2.5 oz	264
raisin nut	1 (4¼ in) 2.3 oz	280
raspberry	1 (4¼ in) 2.5 oz	264
strawberry	1 (4¼ in) 2.5 oz	264

DATES
DRIED
chopped	1 cup	489
deglet noor	10	240
whole	10	228
Bordo		
Diced	2 oz	203
Dole		
Chopped	½ cup	230
Pitted	½ cup	280
Sonoma		
Dried	5-6 (1.4 oz)	110

DEER
(*see* VENISON)

DELI MEATS/COLD CUTS
(*see also* CHICKEN, HAM, MEAT SUBSTITUTES, TURKEY)

beerwurst beef	1 slice (2¾ in x 1/16 in)	20
bologna beef	1 oz	88
braunschweiger pork	1 oz	102
corned beef loaf	1 oz	43
headcheese pork	1 oz	60
liverwurst pork	1 oz	92
olive loaf pork	1 oz	67
pickle & pimiento loaf pork	1 oz	74
Boar's Head		
Bologna Beef	2 oz	150
Bologna Garlic	2 oz	150
Bologna Lowered Sodium	2 oz	150
Bologna Pork & Beef	2 oz	150
Braunschweiger Lite	2 oz	120

FOOD	PORTION	CALS
Boar's Head (CONT.)		
Head Cheese	2 oz	90
Liverwurst Strassburger	2 oz	170
Olive Loaf	2 oz	130
Pastrami	2 oz	90
Prosciutto	1 oz	60
Red Pastrami	2 oz	90
Salami Beef	2 oz	120
Salami Cooked	2 oz	130
Salami Genoa	2 oz	180
Salami Hard	1 oz	110
Spiced Ham	2 oz	120
Carl Buddig		
Beef	1 oz	40
Corned Beef	1 oz	40
Pastrami	1 oz	40
Healthy Choice		
Bologna	1 slice (1 oz)	30
Bologna Beef	1 slice (1 oz)	35
Deli-Thin Bologna	4 slices (1.8 oz)	60
Well-Pack Bologna	1 slice (1 oz)	30
Hebrew National		
Bologna Beef	2 oz	180
Bologna Beef Reduced Fat	2 oz	130
Bologna Lean Chub	2 oz	90
Bologna Midget	2 oz	180
Deli Pastrami	2 oz	80
Deli Express Corned Beef	2 oz	80
Deli Express Tongue Sliced	2 oz	120
Salami Beef	2 oz	170
Salami Beef Reduced Fat	2 oz	110
Salami Sean Chub	2 oz	90
Salami Midget	2 oz	170
Hillshire		
Bologna Large	1 oz	90
Bologna Ring	1 oz	90
Brunschweiger	1 oz	95
Deli Select Corned Beef	1 slice	10
Deli Select Light Bologna	1 slice	12
Deli Select Oven Roasted Cured Beef	1 slice	10
Deli Select Pastrami	1 slice	10
Deli Select Roast Beef	1 slice	10
Deli Select Smoked Beef	1 slice	10
Flavor Pack 90-99% Fat Free Light Bologna	1 slice (0.73 oz)	30

FOOD	PORTION	CALS.
Hillshire (CONT.)		
Flavor Pack 90-99% Fat Free Pastrami	1 slice (0.6 oz)	18
Lunch 'N Munch Bologna/ American/ Snickers	1 pkg (4.25 oz)	490
Lunch 'N Munch Bologna/ American/ Snickers/Hi-C	1 pkg (4.25 oz + 6 fl oz)	590
Lunch 'N Munch Bologna/American	1 pkg (4.5 oz)	480
Lunch 'N Munch Cotto Salami/ Monterey Jack	1 pkg (4.5 oz)	440
Lunch 'N Munch Pepperoni/ American	1 pkg (4.5 oz)	570
Pepperoni	1 oz	110
Salami Hard	1 oz	90
Salami Hard	1 oz	100
Summer Sausage	2 oz	180
Summer Sausage Beef	2 oz	190
Summer Sausage Light	2 oz	150
Summer Sausage w/Cheddar Cheese	2 oz	200
Hormel		
Liverwurst Spread	4 tbsp (2 oz)	130
Pepperoni Chunk	1 oz	140
Pepperoni Sliced	15 slices (1 oz)	140
Pepperoni Twin	1 oz	140
Pillow Pack Genoa Salami	2 oz	160
Pillow Pack Pepperoni	16 slices (1 oz)	140
Jordan's		
Healthy Trim 95% Fat Free Macaroni & Cheese Loaf	2 slices (1.6 oz)	50
Healthy Trim 95% Fat Free Olive Loaf	2 slices (1.6 oz)	50
Healthy Trim 95% Fat Free Pickle & Pepper Loaf	2 slices (1.6 oz)	50
Healthy Trim 97% Fat Free Corned Beef	2 slices (1.6 oz)	45
Healthy Trim Low Fat Cooked Salami	3 slices (2 oz)	70
Healthy Trim Low Fat German Brand Bologna	3 slices (2 oz)	70
Oscar Mayer		
Bologna	1 slice (1 oz)	90
Bologna Beef	1 slice (1 oz)	90
Bologna Garlic	1 slice (1.4 oz)	110
Bologna Wisconsin Made Ring	2 oz	180
Braunschweiger Spread	2 oz	190
Brunschweiger	1 slice (1 oz)	100
Free Bologna	1 slice (1 oz)	20
Head Cheese	1 slice (1 oz)	50
Light Bologna	1 slice (1 oz)	60

FOOD	PORTION	CALS.
Oscar Mayer (CONT.)		
Light Bologna Beef	1 slice (1 oz)	60
Liver Cheese	1 slice (1.3 oz)	120
Lunchables Bologna/American	1 pkg (4.5 oz)	450
Lunchables Deluxe Turkey/Ham	1 pkg (5.1 oz)	360
Lunchables Dessert Jello/Honey Turkey/ Cheddar	1 pkg (5.7 oz)	320
Lunchables Fun Pack Bologna/Wild Cherry	1 pkg (11.2 oz)	530
Lunchables Fun Pack Ham/Fruit Punch	1 pkg (11.2 oz)	450
Lunchables Ham/Swiss	1 pkg (4.5 oz)	320
Lunchables Pepperoni/ American	1 pkg (4.5 oz)	480
Lunchables Salami/American	1 pkg (4.5 oz)	430
Luncheon Loaf Spiced	1 slice (1 oz)	70
New England Brand Sausage	2 slices (1.6 oz)	60
Old Fashioned Loaf	1 slice (1 oz)	70
Olive Loaf	1 slice (1 oz)	70
Pepperoni	15 slices (1 oz)	140
Pickle And Pimiento Loaf	1 slice (1 oz)	80
Salami Cotto	1 slice (1 oz)	70
Salami Cotto Beef	1 slice (1 oz)	60
Salami For Beer	1 slices (1.6 oz)	110
Salami Genoa	3 slices (1 oz)	100
Salami Hard	3 slices (1 oz)	100
Salami Machaich Brand Beef	2 slices (1.6 oz)	120
Sandwich Spread	2 oz	130
Summer Sausage	2 slices (1.6 oz)	140
Summer Sausage Beef	2 slices (1.6 oz)	140
Russer		
Bologna	2 oz	180
Bologna Jalapeno Pepper	2 oz	170
Bologna Wunderbar German Brand	2 oz	190
Bologna Beef	2 oz	180
Bologna Garlic	2 oz	180
Bologna Italian Brand Sweet Red Pepper	2 oz	180
Braunschweiger	2 oz	170
Cooked Salami	2 oz	120
Dutch Brand	2 oz	130
Hot Cooked Salami	2 oz	110
Italian Brand Loaf	2 oz	130
Jalapeno Loaf With Monterey Jack Cheese	2 oz	160
Kielbasa Loaf	2 oz	120
Light Bologna	2 oz	120
Light Bologna Beef	2 oz	120
Light Braunschweiger	2 oz	120

FOOD	PORTION	CALS.
Russer (CONT.)		
Light Old Fashioned Loaf	2 oz	90
Light P&P Loaf	2 oz	100
Light Salami Cooked	2 oz	90
Olive Loaf	2 oz	160
P&P Loaf	2 oz	160
Pepper Loaf	2 oz	90
Polish Loaf	2 oz	140
Sara Lee		
Pastrami Beef	2 oz	100
Peppered Beef	2 oz	70
Shofar		
Salami Beef	2 oz	160
Spam		
Less Salt	2 oz	170
Lite	2 oz	110
Original	2 oz	170
Smoked	2 oz	170
Underwood		
Liverwurst	2.08 oz	180
TAKE-OUT		
corned beef	2 oz	70
corned beef brisket	2 oz	90

DIETING AIDS
(*see* NUTRITION SUPPLEMENTS)

DILL

seed	1 tsp	6
sprigs fresh	5	0
weed dry	1 tsp	3
Watkins		
Liquid Spice	1 tbsp (0.5 oz)	120

DINNER
(*see also* ASIAN FOOD, PASTA DISHES, POT PIES, SPANISH FOOD)

FROZEN

Amy's Organic		
Whole Meals Country Dinner	1 pkg (11 oz)	380
Banquet		
BBQ Style Chicken	1 meal (9 oz)	320
Beef	1 meal (9 oz)	240
Chicken Parmigiana	1 pkg (9.5 oz)	290
Chicken & Dumplings	1 meal (10 oz)	260
Chicken Fried Steak	1 pkg (10 oz)	400

FOOD	PORTION	CALS.
Banquet (CONT.)		
Chicken Nuggets	1 pkg (6.75 oz)	410
Extra Helping All White Chicken	1 meal (18 oz)	820
Extra Helping Chicken Parmigiana	1 meal (19 oz)	650
Extra Helping Chicken Fried Steak	1 meal (18.5 oz)	800
Extra Helping Fried Chicken	1 meal (18 oz)	790
Extra Helping Meatloaf	1 meal (19 oz)	650
Extra Helping Mexican Style	1 meal (22 oz)	820
Extra Helping Salisbury Steak	1 meal (19 oz)	740
Extra Helping Southern Fried Chicken	1 meal (17.5 oz)	750
Extra Helping Turkey Dinner	1 meal (18.8 oz)	560
Family Entree Beef Stew	1 serv (8.13 oz)	160
Family Entree Chicken Parmigiana	1 serv (4.67 oz)	240
Family Entree Chicken & Dumplings	1 serv (7.47 oz)	290
Family Entree Gravy & Sliced Turkey	1 serv (4.8 oz)	100
Family Entree Gravy w/ Charbroiled Beef	1 serv (4.67 oz)	180
Family Entree Onion Gravy w/ Beef	1 serv (4.67 oz)	180
Family Entree Salisbury Steak	1 serv (4.67 oz)	200
Family Entree Veal Parmigiana	1 serv (4.67 oz)	230
Family Entrees Dumplings & Chicken	7 oz	280
Family Entrees Gravy & Sliced Beef	1 serv (5.6 oz)	100
Family Entrees Gravy & Sliced Turkey	6 oz	120
Fried Chicken	1 meal (9 oz)	470
Gravy w/ Beef Patty	1 pkg (9.5 oz)	300
Hot Sandwich Toppers Chicken Ala King	1 pkg (4.5 oz)	100
Hot Sandwich Toppers Creamed Chipped Beef	1 pkg (4 oz)	100
Hot Sandwich Toppers Gravy & Sliced Beef	1 pkg (4 oz)	70
Hot Sandwich Toppers Gravy & Sliced Turkey	1 pkg (5 oz)	90
Hot Sandwich Toppers Salisbury Steak	1 pkg (5 oz)	220
Hot Sandwich Toppers Sloppy Joe	1 meal (4 oz)	140
Meatloaf	1 meal (9.5 oz)	280
Mexican Style Combo Meal	1 pkg (11 oz)	380
Mexican Style Meal	1 pkg (11 oz)	340
Oriental Style Chicken	1 pkg (9 oz)	260
Salisbury Steak	1 meal (9.5 oz)	310
Southern Fried Chicken Meal	1 pkg (8.75 oz)	260
Turkey	1 meal (9.25 oz)	270
Veal Parmagiana	1 pkg (9 oz)	530
Western Style Meal	1 meal (9.5 oz)	210
White Meat Chicken Meal	1 pkg (8.75 oz)	470

FOOD	PORTION	CALS.
Birds Eye		
Easy Recipe Meal Starter Cacciatore as prep	1 serv	280
Easy Recipe Meal Starter Orange Glaze Chicken as prep	1 serv	280
Easy Recipe Meal Starter Southwestern	1 serv	280
Easy Recipe Meal Starter Sweet & Sour as prep	1 serv	280
Budget Gourmet		
Beef Cantonese	1 meal (9.1 oz)	270
Beef Stroganoff	1 meal (8.75 oz)	260
Chicken And Egg Noodles	1 meal (10 oz)	440
Chicken Au Gratin	1 meal (9.1 oz)	230
Chicken Breast Parmigiana	1 pkg (11 oz)	270
Chicken Marsala	1 meal (9 oz)	260
Chicken With Fettucini	1 meal (10 oz)	400
Chinese Style Vegetables & Chicken	1 meal (10 oz)	280
French Recipe Chicken	1 meal (10 oz)	220
Glazed Turkey	1 meal (9 oz)	260
Ham & Asparagus Au Gratin	1 meal (8.7 oz)	300
Herbed Chicken Breast With Fettucini	1 pkg (11 oz)	240
Italian Style Vegetables & Chicken	1 meal (10.25 oz)	310
Mandarin Chicken	1 meal (10 oz)	240
Mesquite Chicken Breast	1 pkg (11 oz)	250
Orange Glazed Chicken	1 meal (9 oz)	270
Oriental Beef	1 meal (10 oz)	290
Oriental Chicken With Vegetables	1 meal (9 oz)	280
Pepper Steak With Rice	1 meal (10 oz)	300
Pot Roast Beef	1 meal (10.5 oz)	230
Roast Chicken With Homestyle Gravy	1 meal (11 oz)	280
Roast Sirloin Supreme	1 meal (9 oz)	320
Sirloin Salisbury Steak	1 meal (11 oz)	280
Sirloin Salisbury Steak	1 meal (9 oz)	220
Sirloin Cheddar Melt	1 meal (9.4 oz)	380
Sirloin Of Beef In Herb Sauce	1 meal (9.5 oz)	250
Sirloin Of Beef In Wine Sauce	1 pkg (11 oz)	280
Sirloin Tips And Country Vegetables	1 meal (10 oz)	290
Special Recipe Sirloin Of Beef	1 meal (11 oz)	250
Stuffed Turkey Breast	1 pkg (11 oz)	250
Swedish Meatballs With Noodles	1 meal (10 oz)	590
Sweet And Sour Chicken	1 meal (10 oz)	340
Teriyaki Beef	1 pkg (10.75 oz)	260
Teriyaki Chicken Breast	1 meal (11 oz)	300

FOOD	PORTION	CALS.
Green Giant		
Create A Meal Broccoli Stir Fry as prep	1⅓ cups (9.9 oz)	290
Create A Meal Cheese & Herb Primavera as prep	1¼ cups (10 oz)	330
Create A Meal Garlic Herb as prep	1¼ cups (10 oz)	340
Create A Meal Hearty Vegetable Stew as prep	1¼ cups (10 oz)	280
Create A Meal Lemon Herb as prep	1½ cups (10 oz)	360
Create A Meal Mushroom & Wine as prep	1¼ cups (10 oz)	390
Create A Meal Vegetable Almond Stir Fry as prep	1⅓ cups (10 oz)	320
Healthy Choice		
Beef & Peppers Cantonese	1 meal (11.5 oz)	270
Beef Pepper Steak Oriental	1 meal (9.5 oz)	250
Beef Tips Francais	1 meal (9.5 oz)	280
Beef Tips With Sauce	1 meal (11 oz)	290
Chicken Cantonese	1 meal (11.25)	210
Chicken Parmigiana	1 meal (11.5 oz)	300
Chicken & Vegetables Marsala	1 meal (11.5 oz)	220
Chicken Bangkok	1 meal (9.5 oz)	270
Chicken Dijon	1 meal (11 oz)	280
Chicken Imperial	1 meal (9 oz)	230
Chicken Picante	1 meal (11.25 oz)	220
Chicken Teriyaki	1 meal (12.25 oz)	270
Classics Beef Broccoli Beijing	1 meal (12 oz)	330
Classics Cacciatore Chicken	1 meal (12.5 oz)	260
Classics Chicken Fransesca	1 meal (12.5 oz)	360
Classics Country Inn Roast Turkey	1 meal (10 oz)	250
Classics Ginger Chicken Hunan	1 meal (12.6 oz)	350
Classics Mesquite Beef Barbecue	1 meal (11 oz)	310
Classics Salisbury Steak	1 meal (11 oz)	260
Classics Sesame Chicken Shanghai	1 meal (12 oz)	310
Classics Shrimp & Vegetables Maria	1 meal (12.5 oz)	260
Country Glazed Chicken	1 meal (8.5 oz)	200
Country Herb Chicken	1 meal (11.5 oz)	270
Country Roast Turkey With Mushroom	1 meal (8.5 oz)	220
Country Turkey & Pasta	1 meal (12.6 oz)	300
Homestyle Turkey With Vegetables	1 meal (9.5 oz)	260
Honey Mustard Chicken	1 meal (9.5 oz)	260
Lemon Pepper Fish	1 meal (10.7 oz)	290
Mandarin Chicken	1 meal (10 oz)	280
Mesquite Chicken Barbecue	1 meal (10.5 oz)	320
Shrimp Marinara	1 meal (10.5 oz)	220
Smoky Chicken Barbecue	1 meal (12.75 oz)	380

FOOD	PORTION	CALS.
Healthy Choice (CONT.)		
Southwestern Glazed Chicken	1 meal (12.5 oz)	300
Sweet & Sour Chicken	1 meal (11.5 oz)	310
Traditional Breast Of Turkey	1 meal (10.5 oz)	280
Traditional Meat Loaf	1 meal (12 oz)	320
Traditional Beef Tips	1 meal (11.25 oz)	260
Tradtional Salisbury Steak	1 meal (11.5 oz)	320
Yankee Pot Roast	1 meal (11 oz)	280
Kid Cuisine		
Chicken Sandwiche	1 pkg (9.43 oz)	480
Chicken Nuggets	1 pkg (9.1 oz)	440
Fish Sticks	1 pkg (8.25 oz)	370
Fried Chicken	1 pkg (10.1 oz)	440
Hot Dogs w/ Buns	6.7 oz	450
Macaroni & Beef	1 pkg (9.6 oz)	370
Le Menu		
Beef Sirloin Tips	11.5 oz	400
Beef Stroganoff	10 oz	430
Chicken Parmigiana	11.75 oz	410
Chicken A La King	10.25 oz	330
Chicken Cordon Bleu	11 oz	460
Chicken In Wine Sauce	10 oz	280
Chopped Sirloin Beef	12.25 oz	430
Entree LightStyle Chicken A La King	8.25 oz	240
Entree LightStyle Chicken Dijon	8 oz	240
Entree LightStyle Empress Chicken	8.25 oz	210
Entree LightStyle Glazed Turkey	8.25 oz	260
Entree LightStyle Herb Roast Chicken	7.75 oz	260
Entree LightStyle Swedish Meatballs	8 oz	260
Entree LightStyle Traditional Turkey	8 oz	200
Ham Steak	10 oz	300
LightStyle Glazed Chicken Breast	10 oz	230
LightStyle Herb Roasted Chicken	10 oz	240
LightStyle Salisbury Steak	10 oz	280
LightStyle Sliced Turkey	10 oz	210
LightStyle Sweet & Sour Chicken	10 oz	250
LightStyle Turkey Divan	10 oz	260
LightStyle Veal Marsala	10 oz	230
Pepper Steak	11.5 oz	370
Salisbury Steak	10.5 oz	370
Sliced Breast Of Turkey w/ Mushroom Gravy	10.5 oz	300
Sweet & Sour Chicken	11.25 oz	400
Veal Parmigiana	11.5 oz	390

FOOD	PORTION	CALS.
Le Menu (CONT.)		
Yankee Pot Roast	10 oz	330
Lean Cuisine		
American Favorite Baked Chicken	1 pkg (8.6 oz)	230
American Favorite Baked Fish	1 pkg (9 oz)	270
American Favorite Beef Pot Roast	1 pkg (9 oz)	210
American Favorite Beef Tips Barbecue	1 pkg (8.75 oz)	290
American Favorite Chicken Medallions w/ Creamy Cheese	1 pkg (9.37 oz)	260
American Favorite Country Vegetables & Beef	1 pkg (9 oz)	210
American Favorite Honey Roasted Chicken	1 pkg (8.5 oz)	290
American Favorite Meatloaf & Whipped Potatoes	1 pkg (9.4 oz)	250
American Favorite Oven Roasted Beef	1 pkg (9.25 oz)	260
American Favorite Roasted Turkey Breast	1 pkg (9.75 oz)	270
American Favorite Salisbury Steak	1 pkg (9.5 oz)	280
American Favorite Scalloped Potatoes w/ Turkey Ham	1 pkg (10 oz)	250
Cafe Classics Chicken Carbonara	1 pkg (9 oz)	280
Cafe Classics Chicken Mediterranean	1 pkg (10.5 oz)	270
Cafe Classics Chicken Breast In Wine Sauce	1 pkg (8.1 oz)	210
Cafe Classics Chicken Parmesan	1 meal (10.9 oz)	220
Cafe Classics Chicken Piccata	1 pkg (9 oz)	270
Cafe Classics Chicken w/ Basil Cream Sauce	1 pkg (8.5 oz)	270
Cafe Classics Glazed Turkey	1 pkg (9 oz)	240
Cafe Classics Grilled Chicken Salsa	1 pkg (8.9 oz)	270
Cafe Classics Herb Roasted Chicken	1 pkg (8 oz)	210
Cafe Classics Honey Mustard Chicken	1 pkg (8 oz)	250
Cafe Classics Mesquite Beef w/ Rice	1 pkg (9 oz)	290
Cafe Classics Sirloin Beef Peppercorn	1 pkg (8.75 oz)	220
Chicken & Vegetables	1 pkg (10.5 oz)	250
Chicken A L'Orange	1 pkg (9 oz)	250
Chicken In Peanut Sauce	1 pkg (9 oz)	290
Fiesta Chicken w/ Rice & Vegetables	1 pkg (8.5 oz)	250
Glazed Chicken w/ Vegetable Rice	1 pkg (8.5 oz)	240
Homestyle Turkey	1 pkg (9.4 oz)	230
Mandarin Chicken	1 pkg (9 oz)	250
Oriental Beef	1 pkg (9.25 oz)	220
Stuffed Cabbage w/ Whipped Potatoes	1 pkg (9.5 oz)	170
Swedish Meatballs w/ Pasta	1 pkg (9.1 oz)	280

FOOD	PORTION	CALS.
Life Choice		
Garden Potato Casserole	1 meal (13.4 oz)	160
Luigino's		
Chicken A La King With Noodles	1 pkg (8 oz)	240
Noodles With Chicken Peas & Carrots	1 cup (6.3 oz)	260
Noodles With Chicken Peas & Carrots	1 pkg (8 oz)	300
Sweet & Sour Chicken With Rice	1 pkg (8 oz)	300
Morton		
Breaded Chicken Pattie	1 meal (6.75 oz)	280
Chicken Nugget	1 meal (7 oz)	320
Fried Chicken	1 meal (9 oz)	420
Meatloaf	1 meal (9 oz)	250
Mexican	1 meal (10 oz)	260
Salisbury Steak	1 meal (9 oz)	210
Turkey	1 meal (9 oz)	230
Veal Parmagiana	1 meal (8.75 oz)	280
Western	1 meal (9 oz)	290
Patio		
Chili	1 cup (8 oz)	260
Ranchera	1 pkg (13 oz)	410
Stouffer's		
Baked Chicken Breast w/ Mashed Potatoes	1 serv (12.2 oz)	330
Beef Stroganoff	1 pkg (9.75 oz)	390
Chicken A La King	1 pkg (9.5 oz)	350
Creamed Chicken	1 pkg (6.5 oz)	260
Creamed Chipped Beef	½ cup (5.5 oz)	160
Creamy Chicken & Broccoli	1 pkg (8.9 oz)	320
Escalloped Chicken & Noodles	1 pkg (10 oz)	430
Fish w/ Macaroni & Cheese	1 serv (9.5 oz)	460
Glazed Chicken w/ Rice	1 serv (11.8 oz)	290
Green Pepper Steak	1 pkg (10.5 oz)	330
Homestyle Beef Pot Roast & Browned Potatoes	1 pkg (8.9 oz)	250
Homestyle Fish Filet w/ Macaroni & Cheese	1 pkg (9 oz)	430
Homestyle Fried Chicken & Whipped Potatoes	1 pkg (7.5 oz)	310
Homestyle Meatloaf & Whipped Potatoes	1 pkg (9.9 oz)	330
Homestyle Roast Turkey w/ Gravy Stuffing & Whipped Potatoes	1 pkg (9.6 oz)	320
Homestyle Salisbury Steak & Gravy & Macaroni & Cheese	1 pkg (9.6 oz)	350
Honestyle Baked Chicken & Gravy & Whipped Potatoes	1 pkg (8.9 oz)	270

FOOD	PORTION	CALS.
Stouffer's (CONT.)		
Meatloaf	1 serv (5.5 oz)	210
Meatloaf w/ Whipped Potatoes	1 serv (11.5 oz)	380
Stuffed Pepper	1 pkg (10 oz)	200
Swedish Meatballs	1 pkg (10.25 oz)	480
Swanson		
Beans & Franks	10.5 oz	440
Beef	11.25 oz	310
Beef In Barbecue Sauce	11 oz	460
Chopped Sirloin Beef	10.75 oz	340
Fish 'n' Chips	10 oz	500
Fried Chicken Dark Meat	9.75 oz	560
Fried Chicken White Meat	10.25 oz	550
Homestyle Chicken Cacciatore	10.95 oz	260
Homestyle Chicken Nibbles	4.25 oz	340
Homestyle Fish & Fries	6.5 oz	340
Homestyle Fried Chicken	7 oz	390
Homestyle Salisbury Steak	10 oz	320
Homestyle Scalloped Potatoes & Ham	9 oz	300
Homestyle Seafood Creole With Rice	9 oz	240
Homestyle Sirloin Tips In Burgundy Sauce	7 oz	160
Homestyle Turkey With Dressing & Potatoes	9 oz	290
Homestyle Veal Parmigiana	10 oz	330
Hungry-Man Boneless Chicken	17.75 oz	700
Hungry-Man Chopped Beef Steak	16.75 oz	640
Hungry-Man Fried Chicken Dark Meat	14.25 oz	860
Hungry-Man Fried Chicken White Meat	14.25 oz	870
Hungry-Man Salisbury Steak	16.5 oz	680
Hungry-Man Sliced Beef	15.25 oz	450
Hungry-Man Turkey	17 oz	550
Hungry-Man Veal Parmigiana	18.25 oz	590
Loin Of Pork	10.75 oz	280
Macaroni & Beef	12 oz	370
Meatloaf	10.75 oz	360
Noodles & Chicken	10.5 oz	280
Salisbury Steak	10.75 oz	400
Swedish Meatballs	8.5 oz	360
Swiss Steak	10 oz	350
Turkey	11.5 oz	350
Veal Parmigiana	12.25 oz	430
Western Style	11.5 oz	430
Tyson		
Beef Champignon	1 pkg (10.5 oz)	370

FOOD	PORTION	CALS.
Tyson (CONT.)		
Chicken Picante	1 pkg (9 oz)	250
Chicken Supreme	1 pkg (9 oz)	230
Francais	1 pkg (9.5 oz)	280
Glazed Chicken With Sauce	1 pkg (9.25 oz)	240
Grilled Chicken	1 pkg (7.75 oz)	220
Grilled Italian Chicken	1 pkg (9 oz)	210
Healthy Portions BBQ Chicken	1 pkg (12.5 oz)	400
Healthy Portions Chicken Marinara	1 pkg (13.75 oz)	340
Healthy Portions Herb Chicken	1 pkg (13.75 oz)	340
Healthy Portions Honey Mustard Chicken	1 pkg (13.75 oz)	390
Healthy Portions Italian Style Chicken	1 pkg (13.75 oz)	310
Healthy Portions Mesquite Chicken	1 pkg (13.25 oz)	330
Healthy Portions Salsa Chicken	1 pkg (13.75 oz)	370
Healthy Portions Sesame Chicken	1 pkg (13.5 oz)	400
Honey Roasted Chicken	1 pkg (9 oz)	220
Kiev	1 pkg (9.25 oz)	450
Marsala	1 pkg (9 oz)	200
Mexquite	1 pkg (9 oz)	320
Picatta	1 pkg (9 oz)	200
Roasted Chicken	1 pkg (9 oz)	200
Sweet & Sour	1 pkg (11 oz)	420
Turkey With Gravy	1 pkg (9.5 oz)	320
Ultra Slim-Fast		
Beef Pepper Steak	12 oz	270
Chicken Fettucini	12 oz	380
Chicken & Vegetable	12 oz	290
Country Style Vegetable & Beef Tips	12 oz	230
Mesquite Chicken	12 oz	360
Roasted Chicken In Mushroom Sauce	12 oz	280
Shrimp Creole	12 oz	240
Shrimp Marinara	12 oz	290
Sweet & Sour Chicken	12 oz	330
Turkey Medallions In Herb Sauce	12 oz	280
Weight Watchers		
Smart One Grilled Salisbury Steak	1 pkg (8.5 oz)	250
Smart Ones Fiesta Chicken	1 pkg (8.5 oz)	210
Smart Ones Honey Mustard Chicken	1 pkg (8.5 oz)	200
Smart Ones Lemon Herb Chicken Piccata	1 pkg (8.5 oz)	190
Smart Ones Pepper Steak	1 pkg (10 oz)	240
Smart Ones Risotto w/ Cheese & Mushrooms	1 pkg (10 oz)	290
Smart Ones Roast Turkey Medallions & Mushrooms	1 pkg (8.5 oz)	180

FOOD	PORTION	CALS.
Weight Watchers (CONT.)		
Smart Ones Shrimp Marinara	1 pkg (9 oz)	180
Smart Ones Stuffed Turkey Breast	1 pkg (10 oz)	260
Smart Ones Swedish Meatballs	1 pkg (9 oz)	300
SHELF-STABLE		
My Own Meal		
Beef Stew	1 pkg (10 oz)	260
Chicken Mediterranean	1 pkg (10 oz)	270
Chicken Noodles	1 pkg (10 oz)	270
Chicken & Black Beans	1 pkg (10 oz)	240
Old World Stew	1 pkg (10 oz)	310
DIP		
Breakstone's		
Bacon & Onion	2 tbsp (1.1 oz)	60
Chesapeake Clam	2 tbsp (1.1 oz)	50
Free Creamy Salsa	2 tbsp (1.1 oz)	20
Free French Onion	2 tbsp (1.1 oz)	25
Free Ranch	2 tbsp (1.1 oz)	25
French Onion	2 tbsp (1.1 oz)	50
Toasted Onion	2 tbsp (1.1 oz)	50
Cheez Whiz		
Medium Cheese & Salsa	2 tbsp (1.2 oz)	100
Mild Cheese & Salsa	2 tbsp (1.2 oz)	100
Chi-Chi's		
Fiesta Bean	2 tbsp (0.9 oz)	35
Fiesta Cheese	2 tbsp (0.9 oz)	40
Durkee		
Sour Cream as prep	2 tbsp	25
Frito-Lay's		
French Onion	2 tbsp (1.1 oz)	60
Jalapeno & Cheddar Cheese	2 tbsp (1.2 oz)	50
Fritos		
Bean	2 tbsp (1.2 oz)	40
Chili Cheese	1.2 oz	45
Hot Bean	2 tbsp (1.2 oz)	40
Guiltless Gourmet		
Black Bean Mild	1 oz	25
Black Bean Spicy	1 oz	25
Pinto Bean	1 oz	25
Hain		
Hot Bean	4 tbsp	70
Mexican Bean	4 tbsp	60
Onion Bean	4 tbsp	70

FOOD	PORTION	CALS.
Hain (CONT.)		
Taco Dip & Sauce	4 tbsp	25
Heluva Good Cheese		
Bacon Horseradish	2 tbsp (1.1 oz)	60
Clam	2 tbsp (1.1 oz)	50
French Onion	2 tbsp (1.1 oz)	50
Homestyle Onion	2 tbsp (1.1 oz)	60
Light French Onion	2 tbsp (1.1 oz)	35
Light Jalapeno Cheddar	2 tbsp (1.1 oz)	40
Ranch	2 tbsp (1.1 oz)	60
Knudsen		
Free Creamy Salsa	2 tbsp (1.1 oz)	20
Free French Onion	2 tbsp (1.1 oz)	25
Free Ranch	2 tbsp (1.1 oz)	25
Kraft		
Avocado	2 tbsp (1.1 oz)	60
Bacon & Horseradish	2 tbsp (1.1 oz)	60
Clam	2 tbsp (1.1 oz)	60
Free French Onion	2 tbsp (1.1 oz)	25
Free Ranch	2 tbsp (1.1 oz)	25
Free Salsa	2 tbsp (1.1 oz)	20
French Onion	2 tbsp (1.1 oz)	60
Green Onion	2 tbsp (1.1 oz)	60
Jalapeno Cheese	2 tbsp (1.1 oz)	60
Premium Sour Cream	2 tbsp (1.1 oz)	50
Premium Sour Cream Bacon & Horseradish	2 tbsp (1.1 oz)	60
Premium Sour Cream Bacon & Onion	2 tbsp (1.1 oz)	60
Premium Sour Cream Creamy Onion	2 tbsp (1.1 oz)	45
Premium Sour Cream French Onion	2 tbsp (1.1 oz)	45
Premium Sour Cream Ranch	2 tbsp (1.1 oz)	50
Ranch	2 tbsp (1.1 oz)	60
Louise's		
Fat Free Honey Mustard	1 oz	40
Fat Free Sour Cream & Onion	1 oz	25
Fat Free White Cheese Peppercorn	1 oz	25
Marzetti		
Blue Cheese Veggie	2 tbsp	200
Lemon Dill Veggie	2 tbsp	140
Light Ranch Veggie	2 tbsp	60
Ranch Veggie	2 tbsp	140
Sour Cream & Onion	2 tbsp	130
Southwestern Veggie	2 tbsp	130
Spinach Veggie	2 tbsp	130

FOOD	PORTION	CALS.
Old El Paso		
Black Bean	2 tbsp (1 oz)	20
Cheese 'n Salsa Medium	2 tbsp (1 oz)	40
Cheese 'n Salsa Mild	2 tbsp (1 oz)	40
Chunky Salsa Medium	2 tbsp (1 oz)	15
Chunky Salsa Mild	2 tbsp (1 oz)	15
Jalapeno	2 tbsp (1 oz)	30
Ruffles		
French Onion	2 tbsp	70
Ranch	2 tbsp (1.2 oz)	70
Snyder's		
Mustard Pretzel	2 tbsp (1.2 oz)	90
Taco Bell		
Fat Free Black Bean	2 tbsp (1.2 oz)	30
Salsa Con Queso Medium	2 tbsp (1.2 oz)	45
Salsa Con Queso Mild	2 tbsp (1.2 oz)	45
Utz		
Fat Free Sour Cream & Onion	2 tbsp (1.1 oz)	30
Jalapeno & Cheddar	2 tbsp (1 oz)	30
Low Fat Desert Garden	2 tbsp (1.1 oz)	40
Low Fat Salsa Con Queso	2 tbsp (1 oz)	40
Mild Cheddar	2 tbsp (1 oz)	45
Sour Cream & Onion	2 tbsp (1 oz)	60
Wise		
Jalapeno Bean	2 tbsp	25
Taco	2 tbsp	12

DOCK

fresh cooked	3½ oz	20
raw chopped	½ cup	15

DOLPHINFISH

fresh baked	3 oz	93

DOUGHNUTS

(*see also* DUNKIN' DONUTS, KRISPY KREME, WINCHELL'S DONUTS)

cake type unsugared	1 (1.6 oz)	198
chocolate glazed	1 (1.5 oz)	175
chocolate sugared	1 (1.5 oz)	175
chocolate coated	1 (1.5 oz)	204
creme filled	1 (3 oz)	307
french cruller glazed	1 (1.4 oz)	169
frosted	1 (1.5 oz)	204
honey bun	1 (2.1 oz)	242
jelly	1 (3 oz)	289

FOOD	PORTION	CALS.
old fashioned	1 (1.6 oz)	198
sugared	1 (1.6 oz)	192
wheat glazed	1 (1.6 oz)	162
wheat sugared	1 (1.6 oz)	162
yeast glazed	1 (2.1 oz)	242
Dolly Madison		
Chocolate Frosted	1 (1.1 oz)	140
Donut Gems Chocolate	4 (2 oz)	260
Donut Gems Crunch	3 (2 oz)	220
Donut Gems Powdered	4 (2 oz)	230
English Cruller	1 (2 oz)	250
Glazed Whirl	1 (1.6 oz)	210
Glazed Yeast	1 (1.5 oz)	190
Old Fashioned	1 (2.1 oz)	280
Plain	1 (1.2 oz)	140
Powdered	1 (1 oz)	120
Dutch Mill		
Cider	1 (2.1 oz)	240
Cinnamon	1 (1.8 oz)	210
Donut Holes Double-Dipped Chocolate	3 (1.4 oz)	220
Donut Holes Shootin' Stars	3 (1.4 oz)	190
Double-Dipped Chocolate	1 (2.1 oz)	280
Glazed	1 (2.1 oz)	250
Glazed Chocolate	1 (2.4 oz)	270
Plain	1 (1.8 oz)	210
Sugared	1 (1.8 oz)	220
Entenmann's		
Crumb Topped	1 (2.1 oz)	260
Devil's Food Crumb	1 (2.1 oz)	250
Rich Frosted	1 (2 oz)	280
Freihofer's		
Assorted	1 (2 oz)	270
Hostess		
Blueberry	1 (1.7 oz)	210
Donettes Crumb	3 (1.5 oz)	170
Donettes Frosted	3 (1.5 oz)	200
Donettes Powdered	3 (1.5 oz)	180
Frosted	1 (1.4 oz)	180
O's Raspberry Filled	1 (2.2 oz)	230
Old Fashioned Glazed	1 (2.1 oz)	260
Plain	1 (1.1 oz)	140
Powdered	1 (1.3 oz)	150
Little Debbie		
Donut Sticks	1 pkg (1.6 oz)	210

FOOD	PORTION	CALS.
Little Debbie (CONT.)		
Donut Sticks	1 pkg (2.5 oz)	320
Donut Sticks	1 pkg (3 oz)	390
Donut Sticks	1 pkg (2 oz)	250
Tastykake		
Mini Plain Glaze	1 pkg (2.5 oz)	260
Mini Powdered Sugar	1 pkg (2.5 oz)	260
Mini Rich Frosted	1 pkg (3 oz)	370

DRESSING
(*see* STUFFING/DRESSING)

DRINK MIXERS
(*see also* SODA, WATER)

whiskey sour mix	2 oz	55
whiskey sour mix as prep	3.6 oz	169
Bacardi		
Margarita Mix w/ rum	8 fl oz	160
Margarita Mix w/o liquor	8 fl oz	100
Pina Colada	8 fl oz	140
Rum Runner	8 fl oz	140
Strawberry Daiquiri w/o liquor	8 fl oz	140
Canada Dry		
Collins Mixer	8 fl oz	120
Sour Mixer	8 fl oz	90
Schweppes		
Collins Mixer	8 fl oz	100
Tabasco		
Bloody Mary Mix	1 serv (8.4 oz)	56
Bloody Mary Mix Extra Spicy	1 serv (8.4 oz)	58

DRUM

freshwater baked	3 oz	130

DUCK

w/ skin roasted	1 cup (4.9 oz)	472
w/ skin w/ bone leg roasted	3 oz	184
w/ skin w/o bone breast roasted	3 oz	172
w/o skin roasted	1 cup (4.9 oz)	281
w/o skin w/ bone leg braised	1 cup (6.1 oz)	310
w/o skin w/o bone breast broiled	1 cup (6.1 oz)	244
wild w/ skin raw	½ duck (9.5 oz)	571
wild w/o skin breast raw	½ breast (2.9 oz)	102

DUMPLING

Pepperidge Farm		
Apple	1 (3 oz)	230
Peach	1 (3 oz)	320

FOOD	PORTION	CALS.
EEL		
fresh cooked	1 fillet (5.6 oz)	375
fresh cooked	3 oz	200
smoked	3.5 oz	330
EGG		
(*see also* EGG DISHES, EGG SUBSTITUTES)		
CHICKEN		
hard cooked	1	77
hard cooked chopped	1 cup	210
poached	1	74
raw	1	75
white only	1	17
EggsPlus		
Fresh	1 (1.8 oz)	70
OTHER POULTRY		
duck preserved hard core	1 (1.8 oz)	80
duck preserved soft core	1 (1.8 oz)	80
duck raw	1 (2.5 oz)	130
duck salted	1 (1.9 oz)	100
goose raw	1 (5 oz)	267
quail raw	1 (9 g)	14
turkey raw	1 (2.7 oz)	135
TAKE-OUT		
scrambled plain	2 (3.3 oz)	199
scrambled w/ whole milk & margarine	1 serv	365
EGG DISHES		
FROZEN		
Downyflake		
Scrambled Eggs With Ham & Hash Browns	1 pkg (6.25 oz)	360
Scrambled Eggs With Ham & Pecan Twirl	1 pkg (6.25 oz)	470
Scrambled Eggs With Hash Browns & Sausage	1 pkg (6.25 oz)	420
Scrambled Eggs With Sausage & Pecan Twirl	1 pkg (6.25 oz)	510
Quaker		
Scrambled Eggs & Sausage With Hash Browns	1 pkg (5.7 oz)	290
Scrambled Eggs & Sausage With Pancakes	1 pkg (5.2 oz)	270
Scrambled Eggs Cheddar Cheese & Fried Potatoes	1 pkg (5.9 oz)	250

FOOD	PORTION	CALS.
Weight Watchers		
Handy Ham & Cheese Omelet	1 (4 oz)	220
TAKE-OUT		
scrambled	2 eggs	202
sunny side up	1	91

EGG ROLLS

(*see also* ASIAN FOODS)

egg roll wrapper fresh	1	83
Chun King		
Chicken	8 (4.4 oz)	270
Pork & Shrimp	8 (4.4 oz)	290
Shrimp	8 (4.4 oz)	260
Empire		
Large	1 (3 oz)	190
Miniature	6 (4.8 oz)	280
Lean Cuisine		
Vegetable	1 pkg (9 oz)	340
Lo-An		
White Meat Chicken	1 (2.7 oz)	140
Luigino's		
Chicken	1 pkg (6 oz)	360
Pork & Shrimp	1 pkg (6 oz)	340
Shrimp	1 pkg (6 oz)	350
Sweet & Sour Chicken	1 pkg (6 oz)	400
Sweet & Sour Pork	1 pkg (6 oz)	360
Szechwan Vegetable	1 pkg (6 oz)	350
Worthington		
Vegetarian Egg Rolls	1 (3 oz)	180
TAKE-OUT		
lobster	1 (4.8 oz)	270
meat & shrimp	1 (4.8 oz)	320
pork & shrimp	1 (5 oz)	300
shrimp	1 (3 oz)	170
spicy pork	1 (3 oz)	200
vegetable	1 (3 oz)	170

EGG SUBSTITUTES

Egg Beaters		
Eggs Substitute	¼ cup	25
Omelette Cheese	½ cup	110
Omelette Vegetable	½ cup	50
Healthy Choice		
Cholesterol Free	¼ cup (2 oz)	25

FOOD	PORTION	CALS.
Morningstar Farms		
Better'n Eggs	¼ cup (2 oz)	20
Breakfast Sandwich Bagel Scramblers Pattie Cheese	1 (5.9 oz)	320
Breakfast Sandwich English Muffin Scramblers Pattie	1 (5.1 oz)	240
Breakfast Sandwich English Muffin Scramblers Pattie Cheese	1 (6 oz)	280
Scramblers	¼ cup (2 oz)	35
Second Nature		
No Cholesterol	2 fl oz	60
No Fat	2 fl oz	40
No Fat With Garden Vegetables	2.5 fl oz	40
Simply Eggs		
Egg Substitute	1.75 fl oz	35
EGGNOG		
eggnog	1 cup	342
eggnog	1 qt	1368
Borden		
Eggnog	4 fl oz	160
Hood		
Fat Free	4 fl oz	100
Golden	4 fl oz	180
Light	4 fl oz	120
Select	4 fl oz	210
EGGPLANT		
CANNED		
Progresso		
Appetizer	2 tbsp (1 oz)	30
FRESH		
cubed cooked	½ cup	13
raw cut up	½ cup (1.4 oz)	11
slices cooked	4 (7 oz)	38
whole peeled raw	1 (1 lb)	117
TAKE-OUT		
baba ghannouj	¼ cup	55
caponata	2 tbsp (1 oz)	30
indian eggplant runi	1 serv	180
ELDERBERRIES		
fresh	1 cup	105
ELK		
roasted	3 oz	124

FOOD	PORTION	CALS.
ENDIVE		
raw chopped	½ cup	4
ENERGY BARS		
(*see* BREAKFAST BARS, CEREAL BARS, GRANOLA BARS, NUTRITION SUPPLEMENTS)		
ENGLISH MUFFIN		
FROZEN		
Weight Watchers		
Sandwich	1 (4 oz)	210
READY-TO-EAT		
apple cinnamon	1	138
granola	1	155
mixed grain	1	155
plain	1	134
plain toasted	1	133
raisin cinnamon	1	138
sourdough	1	134
wheat	1	127
whole wheat	1	134
Arnold		
Extra Crisp	l	130
Sourdough	1	130
Roman Meal		
English Muffin	1 (2.2 oz)	135
Wonder		
Cinnamon Raisin	1 (2.1 oz)	140
Original	1 (2 oz)	130
Sourdough	1 (2 oz)	130
REFRIGERATED		
Roman Meal		
English Muffin	½ muffin (1.1 oz)	66
Honey Nut Oat Bran	½ muffin (1.1 oz)	81
TAKE-OUT		
w/ butter	1 (2.2 oz)	189
w/ cheese & sausage	1 (4 oz)	393
w/ egg cheese & canadian bacon	1 (4.8 oz)	289
w/ egg cheese & sausage	1 (5.8 oz)	487
EPAZOTE		
fresh	1 tbsp (1 g)	tr
fresh sprig	1 (2 g)	1
EPPAW		
raw	½ cup	75

FOOD	PORTION	CALS.

FALAFEL
Casbah
as prep	5	130
Near East		
As Prep	2½ patties	230
TAKE-OUT		
falafel	1 (1.2 oz)	57

FAST FOODS
(*see individual names in Part Two*)

FAT
(*see also* BUTTER, BUTTER BLENDS, BUTTER SUBSTITUTES, MARGARINE, OIL)

chicken	1 cup	1846
chicken	1 tbsp	115
cocoa butter	1 tbsp	120
lard	1 cup (205 g)	1849
lard	1 tbsp (13 g)	115
pork backfat	1 oz	230
pork cooked	1 oz	178
shortening	1 tbsp	113
shortening	1 cup	1812
Crisco		
Butter Flavor	1 tbsp	110
Shortening	1 tbsp	110
Shortening	1 tbsp (0.4 oz)	110
Sticks	1 tbsp (0.4 oz)	110
Sticks Butter Flavor	1 tbsp (0.4 oz)	110
Empire		
Chicken Fat Rendered	1 tbsp (0.5 oz)	120
Wesson		
Shortening	1 tbsp	100

FAT SUBSTITUTES
Soy Is Us
Fat Not! Organic	3 tbsp	66

FAVA BEANS
Progresso
Fava Beans	½ cup (4.6 oz)	110

FEIJOA
fresh	1 (1.75 oz)	25

FENNEL
fresh bulb	1 (8.2 oz)	72

FOOD	PORTION	CALS.
fresh sliced	1 cup	27
leaves	3.5 oz	24
seed	1 tsp	7

FENUGREEK
seed	1 tsp	12

FIBER
Delta
Natural Fiber	½ cup (1 oz)	20

FIDDLEHEAD FERNS
fresh	3.5 oz	34

FIGS
CANNED
in heavy syrup	3	75
in light syrup	3	58
water pack	3	42

DRIED
California	½ cup (3.5 oz)	200
cooked	½ cup	140
whole	10	477

Sonoma
White Misson	3-4 (1.4 oz)	110

FRESH
fig	1 med	50

FIREWEED
leaves chopped	1 cup (0.8 oz)	24

FISH
(*see also individual fish names,* FISH SUBSTITUTES, SUSHI)

CANNED
Holmes
Finest Kippered Snacks drained	1 can (3.2 oz)	135

Port Clyde
Fish Steaks In Louisiana Hot Sauce	1 can (3.75 oz)	150
Fish Steaks In Mustard Sauce	1 can (3.75 oz)	140
Fish Steaks In Soybean Oil With Hot Chilies drained	1 can (3.3 oz)	155
Fish Steaks In Soybean Oil drained	1 can (3.3 oz)	220

FROZEN
Cajun Cookin'
Seafood Gumbo	17 oz	330

Gorton's
Crispy Batter Dipped Fillets	2	290

FOOD	PORTION	CALS.
Gorton's (CONT.)		
Crispy Batter Sticks	4	260
Crunch Fillets	2	230
Crunchy Sticks	4	210
Grilled Fillets Cajun Blackened	1 piece (3.8 oz)	120
Light Recipe Lightly Breaded Fish Fillets	1 fillet	180
Light Recipe Tempura Fillets	1 fillet	200
Microwave Crispy Batter Large Cut Fillets	1	320
Microwave Entree Fillets In Herb Butter	1 pkg	190
Microwave Fillets	2	340
Microwave Larger Cut Fillets	1	320
Microwave Larger Cut Ranch Fillet	1	330
Microwave Sticks	6	340
Potato Crisp Fillets	2	300
Potato Crisp Sticks	4	260
Value Pack Portions	1 portion	180
Value Pack Sticks	4	190
Kineret		
Fish Sticks	5 pieces (4 oz)	280
Van De Kamp's		
Battered Fish Fillets	1 (2.6 oz)	180
Battered Fish Nuggets	8 (4 oz)	280
Battered Fish Portions	2 pieces (5 oz)	350
Battered Fish Sticks	6 (4 oz)	260
Breaded Fillets	2 (3.5 oz)	280
Breaded Fish Portions	3 pieces (4.5 oz)	330
Breaded Fish Sticks	6 (4 oz)	290
Breaded Mini Fish Sticks	13 (3.3 oz)	250
Crisp & Healthy Breaded Fillets	2 (3.5 oz)	150
Crisp & Healthy Fish Sticks	6 (4 oz)	180
Fish 'n Fries	1 pkg (6.6 oz)	380
TAKE-OUT		
fish cake	1 (4.7 oz)	166
jamaican brown fish stew	1 serv	426
mousse	1 serv (3.5 oz)	185
stew	1 cup (7.9 oz)	157

FISH SUBSTITUTES

Loma Linda		
Ocean Platter not prep	⅓ cup (0.9 oz)	90
Worthington		
Fillets	2 (3 oz)	180
Tuno	½ cup (1.9 oz)	80

FLAXSEED

Arrowhead		
Flaxseed	3 tbsp (1 oz)	140

FOOD	PORTION	CALS.
Stone-Buhr		
Flaxseed	1 tsp (1 oz)	150
FLOUNDER		
FRESH		
cooked	3 oz	99
FROZEN		
Gorton's		
Fishmarket Fresh	5 oz	110
Microwave Entree Stuffed	1 pkg	350
Van De Kamp's		
Lightly Breaded Fillets	1 (4 oz)	230
Natural Fillets	1 (4 oz)	110
FLOUR		
buckwheat whole groat	1 cup (4.2 oz)	402
corn masa	1 cup (4 oz)	416
rice brown	1 cup (5.5 oz)	574
rice white	1 cup (5.5 oz)	578
rye dark	1 cup (4.5 oz)	415
rye light	1 cup (3.6 oz)	374
rye medium	1 cup (3.6 oz)	361
triticale whole grain	1 cup (4.6 oz)	439
white all-purpose	1 cup (4.4 oz)	455
white bread	1 cup (4.8 oz)	495
white cake unsifted	1 cup (4.8 oz)	496
white self-rising	1 cup (4.4 oz)	443
white unbleached	1 cup (4.4 oz)	455
whole wheat	1 cup (4.2 oz)	407
All Trump		
Flour	¼ cup (1 oz)	100
Arrowhead		
Kamut	¼ cup (1.2 oz)	110
Pastry	⅓ cup (1.1 oz)	100
Rye Whole Grain	¼ cup (1.6 oz)	160
Spelt	¼ cup (1.2 oz)	100
Teff	¼ cup (1.4 oz)	140
Unbleached White	⅓ cup (1.6 oz)	160
Whole Grain Wheat	¼ cup (1.6 oz)	160
Whole Wheat	¼ cup (1.2 oz)	130
Aunt Jemima		
Self-Rising	3 tbsp	90
General Mills		
Wondra	¼ cup (1 oz)	100

FOOD	PORTION	CALS.
Gold Medal		
All Purpose	¼ cup (1 oz)	100
Better For Bread	¼ cup (1 oz)	100
Better For Bread Wheat Blend	¼ cup (1 oz)	110
Self Rising	¼ cup (1 oz)	100
Supreme Hygluten	¼ cup (1 oz)	100
Unbleached	¼ cup (1 oz)	100
Hodgson Mill		
50/50 Flour	¼ cup (1 oz)	100
Best For Bread	¼ cup (1 oz)	100
Buckwheat	⅓ cup (1.6 oz)	160
Oat Bran Blend	¼ cup (1 oz)	110
Oat Bran Flour	¼ cup (1 oz)	110
Rye	¼ cup (1 oz)	90
Seasoned Flour	¼ cup (1 oz)	90
White	¼ cup (1 oz)	100
Whole Wheat	¼ cup (1 oz)	100
King Arthur		
All Purpose Unbleached	¼ cup (1 oz)	100
La Pina		
Flour	¼ cup (1 oz)	100
Red Band		
All Purpose	¼ cup (1 oz)	100
Bread	¼ cup (1 oz)	100
Self-Rising	¼ cup (1 oz)	100
Robin Hood		
All Purpose	¼ cup (1 oz)	100
Self-Rising	¼ cup (1 oz)	100
Unbleached	¼ cup (1 oz)	100
Whole Wheat	¼ cup (1 oz)	90
Stone Ground Mills		
White Unbleached Organic	¼ cup (1.4 oz)	130
Whole Wheat 100% Stone Ground	3 tbsp (1 oz)	90

FRANKFURTER
(*see* HOT DOG)

FRENCH FRIES
(*see* POTATOES)

FRENCH TOAST
FROZEN

french toast	1 slice (2 oz)	126
Aunt Jemima		
Cinnamon Swirl	2 pieces (4.1 oz)	240

FOOD	PORTION	CALS.
Aunt Jemima (CONT.)		
Slices	2 pieces (4.1 oz)	240
Downyflake		
Extra Thick	1	150
French Toast	2 slices	270
Texas Style & Sausage	1 pkg (4.25 oz)	400
Quaker		
French Toast Sticks & Syrup	1 pkg (5.2 oz)	400
French Toast Wedges & Sausage	1 pkg (5.3 oz)	360
HOME RECIPE		
as prep w/ 2% milk	1 slice	149
as prep w/ whole milk	1 slice	151
TAKE-OUT		
sticks	5 (4.9 oz)	513
w/ butter	2 slices (4.7 oz)	356

FROSTING
(*see* CAKE ICING)

FRUCTOSE
Estee

Fructose	1 tsp	15
Packet	1 pkg	10

FRUIT DRINKS
(*see also individual fruit juice names,* LEMONADE)

FROZEN

Bright & Early		
Fruit Punch	8 fl oz	130
Five Alive		
Berry Citrus	8 fl oz	120
Citrus	8 fl oz	120
Tropical Citrus	8 fl oz	120
Minute Maid		
Berry Punch	8 fl oz	130
Citrus Punch	8 fl oz	120
Fruit Punch	8 fl oz	120
Limeade	8 fl oz	100
Pineapple Orange	8 fl oz	120
Tropical Punch	8 fl oz	120
Seneca		
Cranberry-Apple Juice Cocktail frzn as prep	8 fl oz	140
Raspberry-Cranberry Juice Cocktail frzn as prep	8 fl oz	140

MIX

Crystal Light		
Fruit Punch as prep	1 serv (8 oz)	5

FOOD	PORTION	CALS.
Crystal Light (CONT.)		
Lemon-Lime Drink as prep	1 serv (8 oz)	5
Passion Fruit Pineapple Drink as prep	1 serv (8 oz)	5
Pineapple Orange Drink as prep	1 serv (8 oz)	5
Strawberry Orange Banana as prep	1 serv (8 oz)	5
Strawberry Kiwi as prep	1 serv (8 oz)	5
Watermelon Strawberry as prep	1 serv (8 oz)	5
Kool-Aid		
Cherry as prep	1 serv (8 oz)	60
Grape Berry Splash Drink as prep	1 serv (8 oz)	70
Grape Berry Splash Drink as prep w/ sugar	1 serv (8 oz)	100
Kickin' Kiwi Lime Drink as prep	1 serv (8 oz)	60
Kickin' Kiwi Lime Drink as prep w/ sugar	1 serv (8 oz)	100
Lemon-Lime Drink as prep w/ sugar	1 serv (8 oz)	100
Man-O-Mango Berry Drink as prep w/ sugar	1 serv (8 oz)	100
Mon-O-Mango Berry Drink as prep	1 serv (8 oz)	60
Oh Yeah Orange Pineapple Drink as prep w/ sugar	1 serv (8 oz)	100
Oh Yeah Orange Pineapple Drink as prep	1 serv (8 oz)	60
Pina-Pineapple Drink as prep	1 serv (8 oz)	60
Pina-Pineapple Drink as prep w/ sugar	1 serv (8 oz)	100
Rainbow Punch	8 oz	98
Roarin' Raspberry Cranberry Drink as prep	1 serv (8 oz)	70
Roarin' Raspberry Cranberry Drink as prep w/ sugar	1 serv (8 oz)	100
Slammin' Strawberry Kiwi Drink as prep	1 serv (8 oz)	70
Slammin' Strawberry Kiwi Drink as prep w/ sugar	1 serv (8 oz)	100
Strawberry Raspberry Drink as prep	1 serv (8 oz)	60
Strawberry Raspberry Drink as prep w/ sugar	1 serv (8 oz)	100
Sugar Free Tropical Punch as prep	1 serv (8 oz)	5
Tropical Punch as prep	1 serv (8 oz)	60
Tropical Punch as prep w/ sugar	1 serv (8 oz)	100
Watermelon Cherry Drink as prep	1 serv (8 oz)	60
Watermelon Cherry Drink as prep w/ sugar	1 serv (8 oz)	100
Tang		
Orange Pineapple as prep	1 serv (8 oz)	100
READY-TO-DRINK		
After The Fall		
Amaretto Almond	1 can (12 oz)	170
American Pie Cherry	1 can (12 oz)	190
Apple Apricot	1 cup (8 oz)	100

FOOD	PORTION	CALS.
After The Fall (CONT.)		
Apple Raspberry	1 bottle (10 oz)	110
Apple Strawberry	1 bottle (10 oz)	120
Banana Casablanca	1 bottle (10 oz)	120
Berrymeister	1 can (12 oz)	160
Cranberry Meets Raspberry	1 bottle (10 oz)	120
Georgia Peach Blend	1 bottle (10 oz)	130
Mango Montage	1 bottle (10 oz)	140
Maui Grove	1 bottle (10 oz)	120
Nantucket Ginger Ale	1 can (12 oz)	140
Orange Icicle Cream	1 can (12 oz)	170
Oregon Berry	1 bottle (10 oz)	130
Passion Of The Islands	1 bottle (10 oz)	125
Peach Vanilla	1 can (12 oz)	170
Strawberry Vanilla	1 can (12 oz)	160
Twist O' Strawberry	1 can (12 oz)	190
Vanilla Bean Cream	1 can (12 oz)	170
Apple & Eve		
Apple Cranberry	6 fl oz	80
Apple Grape	6 fl oz	120
Cranberry Grape	6 fl oz	100
Fruit Punch	6 fl oz	78
Raspberry Cranberry	6 fl oz	90
BAMA		
Fruit Punch	8.45 fl oz	130
Boku		
White Grape Raspberry	16 fl oz	120
Capri Sun		
Fruit Punch	1 pkg (7 oz)	100
Maui Punch	1 pkg (7 oz)	100
Mountain Cooler	1 pkg (7 oz)	90
Pacific Cooler	1 pkg (7 oz)	100
Red Berry	1 pkg (7 oz)	100
Safari Punch	1 pkg (7 oz)	100
Strawberry Kiwi Drink	1 pkg (7 oz)	100
Surfer Cooler Drink	1 pkg (7 oz)	100
Coco Lopez		
Mango Kiwi	8 fl oz	130
Crystal Geyser		
Juice Squeeze Citrus Grape	1 bottle (12 fl oz)	145
Juice Squeeze Orange & Passion Fruit	1 bottle (12 fl oz)	130
Juice Squeeze Passion Fruit & Mango	1 bottle (12 fl oz)	125
Juice Squeeze Wild Berry	1 bottle (12 fl oz)	130

FOOD	PORTION	CALS.
Crystal Light		
Fruit Punch	1 serv (8 oz)	5
Kiwi Strawberry	1 serv (8 oz)	5
Orange Strawberry Banana Drink	1 serv (8 oz)	5
Dole		
Cranberry Apple	8 fl oz	120
Fruit Fiesta	8 fl oz	140
Fruit Punch	1 carton (10 oz)	160
Mountain Cherry	8 fl oz	150
Orange Peach Mango	8 oz	120
Orange Strawberry Banana	8 oz	120
Orchard Peach	8 oz	140
Pineapple Orange	8 oz	120
Pineapple Orange Strawberry	8 oz	130
Tropical Fruit	8 oz	160
Everfresh		
Cranberry-Apple Drink	1 can (8 oz)	120
Grape-Strawberry	1 can (8 oz)	120
Kiwi-Strawberry	1 can (8 oz)	120
Mandarin Orange Mango Drink	1 can (8 oz)	120
Orange Banana Strawberry Drink	1 can (8 oz)	120
Tropical Fruit Punch	1 can (8 oz)	120
Wild Blackberry Lime Drink	1 can (8 oz)	120
Five Alive		
Citrus	6 fl oz	90
Citrus	1 bottle (16 fl oz)	120
Citrus	1 can (11.5 fl oz)	170
Citrus Chilled	8 fl oz	120
Fresh Samantha		
Banana Strawberry	1 cup (8 oz)	148
Beta Yet	1 cup (8 oz)	98
Carrot Orange	1 cup (8 oz)	107
Colossal C	1 cup (8 oz)	116
Desperately Seeking C	1 cup (8 oz)	129
Protein Blast	1 cup (8 oz)	156
Spirulina Fruit Blend	1 cup (8 oz)	129
Strawberry Orange	1 cup (8 oz)	120
The Big Bang	1 cup (8 oz)	97
Fruitopia		
Fruit Integration	8 fl oz	110
Hi-C		
Boppin Berry Box	8.45 fl oz	140
Boppin' Berry	8 fl oz	130
Double Fruit Box	8.45 fl oz	130

FOOD	PORTION	CALS.
Hi-C (CONT.)		
Double Fruit Cooler	8 fl oz	130
Ecto Cooler	8 fl oz	130
Ecto Cooler	1 can (11.5 fl oz)	180
Ecto Cooler Box	8.45 fl oz	130
Fruit Punch	8 fl oz	130
Fruit Punch	1 can (11.5 fl oz)	190
Fruit Punch Box	8.45 fl oz	140
Fruity Bubble Gum	8 fl oz	120
Fruity Bubble Gum Box	8.45 fl oz	130
Hula Punch	8 fl oz	120
Hula Punch	1 can (11.5 fl oz)	170
Hula Punch Box	8.45 fl oz	120
Jammin' Apple Box	8.45 fl oz	130
Stompin' Banana Berry	8 fl oz	130
Stompin' Banana Berry Box	8.45 fl oz	130
Wild Berry	8 fl oz	120
Wild Berry Box	8.45 fl oz	130
Hood		
Natural Blenders Apple Cranberry Raspberry	1 cup (8 oz)	130
Natural Blenders Apple Grape Cherry	1 cup (8 oz)	130
Natural Blenders Apple Peach Pear	1 cup (8 oz)	120
Natural Blenders Apple Wild Blueberry Strawberry	1 cup (8 oz)	120
Natural Blenders Pineapple Orange Kiwi	1 cup (8 oz)	120
Juicy Juice		
Apple Grape	1 box (8.45 fl oz)	120
Berry	1 bottle (6 fl oz)	90
Berry	1 box (8.45 fl oz)	130
Punch	1 box (8.45 fl oz)	140
Punch	1 bottle (6 fl oz)	100
Tropical	1 box (8.45 fl oz)	150
Tropical	1 bottle (6 fl oz)	110
Kern's		
Apple Strawberry Nectar	6 fl oz	110
Apricot Pineapple Nectar	6 fl oz	110
Banana Pineapple Nectar	6 fl oz	110
Coconut Pineapple Nectar	6 fl oz	140
Orange Banana Nectar	6 fl oz	110
Strawberry Banana Nectar	6 fl oz	110
Tropical Nectar	6 fl oz	110
Kool-Aid		
Bursts Great Bluedini	1 (7 oz)	100

FOOD	PORTION	CALS.
Kool-Aid (CONT.)		
Bursts Kickin' Kiwi Lime	1 (7 oz)	100
Bursts Oh Yeah Orange Pineapple	1 (7 oz)	100
Bursts Slammin' Strawberry Kiwi	1 (7 oz)	100
Bursts Tropical Punch	1 (7 oz)	100
Splash Grape Berry Punch	1 serv (8 oz)	120
Splash Kiwi Strawberry Drink	1 serv (8 oz)	110
Splash Tropical Punch	1 serv (8 oz)	120
Libby		
Strawberry Banana Nectar	1 can (11.5 fl oz)	220
Mauna La'i		
Island Guava Hawaiian Guava Fruit Juice Drink	8 fl oz	130
Mango & Hawaiian Guava Fruit Juice Drink	8 fl oz	130
Paradise Guava Hawaiian Guava & Passion Fruit Juice Drink	8 fl oz	130
Minute Maid		
Berry Punch Box	8.45 fl oz	130
Berry Punch Chilled	8 fl oz	130
Citrus Punch Chilled	8 fl oz	130
Fruit Punch Box	8.45 fl oz	120
Fruit Punch Chilled	8 fl oz	120
Juices To Go Citrus Punch	1 can (11.5 fl oz)	180
Juices To Go Citrus Punch	1 bottle (10 fl oz)	160
Juices To Go Concord Punch	1 can (11.5 fl oz)	180
Juices To Go Concord Punch	1 bottle (10 fl oz)	160
Juices To Go Concord Punch	1 bottle (16 fl oz)	130
Juices To Go Fruit Punch	1 can (11.5 fl oz)	180
Juices To Go Fruit Punch	1 bottle (10 fl oz)	160
Juices To Go Fruit Punch	1 bottle (16 fl oz)	120
Juices To Go Orange Blend	1 bottle (10 fl oz)	150
Juices To Go Orange Blend	1 can (11.5 fl oz)	170
Naturals Apple Cranberry	8 fl oz	170
Naturals Concord Medley	8 fl oz	130
Naturals Fruit Medley	8 fl oz	120
Naturals Orange Grape Medley	8 fl oz	120
Naturals Tropical Medley	8 fl oz	120
Tropical Punch Box	8.45 fl oz	130
Tropical Punch Chilled	8 fl oz	120
Mott's		
Apple Cranberry Blend	10 fl oz	180
Apple Cranberry From Concentrate as prep	8 fl oz	120
Apple Grape From Concentrate as prep	8 fl oz	120
Apple Raspberry Blend	10 fl oz	140

FOOD	PORTION	CALS.
Mott's (CONT.)		
Apple Raspberry From Concentrate	8.45 fl oz	120
Fruit Basket Apple Raspberry Juice Cocktail as prep	8 fl oz	130
Fruit Basket Tropical Blend Juice Cocktail as prep	8 fl oz	120
Fruit Punch From Concentrate	10 fl oz	170
Fruit Punch From Concentrate	8.45 fl oz	120
Grape Apple	10 fl oz	170
Pineapple Orange	10 fl oz	170
Nantucket Nectars		
Orange Mango	8 fl oz	130
Ocean Spray		
Cran*Grape	8 fl oz	170
Cran*Raspberry	8 fl oz	140
Cran*Strawberry	8 fl oz	140
Cranapple	8 fl oz	160
Cranapple Reduced Calorie	8 fl oz	50
Fruit Punch	8 fl oz	130
Kiwi Strawberry Cooler	8 fl oz	120
Ruby Red & Tangerine Grapefruit Juice Drink	8 fl oz	130
Odwalla		
Boyzenberry Mango	8 fl oz	140
C Monster	16 fl oz	300
Fruitshake Blackberry	8 fl oz	160
Guanaba Dabba Doo!	8 fl oz	130
Lotta Colada	8 fl oz	160
Mango Tango	8 fl oz	150
Mo Beta	16 fl oz	280
Raspberry Smoothie	8 fl oz	140
Strawberry Banana Smoothie	8 fl oz	100
Strawberry Go Man Go	8 fl oz	100
Super Protein	16 fl oz	400
Pek		
Mango Guava Ecstasy	1 bottle (20 fl oz)	110
Passionate Peach Grapefruit	8 fl oz	110
Shasta Plus		
Apple-Strawberry	1 can (11.5 oz)	160
Fruit Punch	1 can (11.5 oz)	160
Pineapple-Cherry	1 can (11.5 oz)	160
Snapple		
Diet Kiwi Strawberry	8 fl oz	13
Fruit Punch	8 fl oz	120

FOOD	PORTION	CALS.
Snapple (CONT.)		
Kiwi Strawberry Cocktail	8 fl oz	130
Melonberry Cocktail	8 fl oz	120
Vitamin Supreme	10 fl oz	150
Squeezit		
Berry B. Wild	1 bottle (7 oz)	110
Blue Raspberry	1 bottle (7 oz)	110
Cherry Cola	1 bottle (7 oz)	110
Chucklin' Cherry	1 bottle (7 oz)	110
Green Apple	1 bottle (7 oz)	110
Grumpy Grape	1 bottle (7 oz)	110
Lemon Lime	1 bottle (7 oz)	110
Rockin' Red Puncher	1 bottle (7 oz)	110
Smarty Arty Orange	1 bottle (7 oz)	110
Strawberry	1 bottle (7 oz)	110
Tropical Punch	1 bottle (7 oz)	110
Watermelon	1 bottle (7 oz)	110
Tropicana		
Berry Punch	8 fl oz	130
Citrus Punch	8 fl oz	140
Fruit Punch	8 oz	130
Fruit Punch	1 container (10 fl oz)	160
Orange Pineapple	8 fl oz	110
Tangerine Orange Juice	8 fl oz	110
Tropics Orange Strawberry Banana	8 fl oz	110
Tropics Orange Kiwi Passion	8 fl oz	100
Tropics Orange Peach Mango	8 fl oz	110
Tropics Orange Pineapple	8 fl oz	110
Twister Apple Raspberry Blackberry	1 bottle (10 fl oz)	160
Twister Citrus Punch	1 bottle (10 oz)	180
Twister Cranberry Punch	1 bottle (10 oz)	170
Twister Fruit Punch	1 bottle (10 oz)	170
Twister Light Orange Strawberry Banana	1 bottle (10 oz)	45
Twister Orange Cranberry	1 bottle (10 fl oz)	160
Twister Orange Strawberry Banana	1 bottle (10 oz)	160
Twister Ruby Red Tangerine	1 bottle (10 oz)	160
Twister Strawberry Kiwi	1 bottle (10 oz)	160
Veryfine		
Apple Cherryberry	8 fl oz	130
Apple Cranberry	1 bottle (10 oz)	190
Apple Quenchers Black Cherry White Grape	8 fl oz	120
Apple Quenchers Cranberry Tangerine	8 fl oz	120
Apple Quenchers Peach Kiwi	8 fl oz	130

FOOD	PORTION	CALS.
Veryfine (CONT.)		
Apple Quenchers Peach Plum	8 fl oz	130
Apple Quenchers Pear Passionfruit	8 fl oz	120
Apple Quenchers Raspberry Cherry	8 fl oz	120
Apple Quenchers Raspberry Lime	8 fl oz	120
Apple Quenchers Strawberry Banana	8 fl oz	120
Chillers Arctic Mango Tangerine	8 fl oz	110
Chillers Freezing Fruit Punch	8 fl oz	130
Chillers Lemon Lime Blizzard	8 fl oz	120
Chillers Shivering Strawberry Melon	1 can (11.5 oz)	160
Chillers Tropical Freeze	8 fl oz	120
Cranberry Raspberry	8 fl oz	160
Fruit Punch	1 bottle (10 oz)	170
Juice-Ups Berry	8 fl oz	140
Juice-Ups Fruit Punch	8 fl oz	140
Juice-Ups Orange Punch	8 fl oz	140
Orange Strawberry	8 fl oz	120
Papaya Punch	1 bottle (10 oz)	160
Pineapple Orange	1 bottle (10 oz)	160
Strawberry Banana	1 can (1l.5 oz)	160
Strawberry Banana Punch	1 can (11.5 oz)	190

FRUIT MIXED
(see also individual fruit names)

CANNED

fruit cocktail in heavy syrup	½ cup	93
fruit cocktail juice pack	½ cup	56
fruit cocktail water pack	½ cup	40
fruit salad in heavy syrup	½ cup	94
fruit salad in light syrup	½ cup	73
fruit salad juice pack	½ cup	62
fruit salad water pack	½ cup	37
tropical fruit salad in heavy syrup	½ cup	110
Del Monte		
Fruit Cocktail Fruit Naturals	½ cup (4.4 oz)	60
Fruit Cocktail In Heavy Syrup	½ cup (4.5 oz)	100
Fruit Cocktail Lite	½ cup (4.4 oz)	60
Lite Mixed Fruits Chunky	½ cup (4.4 oz)	60
Mixed Fruits Chunky Fruit Naturals	½ cup (4.4 oz)	60
Mixed Fruits Chunky In Heavy Syrup	½ cup (4.5 oz)	100
Orchard Select California Mixed	½ cup (4.4 oz)	80
Snack Cups Mixed Fruit Fruit Naturals	1 serv (4.5 oz)	60
Snack Cups Mixed Fruit Fruit Naturals EZ-Open Lid	1 serv (4.5 oz)	60

FOOD	PORTION	CALS.
Del Monte (CONT.)		
Snack Cups Mixed Fruit In Heavy Syrup	1 serv (4.5 oz)	100
Snack Cups Mixed Fruit In Heavy Syrup EZ-Open Lid	1 serv (4.2 oz)	90
Snack Cups Mixed Fruit Lite	1 serv (4.5 oz)	60
Snack Cups Mixed Fruit Lite EZ-Open Lid	1 serv (4.5 oz)	60
Dole		
Tropical Fruit Salad	½ cup	70
Hunt's		
Fruit Cocktail	½ cup (4.5 oz)	90
Libby		
Chunky Mixed Lite	½ cup (4.3 oz)	60
Fruit Cocktail Lite	½ cup (4.3 oz)	60
Mott's		
Fruitsations Mixed Berry	1 pkg (4 oz)	90
DRIED		
Del Monte		
Mixed	⅓ cup (1.4 oz)	110
Planters		
Fruit'n Nut Mix	1 oz	140
Sonoma		
Diced	⅓ cup (1.4 oz)	120
Mixed Fruit	5-8 pieces (1.4 oz)	120
FROZEN		
Big Valley		
Burst O' Berries	⅔ cup (4.9 oz)	70
California Tropics	⅔ cup (4.9 oz)	60
Cup A Fruit	1 pkg (4 oz)	50
Mixed	4.9 oz	60
Birds Eye		
Mixed Fruit	½ cup (4.4 oz)	90
FRUIT SNACKS		
fruit leather	1 bar (0.8 oz)	81
fruit leather pieces	1 oz	97
fruit leather pieces	1 pkg (0.9 oz)	92
fruit leather rolls	1 lg (0.7 oz)	73
fruit leather rolls	1 sm (0.5 oz)	49
Brock		
Beauty & The Beast	1 pkg (0.9 oz)	90
Cinderella	1 pkg (0.9 oz)	90
Dinosaurs	1 pkg (0.9 oz)	90
Ninja Trolls	1 pkg (0.9 oz)	90
Sharks	1 pkg (0.9 oz)	90

FOOD	PORTION	CALS.
Del Monte		
Sierra Trail Mix	¼ cup (1.2 oz)	150
Sierra Trail Mix	1 pkg (1 oz)	120
Sierra Trail Mix	1 pkg (0.9 oz)	110
Favorite Brands		
Cherry Fruit Snack	1 pkg (0.9 oz)	80
Creepy Crawler Fruit Snacks	1 pkg (0.9 oz)	80
Dinosaur Fruit Snack	1 pkg (0.9 oz)	80
Grape Fruit Snack	1 pkg (0.9 oz)	80
Space Alien Fruit Snack	1 pkg (0.9 oz)	80
Sports Fruit Snacks	1 pkg (0.9 oz)	80
Strawberry Fruit Snack	1 pkg (0.9 oz)	80
Teenage Mutant Ninja Turtle Fruit Snacks	1 pkg (0.9 oz)	80
The Mega Roll Strawberry	1 pkg (1 oz)	110
The Roll Cherry	1 pkg (0.75 oz)	80
The Roll Strawberry	1 pkg (0.75 oz)	80
Troll Fruit Snacks	1 pkg (0.9 oz)	80
Zoo Animal Fruit Snacks	1 pkg (0.9 oz)	80
General Mills		
Fruit Snacks All Flavors	1 pkg (0.9 oz)	80
Health Valley		
Bakes Apple	1 bar	70
Bakes Date	1 bar	70
Bakes Raisin	1 bar	70
Fruit Bars Apple	1	140
Fruit Bars Apricot	1	140
Fruit Bars Raisin	1	140
Seneca		
Apple Chips	12 chips (1 oz)	140
Sensible Foods		
Crackin' Fruit Cherry Berry	1 pkg (0.6 oz)	51
Crackin' Fruit Tropical Fruit	1 pkg (0.6 oz)	65
Sonoma		
Trail Mix	¼ cup (1.4 oz)	160
Sovex		
Fruit Bites Jungle Pals	1 pkg (0.9 oz)	90
Stretch Island		
Fruit Leather Berry Blackberry	2 pieces (1 oz)	90
Fruit Leather Chunky Cherry	2 pieces (1 oz)	90
Fruit Leather Great Grape	2 pieces (1 oz)	90
Fruit Leather Organic Apple	2 pieces (1 oz)	90
Fruit Leather Organic Grape	2 pieces (1 oz)	90
Fruit Leather Organic Raspberry	2 pieces (1 oz)	90
Fruit Leather Rare Raspberry	2 pieces (1 oz)	90

FOOD	PORTION	CALS.
Stretch Island (CONT.)		
Fruit Leather Snappy Apple	2 pieces (1 oz)	90
Fruit Leather Tangy Apricot	2 pieces (1 oz)	90
Fruit Leather Truly Tropical	2 pieces (1 oz)	90
Sunbelt		
Fruit Boosters Apple	1 (1.3 oz)	130
Fruit Boosters Blueberry	1 (1.3 oz)	130
Fruit Boosters Strawberry	1 (1.3 oz)	130
Fruit Jammers	1 (1 oz)	100
Weight Watchers		
Apple & Cinnamon	1 pkg (0.5 oz)	50
Apple Chips	1 pkg (0.75 oz)	70
Peach & Strawberry	1 pkg (0.5 oz)	50

GARBANZO
(*see* CHICKPEAS)

GARLIC
clove	1	4
powder	1 tsp	9
Watkins		
Garlic & Chive Seasoning	1 tbsp (7 g)	25
Garlic Lover's Herb Blend	¼ tsp (0.5 oz)	0
Liquid Spice	1 tbsp (0.5 oz)	120

GEFILTE FISH
sweet	1 piece (1.5 oz)	35

GELATIN
MIX
low calorie	½ cup	8
mix as prep	½ cup (4.7 oz)	80
mix as prep	1 pkg 4 serv (19 oz)	319
mix not prep	1 pkg (3 oz)	324
mix w/ fruit as prep	½ cup (3.7 oz)	73
mix w/ fruit as prep	1 pkg 8 serv (19 oz)	588
powder unsweetened	1 pkg (7 g)	23
powder unsweetened	1 oz	94
Emes		
Kosher-Jel	½ cup (4 fl oz)	60
Kosher-Jel Plain	1 tbsp (7 g)	21
Jell-O		
1-2-3-Brand Strawberry as prep	⅔ cup (5.2 oz)	130
Apricot as prep	½ cup (5 oz)	80
Berry Black as prep	½ cup (5 oz)	80
Berry Blue as prep	½ cup (5 oz)	80

FOOD	PORTION	CALS.
Jell-O (CONT.)		
Black Cherry as prep	½ cup (5 oz)	80
Cherry as prep	½ cup (5 oz)	80
Cranberry Raspberry as prep	½ cup (5 oz)	80
Cranberry Strawberry as prep	½ cup (5 oz)	80
Cranberry as prep	½ cup (5 oz)	80
Grape as prep	½ cup (5 oz)	80
Lemon as prep	½ cup (5 oz)	80
Lime as prep	½ cup (5 oz)	80
Mango as prep	½ cup (5 oz)	80
Mixed Fruit as prep	½ cup (5 oz)	80
Orange as prep	½ cup (5 oz)	80
Peach as prep	½ cup (5 oz)	80
Peach Passion Fruit as prep	½ cup (5 oz)	80
Pineapple as prep	½ cup (5 oz)	80
Raspberry as prep	½ cup (5 oz)	80
Sparkling White Grape as prep	½ cup (5 oz)	80
Strawberry Banana as prep	½ cup (5 oz)	80
Strawberry Kiwi as prep	½ cup (5 oz)	80
Strawberry as prep	½ cup (5 oz)	80
Sugar Free Cherry as prep	½ cup (4.2 oz)	10
Sugar Free Cranberry as prep	½ cup (4.2 oz)	10
Sugar Free Lemon	½ cup (4.2 oz)	10
Sugar Free Lime as prep	½ cup (4.2 oz)	10
Sugar Free Mixed Fruit as prep	½ cup (4.2 oz)	10
Sugar Free Orange as prep	½ cup (4.2 oz)	10
Sugar Free Raspberry as prep	½ cup (4.2 oz)	10
Sugar Free Strawberry Banana as prep	½ cup (4.2 oz)	10
Sugar Free Strawberry as prep	½ cup (4.2 oz)	10
Sugar Free Strawberry Kiwi as prep	½ cup (4.2 oz)	10
Sugar Free Watermelon as prep	½ cup (4.2 oz)	10
Watermelon as prep	½ cup (5 oz)	80
Wild Strawberry as prep	½ cup (5 oz)	80
Kojel		
Diet	1 serv	10
Royal		
Apple	½ cup	80
Blackberry	½ cup	80
Cherry	½ cup	80
Cherry Sugar Free	½ cup	8
Concord Grape	½ cup	80
Fruit Punch	½ cup	80
Lemon	½ cup	80
Lemon-Lime	½ cup	80

FOOD	PORTION	CALS.
Royal (CONT.)		
Lime	½ cup	80
Lime Sugar Free	½ cup	8
Mixed Berry	½ cup	80
Orange	½ cup	80
Orange Sugar Free	½ cup	10
Peach	½ cup	80
Pineapple	½ cup	80
Raspberry	½ cup	80
Raspberry Sugar Free	½ cup	8
Strawberry	½ cup	80
Strawberry Banana Sugar Free	½ cup	8
Strawberry Orange	½ cup	80
Strawberry Sugar Free	½ cup	8
Tropical Fruit	½ cup	80
READY-TO-EAT		
Del Monte		
Gel Snack Cups Blue Berry	1 serv (3.5 oz)	70
Gel Snack Cups Cherry	1 serv (3.5 oz)	70
Gel Snack Cups Orange	1 serv (3.5 oz)	70
Gel Snack Cups Strawberry	1 serv (3.5 oz)	70
Handi-Snacks		
Gels Blue Raspberry	1 serv (4 oz)	80
Gels Cherry	1 serv (4 oz)	80
Gels Orange	1 serv (3.5 oz)	80
Gels Strawberry	1 serv (3.5 oz)	80
Hunt's		
Snack Pack Juicy Gels Cherry	1 (4 oz)	100
Snack Pack Juicy Gels Lemon Lime	1 (4 oz)	100
Snack Pack Juicy Gels Mixed Fruit	1 (4 oz)	100
Snack Pack Juicy Gels Orange	1 (4 oz)	100
Snack Pack Juicy Gels Strawberry	1 (4 oz)	100
Jell-O		
Berry Black	1 serv (3.5 oz)	70
Berry Blue	1 serv (3.5 oz)	70
Cherry	1 serv (3.5 oz)	70
Orange	1 serv (3.5 oz)	70
Orange Strawberry Banana	1 serv (3.5 oz)	70
Raspberry	1 serv (3.5 oz)	70
Rhymin' Lymon	1 serv (3.5 oz)	70
Strawberry	1 serv (3.5 oz)	70
Strawberry Kiwi	1 serv (3.5 oz)	10
Sugar Free Orange	1 serv (3.2 oz)	10
Sugar Free Raspberry	1 serv (3.2 oz)	10

FOOD	PORTION	CALS.
Jell-O (CONT.)		
Sugar Free Strawberry	1 serv (3.2 oz)	10
Tropical Berry	1 serv (3.5 oz)	10
Tropical Fruit Punch	1 serv (3.5 oz)	70
Wild Watermelon	1 serv (3.5 oz)	70
Kozy Shack		
Gel Treat Cherry	1 pkg (4 oz)	100
Gel Treat Lemon Lime	1 pkg (4 oz)	100
Gel Treat Orange	1 pkg (4 oz)	100
Gel Treat Strawberry	1 pkg (4 oz)	100
Gel Treat Sugar Free Orange	1 pkg (4 oz)	10
Gel Treat Sugar Free Strawberry	1 pkg (4 oz)	10

GIBLETS

capon simmered	1 cup (5 oz)	238
chicken floured & fried	1 cup (5 oz)	402
chicken simmered	1 cup (5 oz)	228
turkey simmered	1 cup (5 oz)	243

GINGER

ground	1 tsp (1.8 g)	6
root fresh	¼ cup	17
root fresh	5 slices	8
root fresh sliced	¼ cup	17

GINKGO NUTS

canned	1 oz	32
dried	1 oz	99

GIZZARDS

chicken simmered	1 cup (5 oz)	222
turkey simmered	1 cup (5 oz)	236
Shady Brook		
Turkey	4 oz	130

GOAT

roasted	3 oz	122

GOOSE

w/ skin roasted	½ goose (1.7 lbs)	2362
w/ skin roasted	6.6 oz	574
w/o skin roasted	5 oz	340
w/o skin roasted	½ goose (1.3 lbs)	1406

GOOSEBERRIES

canned in light syrup	½ cup	93
fresh	1 cup	67

FOOD	PORTION	CALS.

GRANOLA BARS

(*see also* CEREAL BARS, NUTRITION SUPPLEMENTS)

FOOD	PORTION	CALS.
almond	1 (0.8 oz)	117
almond	1 (1 oz)	140
chewy chocolate coated chocolate chip	1 (1 oz)	132
chewy chocolate coated chocolate chip	1 (1.25 oz)	165
chewy chocolate coated peanut butter	1 (1 oz)	144
chewy chocolate coated peanut butter	1 (1.3 oz)	187
chewy raisin	1 (1 oz)	127
chewy raisin	1 (1.5 oz)	191
chocolate chip	1 (0.8 oz)	103
chocolate chip	1 (1 oz)	124
chocolate chip chewy	1 (1 oz)	119
chocolate chip chewy	1 (1.5 oz)	178
chocolate chip graham & marshmallow chewy	1 (1 oz)	121
nut & raisin chewy	1 (1 oz)	129
peanut	1 (1 oz)	136
peanut	1 (0.8 oz)	113
peanut butter	1 (0.8 oz)	114
peanut butter	1 (1 oz)	137
peanut butter chewy	1 (1 oz)	121
peanut butter & chocolate chip chewy	1 (1 oz)	122
plain	1 (1 oz)	134
plain	1 (0.9 oz)	115
plain chewy	1 (1 oz)	126
Carnation		
Chocolate Chunk	1 (1.26 oz)	140
Honey & Oats	1 (1.26 oz)	130
Fi-Bar		
Coconut	1	120
Peanut Butter	1	130
Grist Mill		
Chewy Apple Cinnamon	1 (1 oz)	120
Chewy Chocolate Chip	1 (1 oz)	130
Chewy Chunky Nut & Raisin	1 (1 oz)	130
Chewy Peanut Butter	1 (1 oz)	130
Chewy Peanut Butter Chocolate	1 (1 oz)	130
Chocolate Snack Chocolate Chip	1 (1.2 oz)	180
Chocolate Snack Nutty Fudge	1 (1.3 oz)	190
Crunchy Cinnamon	1 (0.8 oz)	110
Crunchy Oats 'N Honey	1 (0.8 oz)	110
Health Valley		
Blueberry	1	140

FOOD	PORTION	CALS.
Health Valley (CONT.)		
Chocolate Chip	1	140
Date Almond	1	140
Raisin	1	140
Raspberry	1	140
Strawberry	1	140
Kudos		
Chocolate Chunk	1 (0.7 oz)	90
Chocolate Coated Chocolate Chip	1 (1 oz)	120
Chocolate Coated Milk & Cookies	1 (1 oz)	130
Chocolate Coated Nutty Fudge	1 (1 oz)	130
Chocolate Coated Peanut Butter	1 (1 oz)	130
Low Fat Blueberry	1 (0.7 oz)	90
Low Fat Strawberry	1 (0.7 oz)	80
Nature Valley		
Crunchy Cinnamon	2 bars (1.6 oz)	200
Crunchy Oats'n Honey	2 bars (1.6 oz)	200
Crunchy Peanut Butter	2 bars (1.6 oz)	200
Low Fat Chewy Apple Brown Sugar	1 bar (1 oz)	110
Low Fat Chewy Chocolate Chip	1 bar (1 oz)	110
Low Fat Chewy Honey Nut	1 bar (1 oz)	110
Low Fat Chewy Oatmeal Raisin	1 bar (1 oz)	110
Low Fat Chewy Orchard Blend	1 bar (1 oz)	110
Low Fat Chewy Triple Berry	1 bar (1 oz)	110
Nature's Choice		
Carob Chip	1 bar (0.7 oz)	80
Cinnamon & Raisin	1 bar (0.7 oz)	80
Oats 'n Honey	1 bar (0.7 oz)	80
Peanut Butter	1 bar (0.7 oz)	80
Sunbelt		
Chewy Chocolate Chip	1 (1.25 oz)	160
Chewy Chocolate Chip	1 (1.8 oz)	220
Chewy Oats & Honey	1 (1 oz)	130
Chewy Oats & Honey	1 (1.7 oz)	210
Chewy With Almonds	1 (1 oz)	130
Chewy With Almonds	1 (1.5 oz)	190
Chewy With Raisins	1 (1.2 oz)	150
Fudge Dipped Chewy Chocolate Chip	1 (1.5 oz)	190
Fudge Dipped Chewy Macaroo	1 bar (2 oz)	280
Fudge Dipped Chewy Macaroo	1 (1.4 oz)	200
Fudge Dipped Chewy With Peanuts	1 bar (1.5 oz)	210
Fudge Dipped Chewy With Peanuts	1 (2 oz)	270
GRANOLA CEREAL		
(*see also* GRANOLA BARS)		
granola	½ cup (2.1 oz)	285

FOOD	PORTION	CALS.
Good Shepherd		
Crunchy	1 oz	130
Honey Almond	1 oz	120
Organic 5 Grain Muesli	1 oz	160
Organic Brown Rice	1 oz	130
Organic Wheat Free	1 oz	90
Organic Wheat Free Apple Cinnamon	1 oz	125
Organic Wheat Free Blueberry Amaranth	1 oz	110
Organic Wheat Free Strawberry Amaranth	1 oz	110
Grist Mill		
Low-Fat With Raisins	⅔ cup (1.9 oz)	220
Health Valley		
98% Fat Free Date Almond	⅔ cup	180
98% Fat Free Raisin Cinnamon	⅔ cup	180
98% Fat Free Tropical	⅔ cup	180
O's Almond	¾ cup	120
O's Apple Cinnamon	¾ cup	120
O's Honey Crunch	¾ cup	120
Kellogg's		
Low Fat	½ cup (1.7 oz)	190
Low Fat With Raisins	⅔ cup (2.1 oz)	220
Nature Valley		
Low Fat Fruit	⅔ cup (1.9 oz)	210
Stone-Buhr		
Hot Apple	⅓ cup (1.6 oz)	153
Sunbelt		
Banana Nut	1.9 oz	250
Fruit & Nut	1.9 oz	230
Low Fat	1.9 oz	200
Uncle Roy's		
Cashew Raisin	½ cup (1.6 oz)	180
Fat Free Apple Cinnamon	½ cup (1.6 oz)	175
Fat Free Wild Cherry	½ cup (1.6 oz)	175
Fruit & Nut	½ cup (1.6 oz)	175
Low Fat Berries Jubilee	½ cup (1.6 oz)	175
Low Fat Crispy	½ cup (1.4 oz)	160
Low Fat Luscious Raspberry	½ cup (1.6 oz)	175
Low Fat True Blueberry	½ cup (1.6 oz)	175
Maple Date Nut	½ cup (1.6 oz)	180
Nut Butter & Almonds	½ cup (1.6 oz)	195
Organic Golden Honey	½ cup (1.6 oz)	190
Organic Maple Nut'N Rice	½ cup (1.4 oz)	170

FOOD	PORTION	CALS.
Uncle Roy's (CONT.)		
Organic Maple Raisin	½ cup (1.6 oz)	190

GRAPE JUICE

FOOD	PORTION	CALS.
BAMA		
Juice	8.45 fl oz	120
Bright & Early		
Frozen	8 fl oz	140
Capri Sun		
Drink	1 pkg (7 oz)	100
Everfresh		
Juice	1 can (8 oz)	150
Hi-C		
Box	8.45 fl oz	130
Drink	8 fl oz	130
Drink	1 can (11.5 fl oz)	180
Juicy Juice		
Drink	1 bottle (6 fl oz)	90
Drink	1 box	130
Kool-Aid		
Bursts Grape Drink	1 (7 oz)	100
Drink as prep w/ sugar	1 serv (8 oz)	100
Drink Mix as prep	1 serv (8 oz)	60
Sugar Free Drink Mix as prep	1 serv (8 oz)	5
Minute Maid		
Chilled	8 fl oz	130
Grape Punch frzn	8 fl oz	130
Punch Chilled	8 fl oz	130
Mott's		
Drink	10 fl oz	170
Fruit Basket Cocktail as prep	8 fl oz	130
Seneca		
Blush Grape Juice frzn as prep	8 fl oz	170
Fortified With Vitamin C frzn as prep	8 fl oz	170
Sweetened frzn as prep	8 fl oz	140
White Grape Juice frzn as prep	8 fl oz	140
Shasta Plus		
Grape Drink	1 can (11.5 oz)	160
Sippin' Pak		
100% Pure	8.45 fl	130
Snapple		
Grapeade	8 fl oz	120
Veryfine		
100% Juice	1 bottle (10 oz)	200

FOOD	PORTION	CALS.
Veryfine (CONT.)		
Chillers Glacial Grape	1 can (11.5 oz)	160
Grape Drink	1 bottle (10 oz)	160
Juice-Ups	8 fl oz	130
GRAPE LEAVES		
canned	1 (4 g)	3
fresh raw	1 (3 g)	3
Cedar's		
Grape Leaves Stuffed With Rice	6 pieces (4.9 oz)	180
GRAPEFRUIT		
CANNED		
juice pack	½ cup	46
FRESH		
pink	½ fruit	37
pink sections	1 cup	69
red	½ fruit	37
red sections	1 cup	69
white	½ fruit	39
white sections	1 cup	76
Dole		
Grapefruit	½ fruit	50
GRAPEFRUIT JUICE		
fresh	1 cup	96
After The Fall		
Pink	1 bottle (10 oz)	100
Apple & Eve		
Made In The Shade Ruby Red	8 fl oz	130
Crystal Geyser		
Juice Squeeze	1 bottle (12 fl oz)	150
Del Monte		
Juice	8 fl oz	100
Everfresh		
Juice	1 can (8 oz)	90
Ruby Red Cocktail	1 can (8 oz)	130
Fresh Samantha		
Juice	1 cup (8 oz)	101
Hood		
Select	1 cup (8 oz)	100
Minute Maid		
Frozen	8 fl oz	100
Juices To Go	1 can (11.5 fl oz)	140
Juices To Go	1 bottle (10 fl oz)	120

FOOD	PORTION	CALS.
Minute Maid (CONT.)		
Juices To Go	1 bottle (16 fl oz)	100
Juices To Go Pink Cocktail	1 bottle (10 fl oz)	140
Juices To Go Pink Cocktail	1 bottle (16 fl oz)	110
Juices to Go Pink Cocktail	8 fl oz	160
Mott's		
From Concentrate as prep	8 fl oz	120
Ocean Spray		
100% Juice	8 oz	100
Pink Juice Cocktail	8 oz	110
Ruby Red Drink	8 oz	130
Odwalla		
Juice	8 fl oz	90
Snapple		
Juice	10 fl oz	110
Pink Grapefruit Cocktail	8 fl oz	120
Tree Of Life		
Juice	8 fl oz	100
Tropicana		
Golden	8 oz	90
Ruby Red	8 oz	90
Season's Best	8 oz	90
Twister Pink	1 bottle (10 oz)	140
W/ Double Vitamin C	8 fl oz	110
Veryfine		
100% Juice	1 bottle (10 oz)	110
Pink	1 bottle (10 oz)	150
Ruby Red	8 fl oz	120

GRAPES

fresh	10	36
Dole		
Fresh	1½ cup	85

GRAVY
(*see also* SAUCE)
CANNED
Franco-American

Au Jus	2 oz	10
Beef	2 oz	25
Chicken	2 oz	45
Chicken Giblet	2 oz	30
Cream	2 oz	35
Mushroom	2 oz	25
Pork	2 oz	40

FOOD	PORTION	CALS.
Franco-American (CONT.)		
Turkey	2 oz	30
Gravymaster		
Seasoning	¼ tsp	3
Rudy's Farm		
Sausage Gravy	¼ cup (2 oz)	50
MIX		
Cajun King		
Oil-Less Roux And Gravy Mix	3.5 oz	394
Durkee		
Au Jus as prep	¼ cup	5
Brown as prep	¼ cup	10
Brown Herb as prep	¼ cup	15
Brown Mushroom as prep	¼ cup	15
Brown Onion as prep	¼ cup	15
Chicken as prep	¼ cup	20
Country as prep	¼ cup	35
Homestyle as prep	¼ cup	15
Mushroom as prep	¼ cup	15
Onion as prep	¼ cup	10
Pork as prep	¼ cup	10
Sausage as prep	¼ cup	35
Swiss Steak as prep	¼ cup	15
Turkey as prep	¼ cup	20
French's		
Au Jus as prep	¼ cup	5
Brown as prep	¼ cup	10
Chicken as prep	¼ cup	25
Country as prep	¼ cup	35
Herb Brown as prep	¼ cup	15
Homestyle as prep	¼ cup	10
Mushroom as prep	¼ cup	10
Onion	¼ cup	15
Pork as prep	¼ cup	10
Sausage as prep	¼ cup	35
Turkey as prep	¼ cup	20
Hain		
Brown	¼ pkg	16
Loma Linda		
Gravy Quik Brown	1 tbsp (5 g)	20
Gravy Quik Chicken	1 tbsp (5 g)	20
Quik Gravy Country	1 tbsp (5 g)	25
Quik Gravy Mushroom	1 tbsp (5 g)	15
Quik Gravy Onion	1 tbsp (5 g)	20

FOOD	PORTION	CALS.
Pillsbury		
Brown	¼ cup	15
Chicken	¼ cup	25
Home Style	¼ cup	15

GREAT NORTHERN BEANS
CANNED
Allen

Great Northern	½ cup (4.5 oz)	100
Green Giant		
Great Northern	½ cup (4.4 oz)	100
Trappey		
With Sausage	½ cup (4.5 oz)	100

DRIED
Bean Cuisine

Dried	½ cup	115
Hurst		
HamBeens w/ Ham	3 tbsp (1.2 oz)	120

GREEN BEANS
CANNED
Allen

Cut	½ cup (4.2 oz)	30
Cut No Added Salt	½ cup (4.2 oz)	15
French Style	½ cup (4.2 oz)	25
Italian	½ cup (4.2 oz)	35
Shell Outs	½ cup (4.5 oz)	30
Alma		
Cut	½ cup (4.2 oz)	30
Crest Top		
Cut	½ cup (4.2 oz)	30
Del Monte		
Cut	½ cup (4.3 oz)	20
Cut 50% Less Salt	½ cup (4.3 oz)	20
Cut Italian	½ cup (4.3 oz)	30
Cut No Salt Added	½ cup (4.3 oz)	20
French Style	½ cup (4.3 oz)	20
French Style 50% Less Salt	½ cup (4.3 oz)	20
French Style No Salt Added	½ cup (4.3 oz)	20
French Style Seasoned	½ cup (4.3 oz)	20
Whole	½ cup (4.3 oz)	20
GaBelle		
Cut	½ cup (4.2 oz)	30
Green Giant		
Cut	½ cup (4.2 oz)	20

FOOD	PORTION	CALS.
Green Giant (CONT.)		
Cut 50% Less Sodium	½ cup (4.2 oz)	20
French Style	½ cup (4.1 oz)	20
Kitchen Sliced	½ cup (4.2 oz)	20
Whole	½ cup (4.1 oz)	25
Seneca		
Cut	½ cup	20
Cuts Natural Pack	½ cup	25
French	½ cup	20
French Natural Pack	½ cup	25
Whole	½ cup	20
Sunshine		
Cut	½ cup (4.2 oz)	30
Italian	½ cup (4.2 oz)	35
FRESH		
cooked	½ cup	22
raw	½ cup	17
FROZEN		
Birds Eye		
French w/ Toasted Almonds	¾ cup (4.1 oz)	80
Fresh Like		
Cut	3.5 oz	29
French	3.5 oz	29
Italian	3.5 oz	35
Whole	3.5 oz	29
Green Giant		
Cut	¾ cup (2.8 oz)	25
Harvest Fresh & Almonds	⅔ cup (2.8 oz)	60
Harvest Fresh Cut	⅔ cup (2.9 oz)	25
Stouffer's		
Green Bean Mushroom Casserole	1 serv (4 oz)	130
Tree Of Life		
Green Beans	⅔ cup (2.8 oz)	25
GREENS		
CANNED		
Allen		
Mixed	½ cup (4.2 oz)	30
Sunshine		
Mixed	½ cup (4.2 oz)	30
GROUNDCHERRIES		
fresh	½ cup	37
GROUPER		
cooked	3 oz	100

FOOD	PORTION	CALS.
GUANABANA JUICE		
Libby		
Nectar	1 can (11.5 fl oz)	210
GUAVA		
fresh	1	45
guava sauce	½ cup	43
GUAVA JUICE		
Kern's		
Nectar	6 fl oz	110
Libby		
Nectar	1 can (11.5 fl oz)	220
Snapple		
Guava Mania	8 fl oz	110
GUINEA HEN		
w/ skin raw	½ hen (12.1 oz)	545
HADDOCK		
FRESH		
cooked	3 oz	95
roe raw	3½ oz	130
FROZEN		
Gorton's		
Fishmarket Fresh	5 oz	110
Microwave Entree Haddock In Lemon Butter	1 pkg	360
Van De Kamp's		
Battered Fillets	2 (4 oz)	260
Breaded Fillets	2 (3.5 oz)	280
Lightly Breaded Fillets	1 (4 oz)	220
SMOKED		
smoked	1 oz	33
TAKE-OUT		
breaded & fried	1 piece (3.5 oz)	187
HALIBUT		
FRESH		
atlantic & pacific cooked	3 oz	119
atlantic & pacific raw	3 oz	93
greenland baked	3 oz	203
FROZEN		
Van De Kamp's		
Battered Fillets	3 (4 oz)	300

FOOD	PORTION	CALS.

HALVA
(*see* SESAME)

HAM
(*see also* HAM DISHES, PORK, TURKEY)

FOOD	PORTION	CALS.
boneless 11% fat roasted	3 oz	151
canned extra lean roasted	3 oz	116
canned extra lean roasted	1 cup	190
canned extra lean 4% fat	3 oz	116
center slice country style lean roasted	4 oz	220
patty cooked	1 patty (2 oz)	203
sliced extra lean 5% fat	1 oz	37
sliced regular 11% fat	1 oz	52
steak boneless extra lean	1 (2 oz)	69
Alpine Lace		
Boneless Cooked	2 oz	60
Boar's Head		
Black Forest Smoked	2 oz	60
Cappy	2 oz	60
Deluxe	2 oz	60
Deluxe Lowered Sodium	2 oz	50
Fresh Roasted Seasoned	2 oz	80
Maple Glazed Honey	2 oz	60
Pepper	2 oz	60
Sweet Slice Smoked	3 oz	110
Virgina	2 oz	60
Virginia Smoked	2 oz	60
Carl Buddig		
Ham	1 oz	50
Honey Ham	1 oz	50
Healthy Choice		
Baked Cooked	3 slices (2.2 oz)	70
Cooked	3 slices (2.2 oz)	70
Deli-Thin Baked Cooked With Natural Juices	6 slices (2 oz)	60
Deli-Thin Cooked	6 slices (2 oz)	60
Deli-Thin Honey With Natural Juices	6 slices (2 oz)	60
Deli-Thin Smoked With Natural Juices	6 slices (2 oz)	60
Fresh-Trak Cooked	1 slice (1 oz)	30
Fresh-Trak Honey	1 slice (1 oz)	30
Honey Boneless	3 oz	100
Smoked	3 slices (2.2 oz)	70
Variety Pack Regular	3 slices (2.2 oz)	70
Hillshire		
Brown Sugar	1 oz	40

FOOD	PORTION	CALS.
Hillshire (CONT.)		
Cooked Ham	1 oz	30
Deli Select Baked Ham	1 slice	10
Deli Select Brown Sugar Baked	1 slice	10
Deli Select Cajun Ham	1 slice	10
Deli Select Honey Ham	1 slice	10
Deli Select Lower Salt	1 slice	10
Deli Select Smoked Ham	1 slice	10
Flavor Pack 90-99% Fat Free Brown Sugar Baked	1 slice (0.6 oz)	20
Flavor Pack 90-99% Fat Free Honey Ham	1 slice (0.6 oz)	20
Flavor Pack 90-99% Fat Free Smoked	1 slice (0.6 oz)	20
Genuine Baked	1 oz	35
Honey Ham	1 oz	40
Lower Salt	1 oz	30
Lunch 'N Munch Cooked Ham/Swiss	1 pkg (4.5 oz)	360
Lunch 'N Munch Cooked Ham/Swiss Oreo	1 pkg (4.125 oz)	370
Lunch 'N Munch Cooked Ham/Swiss Snickers/Hi-C	1 pkg (4.25 oz + 6 fl oz)	470
Lunch 'N Munch Honey Ham/ Cheddar/ Snickers/Hi-C	1 pkg (4.25 oz + 6 fl oz)	500
Hormel		
Black Label Canned (refrigerated)	3 oz	100
Black Label Canned (shelf stable)	3 oz	110
Cure 81 Half Ham	3 oz	100
Curemaster	3 oz	80
Deviled Ham	4 tbsp (2 oz)	150
Ham & Cheese Patties	1 patty (2 oz)	190
Ham Patties	1 (2 oz)	180
Light & Lean 97 Sliced	1 slice (1 oz)	25
Primissimo Proscuitti	2 oz	120
Spiral Cure 81	3 oz	150
Jordan's		
Healthy Trim 97% Fat Free Cooked	1 slice (1 oz)	30
Healthy Trim 97% Fat Free EZ Serve	1 slice (1 oz)	30
Healthy Trim 97% Fat Free Virginia	1 slice (1 oz)	30
Krakus		
Ham	1 oz	25
Louis Rich		
Carving Board Baked	2 slices (1.6 oz)	50
Carving Board Honey Glazed Thin	6 slices (2.1 oz)	70
Carving Board Honey Glazed Traditional	2 slices (1.6 oz)	50
Carving Board Smoked	1 slice (1.6 oz)	45
Dinner Slices Baked	1 slice (3.3 oz)	80

FOOD	PORTION	CALS.
Mr. Turkey		
Deli Cuts Honey Cured	3 slices	35
Oscar Mayer		
Baked	3 slices (2.2 oz)	70
Boiled	3 slices (2.2 oz)	60
Chopped	1 slice (1 oz)	50
Dinner Slice	3 oz	80
Dinner Steaks	1 (2 oz)	60
Free Baked	3 slices (1.6 oz)	35
Free Honey	3 slices (1.6 oz)	35
Free Smoked	3 slices (1.6 oz)	35
Ham & Cheese Loaf	1 slice (1 oz)	70
Honey	3 slices (2.2 oz)	70
Lower Sodium	3 slices (2.2 oz)	70
Lunchables Cookies/Ham/ Swiss	1 pkg (4.2 oz)	360
Lunchables Dessert Chocolate Pudding/ Ham/ American	1 pkg (6.2 oz)	390
Lunchables Ham/Cheddar	1 pkg (4.5 oz)	340
Smoked	3 slices (2.2 oz)	60
Russer		
Baked	2 oz	70
Canadian Brand Maple	2 oz	70
Chopped	2 oz	130
Cooked Ham	2 oz	60
Ham & Cheese Loaf	2 oz	120
Honey & Maple Cured	2 oz	70
Honey Cured	2 oz	60
Hot	2 oz	70
Light Cooked	2 oz	60
Light Smoked	2 oz	60
Smoked Virginia	2 oz	70
Spiced	2 oz	160
Sara Lee		
Bavarian Brand Baked	2 oz	80
Bavarian Brand Baked Honey	2 oz	80
Golden Cure Smoked	2 oz	80
Honey Ham	2 oz	60
Honey Roasted	2 oz	90
Spam		
Spread	4 tbsp (2 oz)	140
Spreadables		
Ham Salad	¼ can	100
Underwood		
Deviled	2.08 oz	220

FOOD	PORTION	CALS.
Underwood (CONT.)		
Deviled Light	2.08 oz	120
Deviled Smoked	2.08 oz	190

HAM DISHES
FROZEN
Croissant Pocket

Stuffed Sandwich Ham & Cheddar	1 piece (4.5 oz)	360
Hot Pocket		
Stuffed Sandwich Ham & Cheese	1 (4.5 ox)	340

HAMBURGER
(*see also* BEEF)

Jimmy Dean		
Burger	1 (2 oz)	220
Flamed Broiled Cheeseburger	1 (6.3 oz)	540
Mini Cheeseburger	2 (3 oz)	270
Kid Cuisine		
Beef Patty Sandwich w/ Cheese	1 (8.5 oz)	410
Rudy's Farm		
Mild Burger	1 (3 oz)	360
White Castle		
Cheeseburger	2 (3.6 oz)	310
Hamburger	2 (3.2 oz)	270

TAKE-OUT

double patty w/ bun	1 reg	544
double patty w/ cheese & bun	1 reg	457
double patty w/ cheese & double bun	1 reg	461
double patty w/ cheese ketchup mayonnaise onion pickle tomato & bun	1 reg	416
double patty w/ ketchup mayonnaise onion pickle tomato & bun	1 reg	649
double patty w/ ketchup cheese mayonnaise mustard pickle tomato & bun	1 lg	706
double patty w/ ketchup mustard mayonnaise onion pickle tomato & bun	1 lg	540
double patty w/ ketchup mustard onion pickle & bun	1 reg	576
single patty w/ bacon ketchup cheese mustard onion pickle & bun	1 lg	609
single patty w/ bun	1 lg	400
single patty w/ bun	1 reg	275
single patty w/ cheese & bun	1 lg	608
single patty w/ cheese & bun	1 reg	320
single patty w/ ketchup cheese ham mayonnaise pickle tomato & bun	1 lg	745

FOOD	PORTION	CALS.
single patty w/ ketchup mustard mayonnaise onion pickle tomato & bun	1 reg	279
triple patty w/ cheese & bun	1 lg	769
triple patty w/ ketchup mustard pickle & bun	1 lg	693

HAZELNUTS
dried blanched	1 oz	191
dried unblanched	1 oz	179
dry roasted unblanched	1 oz	188
oil roasted unblanched	1 oz	187
Crumpy		
Chocolate Hazelnut Spread	1 tbsp (0.5 oz)	80

HEART
beef simmered	3 oz	148
chicken simmered	1 cup (5 oz)	268
lamb braised	3 oz	158
pork braised	1 cup	215
pork braised	1	191
turkey simmered	1 cup (5 oz)	257
veal braised	3 oz	158

HEARTS OF PALM
canned	1 (1.2 oz)	9
canned	1 cup (5.1 oz)	41

HERBAL TEA
(*see* TEA/HERBAL TEA)

HERBS/SPICES
(*see also individual names*)
curry powder	1 tsp	6
poultry seasoning	1 tsp	5
pumpkin pie spice	1 tsp	6
Ac'cent		
Flavor Enhancer	½ tsp	5
Herbal All Purpose Seasoning	½ tsp	0
Chi-Chi's		
Seasoning Mix	1 tsp (3 g)	10
Lawry's		
Seasoning Blend Sloppy Joe	1 pkg	126
McIlhenny		
Crab Boil	3 oz	378
Mrs. Dash		
Extra Spicy	⅛ tsp (0.02 oz)	2
Garlic & Herb	⅛ tsp (0.02 oz)	2

FOOD	PORTION	CALS.

Mrs. Dash (CONT.)

Lemon & Herb	⅛ tsp (0.02 oz)	2
Low Pepper No Garlic	⅛ tsp (0.02 oz)	2
Original Blend	⅛ tsp (0.02 oz)	2
Table Blend	⅛ tsp (0.02 oz)	2

Watkins

Apple Bake Seasoning	¼ tsp (0.5 g)	0
Barbecue Spice	¼ tsp (0.5 g)	0
Bean Soup Seasoning	¾ tsp (2 g)	5
Beef Jerky Seasoning	2 tsp (6 g)	15
Chicken Seasoning	½ tsp (1 g)	0
Cole Slaw Seasoning	½ tsp (1.5 g)	5
Egg Sensations	1 tsp (3 g)	10
Fajita Seasoning	½ tsp (3 g)	10
Grill Seasoning	¼ tsp (1 g)	0
Ground Beef Seasoning	⅛ tsp (0.5 g)	0
Italian Blend	1 tsp (3 g)	1
Meat Tenderizer	⅛ tsp (0.5 g)	0
Meatloaf Seasoning	½ tsp (5 g)	15
Mexican Blend	½ tbsp (4 g)	15
Omelet & Souffle Seasoning	¾ tsp (2 g)	5
Oriental Ginger Garlic Liquid Spice Blend	1 tbsp (0.5 oz)	120
Potato Salad Seasoning	¼ tsp (1 g)	0
Pumpkin Pie Spice	¼ tsp (0.5 g)	0
Smokehouse Liquid Blend	1 tbsp (0.5 oz)	120
Soup & Vegetable Seasoning	¼ tsp (0.5 g)	0
Spanish Seasoning Blend	¼ tsp (0.5 oz)	0

HERRING

atlantic cooked	3 oz	172
pacific baked	3 oz	213
roe canned	3.5 oz	118
roe raw	3.5 oz	130
smoked	3.5 oz	210

TAKE-OUT

atlantic kippered	1 fillet (1.4 oz)	87
atlantic pickled	0.5 oz	39
fried	1 serv (3.5 oz)	233

HICKORY NUTS

dried	1 oz	187

HOMINY

CANNED

white	1 cup (5.6 oz)	482

FOOD	PORTION	CALS.
Allen		
Golden	½ cup (4.5 oz)	120
Mexican	½ cup (4.5 oz)	120
White	½ cup (4.5 oz)	100
Uncle William		
Golden	½ cup (4.5 oz)	120
Mexican	½ cup (4.5 oz)	120
White	½ cup (4.5 oz)	100
Van Camp's		
Golden	½ cup (4.3 oz)	80
White	½ cup (4.3 oz)	80

HONEY

FOOD	PORTION	CALS.
honey	1 cup (11.9 oz)	1031
honey	1 tbsp (0.7 oz)	64
Burleson's		
Clover	1 tbsp	60
Creamed	1 tbsp	60
Natural	1 tbsp	60
Pure	1 tbsp	60
Raw	1 tbsp	60
Rocky Mountain Clover	1 tbsp	60
Tree Of Life		
Alfalfa	1 tbsp (0.7 oz)	60
Avocado	1 tbsp (0.7 oz)	60
Buckwheat	1 tbsp (0.7 oz)	60
Clover	1 tbsp (0.7 oz)	60
Honeybear Wildflower	1 tbsp (0.7 oz)	60
Orange	1 tbsp (0.7 oz)	60
Tupelo	1 tbsp (0.7 oz)	60
Wildflower	1 tbsp (0.7 oz)	60

HONEYDEW
FRESH

FOOD	PORTION	CALS.
cubed	1 cup	60
wedge	1/10	46
Dole		
Honeydew	1/10	50

FROZEN
Big Valley

FOOD	PORTION	CALS.
Balls	¾ cup (4.9 oz)	45

HORSE

FOOD	PORTION	CALS.
roasted	3 oz	149

FOOD	PORTION	CALS

HORSERADISH
Boar's Head
Horseradish	1 tsp (5 g)	5

Hebrew National
White	1 tbsp	7

Heluva Good Cheese
Horseradish	1 tsp (5 g)	0

Kraft
Cream Style	1 tsp (5 g)	0
Horseradish Sauce	1 tsp (5 g)	20
Prepared	1 tsp (5 g)	0

Rosoff's
Red	1 tbsp (0.5 oz)	8
White	1 tbsp (0.5 oz)	7

Schorr's
Red	1 tbsp (0.5 oz)	8
White	1 tbsp (0.5 oz)	7

HOT CAKES
(*see* PANCAKES)

HOT COCOA
(*see* COCOA)

HOT DOG
(*see also* MEAT SUBSTITUTES, SAUSAGE, SAUSAGE SUBSTITUTES)
Applegate Farms
Chicken Natural Uncured	1 (1.5 oz)	120
Natural Turkey	1 (1.5 oz)	120

Boar's Head
Beef	1 (1.6 oz)	120
Beef Lite	1 (1.6 oz)	90
Pork & Beef	1 (2 oz)	150

Empire
Chicken	1 (2 oz)	100
Turkey	1 (2 oz)	90

Healthy Choice
Beef	1 (1.8 oz)	60
Bunsize	1 (2 oz)	70
Franks	1 (1.6 oz)	50
Jumbo	1 (2 oz)	70

Hebrew National
Beef	1 (1.7 oz)	150
Cocktail Beef	6 (1.8 oz)	160
Dinner Beef	1 (4 oz)	350

FOOD	PORTION	CALS.
Hebrew National (CONT.)		
Reduced Fat Beef	1 (1.7 oz)	120
Hillshire		
Franks Bun Size Beef	2 oz	180
Light & Mild Franks Jumbo	1 link	110
Light & Mild Wieners	1 link	90
Lit'l Franks Beef	2 oz	180
Lit'l Wieners	2 oz	180
Weiners Natural Casing	2 oz	180
Wieners Bun Size	2 oz	180
Hormel		
Fat Free	1 (1.8 oz)	45
Fat Free Beef	1 (1.8 oz)	45
Jordan's		
Healthy Trim Low Fat	1 (1.8 oz)	70
Healthy Trim Low Fat Skinless	1 (1.8 oz)	70
Louis Rich		
Bun Length	1 (2 oz)	110
Cheese	1 (1.6 oz)	90
Franks	1 (1.6 oz)	80
Mr. Turkey		
Bun Size	1	130
Cheese	1	140
Hot Dog	1	110
Oscar Mayer		
Beef	1 (1.6 oz)	140
Big & Juicy Franks Deli Style	1 (2.7 oz)	230
Big & Juicy Franks Original	1 (2.7 oz)	240
Big & Juicy Franks Quarter Pound	1 (4 oz)	350
Big & Juicy Weiners Hot 'N Spicy	1 (2.7 oz)	220
Big & Juicy Wieners Smokie Links	1 (2.7 oz)	220
Big & Juicy Wieners Original	1 (2.7 oz)	240
Bun-Length Beef	1 (2 oz)	180
Cheese	1 (1.6 oz)	140
Free Beef	1 (1.8 oz)	40
Free Turkey & Beef	1 (1.8 oz)	35
Jumbo Beef	1 (2 oz)	180
Light Beef	1 (2 oz)	110
Wieners	1 (1.6 oz)	150
Wieners Bun-Length	1 (2 oz)	190
Wieners Jumbo	1 (2 oz)	180
Wieners Light	1 (2 oz)	110
Wieners Little	6 (2 oz)	180

FOOD	PORTION	CALS.
Russer		
Lil'Salt Deli Franks	1 (2.67 oz)	160
Shofar		
Kosher Beef	1 (1.8 oz)	150
Kosher Beef Reduced Fat Reduced Sodium	1 (1.8 oz)	120
Tyson		
Chicken Cheese	1	145
Chicken Hot Dog	1	115
Wampler Longacre		
Chicken	1 (2 oz)	130
Chicken	1 (1.6 oz)	110
Turkey	1 (2 oz)	130
Turkey	1 (1.6 oz)	110
TAKE-OUT		
corndog	1	460
w/ bun chili	1	297
w/ bun plain	1	242

HUMMUS

hummus	1 cup	420
Athenos		
Roasted Red Pepper	2 tbsp (1.1 oz)	60
Casbah		
Mix as prep	¼ cup	120
Cedar's		
No Salt Added Hommus Tahini	2 tbsp (1 oz)	50
TAKE-OUT		
hummus	⅓ cup	140

HYACINTH BEANS

dried cooked	1 cup	228

ICE CREAM AND FROZEN DESSERTS

(*see also* ICES AND ICE POPS, PUDDING POPS, SHERBET, YOGURT FROZEN)

chocolate	½ cup (4 fl oz)	143
dixie cup chocolate	1 (3.5 fl oz)	125
dixie cup strawberry	1 (3.5 fl oz)	112
dixie cup vanilla	1 (3.5 fl oz)	116
freeze dried ice cream chocolate strawberry & vanilla	1 pkg (0.75 oz)	158
french vanilla soft serve	½ gal	3014
french vanilla soft serve	½ cup (4 fl oz)	185
strawberry	½ cup (4 fl oz)	127
vanilla	½ cup (4 fl oz)	132

FOOD	PORTION	CALS.
vanilla light	½ cup (2.3 oz)	92
vanilla rich	½ cup (2.6 oz)	178
vanilla soft serve	½ cup	111
3 Musketeers		
Single Chocolate	1 (2 fl oz)	160
Single Vanilla	1 (2 fl oz)	160
Snack Chocolate	1 (0.72 fl oz)	60
Snack Vanilla	1 (0.72 fl oz)	60
Ben & Jerry's		
Banana Walnut	½ cup (3.9 oz)	290
Butter Pecan	½ cup (3.9 oz)	310
Cherry Garcia	½ cup (3.7 oz)	240
Cherry Vanilla	½ cup (3.9 oz)	240
Chocolate Chip Cookie Dough	½ cup (3.7 oz)	270
Chocolate Fudge Brownie	½ cup (3.7 oz)	250
Chunky Monkey	½ cup (3.7 oz)	280
Coconut Almond	½ cup (3.7 oz)	260
Coconut Almond Fudge Chip	½ cup (3.8 oz)	320
Coffee Almond Fudge	½ cup (3.7 oz)	290
Coffee Toffee Crunch	½ cup (3.7 oz)	280
English Toffee Crunch	½ cup (4 oz)	310
Mint Chocolate Cookie	½ cup (3.8 oz)	260
New York Super Fudge Chunk	½ cup (3.7 oz)	290
No Fat Strawberry	½ cup (3.3 oz)	140
No Fat Vanilla Fudge Swirl	½ cup (3.1 oz)	150
Peanut Butter Cup	½ cup (4.1 oz)	370
Pop Chocolate Chip Cookie Dough	1 (4.1 oz)	450
Pop English Toffee Crunch	1 (3.7 oz)	340
Pop Vanilla	1 (3.9 oz)	360
Rain Forest Crunch	½ cup (3.7 oz)	300
Smooth Aztec Harvest Coffee	½ cup (3.8 oz)	230
Smooth Deep Dark Chocolate	½ cup (3.9 oz)	260
Smooth Double Chocolate Fudge	½ cup (4.1 oz)	280
Smooth Mocho Fudge	½ cup (4 oz)	270
Smooth Vanilla	½ cup (3.8 oz)	230
Smooth Vanilla Bean	½ cup (3.8 oz)	230
Smooth Vanilla Caramel Fudge	½ cup (4.1 oz)	280
Smooth White Russian	½ cup (3.8 oz)	240
Vanilla	½ cup (3.7 oz)	230
Wavy Gravy	½ cup (4.1 oz)	330
Bon Bons		
Vanilla With Milk Chocolate Coating	8 pieces	330
Vanilla With Milk Chocolate Coating	5 pieces	200

FOOD	PORTION	CALS.
Borden		
Buttered Pecan	½ cup	180
Chocolate Swirl	½ cup	130
Dutch Chocolate Olde Fashioned Recipe	½ cup	130
Fat Free Black Cherry	½ cup	90
Fat Free Chocolate	½ cup	100
Fat Free Peach	½ cup	90
Fat Free Strawberry	½ cup	90
Fat Free Vanilla	½ cup	90
Ice Milk Chocolate	½ cup	100
Ice Milk Strawberry	½ cup	90
Ice Milk Vanilla	½ cup	90
Strawberries 'N Cream Olde Fashioned Recipe	½ cup	130
Strawberry	½ cup	130
Sundae Cone	1	210
Vanilla Olde Fashioned Recipe	½ cup	130
Bounty		
Cherry/Dark	1 (0.84 fl oz)	70
Coconut/Dark	1 (0.84 fl oz)	70
Coconut/Milk	1 (0.84 fl oz)	70
Breyers		
Butter Pecan	½ cup (2.4 oz)	180
Caramel Praline Crunch	½ cup (2.6 oz)	180
Cherry Vanilla	½ cup (2.4 oz)	150
Chocolate	½ cup (2.4 oz)	160
Chocolate Chip	½ cup (2.4 oz)	170
Chocolate Chip Cookie Dough	½ cup (2.5 oz)	180
Chocolate Rainbow	½ cup (2.4 oz)	120
Coffee	½ cup (2.4 oz)	150
Cookies N Cream	½ cup (2.4 oz)	170
Creamsicle	½ cup (2.8 oz)	130
Double Chocolate Fudge	½ cup (2.6 oz)	150
Fat Free Caramel Praline	½ cup (2.5 oz)	120
Fat Free Chocolate	½ cup (2.4 oz)	90
Fat Free Mint Cookies N Cream	½ cup (2.4 oz)	100
Fat Free Strawberry	½ cup (2.4 oz)	90
Fat Free Take Two Vanilla Strawberry	½ cup (2.4 oz)	80
Fat Free Vanilla	½ cup (2.4 oz)	90
Fat Free Vanilla Chocolate Strawberry	½ cup (2.4 oz)	90
Fat Free Vanilla Fudge Twirl	½ cup (2.5 oz)	100
French Vanilla	½ cup (2.4 oz)	160
Fruit Rainbow	½ cup (2.4 oz)	140
Hershey w/ Almonds	½ cup (2.7 oz)	190

FOOD	PORTION	CALS.
Breyers (CONT.)		
Light Butter Pecan	½ cup (2.3 oz)	120
Light Caramel Praline Pecan	½ cup (3 oz)	180
Light French Chocolate	½ cup (2.4 oz)	150
Light Mint Chocolate Chip	½ cup (2.4 oz)	140
Light Vanilla	½ cup (2.4 oz)	130
Light Vanilla Chocolate Strawberry	½ cup (2.4 oz)	120
Light Low Fat Brown Marble Fudge	½ cup (2.6 oz)	130
Light Low Fat French Vanilla	½ cup (2.3 oz)	110
Light Low Fat Swiss Almond Fudge	½ cup (2.5 oz)	130
Low Fat Butter Pecan	½ cup (2.6 oz)	150
Low Fat Vanilla	½ cup (2.6 oz)	120
Low Fat Vanilla Chocolate Strawberry	½ cup (2.6 oz)	120
Mint Chocolate Chip	½ cup (2.4 oz)	170
No Sugar Added Fudge Twirl	½ cup (2.6 oz)	100
No Sugar Added Mint Chocolate Chip	½ cup (2.4 oz)	100
No Sugar Added Vanilla	½ cup (2.4 oz)	90
No Sugar Added Vanilla Chocolate Strawberry	½ cup (2.4 oz)	90
Peach	½ cup (2.4 oz)	130
Peanut Butter Cup	½ cup (2.7 oz)	210
Rocky Road	½ cup (2.5 oz)	180
Soft'N Creamy Vanilla	½ cup (2.3 oz)	150
Soft'N Creamy Vanilla Chocolate Strawberry	½ cup (2.3 oz)	150
Strawberry	½ cup (2.4 oz)	130
Take Two Vanilla Chocolate	½ cup (2.5 oz)	160
Take Two Vanilla Orange Sherbet	½ cup (2.7 oz)	130
Vanilla	½ cup (2.4 oz)	150
Vanilla Chocolate Strawberry	½ cup (2.4 oz)	150
Vanilla Fudge Twirl	½ cup (2.6 oz)	160
Viennetta Cappuccino	½ cup (2.4 oz)	190
Viennetta Chocolate	½ cup (2.4 oz)	190
Viennetta Vanilla	½ cup (2.4 oz)	190
Butterfinger		
Bar	1 (2.5 oz)	170
Nuggets	8	340
California Joe		
Soft Serve Chocolate	½ cup (2.5 oz)	72
Soft Serve Vanilla	½ cup (2.5 oz)	70
Cool Creations		
Cookies & Cream Sandwich	1 (3.5 oz)	240
Mini Sandwich	1 (2.3 oz)	110

FOOD	PORTION	CALS.
DoveBar		
Almond	1 (3.67 fl oz)	335
Bite Size Almond Praline	1 (0.75 fl oz)	80
Bite Size Cherry Royale	1 (0.75 fl oz)	70
Bite Size Classic Vanilla	1 (0.75 fl oz)	70
Bite Size French Vanilla	1 (0.75 fl oz)	70
Bite Size Mint Supreme	1 (0.75 fl oz)	80
Caramel Pecan	1 (3.67 fl oz)	350
Chocolate Milk Chocolate	1 (3.8 fl oz)	340
Coffee Cashew	1 (3.67 fl oz)	335
Crunchy Cookie	1 (3.8 fl oz)	340
Peanut	1 (3.8 fl oz)	380
Single Vanilla/Dark	1 (2 fl oz)	200
Vanilla Dark Chocolate	1 (3.8 fl oz)	340
Vanilla Milk Chocolate	1 (3.8 fl oz)	340
Drumstick		
Cone Chocolate	1 (4.6 oz)	340
Cone Chocolate Dipped	1 (4.6 oz)	340
Cone Vanilla	1 (4.6 oz)	350
Cone Vanilla Caramel	1 (4.6 oz)	360
Cone Vanilla Fudge	1 (4.6 oz)	370
Eagle Brand		
Vanilla	½ cup	150
Edy's		
American Dream Chocolate	3 oz	90
American Dream Chocolate Chip	3 oz	100
American Dream Cookies'N'Cream	3 oz	100
American Dream Mocha Almond Fudge	3 oz	110
American Dream Rocky Road	3 oz	110
American Dream Strawberry	3 oz	70
American Dream Toasted Almond	3 oz	110
American Dream Vanilla	3 oz	80
American Dream Vanilla Chocolate Strawberry	3 oz	80
Light Almond Praline	4 oz	140
Light Banana-Politan	4 oz	110
Light Butter Pecan	4 oz	140
Light Cafe Au Lait	4 oz	110
Light Candy Bar	4 oz	140
Light Chocolate Chip	4 oz	120
Light Chocolate Fudge Mousse	4 oz	130
Light Cookies'N'Cream	4 oz	120
Light Dreamy Caramel Cream	4 oz	140
Light Malt Ball 'N' Fudge	4 oz	140

FOOD	PORTION	CALS.
Edy's (cont.)		
Light Marble Fudge	4 oz	120
Light Mocha Almond Fudge	4 oz	140
Light Peanut Butter & Chocolate	4 oz	130
Light Raspberry Truffle	4 oz	110
Light Rocky Road	4 oz	130
Light Strawberry	4 oz	110
Light Vanilla	4 oz	100
Vanilla Chocolate Strawberry	4 oz	110
Fi-Bar		
Banana Cream	1 bar	93
Cocoa-Fudge 'N Cream	1 bar	93
Raspberries 'N Cream	1 bar	93
Wildberry Cream	1 bar	93
Flintstones		
Cool Cream	1 (2.75 oz)	90
Push-Up	1 (2.75 oz)	100
Friendly's		
Black Raspberry	½ cup	150
Chocolate Almond Chip	½ cup	170
Forbidden Chocolate	½ cup	150
Fudge Nut Brownie	½ cup	200
Heath English Toffee	½ cup (2.7 oz)	190
Purely Pistachio	½ cup	160
Vanilla	½ cup	150
Vanilla Chocolate Strawberry	½ cup	150
Vienna Mocha Chunk	½ cup	180
Good Humor		
Banana Bob	1 (3 fl oz)	155
Bar Classic Toasted Almond	1 (3.1 fl oz)	170
Bar Classic Vanilla	1 (3.1 fl oz)	190
Bar Classic Almond	1 (3.1 fl oz)	210
Bar Sidewalk Sundae	1	280
Bubble O'Bill	1 (3.6 fl oz)	170
Bubble Play	1	110
Chip Burrrger	1 (4.7 oz)	320
Chip Sandwich	1 (4.7 fl oz)	320
Choco Taco	1 (4.4 fl oz)	320
Chocolate Eclair Classic	1 (3.1 fl oz)	170
Classic Candy Center Crunch Vanilla	1	280
Colonel Crunch Chocolate	1 (3.1 oz)	160
Colonel Crunch Strawberry	1 (3.1 oz)	170
Combo Cup	1 (6.2 fl oz)	200
Cone Olde Nut Sundae	1 (3.9 oz)	230

FOOD	PORTION	CALS.
Good Humor (CONT.)		
Cone Sidewalk Sundae	1 (4.2 oz)	270
Creamee Burrrger	1 (4.7 oz)	310
Crunch Classic Candy Center	1 (3.1 fl oz)	260
Dinosaur Bar	1	110
Far Frog	1 (3.6 fl oz)	150
Fun Box Ice Cream Sandwich	1 (3.1 fl oz)	160
King Cone	1 (5.7 fl oz)	300
King Cone Classic Vanilla	1 (4.8 oz)	300
King Cone Strawberry	1 (5.7 oz)	250
Light Chocolate Chocolate Chip	½ cup (2.4 oz)	130
Light Chocolate Chip	½ cup (2.4 oz)	130
Light Coffee	½ cup (2.4 oz)	110
Light Cookies N'Cream	½ cup (2.4 oz)	130
Light Heavenly Hash	½ cup (2.4 oz)	140
Light Praline Almond Crunch	½ cup (2.4 oz)	130
Light Toffee Bar Crunch	½ cup (2.4 oz)	130
Light Vanilla	½ cup (2.4 oz)	110
Light Vanilla Chocolate Strawberry	½ cup (2.4 oz)	110
Light Vanilla Fudge	½ cup (2.6 oz)	120
Magnum Almond	1 (4.2 fl oz)	270
Magnum Chocolate	1 (4.2 fl oz)	260
Number One Bar	1 (4.1 fl oz)	190
Popsicle Ice Cream Bar	1 (3.1 fl oz)	160
Popsicle Ice Cream Sandwich	1 (3.6 fl oz)	190
Sandwich Classic Chip Cookie	1 (4.1 fl oz)	300
Sandwich Giant Neapolitan	1 (5.2 fl oz)	260
Sandwich Giant Vanilla	1 (5.2 fl oz)	240
Sandwich Ice Cream	1	190
Sandwich Sidewalk Sundae	1 (3.1 oz)	160
Sandwich Sprinkle	1 (3.1 fl oz)	180
Strawberry Shortcake Bar Classic	1 (3.1 fl oz)	160
Sundae Twist Cup	1	160
Toffee Taco	1 (4.4 fl oz)	300
WWF Bar	1 (3.7 fl oz)	200
X-Men Bar	1 (3 fl oz)	150
Haagen-Dazs		
Baileys Original Irish Cream	½ cup (3.6 oz)	280
Brownies A La Mode	½ cup (3.7 oz)	280
Butter Pecan	½ cup (3.7 oz)	320
Cappuccino Commotion	½ cup (3.6 oz)	310
Caramel Cone Explosion	½ cup (3.6 oz)	310
Chocolate	½ cup (3.7 oz)	270
Chocolate Chocolate Chip	½ cup (3.7 oz)	300

FOOD	PORTION	CALS.
Haagen-Dazs (CONT.)		
Coffee	½ cup (3.7 oz)	270
Cookie Dough Dynamo	½ cup (3.6 oz)	300
Cookies & Cream	½ cup (3.6 oz)	270
DiSaronno Amaretto	½ cup (3.6 oz)	260
Macadamia Brittle	½ cup (3.7 oz)	300
Multi Pack Bars Caramel Cone Explosion	1 (3.1 oz)	330
Multi Pack Bars Chocolate & Dark Chocolate	1 (3.2 oz)	320
Multi Pack Bars Coffee & Almond Crunch	1 (3 oz)	290
Multi Pack Bars Iced Cappuccino Explosion	1 (2.9 oz)	290
Multi Pack Bars Triple Brownie Overload	1 (3 oz)	320
Multi Pack Bars Vanilla & Almonds	1 (3 oz)	300
Multi Pack Bars Vanilla & Dark Chocolate	1 (3.2 oz)	320
Multi Pack Bars Vanilla & Milk Chocolate	1 (3 oz)	280
Peanut Butter Burst	½ cup (3.6 oz)	330
Rum Raisin	½ cup (3.7 oz)	270
Single Pack Bars Caramel Cone Explosion	1 (3.3 oz)	350
Single Pack Bars Chocolate & Dark Chocolate	1 (3.9 oz)	400
Single Pack Bars Coffee & Almond Crunch	1 (3.7 oz)	360
Single Pack Bars Cookie Dough Dynamo	1 (3.5 oz)	380
Single Pack Bars Iced Cappuccino	1 (3.4 oz)	330
Single Pack Bars Triple Brownie Overload	1 (3.5 oz)	380
Single Pack Bars Vanilla & Almonds	1 (3.7 oz)	370
Single Pack Bars Vanilla & Dark Chocolate	1 (3.9 oz)	400
Single Pack Bars Vanilla & Milk Chocolate	1 (3.5 oz)	330
Strawberry	½ cup (3.7 oz)	250
Strawberry Cheesecake Craze	½ cup (3.7 oz)	290
Triple Brownie Overload	½ cup (3.5 oz)	300
Vanilla	½ cup (3.7 oz)	270
Vanilla Fudge	½ cup (3.7 oz)	280
Vanilla Swiss Almond	½ cup (3.7 oz)	310
Healthy Choice		
Black Forest	½ cup (2.5 oz)	120
Bordeaux Cherry Chocolate Chip	½ cup (2.5 oz)	110
Butter Pecan Crunch	½ cup (2.5 oz)	120
Cappuccino Chocolate Chunk	½ cup (2.5 oz)	120
Cookies 'N Cream	½ cup (2.5 oz)	120
Double Fudge Swirl	½ cup (2.5 oz)	120
Fudge Brownie	½ cup (2.5 oz)	120
Malt Caramel Cone	½ cup (2.5 oz)	120
Mint Chocolate Chip	½ cup (2.5 oz)	120

FOOD	PORTION	CALS.
Healthy Choice (CONT.)		
Peanut Butter Cookie Dough 'N Fudge	½ cup (2.5 oz)	120
Praline & Caramel	½ cup (2.5 oz)	130
Rocky Road	½ cup (2.5 oz)	140
Vanilla	½ cup	100
Heath		
Bar	1 (2.5 oz)	160
Nuggets	8	180
Hood		
Bar Orange Cream	1 bar (1.8 oz)	90
Bar Vanilla	1 bar (1.6 oz)	160
Caramel Butterscotch Blast	½ cup (2.3 oz)	160
Chocolate	½ cup (2.3 oz)	140
Chocolate Chip	½ cup (2.3 oz)	160
Chocolate Eclair	1 bar (1.6 oz)	150
Christmas Tree	½ cup (2.3 oz)	140
Coffee	½ cup (2.3 oz)	140
Cookie Dough Delight	½ cup (2.3 oz)	160
Cookies N Cream	½ cup (2.3 oz)	160
Cooler Cups	1 (2.1 oz)	80
Crispy Bar	1 (1.9 oz)	180
Egg Nog	½ cup (2.3 oz)	130
Fabulous Fudge & Peanut Butter Swirled Fudge Bars	1 bar (2.1 oz)	110
Fabulous Fudgies Assorted Bars	1 bar (2.1 oz)	100
Fat Free Chocolate Passion	½ cup (2.5 oz)	100
Fat Free Classic Harlequin	½ cup (2.5 oz)	100
Fat Free Double Brownie Sundae	½ cup (2.5 oz)	120
Fat Free Heavenly Hash	½ cup (2.5 oz)	120
Fat Free Mississippi Mud Pie	½ cup (2.5 oz)	130
Fat Free Praline Pecan Delight	½ cup (2.5 oz)	120
Fat Free Raspberry Blush	½ cup (2.5 oz)	120
Fat Free Super Strawberry Swirl	½ cup (2.5 oz)	100
Fat Free Vanilla Fudge Twist	½ cup (2.5 oz)	120
Fat Free Very Vanilla	½ cup (2.5 oz)	100
Fudge Bars	1 bar (2.7 oz)	100
Grasshopper Pie	½ cup (2.3 oz)	160
Heavenly Hash	½ cup (2.3 oz)	140
Hendrie's Cherry Chocolate Dips	1 bar (1.3 oz)	120
Hoodsie Cup Vanilla & Chocolate	1 (1.7 oz)	100
Light Almond Praline Delight	½ cup (2.4 oz)	110
Light Brownie Nut Sundae	½ cup (2.4 oz)	140
Light Caribbean Coffee Royale	½ cup (2.4 oz)	110
Light Chocolate Almond Chip Sundae	½ cup (2.4 oz)	140

FOOD	PORTION	CALS.
Hood (CONT.)		
Light Chocolate Chocolate Chip Cookie Dough	½ cup (2.4 oz)	140
Light Cookies N Cream	½ cup (2.4 oz)	130
Light Heath Toffee Chunk Swirl	½ cup (2.4 oz)	140
Light Heavenly Hash	½ cup (2.4 oz)	130
Light Maple Sugar Shack	⅓ cup (2.4 oz)	130
Light Massachusetts Mud Pie	½ cup (2.4 oz)	140
Light Raspberry Swirl	½ cup (2.4 oz)	120
Light Strawberry Supreme	½ cup (2.4 oz)	110
Light Triple Nut Cluster Sundae	½ cup (2.4 oz)	140
Light Vanilla	½ cup (2.4 oz)	110
Light Vanilla Chocolate Strawberry	½ cup (2.4 oz)	110
Low Fat No Sugar Added Caramel Swirl	½ cup (2.4 oz)	120
Low Fat No Sugar Added Chocolate Supreme	½ cup (2.4 oz)	120
Low Fat No Sugar Added Mocha Fudge	½ cup (2.4 oz)	110
Low Fat No Sugar Added Raspberry Swirl	½ cup (2.4 oz)	110
Low Fat No Sugar Added Vanilla	½ cup (2.4 oz)	100
Maple Walnut	½ cup (2.3 oz)	160
Rockets	1 (2 oz)	120
Sandwich Light	1 (2.2 oz)	160
Sandwich Vanilla	1 (2.2 oz)	180
Sports Bar	1 (2.9 oz)	250
Spumoni	½ cup (2.3 oz)	140
Strawberry	½ cup (2.3 oz)	130
Super Sortment Chocolate & Banana Fudge Bar	1 bar (2.1 oz)	100
Super Sortment Root Beer Float & Orange Cream Bar	1 bar (1.5 oz)	70
Vanilla	½ cup (2.3 oz)	140
Vanilla Chocolate Patchwork	½ cup (2.3 oz)	140
Vanilla Chocolate Strawberry	½ cup (2.3 oz)	140
Vanilla Fudge	½ cup (2.3 oz)	140
Klondike		
Almond Bar	1 (5.2 fl oz)	310
Caramel Crunch	1 (5.2 fl oz)	300
Chocolate Chocolate Bar	1 (5.2 fl oz)	280
Coffee Bar	1 (5.2 fl oz)	290
Dark Chocolate Bar	1 (5.2 fl oz)	290
Gold Bar	1 (5.2 fl oz)	340
Krispy Bar	1 (5.2 fl oz)	300
Krunch	1 (3.1 fl oz)	200
Lite Bar	1 (2.3 fl oz)	110

FOOD	PORTION	CALS.
Klondike (CONT.)		
Lite Bar Caramel	1 (2.4 fl oz)	120
Movie Bites Chocolate	8 pieces (4.6 fl oz)	340
Movie Bites Vanilla	8 pieces (4.6 fl oz)	320
Original Bar	1 (5.2 fl oz)	290
Sandwich Chocolate	1 (5.2 fl oz)	270
Sandwich Lite	1 (2.9 fl oz)	100
Sandwich Vanilla	1 (5.2 fl oz)	250
Mars		
Almond Bar	1 (1.85 fl oz)	210
Meadow Gold		
Sundae Cone	1	210
Milky Way		
Single Chocolate/Milk	1 (2 fl oz)	210
Snack Chocolate/Milk	1 (0.72 fl oz)	70
Snack Vanilla/Dark	1 (0.72 fl oz)	70
Mocha Mix		
Berry Berry Berry	½ cup	140
Dutch Chocolate	½ cup (2.3 oz)	140
Mocha Almond Fudge	½ cup (2.3 oz)	150
Neapolitan	½ cup (2.3 oz)	140
Strawberry Swirl	½ cup (2.3 oz)	140
Vanilla	½ cup (2.3 oz)	140
Nestle Crunch		
Chocolate	1 bar (3 oz)	200
Cones	1 (4.6 oz)	300
Crunch King	1 (4 oz)	270
Nuggets	8 pieces	140
Reduced Fat	1 (2.5 oz)	130
Vanilla	1 bar (3 oz)	200
Perry's		
No Fat No Sugar Added Caramel	½ cup (2.8 oz)	90
No Fat No Sugar Added Chocolate	½ cup (2.6 oz)	80
No Fat No Sugar Added Peach	½ cup (2.9 oz)	90
No Fat No Sugar Added Strawberry	½ cup (2.8 oz)	90
No Fat No Sugar Added Vanilla	½ cup (2.6 oz)	80
Rice Dream		
Bar Chocolate	1	270
Bar Chocolate Nutty	1	330
Bar Strawberry	1	260
Bar Vanilla	1	275
Bar Vanilla Nutty	1	330
Cappuccino	½ cup	130
Carob	½ cup	130

FOOD	PORTION	CALS.
Rice Dream (CONT.)		
Carob Almond	½ cup	140
Carob Chip	½ cup	140
Carob Chip Mint	½ cup	140
Cocoa Marble Fudge	½ cup	140
Dream Pie Chocolate	1	380
Dream Pie Mint	1	380
Dream Pie Mocha	1	380
Dream Pie Vanilla	1	380
Lemon	½ cup	130
Peanut Butter Fudge	½ cup	160
Strawberry	½ cup	130
Vanilla	½ cup	130
Vanilla Fudge	½ cup	140
Vanilla Swiss Almond	½ cup	140
Wildberry	½ cup	130
Sealtest		
American Glory	½ cup (2.4 oz)	130
Butter Pecan	½ cup (2.4 oz)	160
Candy Cane Crunch	½ cup (2.4 oz)	150
Chocolate	½ cup (2.4 oz)	140
Chocolate Butter Pecan	½ cup (2.4 oz)	150
Chocolate Chip	½ cup (2.4 oz)	150
Coconut Chocolate	½ cup (2.4 oz)	160
Coffee	½ cup (2.4 oz)	140
Cupid's Scoops	½ cup (2.5 oz)	140
Dessert Bar Free Chocolate Fudge	1	90
Dessert Bar Free Vanilla Strawberry Swirl	1	80
Dessert Bar Free Vanilla Fudge	1	80
Free Black Cherry	½ cup	100
Free Chocolate	½ cup	100
Free Peach	½ cup	100
Free Strawberry	½ cup	100
Free Vanilla	½ cup	100
Free Vanilla Fudge Royale	½ cup	100
Free Vanilla Strawberry Royale	½ cup	100
French Vanilla	½ cup (2.4 oz)	140
Fudge Royale	½ cup (2.5 oz)	150
Heavenly Hash	½ cup (2.4 oz)	150
Maple Walnut	½ cup (2.4 oz)	160
Strawberry	½ cup (2.4 oz)	130
Triple Chocolate Passion	½ cup (2.5 oz)	160
Vanilla	½ cup (2.4 oz)	140
Vanilla Chocolate Strawberry	½ cup (2.4 oz)	140

FOOD	PORTION	CALS.
Sealtest (CONT.)		
Vanilla With Orange Sherbet	½ cup (2.7 oz)	130
Snickers		
Single	1 (2 fl oz)	220
Snack	1 (1 fl oz)	110
Starbucks		
Biscotti Bliss	½ cup	240
Caffe Almond Fudge	½ cup	260
Caffe Almond Roast	1 bar	280
Dark Roast Expresso Swirl	½ cup	220
Frappuccino	1 bar (2.8 oz)	110
Italian Roast Coffee	½ cup	230
Javachip	½ cup	250
Low Fat Latte	½ cup	170
Low Fat Mocha Mambo	½ cup	170
Vanilla Mochachip	½ cup	270
Tofu Ice Creme		
Carob	4 fl oz	190
Vanilla	4 fl oz	190
Tofutti		
Cuties Chocolate	1 (1.4 oz)	130
Cuties Vanilla	1 (1.4 oz)	121
Frutti Vanilla Apple Orchard	4 fl oz	100
Turkey Hill		
Black Cherry	½ cup (2.3 oz)	140
Butter Pecan	½ cup (2.3 oz)	170
Choco Mint Chip	½ cup (2.3 oz)	160
Cookies 'N Cream	½ cup (2.3 oz)	160
Lite Butter Pecan	½ cup (2.3 oz)	130
Lite Choco Mint Chip	½ cup (2.3 oz)	140
Lite Cookies 'N Cream	½ cup (2.3 oz)	130
Lite Vanilla & Chocolate	½ cup (2.3 oz)	110
Lite Vanilla Bean	½ cup (2.3 oz)	110
Neapolitan	½ cup (2.3 oz)	150
Rocky Road	½ cup (2.3 oz)	170
Tin Roof Sundae	½ cup (2.3 oz)	160
Vanilla	½ cup (2.3 oz)	140
Vanilla & Chocolate	½ cup (2.3 oz)	150
Vanilla Bean	½ cup (2.3 oz)	140
Ultra Slim-Fast		
Bar Fudge	1	90
Bar Vanilla Cookie Crunch	1	90
Chocolate	4 oz	100
Chocolate Fudge	4 oz	120

FOOD	PORTION	CALS.
Ultra Slim-Fast (CONT.)		
Peach	4 oz	100
Pralines & Caramel	4 oz	120
Sandwich Vanilla	1	140
Sandwich Vanilla Chocolate	1	140
Sandwich Vanilla Oatmeal	1	150
Vanilla	4 oz	90
Vanilla Fudge Cookie	4 oz	110
Weight Watchers		
Chocolate Chip Cookie Dough Sundae	1 (2.64 oz)	190
Chocolate Mousse	1 bar	40
Chocolate Treat	1 bar	100
English Toffee Crunch	1 bar	110
Orange Vanilla Treat	1 bar	40
Vanilla Sandwich	1 bar	150
TAKE-OUT		
cone vanilla light soft serve	1 (4.6 oz)	164
gelato chocolate hazelnut	½ cup (5.3 oz)	370
gelato vanilla	½ cup (3 oz)	211
sundae caramel	1 (5.4 oz)	303
sundae hot fudge	1 (5.4 oz)	284
sundae strawberry	1 (5.4 oz)	269

ICE CREAM CONES AND CUPS

sugar cone	1	40
wafer cone	1	17
Comet		
Cups	1 (5 g)	20
Sugar Cones	1 (12 g)	50
Waffle Cone	1 (17 g)	70
Dutch Mill		
Chocolate Covered Wafer Cups	1 (0.5 oz)	80
Frookie		
Chocolate Crunch	1 (0.4 oz)	50
Honey Crunch	1 (0.4 oz)	45
Oreo		
Chocolate Cones	1 (13 g)	50
Teddy Grahams		
Cinnamon Cones	1 (0.5 oz)	60

ICE CREAM TOPPINGS
(*see also* SYRUP)

butterscotch	2 tbsp (1.4 oz)	103
caramel	2 tbsp (1.4 oz)	103
marshmallow cream	1 oz	88

FOOD	PORTION	CALS.
marshmallow cream	1 jar (7 oz)	615
pineapple	2 tbsp (1.5 oz)	106
pineapple	1 cup (11.5 oz)	861
strawberry	2 tbsp (1.5 oz)	107
strawberry	1 cup (11.5 oz)	863
walnuts in syrup	2 tbsp (1.4 oz)	167
Ben & Jerry's		
Hot Fudge	(1.3 oz)	140
Crumpy		
Chocolate Hazelnut Spread	1 tbsp (0.5 oz)	80
Hershey		
Chocolate Shoppe Candy Bar Sprinkles York	2 tbsp (1.1 oz)	170
Kraft		
Butterscotch	2 tbsp (1.4 oz)	130
Caramel	2 tbsp (1.4 oz)	120
Chocolate	2 tbsp (1.4 oz)	110
Hot Fudge	2 tbsp (1.4 oz)	140
Pineapple	2 tbsp (1.4 oz)	110
Strawberry	2 tbsp (1.4 oz)	110
Marzetti		
Caramel Apple	2 tbsp	60
Caramel Apple Reduced Fat	2 tbsp	30
Peanut Butter Caramel	2 tbsp	60
Planters		
Nut	2 tbsp (0.5 oz)	100

ICED TEA
(*see also* TEA/HERBAL TEA)

MIX

FOOD	PORTION	CALS.
Bigelow		
Nice Over Ice	5 fl oz	1
Celestial Seasonings		
Iced Delight	8 fl oz	4
Crystal Light		
Decaffeinated as prep	1 serv (8 oz)	5
Iced Tea as prep	1 serv (8 oz)	5
Peach Tea as prep	1 serv (8 oz)	5
Raspberry Tea as prep	1 serv (8 oz)	5
Lipton		
100% Tea Decaffeinated as prep	1 serv	0
100% Tea Unsweetened as prep	1 serv	0
100% Tea as prep	1 serv	0
Calorie Free as prep	1 serv	0

FOOD	PORTION	CALS.
Lipton (CONT.)		
Decaffeinated Ice Tea Brew as prep	1 serv (8 oz)	0
Decaffeinated Lemon as prep	1 serv	90
Diet Decaffeinated Lemon as prep	1 serv	5
Diet Lemon as prep	1 serv	5
Diet Peach as prep	1 serv	5
Diet Raspberry as prep	1 serv	5
Diet Tea & Lemondage as prep	1 serv	10
Herbal Iced Collection	1 tea bag	0
Ice Tea Brew as prep	1 serv (8 oz)	0
Lemon as prep	1 serv	90
Lemon as prep	1 pkg (0.5 oz)	50
Natrual Brew Tropical as prep	1 serv	90
Natural Brew 100% Tea Decaffeinated as prep	1 serv	0
Natural Brew 100% Tea as prep	1 serv	0
Natural Brew Diet Lemon as prep	1 serv	5
Natural Brew Diet Peach as prep	1 serv	5
Natural Brew Diet Tropical as prep	1 serv	5
Natural Brew Unsweetened Lemon as prep	1 serv	0
Peach as prep	1 serv	90
Rasberry as prep	1 serv	90
Tea & Lemonade as prep	1 serv	90
Nestea		
Peach as prep	8 oz	88
Raspberry as prep	8 oz	88
READY-TO-DRINK		
Arizona		
Lemon	1 bottle (16 oz)	180
Raspberry	8 fl oz	95
Clearly Canadian		
Clearly Tea Original	8 fl oz	80
Clearly Tea Tangy Lemon	8 fl oz	80
Crystal Light		
Lemon	1 serv (8 oz)	5
Peach Tea	1 serv (8 oz)	5
Raspberry Tea	1 serv (8 oz)	5
Lipton		
Carribean Cooler	1 can (12 oz)	130
Diet Lemon	8 oz	0
Diet Lemon	1 bottle (16 oz)	10
Green Tea & Passion Fruit	1 bottle (16 oz)	160
Lemon	8 oz	80
Lemon	1 can (12 oz)	120

FOOD	PORTION	CALS.
Lipton (CONT.)		
Lemon	1 bottle (16 oz)	180
Natural Lemon	1 box (8 oz)	100
Peach	8 oz	80
Peach	1 bottle (16 oz)	220
Raspberry	8 oz	80
Raspberry	1 bottle (16 oz)	220
Raspberry Blast	1 can (12 oz)	130
Southern Style Extra Sweet No Lemon	1 bottle (16 oz)	240
Southern Style Lemon	1 bottle (16 oz)	200
Southern Style Sweetened No Lemon	1 bottle (16 oz)	200
Sweet	8 oz	80
Sweetened No Lemon	1 bottle (16 oz)	140
Sweetened Lemon	8 oz	80
Tangerine Twist	1 can (12 oz)	120
Tea & Lemonade	1 bottle (16 oz)	220
Unsweetened No Lemon	1 bottle (16 oz)	0
Nestea		
With Sugar & Lemon	1 bottle (16 fl oz)	176
With Sugar & Lemon	1 can (11.5 fl oz)	127
Royal Mistic		
Diet	12 fl oz	8
Lemon	12 fl oz	144
Orange	12 fl oz	144
Wild Berry	12 fl oz	144
Schweppes		
Ice Tea	8 fl oz	90
Snapple		
Cranberry	8 fl oz	110
Diet	8 fl oz	0
Diet Peach	8 fl oz	0
Diet Raspberry	8 fl oz	0
Lemon	8 fl oz	110
Mango	8 fl oz	110
Mint	8 fl oz	120
Old Fashioned	8 fl oz	80
Orange	8 fl oz	110
Peach	8 fl oz	110
Raspberry	8 fl oz	120
Strawberry	8 fl oz	100
Turkey Hill		
Diet Decaffeinated	1 cup (8 oz)	0
Raspberry Cooler	1 cup (8 oz)	110

FOOD	PORTION	CALS.
Turkey Hill (cont.)		
Regular	1 cup (8 oz)	90

ICES AND ICE POPS

(*see also* ICE CREAM AND FROZEN DESSERTS, PUDDING POPS, SHERBET, YOGURT FROZEN)

FOOD	PORTION	CALS.
fruit & juice bar	1 (3 fl oz)	75
gelatin pop	1 (1.5 oz)	31
ice coconut pineapple	½ cup (4 fl oz)	109
ice fruit w/ Equal	1 bar (1.7 oz)	12
ice lime	½ cup (4 fl oz)	75
ice pop	1 (2 fl oz)	42
Cool Creations		
10 Pack	1 pop (2 oz)	60
Lion King Cone	1 (4 oz)	280
Mickey Mouse Bar	1 (2.5 oz)	110
Mickey Mouse Bar	1 (4 oz)	170
Surprise Pops	1 (2 oz)	60
Dole		
Fruit 'N Juice Coconut	1 bar (4 oz)	210
Fruit 'N Juice Lemonade	1 bar (4 oz)	120
Fruit 'N Juice Lime	1 bar (4 oz)	110
Fruit 'N Juice Peach Passion	1 bar (2.5 oz)	70
Fruit 'N Juice Pineapple Coconut	1 bar (4 oz)	140
Fruit 'N Juice Pineapple Orange Banana	1 bar (2.5 oz)	70
Fruit 'N Juice Pineapple Orange Banana	1 bar (4 oz)	110
Fruit 'N Juice Raspberry	1 bar (2.5 oz)	70
Fruit 'N Juice Strawberry	1 bar (4 oz)	110
Fruit 'N Juice Strawberry	1 bar (2.5 oz)	70
Fruit Juice Grape	1 bar (1.75 oz)	45
Fruit Juice No Sugar Added Grape	1 bar (1.75 oz)	25
Fruit Juice No Sugar Added Strawberry	1 bar (1.75 oz)	25
Fruit Juice Raspberry	1 bar (1.75 oz)	45
Fruit Juice Raspberry	1 bar (1.75 oz)	25
Fruit Juice Strawberry	1 bar (1.75 oz)	45
Fi-Bar		
Juice Bar Lemoney-Lime	1 bar	63
Juice Bar Strawberry Nectar	1 bar	63
Juice Bar Tropical Delight	1 bar	63
Flintstones		
Rock Pops	1 (3.5 oz)	80
Frozfruit		
Banana Cream	1 bar (4 oz)	150
Cantaloupe	1 bar (4 oz)	60

FOOD	PORTION	CALS.
Frozfruit (CONT.)		
Cappuccino Cream	1 bar (3 oz)	140
Cherry	1 bar (4 oz)	70
Coconut Cream	1 bar (4 oz)	170
Kiwi Strawberry	1 bar (4 oz)	90
Lemon	1 bar (4 oz)	90
Lemon Iced Tea	1 bar (4 oz)	80
Lime	1 bar (4 oz)	90
Orange	1 bar (4 oz)	90
Pina Colada Cream	1 bar (4 oz)	170
Pineapple	1 bar (4 oz)	80
Raspberry	1 bar (4 oz)	80
Strawberry	1 (4 oz)	80
Strawberry Banana Cream	1 bar (4 oz)	140
Strawberry Cream	1 bar (4 oz)	130
Tropical	1 bar (4 oz)	90
Watermelon	1 bar (4 oz)	50
Good Humor		
Big Stick Cherry Pineapple	1 (3.6 fl oz)	50
Big Stick Popsicle	1 (3.6 fl oz)	50
Calippo Cherry	1 (3.8 fl oz)	100
Calippo Grape Lemon	1 (3.9 fl oz)	90
Calippo Orange	1 (3.9 fl oz)	90
Citrus Bites	1 (1.8 fl oz)	35
Creamsicle Orange	1 (1.8 fl oz)	70
Creamsicle Orange	1 (2.8 fl oz)	110
Creamsicle Orange Raspberry	1 (2.6 fl oz)	100
Creamsicle Sugar Free	1 (1.8 fl oz)	25
Flinstones Push-Up Yabba Dabba Doo Orange	1 (2.75 fl oz)	90
Fudgsicle Bar	1 (2.8 fl oz)	90
Fudgsicle Pop	1 (1.8 fl oz)	60
Fudgsicle Sugar Free	1 (1.8 fl oz)	40
Fun Box Fudge Bar	1 (2.3 fl oz)	80
Fun Box Pops	1 (2 fl oz)	35
Fun Box Twin Box Cherry	1 (2.6 fl oz)	50
Fun Box Twin Pop Banana	1 (2.6 fl oz)	50
Fun Box Twin Pop Blue Raspberry	1 (2.6 fl oz)	50
Fun Box Twin Pop Cherry Lemon	1 (2.6 fl oz)	50
Fun Box Twin Pop Orange Cherry Grape	1 (2.6 oz)	50
Fun Box Twin Pop Root Beer	1 (2.6 fl oz)	50
Garfield Bar	1 (3.9 fl oz)	90
Great White	1 (3.1 fl oz)	70
Hyperstripe	1 (2.8 fl oz)	80

FOOD	PORTION	CALS.
Good Humor (CONT.)		
Ice Stripe Cherry Orange	1 (1.5 fl oz)	35
Jumbo Jet Star	1 (4.7 fl oz)	80
Laser Blazer	1 (2.6 oz)	70
Popsicle All Natural	1 (1.8 fl oz)	45
Popsicle Orange Cherry Grape	1 (1.8 fl oz)	45
Popsicle Rainbow Pops	1 (1.8 fl oz)	45
Popsicle Rootbeer Banana Lime	1 (1.8 fl oz)	45
Popsicle Strawberry Raspberry Wildberry	1 (1.8 fl oz)	45
Popsicle Supersicle Traffic Signal	1	80
Popsicle Twin Pop Cherry	1 (2.6 fl oz)	70
Popsicle Twin Pop Orange Cherry Grape Lime	1 (2.6 fl oz)	70
Snow Cone	1	60
Snowfruit Coconut Bar	1 (3.75 fl oz)	150
Snowfruit Orange Bar	1	140
Snowfruit Strawberry Bar	1	120
Snowfruit Tropical Fruit Bar	1	110
Sugar Free Pop Orange Cherry Grape	1 (1.8 fl oz)	15
Super Mario Bar	1	120
Supersicle Cherry Banana	1 (4.7 fl oz)	80
Supersicle Cherry Cola	1 (4.7 fl oz)	80
Supersicle Double Fudge	1 (4.7 fl oz)	150
Supersicle Firecracker	1 (4.7 fl oz)	90
Supersicle Firecracker Jr.	1	72
Supersicle Sour Tower	1	80
Swirl Bubble Gum	1 (2.7 fl oz)	55
Swirl Cherry Banana	1 (2.7 fl oz)	55
Torpedo Cherry	1 (1.8 fl oz)	35
Twister Blue Raspberry Cherry Cherry Cola Cherry	1 (1.8 fl oz)	45
Twister Cherry Lemon Orange Lemon	1 (1.8 fl oz)	45
Vampire's Deadly Secret	1 (2.8 fl oz)	100
Watermelon Bar	1 (3.6 fl oz)	80
Haagen-Dazs		
Sorbet Banana Strawberry	½ cup (4 oz)	140
Sorbet Chocolate	½ cup (4 oz)	130
Sorbet Manago	½ cup (4 oz)	120
Sorbet Orchard Peach	½ cup (4 oz)	140
Sorbet Raspberry	½ cup (4 oz)	120
Sorbet Strawberry	½ cup (4 oz)	130
Sorbet Zesty Lemon	½ cup (4 oz)	130
Sorbet & Cream Orange	½ cup (3.7 oz)	200
Sorbet & Cream Raspberry	½ cup (3.7 oz)	190

FOOD	PORTION	CALS.
Haagen-Dazs (CONT.)		
Sorbet Bar Chocolate	1 (2.7 oz)	80
Sorbet Bar Wild Berry	1 (2.7 oz)	90
Hershey		
Orange Blossom	1 bar (1.6 oz)	90
Hood		
Hendrie's Sizzle'N Sour Stix	1 bar (2 oz)	80
Hoodsie Pop	1 (3.3 oz)	60
Natural Blenders Pineappple	1 bar (1 oz)	60
Natural Blenders Raspberry	1 bar (1 oz)	60
Natural Blenders Strawberry	1 bar (1 oz)	60
Pop Banana	1 (3.3 oz)	60
Pop Blue Raspberry	1 (3.3 oz)	60
Pop Cherry	1 (3.3 oz)	60
Pop Grape	1 (3.3 oz)	60
Pop Orange	1 (3.3 oz)	60
Pop Root Beer	1 (3.3 oz)	60
Super Sortment Juice Bars	1 bar (1.9 oz)	40
Lifesavers		
Ice Pops	1	35
Ice Pops	1 (1.75 oz)	35
Mr. Freeze		
Assorted	2 bars (3 oz)	45
Tropical	2 bars (3 oz)	45
Natural Choice		
Organic Banana	½ cup (3.6 oz)	110
Organic Blueberry	½ cup (3.6 oz)	100
Organic Kiwi	½ cup (3.6 oz)	110
Organic Mango	½ cup (3.6 oz)	110
Organic Strawberry	½ cup (3.6 oz)	110
Organic Strawberry Kiwi	½ cup (3.6 oz)	110
Sunkist		
Orange Juice Bar	1 (3.4 fl oz)	80
Wildberry	1 (3.4 fl oz)	120
Tofutti		
Frutti Apricot Mango	4 fl oz	100
Frutti Three Berry	4 fl oz	100

ICING
(*see* CAKE ICING)

INSTANT BREAKFAST
(*see* BREAKFAST DRINKS)

JALAPENO
(*see* PEPPERS)

JAM/JELLY/PRESERVES

all flavors jam	1 tbsp (0.7 oz)	48

FOOD	PORTION	CALS.
all flavors jam	1 pkg (0.5 oz)	34
all flavors jelly	1 tbsp (0.7 oz)	52
all flavors jelly	1 pkg (0.5 oz)	38
all flavors preserve	1 pkg (0.5 oz)	34
all flavors preserve	1 tbsp (0.7 oz)	48
apple butter	1 tbsp (0.6 oz)	33
apple butter	1 cup (9.9 oz)	519
apple jelly	1 tbsp (0.7 oz)	52
apple jelly	1 pkg (0.5 oz)	38
linganberry jam	0.5 oz	23
orange marmalade	1 pkg (0.5 oz)	34
orange marmalade	1 tbsp (0.7 oz)	49
strawberry jam	1 pkg (0.5 oz)	34
strawberry jam	1 tbsp (0.7 oz)	48
strawberry preserve	1 pkg (0.5 oz)	34
strawberry preserve	1 tbsp (0.7 oz)	48
BAMA		
Apple Butter	2 tsp	25
Apple Jelly	2 tsp	30
Grape Jelly	2 tsp	30
Peach Preserves	2 tsp	30
Red Plum Jam	2 tsp	30
Strawberry Preserves	2 tsp	30
Estee		
Fruit Spread Apple Spice	1 tbsp	16
Fruit Spread Apricot	1 tbsp	16
Fruit Spread Grape	1 tbsp	16
Fruit Spread Peach	1 tbsp	16
Fruit Spread Red Raspberry	1 tbsp	16
Fruit Spread Strawberry	1 tbsp	16
Harvest Moon		
Apricot Fruit Spread	1 tbsp (0.6 oz)	35
Blueberry Fruit Spread	1 tbsp (0.6 oz)	35
Cherry Fruit Spread	1 tbsp (0.6 oz)	35
Grape Fruit Spread	1 tbsp (0.6 oz)	35
Peach Fruit Spread	1 tbsp (0.6 oz)	35
Raspberry Fruit Spread	1 tbsp (0.6 oz)	35
Strawberry Fruit Spread	1 tbsp (0.6 oz)	35
Red Wing		
Apple Jelly	1 tbsp (0.7 oz)	50
Apple Blackberry Jelly	1 tbsp (0.7 oz)	50
Apple Cherry Jelly	1 tbsp (0.7 oz)	50
Apple Currant Jelly	1 tbsp (0.7 oz)	50
Apple Grape Jelly	1 tbsp (0.7 oz)	50

FOOD	PORTION	CALS.
Red Wing (CONT.)		
Apple Raspberry Jelly	1 tbsp (0.7 oz)	50
Apple Strawberry Jelly	1 tbsp (0.7 oz)	50
Black Raspberry Jelly	1 tbsp (0.7 oz)	50
Blackberry Jelly	1 tbsp (0.7 oz)	50
Cherry Jelly	1 tbsp (0.7 oz)	50
Concord Grape Jelly	1 tbsp (0.7 oz)	50
Crabapple Jelly	1 tbsp (0.7 oz)	50
Cranberry Jelly	1 tbsp (0.7 oz)	50
Cranberry Grape Jelly	1 tbsp (0.7 oz)	50
Currant Jelly	1 tbsp (0.7 oz)	50
Damson Plum Jelly	1 tbsp (0.7 oz)	50
Elderberry Jelly	1 tbsp (0.7 oz)	50
Grape Jelly	1 tbsp (0.7 oz)	50
Mint Jelly	1 tbsp (0.7 oz)	50
Mint Apple Jelly	1 tbsp (0.7 oz)	50
Mixed Fruit Jelly	1 tbsp (0.7 oz)	50
Red Plum Jelly	1 tbsp (0.7 oz)	50
Red Raspberry Jelly	1 tbsp (0.7 oz)	50
Strawberry Jelly	1 tbsp (0.7 oz)	50
Strawberry Apple Jelly	1 tbsp (0.7 oz)	50
Tabasco		
Spicy Pepper Jelly	1 tbsp (0.6 oz)	50
Tree Of Life		
Apricot Fruit Spread	1 tbsp (0.6 oz)	45
Blueberry Fruit Spread	1 tbsp (0.6 oz)	35
Cherry Fruit Spread	1 tbsp (0.6 oz)	40
Grape Fruit Spread	1 tbsp (0.6 oz)	35
Peach Fruit Spread	1 tbsp (0.6 oz)	45
Raspberry Fruit Spread	1 tbsp (0.6 oz)	30
Strawberry Fruit Spread	1 tbsp (0.6 oz)	35
Whistling Wings		
Blueberry Jam	1 oz	50
Raspberry Jam	1 oz	60

JAPANESE FOOD
(*see* ASIAN FOOD, SUSHI)

JELLY
(*see* JAM/JELLY/PRESERVE)

JERUSALEM ARTICHOKE
(*see* ARTICHOKE)

JAVA PLUM

fresh	1 cup	82
fresh	3	5

FOOD	PORTION	CALS.
KALE		
FRESH		
chopped cooked	½ cup	21
raw chopped	½ cup	21
Dole		
Chopped	½ cup	17
KETCHUP		
ketchup	1 pkg (0.2 oz)	6
low sodium	1 tbsp	16
Del Monte		
Ketchup	1 tbsp (0.5 oz)	15
Estee		
Ketchup	1 tbsp	15
Hain		
Natural	1 tbsp	16
Natural No Salt Added	1 tbsp	16
Healthy Choice		
Ketchup	1 tbsp (0.5 oz)	9
Hunt's		
Ketchup	1 tbsp (0.6 oz)	16
No Salt Added	1 tbsp (0.6 oz)	16
McIlhenny		
Spicy	1 tbsp (0.6 oz)	20
Muir Glen		
Organic	1 tbsp (0.6 oz)	15
Red Wing		
Extra Fancy	1 tbsp (0.6 oz)	20
Tree Of Life		
Ketchup	1 tbsp (0.5 oz)	10
Salsa Ketchup	1 tbsp (0.5 oz)	10
KIDNEY		
beef simmered	3 oz	122
lamb braised	3 oz	117
pork cooked	1 cup	211
pork cooked	3 oz	128
veal braised	3 oz	139
KIDNEY BEANS		
CANNED		
B&M		
Red Baked Beans	½ cup (4.6 oz)	170
Eden		
Organic	½ cup (4.6 oz)	100

FOOD	PORTION	CALS.
Friend's		
Red Baked Beans	½ cup (4.6 oz)	160
Goya		
Spanish Style	7.5 oz	140
Green Giant		
Dark Red	½ cup (4.5 oz)	110
Light Red	½ cup (4.5 oz)	110
Hunt's		
Red	½ cup (4.5 oz)	94
Progresso		
Red	½ cup (4.6 oz)	110
Trappey		
Dark Red	½ cup (4.5 oz)	130
Light Red	½ cup (4.5 oz)	120
Light Red New Orleans Style With Bacon	½ cup (4.5 oz)	110
Light Red With Jalapeno	½ cup (4.5 oz)	110
With Chili Gravy	½ cup (4.5 oz)	110
Van Camp's		
Dark Red	½ cup (4.6 oz)	90
Light Red	½ cup (4.6 oz)	90
DRIED		
Arrowhead		
Red	¼ cup (1.6 oz)	160
SPROUTS		
cooked	1 lb	152
raw	½ cup	27
KIWI JUICE		
After The Fall		
Kiwi Bear	1 cup (8 oz)	100
KIWIS		
fresh	1 med	46
Dole		
Fresh	2	90
Sonoma		
Dried	7-8 pieces (1 oz)	90
KNISH		
Joshua's		
Coney Island Potato	1 (4.6 oz)	280
TAKE-OUT		
cheese & blueberry	1 (7 oz)	378
cheese & cherry	1 (7 oz)	378
everything	1 (7 oz)	221

FOOD	PORTION	CALS.
kashe	1 (7 oz)	270
potato	1 lg (7 oz)	332
potato	1 med (3.5 oz)	166
potato w/ broccoli & cheese	1 (7 oz)	312
potato w/ spinach & mushroom	1 (7 oz)	214

KOHLRABI
raw sliced	½ cup	19
sliced cooked	½ cup	24

KUMQUATS
fresh	1	12

LAMB
FRESH
cubed lean only braised	3 oz	190
cubed lean only broiled	3 oz	158
ground broiled	3 oz	240
leg lean & fat Choice roasted	3 oz	219
loin chop w/ bone lean & fat Choice broiled	1 chop (2.3 oz)	201
loin chop w/ bone lean only Choice broiled	1 chop (1.6 oz)	100
rib chop lean & fat Choice broiled	3 oz	307
rib chop lean only Choice broiled	3 oz	200
shank lean & fat Choice braised	3 oz	206
shank lean & fat Choice roasted	3 oz	191
shoulder chop w/ bone lean & fat Choice braised	1 chop (2.5 oz)	244
shoulder chop w/ bone lean only Choice braised	1 chop (1.9 oz)	152
sirloin lean & fat Choice roasted	3 oz	248

LAMBSQUARTERS
chopped cooked	½ cup	29

LECITHIN
(*see* SOY)

LEEKS
chopped cooked	¼ cup	8
cooked	1 (4.4 oz)	38
freeze dried	1 tbsp	1
raw chopped	¼ cup	16

LEMON
fresh	1 med	22
peel	1 tbsp	0
wedge	1	5

FOOD	PORTION	CALS.
Dole		
Fresh	1	18
LEMON EXTRACT		
Virginia Dare		
Extract	1 tsp	22
LEMON GRASS		
fresh	1 cup (2.4 oz)	66
fresh	1 tbsp (5 g)	5
LEMON JUICE		
bottled	1 tbsp	3
fresh	1 tbsp	4
frzn	1 tbsp	3
After The Fall		
Spicy Lemon	1 can (12 oz)	150
Realemon		
Juice	1 fl oz	6
LEMONADE		
FROZEN		
Bright & Early		
Lemonade	8 fl oz	120
Minute Maid		
Country Style	8 fl oz	120
Cranberry Lemonade	8 fl oz	80
Lemonade	8 fl oz	110
Pink	8 fl oz	120
Raspberry	8 fl oz	120
Seneca		
as prep	8 fl oz	110
MIX		
Country Time		
Lem'n Berry Sippers Cranberry Raspberry Lemonade as prep	1 serv (8 oz)	90
Lem'n Berry Sippers Raspberry Lemonade as prep	1 serv (8 oz)	90
Lem'n Berry Sippers Strawberry Lemonade as prep	1 serv (8 oz)	90
Lem'n Berry Sippers Wildberry Lemonade as prep	1 serv (8 oz)	90
Lem'n Berry Sippers Sugar Free Strawberry Lemonade as prep	1 serv (8 oz)	5
Lemonade as prep	1 serv (8 oz)	70
Pink as prep	1 serv (8 oz)	70

FOOD	PORTION	CALS.
Country Time (CONT.)		
Sugar Free Pink as prep	1 serv (8 oz)	5
Sugar Free as prep	1 serv (8 oz)	5
Crystal Light		
Lemonade as prep	1 serv (8 oz)	5
Pink as prep	1 serv (8 oz)	5
Kool-Aid		
Lemonade as prep	1 serv (8 oz)	70
Mix as prep w/ sugar	1 serv (8 oz)	100
Pink as prep w/ sugar	1 serv (8 oz)	100
Soarin' Strawberry Lemonade as prep	1 serv (8 oz)	70
Soarin' Strawberry Lemonade as prep w/ sugar	1 serv (8 oz)	100
Sugar Free Soarin' Strawberry Lemonade as prep	1 serv (8 oz)	5
Sugar Free Mix as prep	1 serv (8 oz)	5
READY-TO-DRINK		
After The Fall		
Apple Raspberry	1 bottle (10 oz)	120
Crystal Geyser		
Juice Squeeze Pink	1 bottle (12 fl oz)	140
Crystal Light		
Lemonade	1 serv (8 oz)	5
Pink	1 serv (8 oz)	5
Diet Rite		
Salt/Sodium Free	8 fl oz	2
Everfresh		
Lemonade	1 can (8 oz)	120
Ruby Red	1 can (8 oz)	110
Fruitopia		
Lemonade	8 fl oz	120
Minute Maid		
Chilled	8 fl oz	110
Cranberry Chilled	8 fl oz	120
Juices To Go	1 bottle (16 fl oz)	110
Juices To Go	1 can (11.5 fl oz)	160
Juices To Go Cranberry Lemonade	1 bottle (16 fl oz)	110
Juices To Go Raspberry Lemonade	1 bottle (16 fl oz)	120
Pink Chilled	8 fl oz	110
Raspberry Chilled	8 fl oz	120
Mott's		
Lemonade	10 fl oz	160
Nehi		
Lemonade	8 fl oz	130

FOOD	PORTION	CALS.
Newman's Own		
Lemonade	1 bottle (10 oz)	140
Roadside Virginia	8 fl oz	110
Odwalla		
Honey	8 fl oz	70
Strawberry	8 fl oz	150
Royal Mistic		
Lemonade Limeade	16 fl oz	230
Tropical Pink	16 fl oz	230
Santa Cruz		
Organic	8 oz	100
Shasta Plus		
Lemonade	1 can (11.5 oz)	160
Snapple		
Diet Pink	8 fl oz	13
Lemonade	8 fl oz	110
Pink	8 fl oz	110
Strawberry	8 fl oz	110
Turkey Hill		
Lemonade	8 fl oz	110
Veryfine		
Chillers	1 can (11.5 oz)	190
Chillers Cherry	8 fl oz	120
Chillers Peach	8 fl oz	120
Chillers Pink	1 can (11.5 oz)	180
Chillers Strawberry	1 can (11.5 oz)	170

LENTILS
CANNED
Eden

Organic w/ Sweet Onion & Bay Leaf	½ cup (4.6 oz)	90

FROZEN
Natural Touch

Lentil Rice Loaf	1 in slice (3.2 oz)	170

MIX
Casbah

Pilaf as prep	1 cup	200

SPROUTS

raw	½ cup	40

TAKE-OUT

indian sambar	1 serv	236

LETTUCE
(*see also* SALAD)

bibb	1 head (6 oz)	21

FOOD	PORTION	CALS.
boston	2 leaves	2
boston	1 head (6 oz)	21
iceberg	1 leaf	3
iceberg	1 head (19 oz)	70
looseleaf shredded	½ cup	5
romaine shredded	½ cup	4
Dole		
Butter	1 head	21
Iceberg	⅙ med head	20
Leaf shredded	1½ cup	12
Romaine shredded	1½ cups	18
Western Express		
Heart's Of Romaine	6 leaves (3 oz)	20

LIMA BEANS
CANNED
Allen		
Green	½ cup (4.5 oz)	120
Green & White	½ cup (4.5 oz)	110
Del Monte		
Green	½ cup (4.4 oz)	80
East Texas Fair		
Green	½ cup (4.5 oz)	120
Seneca		
Limas	½ cup	80
Trappey		
Baby Green With Bacon	½ cup (4.5 oz)	120

DRIED
Hurst		
HamBeens Baby Limas w/ Ham	1 serv	120
HamBeens Large Limas w/ Ham	1 serv	120

FROZEN
Birds Eye		
Baby	½ cup (3.3 oz)	130
Fordhook	½ cup (3.3 oz)	100
Fresh Like		
Baby	3.5 oz	138
Green Giant		
Butter Sauce	⅔ cup (3.6 oz)	120
Harvest Fresh Baby	½ cup (2.7 oz)	80

LIME
fresh	1	20

LIME JUICE
bottled	1 tbsp	3
fresh	1 tbsp	4

FOOD	PORTION	CALS.
After The Fall		
Caribbean Lime	1 can (12 oz)	170
Key West	1 cup (8 oz)	100
Odwalla		
Summertime Lime	8 fl oz	90
Realime		
Juice	1 oz	6

LING
fresh baked	3 oz	95

LIQUOR/LIQUEUR
(*see also* BEER AND ALE, CHAMPAGNE, DRINK MIXERS, MALT, WINE, WINE COOLERS)

anisette	0.7 oz	74
apricot brandy	0.7 oz	64
aquavit	3.5 oz	229
bloody mary	5 oz	116
bourbon & soda	4 oz	105
coffee liqueur	1.5 oz	174
coffee w/ cream liqueur	1.5 oz	154
cognac	3.5 oz	233
creme de menthe	1.5 oz	186
daiquiri	2 oz	111
gin	1.5 oz	110
gin & tonic	7.5 oz	171
gin ricky	4 oz	150
long island ice tea	1 serv (7.5 oz)	159
manhattan	2 oz	128
martini	2.5 oz	156
pina colada	4.5 oz	262
planter's punch	3.5 oz	175
rum	1.5 oz	97
screwdriver	7 oz	174
tequila sunrise	5.5 oz	189
tom collins	7.5 oz	121
vodka	1.5 oz	97
whiskey	1.5 oz	105
whiskey sour	3 oz	123
whiskey sour mix not prep	1 pkg (0.6 oz)	64

LIVER
(*see also* PATE)

beef braised	3 oz	137
beef pan-fried	3 oz	184

FOOD	PORTION	CALS.
chicken stewed	1 cup (5 oz)	219
duck raw	1 (1.5 oz)	60
goose raw	1 (3.3 oz)	125
lamb braised	3 oz	187
lamb fried	3 oz	202
pork braised	3 oz	140
turkey simmered	1 cup (5 oz)	237
veal braised	3 oz	140
veal fried	3 oz	208
Shady Brook		
Turkey	4 oz	160

LOBSTER
(*see also* CRAYFISH)
CANNED
Progresso

Rock Lobster Sauce	½ cup (4.3 oz)	100

FRESH

northern cooked	1 cup	142
northern cooked	3 oz	83
spiny steamed	1 (5.7 oz)	233
spiny steamed	3 oz	122

FROZEN
Cajun Cookin'

Crawfish Etouffee	12 oz	390

LOGANBERRIES

frzn	1 cup	80

LONGANS

fresh	1	2

LOQUATS

fresh	1	5

LOTUS

root raw sliced	10 slices	45
root sliced cooked	10 slices	59
seeds dried	1 oz	94

LOX
(*see* SALMON)

LUPINES

dried cooked	1 cup	197

LYCHEES

fresh	1	6

FOOD	PORTION	CALS.
MACADAMIA NUTS		
dried	1 oz	199
oil roasted	1 oz	204
MacFarms of Hawaii		
Chocolate Covered	¼ cup (1.3 oz)	210
Dry Roasted Salted	¼ cup (1.3 oz)	220
Kona Coffee Dark Chocolate Covered	¼ cup (1.3 oz)	210
Mauna Loa		
Candy Glazed	1 oz	170
Chocolate Covered	1 oz	170
Honey Roasted	1 oz	200
Macadamia Nut Brittle	1 oz	150
Roasted & Salted	1 oz	210
MACARONI		
(*see* PASTA)		
MACE		
ground	1 tsp	8
MACKEREL		
CANNED		
jack	1 can (12.7 oz)	563
jack	1 cup	296
FRESH		
atlantic cooked	3 oz	223
jack baked	3 oz	171
king baked	3 oz	114
pacific baked	3 oz	171
spanish cooked	3 oz	134
SMOKED		
atlantic	3.5 oz	296
MALANGA		
fresh	½ cup	137
MALT		
nonalcoholic	12 fl oz	32
Bartles & Jaymes		
Malt Cooler Berry	12 fl oz	210
Malt Cooler Black Cherry	12 fl oz	190
Malt Cooler Light Berry	12 fl oz	140
Malt Cooler Mandarin Lemon	12 fl oz	210
Malt Cooler Margarita	12 fl oz	250
Malt Cooler Original	12 fl oz	180
Malt Cooler Peach	12 fl oz	200

FOOD	PORTION	CALS.
Bartles & Jaymes (CONT.)		
Malt Cooler Pina Colada	12 fl oz	270
Malt Cooler Planter's Punch	12 fl oz	220
Malt Cooler Red Sangria	12 fl oz	190
Malt Cooler Strawberry	12 fl oz	200
Malt Cooler Strawberry Daiquiri	12 fl oz	220
Malt Cooler Tropical	12 fl oz	220
MALTED MILK		
chocolate as prep w/ milk	1 cup	229
chocolate flavor powder	3 heaping tsp (¾ oz)	79
natural flavor as prep w/ milk	1 cup	237
natural flavor powder	3 heaping tsp (¾ oz)	87
Carnation		
Chocolate	3 tbsp (0.7 oz)	90
Original	3 tbsp (0.7 oz)	90
MAMMY-APPLE		
fresh	1	431
MANGO		
fresh	1	135
DRIED		
Rainforest Farms		
Slices	6 slices (1.3 oz)	140
Sonoma		
Pieces	8 pieces (2 oz)	180
MANGO JUICE		
After The Fall		
Hawaiian Mango	1 can (12 oz)	180
Mango Ginger	1 can (12 oz)	150
Fresh Samantha		
Mango Mama	1 cup (8 oz)	125
Kern's		
Nectar	6 fl oz	100
Libby		
Nectar	1 can (11.5 fl oz)	210
Snapple		
Diet Mango Madness	8 fl oz	13
Mango Madness Cocktail	8 fl oz	110
Tang		
Drink Mix as prep	1 serv (8 oz)	100
MARGARINE		
(*see also* BUTTER BLENDS, BUTTER SUBSTITUTES)		
Fleischmann's		
Stick	1 tbsp	100

FOOD	PORTION	CALS.
Fleischmann's (CONT.)		
Stick Light Corn Oil	1 tbsp	80
Stick Sweet Unsalted	1 tbsp	100
Hain		
Stick Safflower	1 tbsp	100
Stick Safflower Unsalted	1 tbsp	100
Tub Safflower	1 tbsp	100
Hollywood		
Safflower	1 tbsp	100
Safflower Unsalted Sweet	1 tbsp	100
Soft Spread	1 tbsp	90
Land O'Lakes		
Stick	1 tbsp (0.5 oz)	90
Stick With Sweet Cream	1 tbsp (0.5 oz)	90
Stick With Sweet Cream Unsalted	1 tbsp (0.5 oz)	90
Tub	1 tbsp (0.5 oz)	80
Tub With Sweet Cream	1 tbsp (0.5 oz)	80
Nucanola		
Stick	1 tbsp	90
Parkay		
Squeeze	1 tbsp (0.5 oz)	80
Stick	1 tbsp (0.5 oz)	90
Stick ⅓ Less Fat	1 tbsp (0.5 oz)	70
Tub	1 tbsp (0.5 oz)	60
Tub Light	1 tbsp (0.5 oz)	50
Tub Soft	1 tbsp (0.5 oz)	100
Tub Soft Diet	1 tbsp (0.5 oz)	50
Whipped	1 tbsp (0.3 oz)	70
Promise		
Spread Soft	1 tbsp	80
Spread Stick	1 tbsp	90
Spread Light Soft	1 tbsp	50
Spread Light Stick	1 tbsp	50
Ultra Soft	1 tbsp	30
Ultra Spread Fat Free	1 tbsp	5
Smart Balance		
No Trans Fat	1 tbsp (0.5 oz)	120
No Trans Fat Light	1 tbsp (0.5 oz)	45
No Trans Fat Spread	1 tbsp (0.5 oz)	80
Smart Beat		
Light Unsalted	1 tbsp (0.5 oz)	25
Squeeze Fat Free	1 tbsp (0.5 oz)	5
Super Light Trans Fat Free	1 tbsp (0.5 oz)	20
Tub	1 tbsp	25

FOOD	PORTION	CALS.
Smart Beat (CONT.)		
Tub Unsalted	1 tbsp	25
Tree Of Life		
Canola Soft	1 tbsp (0.5 oz)	100
Stick 100% Soy	1 tbsp (0.5 oz)	100
Stick 100% Soy Salt Free	1 tbsp (0.5 oz)	100
Stick Canola Soy	1 tbsp (0.5 oz)	100
Stick Canola Soy Salt Free	1 tbsp (0.5 oz)	100
Weight Watchers		
Light	1 tbsp	45
Light Sodium Free	1 tbsp	45

MARINADE
(*see* SAUCE)

MARJORAM
dried	1 tsp	2

MARSHMALLOW
marshmallow	1 reg (0.3 oz)	23
marshmallow	1 cup (1.6 oz)	146
Campfire		
Large	2	40
Miniature	24	40
Joyva		
Twists Chocolate Covered	2 (1.5 oz)	190
Just Born		
Peeps	5 (1.5 oz)	160

MATZO
egg	1 (1 oz)	111
egg & onion	1 (1 oz)	111
plain	1 (1 oz)	112
whole wheat	1 (1 oz)	99
Goodman's		
Matzo Ball Mix 50% Less Salt	2 tbsp (0.5 oz)	50
Matzo Ball Mix as prep	2 tbsp (0.5 oz)	60
Horowitz Margareten		
Egg Milk Chocolate Coated	1 oz	97
Manischewitz		
Egg Dark Chocolate Coated	½ matzo (1 oz)	97
Streit's		
Dietetic	1 (1 oz)	100
Lightly Salted	1 (1 oz)	110
Matzoh Meal	¼ cup (1 oz)	110
Passover	1 (1 oz)	110

FOOD	PORTION	CALS.
Streit's (CONT.)		
Unsalted	1 (0.9 oz)	100
Whole Wheat	1 (1 oz)	110

MAYONNAISE

(*see also* MAYONNAISE TYPE SALAD DRESSING, RELISH)

FOOD	PORTION	CALS.
BAMA		
Mayonnaise	1 tbsp	100
Bennett's		
Mayonnaise	1 tbsp	110
Hain		
Canola	1 tbsp	100
Canola	1 tbsp	60
Cold Processed	1 tbsp	110
Eggless No Salt Added	1 tbsp	110
Light Low Sodium	1 tbsp	60
Real No Salt Added	1 tbsp	110
Safflower	1 tbsp	110
Hollywood		
Canola	1 tbsp	100
Mayonnaise	1 tbsp	110
Safflower	1 tbsp	100
Kraft		
Fat Free	1 tbsp (0.6 oz)	10
Light	1 tbsp (0.5 oz)	50
Real	1 tbsp (0.5 oz)	100
McIlhenny		
Spicy	1 tbsp (0.5 oz)	108
Red Wing		
"H" Style	1 tbsp (0.5 oz)	110
Smart Beat		
Canola Oil	1 tbsp	40
Corn Beat	1 tbsp	40
Fat Free	1 tbsp	10
Weight Watchers		
Fat Free	1 tbsp	10
Light	1 tbsp	25
Light Low Sodium	1 tbsp	25

MAYONNAISE TYPE SALAD DRESSING

(*see also* MAYONNAISE, RELISH)

FOOD	PORTION	CALS.
BAMA		
Dressing	1 tbsp	50
Miracle Whip		
Free	1 tbsp (0.5 oz)	15

FOOD	PORTION	CALS.
Miracle Whip (CONT.)		
Light	1 tbsp (0.5 oz)	35
Salad Dressing	1 tbsp (0.6 oz)	70
Nayonaise		
Cholesterol Free	1 tbsp (0.5 oz)	35
Fat Free	1 tbsp (0.5 oz)	11
Spin Blend		
Cholesterol Free	1 tbsp	40
Dressing	1 tbsp	60
Weight Watchers		
Fat Free Whipped Dressing	1 tbsp	15

MEAT STICKS

FOOD	PORTION	CALS.
jerky beef	1 oz	96
jerky beef	1 lg piece (0.7 oz)	67
smoked	1 (0.7 oz)	109
smoked	1 oz	156
Jack Link's		
Kippered Beefsteak Teriyaki	1 oz	80
Pemmican		
Original Tender Kippered Beef Steak	1	110
Peppered Tender Kippered Beef Steak	1	110
Rustlers Roundup		
Beef Jerky	1 serv (5 g)	20
Flamin' Hot	1 serv (8 g)	40
Smoky Steak	1 serv (0.8 oz)	60
Spicy	1 serv (0.5 oz)	70
Slim Jim		
Spicy	1 (4½ in) (0.3 oz)	50
Spicy Big	1 (.44 oz)	70
Spicy Giant	1 (0.97 oz)	150
Spicy Super	1 (0.64 oz)	100

MEAT SUBSTITUTES

(*see also* BACON SUBSTITUTES, CHICKEN SUBSTITUTES, SAUSAGE SUBSTITUTES, TURKEY SUBSTITUTES)

FOOD	PORTION	CALS.
Amy's Organic		
Veggie Burger California	1 (2.5 oz)	100
Veggie Burger Chicago	1 (2.5 oz)	100
Veggie Burger Texas	1 (2.5 oz)	130
Whole Meals Veggie Loaf	1 pkg (10 oz)	260
Boca Burgers		
Chef Max's Original	1 patty (2.5 oz)	110
Hint of Garlic	1 patty (2.5 oz)	110
Vegan Original	1 patty (2.5 oz)	84

FOOD	PORTION	CALS.
Gardenburger		
Classic Greek	1 (2.5 oz)	120
Fire Roasted Vegetable	1 (2.5 oz)	120
Hamburger Style	1 (2.5 oz)	90
Hamburger Style w/ Cheese	1 (2.5 oz)	110
Savory Mushroom	1 (2.5 oz)	120
Green Giant		
Southwestern Style	1 patty (3.2 oz)	140
Harvest Burgers		
For Recipes	⅔ cup (2.1 oz)	90
Italian Style	1 patty (3.2 oz)	140
Original	1 (3 oz)	140
Harvest Direct		
TVP Beef Chunks	3.5 oz	280
TVP Beef Chunks Flavored	3.5 oz	250
TVP Beef Strips	3.5 oz	280
TVP Ground Beef	3.5 oz	280
TVP Ground Beef Flavored	3.5 oz	250
Ken & Robert's		
Veggie Burger	1 (62 g)	110
Knox Mountain Farm		
Wheat Balls Mix	1 serv (¹/₁₀ pkg)	110
Lightlife		
American Grill	2.75 oz	110
Barbecue Grill	2.75 oz	130
Smart Deli Slices	2 slices (1.5 oz)	44
Smart Dogs	1 (1.5 oz)	40
Smart Dogs To Go	1 (5 oz)	115
Vegetarian Sloppy Joe	4.3 oz	130
Loma Linda		
Big Franks	1 (1.8 oz)	110
Big Franks Low Fat	1 (1.8 oz)	80
Corn Dogs	1 (2.5 oz)	200
Dinner Cuts	2 pieces (3.2 oz)	90
Nuteena	⅜ in slice (1.9 oz)	160
Patty Mix not prep	⅓ cup (0.9 oz)	90
Redi-Burger	⅝ in slice (3 oz)	120
Sandwich Spread	¼ cup (1.9 oz)	80
Savory Dinner Loaf Mix not prep	⅓ cup (0.9 oz)	90
Swiss Stake	1 piece (3.2 oz)	120
Tender Bits	6 pieces (3 oz)	110
Tender Rounds	6 pieces (2.8 oz)	120
Vege-Burger	¼ cup (1.9 oz)	70
Vita Burger Chunks not prep	¼ cup (0.7 oz)	70

FOOD	PORTION	CALS.
Loma Linda (CONT.)		
Vita Burger Granules	3 tbsp (0.7 oz)	70
Midland Harvest		
Burger n' Loaf Chili w/o Beans	0.8 oz	90
Burger n' Loaf Herbs & Spice	3.2 oz	140
Burger n' Loaf Italian	3.2 oz	140
Burger n' Loaf Original	3.2 oz	140
Burger n' Loaf Sloppy Joe w/o Sauce	0.8 oz	80
Burger n' Loaf Taco	2.7 oz	90
Morningstar Farms		
Better'n Burger	1 (2.7 oz)	70
Burger Style Recipe Crumbles	⅔ cup (1.9 oz)	90
Deli Franks	1 (1.6 oz)	110
Garden Grille	1 patty (2.5 oz)	120
Garden Veggie Patties	1 patty (2.4 oz)	100
Ground Meatless	½ cup (1.9 oz)	60
Prime Patties	1 (2.7 oz)	110
Quarter Prime	1 patty (3.4 oz)	140
Southwestern Veggie Burger Kit	¼ pkg (0.9 oz)	90
Spicy Black Bean Burger	1 (2.7 oz)	110
Natural Touch		
Dinner Entree	1 patty (3 oz)	220
Garden Veggie Pattie	1 (2.4 oz)	110
Loaf Mix not prep	4 tbsp (1 oz)	100
Okara Pattie	1 (2.2 oz)	110
Original Veggie Burger Kit not prep	¼ pkg (0.8 oz)	80
Southwestern Veggie Burger Kit not prep	¼ pkg (0.9 oz)	90
Spicy Black Bean Burger	1 (2.7 oz)	100
Stroganoff Mix not prep	4 tbsp (0.8 oz)	90
Taco Mix not prep	3 tbsp (0.6 oz)	90
Vegan Burger	1 (2.7 oz)	70
Vegan Burger Crumbles	½ cup (1.9 oz)	60
Vege Frank	1 (1.6 oz)	100
NewMenu		
VegiBurger	1 patty (3 oz)	110
VegiDogs	1 (1.5 oz)	45
Quorn		
Burger	1 patty (3 oz)	100
Sovex		
Better Than Burger?	½ cup (1.9 oz)	165
Soy Is Us		
Beef Not!	½ cup (1.75 oz)	140
Trader Joe's		
French Village Burger Champignon No Soy No Preservatives	1 patty (3.4 oz)	190

FOOD	PORTION	CALS.
Veggie Patch		
Burgeriffics	1 (2.5 oz)	110
Perfectly Franks	1 (1.7 oz)	70
Veggie Rounds	1 (2.5 oz)	120
Veggitinos Meatballs	5 (2.8 oz)	120
White Wave		
Meatless Healthy Franks	1 (1.5 oz)	90
Meatless Jumbo Franks	1 (3 oz)	170
Meatless Sandwich Slices Beef	2 slices (1.6 oz)	90
Meatless Sandwich Slices Bologna	2 slices (1.6 oz)	120
Meatless Sandwich Slices Pastrami	2 slices (1.6 oz)	90
Meatless Healthy Franks	1 (1.5 oz)	90
Veggie Burger	1 patty (2.5 oz)	110
Worthington		
Beef Style Meatless	⅜ in slice (1.9 oz)	110
Bolono	3 slices (2 oz)	80
Choplets	2 slices (3.2 oz)	90
Corn Beef Meatless	4 slices (2 oz)	140
Country Stew	1 cup (8.4 oz)	210
Dinner Roast	¾ in slice (3 oz)	180
FriPats	1 patty (2.2 oz)	60
Granburger not prep	3 tbsp (0.6 oz)	60
Multigrain Cutlet	2 slices (3.2 oz)	100
Numete	⅜ in slice (1.9 oz)	130
Prime Stakes	1 piece (3.2 oz)	140
Prosage Patties	1 (1.3 oz)	100
Prosage Roll	⅝ in slice (1.9 oz)	140
Protose	⅜ in slice (1.9 oz)	130
Salami Meatless	3 slices (2 oz)	130
Savory Slices	3 slices (2.9 oz)	150
Smoked Beef Meatless	6 slices (2 oz)	120
Stakelets	1 piece (2.5 oz)	140
Veelets	1 patty (2.5 oz)	180
Vegetable Skallops	½ cup (3 oz)	90
Vegetable Steaks	2 pieces (2.5 oz)	80
Vegetarian Burger	¼ cup (1.9 oz)	60
Veja Links Low Fat	1 (1.1 oz)	40
Wham	2 slices (1.6 oz)	80
Zoglo's		
Crispy Vegetarian Cutlets	1 (3.5 oz)	200
Savory Vegetarian Kebabs	1 serv (2.8 oz)	135
Tender Vegetarian Burgers	1 (2.6 oz)	150
Vegetable Patties	1 (2.6 oz)	130

FOOD	PORTION	CALS.
Zoglo's (CONT.)		
Vegetarian Franks	1 (2.6 oz)	125

MELON
(*see also individual fruit names*)
FROZEN
Big Valley
| Mixed | ¾ cup (4.9 oz) | 40 |

MEXICAN FOOD
(*see* SALSA, SAUCE, SPANISH FOOD, TORTILLA)

MILK
(*see also* CHOCOLATE, COCOA, MILK DRINKS, MILKSHAKE)
CANNED
Carnation
Evaporated	2 tbsp	40
Evaporated Lowfat	2 tbsp	25
Lite Evaporated Skimmed	½ cup (4 fl oz)	100
Sweetened Condensed	2 tbsp	130
Eagle
| Sweetened Condensed | ⅓ cup | 320 |
Pet
Evaporated	½ cup	170
Evaporated Filled	½ cup	150
Evaporated Light Skimmed	½ cup	100
DRIED
Carnation
| Nonfat | ⅓ cup dry | 80 |
Nutra/Balance
| Lactose Reduced as prep | 8 oz | 80 |
Saco
| Cultured Buttermilk | 4 tbsp (0.8 oz) | 80 |
Sanalac
| As Prep | 8 oz | 80 |
REFRIGERATED
goat	1 cup	168
indian buffalo	1 cup	236
nonfat	1 cup	86
sheep	1 cup	264
whole	1 cup	150
BodyWise
| Nonfat | 8 fl oz | 100 |
Borden
| Acidophilus 1% | 8 fl oz | 100 |

FOOD	PORTION	CALS.
Borden (CONT.)		
Buttermilk Lowfat Golden Churn	8 fl oz	120
Hi-Calcium	8 fl oz	150
Hi-Protein 2%	8 fl oz	140
Milk	8 fl oz	150
Skim	8 fl oz	90
Skim-line	8 fl oz	100
CaliMilk		
CalciMilk	8 fl oz	102
Cool Cow		
Low Fat	1 cup (8 oz)	110
Farmland		
1%	8 fl oz	100
2%	8 fl oz	130
Cholesterol Reduced	8 oz	150
Easylac 1%	8 fl oz	100
Easylac Nonfat	8 fl oz	90
Skim	8 fl oz	80
Skim Plus	8 fl oz	110
Friendship		
Buttermilk	8 fl oz	120
Hood		
1%	1 cup (8 oz)	110
Better Taste 2%	1 cup (8 oz)	130
Buttermilk	1 cup (8 oz)	90
Whole	1 cup (8 oz)	150
Lactaid		
1%	8 fl oz	102
Nonfat	8 fl oz	86
Nuform		
1%	1 cup (8 oz)	120
Skim	1 cup (8 oz)	100
Silovet		
Skim	1 cup (8 oz)	90
Viva		
2%	8 fl oz	120
Skim	8 fl oz	100
SHELF-STABLE		
Parmalat		
1%	1 cup (8 oz)	110
2%	1 cup (8 oz)	130
Skim	1 cup (8 oz)	90

FOOD	PORTION	CALS.
Parmalat (cont.)		
Whole	1 cup (8 oz)	160

MILK DRINKS
(*see also* BREAKFAST DRINKS, CHOCOLATE, COCOA, MILKSHAKES)

FOOD	PORTION	CALS.
Body Wise		
Chocolate Nonfat Milk	1 cup (8 fl oz)	180
Borden		
Chocolate Lowfat Dutch Brand	8 fl oz	180
Bosco		
Chocolate Milk	1 cup (8 fl oz)	230
Hood		
Chocolate Lowfat	1 cup (8 oz)	150
Horizon		
Organic 1% Chocolate Milk	1 cup (8 oz)	160
Lactaid		
Chocolate Milk 1%	8 fl oz	158
Meadow Gold		
Chocolate Milk	8 fl oz	210
Parmalat		
Chocolate 2%	1 box (8 oz)	180
Quik		
Banana Powder	2 tbsp (0.8 oz)	90
Cookies n Cream Powder	2 tbsp (0.8 oz)	100
Strawberry Powder	2 tbsp (0.8 oz)	90

MILK SUBSTITUTES
(*see also* COFFEE WHITENERS)

FOOD	PORTION	CALS.
Better Than Milk		
Carob	8 fl oz	130
Chocolate	8 fl oz	125
Light	8 fl oz	80
Natural	8 fl oz	90
EdenBlend		
Original	8 fl oz	120
Edensoy		
Carob	8 fl oz	150
Extra Original	8 oz	130
Extra Original	8 fl oz	130
Extra Vanilla	8 fl oz	150
Original	8 oz	130
Vanilla	8 oz	150
Health Valley		
Soo Moo	1 cup	110

FOOD	PORTION	CALS.
Rice Dream		
Carob Lite	8 fl oz	150
Chocolate	8 fl oz	190
Chocolate	8 fl oz	190
Lite Organic Original	8 fl oz	130
Lite Vanilla	8 fl oz	130
Vegelicious		
Milk	8 fl oz	100
Vitamite		
Non-Dairy 2% Fat	1 cup (8 oz)	110
Non-Diary Nonfat	1 cup (8 oz)	90
Vitasoy		
Carob Supreme	8 fl oz	210
Cocoa Light	8 fl oz	130
Original Creamy	8 fl oz	160
Original Light	8 fl oz	90
Rich Cocoa	8 fl oz	210
Vanilla Light	8 fl oz	110
Vanilla Delite	8 fl oz	190
Westsoy		
Cocoa Lite	8 fl oz	140
Plain Lite	8 fl oz	100
Vanilla Lite	8 fl oz	110

MILKFISH
baked	3 oz	162

MILKSHAKE
D'Frosta Shake		
Vanilla	1 serv (13.5 oz)	340
Freeze Flip		
Fruit Shake No Fat Lactose Free Black Raspberry	1 serv (6 oz)	150
Frostee		
Chocolate	8 fl oz	200
Strawberry	8 fl oz	180
Hood		
Shake Up Chocolate	1 cup (8 oz)	240
Shake Up Strawberry	1 cup (8 oz)	220
Shake Up Vanilla	1 cup (8 oz)	220
Milky Way		
Shake	1 (10 fl oz)	390
Parmalat		
Shake A Shake Chocolate	1 box (6 oz)	180
Shake A Shake Orange Vanilla	1 box (6 oz)	110

FOOD	PORTION	CALS.
Parmalat (CONT.)		
Shake A Shake Vanilla	1 box (6 oz)	170
Weight Watchers		
Chocolate Fudge Shake Mix as prep	1 pkg	80

MILLET
cooked	1 cup (6.1 oz)	207

MINERAL WATER
(*see* WATER)

MISO
miso	½ cup	284
Eden		
Genmai Miso Organic	1 tbsp (0.5 oz)	25
Hacho Miso Organic	1 tbsp (0.5 oz)	35
Kome Miso Organic	1 tbsp (0.6 oz)	25
Mugi Miso Organic	1 tbsp (0.6 oz)	25
Shiro Miso Organic	1 tbsp (0.6 oz)	35

MOLASSES
blackstrap	1 tbsp (0.7 oz)	47
blackstrap	1 cup (11.5 oz)	771
molasses	1 tbsp (0.7 oz)	53
molasses	1 cup (11.5 oz)	873
Brer Rabbit		
Dark	2 tbsp	110
Light	2 tbsp	110
McIlhenny		
Molasses	1 tbsp (0.7 oz)	66
Tree Of Life		
Blackstrap	1 tbsp (0.5 oz)	45

MONKFISH
baked	3 oz	82

MOOSE
roasted	3 oz	114

MOTH BEANS
dried cooked	1 cup	207

MOUSSE
FROZEN
Sara Lee
Chocolate Mint Mousse	⅕ pkg (4.3 oz)	440

FOOD	PORTION	CALS.
Weight Watchers		
Chocolate Mousse	1 (2.75 oz)	190
MIX		
Royal		
Chocolate Mousse No-Bake	⅛ pie	130
TAKE-OUT		
chocolate	½ cup (7.1 oz)	447

MUFFIN
FROZEN

FOOD	PORTION	CALS.
Pepperidge Farm		
Blueberry	1 (2 oz)	180
Bran w/ Raisins	1 (2 oz)	180
Corn	1 (2 oz)	190
Orange Cranberry	1 (2 oz)	180
Sara Lee		
Blueberry	1 (2.2 oz)	220
Corn	1 (2.2 oz)	260
Oat Bran	1	210
Weight Watchers		
Chocolate Chocolate Chip	1 (2.5 oz)	190
Fat Free Banana	1 (2.5 oz)	170
Fat Free Blueberry	1 (2.5 oz)	160
HOME RECIPE		
blueberry as prep w/ 2% milk	1 (2 oz)	163
blueberry as prep w/ whole milk	1 (2 oz)	165
corn as prep w/ 2% milk	1 (2 oz)	180
corn as prep w/ whole milk	1 (2 oz)	183
plain as prep w/ 2% milk	1 (2 oz)	169
plain as prep w/ whole milk	1 (2 oz)	172
wheat bran as prep w/ 2% milk	1 (2 oz)	161
wheat bran as prep w/ whole milk	1 (2 oz)	164
MIX		
blueberry	1 (1.75 oz)	149
corn	1 (1.75 oz)	160
wheat bran as prep	1 (1.75 oz)	138
Arrowhead		
Bran	⅓ cup (1.4 oz)	150
Oat Bran Wheat Free	⅓ cup (1.5 oz)	160
Flako		
Corn	⅓ cup (1.4 oz)	160
Gold Medal		
Banana Nut	1	170
Caramel Nut	1	170

FOOD	PORTION	CALS.
Gold Medal (CONT.)		
Corn	1	160
Hain		
Oat Bran Apple Cinnamon	1	140
Oat Bran Banana Nut	1	140
Oat Bran Raspberry Spice	1	140
Jiffy		
Apple Cinnamon as prep	1	190
Banana Nut as prep	1	180
Blueberry as prep	1	190
Bran With Dates as prep	1	170
Corn as prep	1	180
Honey Date as prep	1	170
Oatmeal as prep	1	180
Robin Hood		
Apple Cinnamon	1	170
Banana Nut	1	170
Blueberry	1	160
Caramel Nut	1	170
Sweet Rewards		
Fat Free Apple Cinnamon	1	120
Fat Free Wild Blueberry	1	120
Low Fat Recipe Apple Cinnamon	1	130
Low Fat Recipe Wild Blueberry	1	120
Wanda's		
Blue Corn	¼ cup mix per serv (1.2 oz)	130
READY-TO-EAT		
blueberry	1 (2 oz)	158
corn	1 (2 oz)	174
oat bran wheat free	1 (2 oz)	154
toaster type blueberry	1	103
toaster type corn	1	114
toaster type wheat bran w/ raisins	1 (1.3 oz)	106
Arnold		
Bran'nola	1 (2.3 oz)	160
Raisin	1 (2.3 oz)	160
Dolly Madison		
Blueberry	1 (1.75 oz)	170
Mega Banana Nut	1 (5.9 oz)	620
Mega Blueberry	1 (5.9 oz)	590
Mega Chocolate Chip	1 (5.9 oz)	620
Mega Cranberry Orange	1 (5.9 oz)	590
Mega Cream Cheese	1 (5.9 oz)	620

FOOD	PORTION	CALS.
Dutch Mill		
Apple Oat Bran	1 (2 oz)	180
Banana Walnut	1 (2 oz)	220
Carrot	1 (2 oz)	190
Corn	1 (2 oz)	190
Cranberry Orange	1 (2 oz)	170
Raisin Bran	1 (2 oz)	230
Entenmann's		
Blueberry	1 (2 oz)	200
Freihofer's		
Corn Toasters	1 (1.3 oz)	130
Hostess		
Banana Bran Low Fat	1 (2.7 oz)	240
Blueberry Low Fat	1 (2.7 oz)	230
Hearty Banana Nut	1 (5.9 oz)	620
Hearty Blueberry	1 (5.9 oz)	590
Hearty Chocolate Chip	1 (5.9 oz)	620
Hearty Cranberry Orange	1 (5.9 oz)	590
Hearty Cream Cheese	1 (5.9 oz)	620
Mini Banana Walnut	3 (1.2 oz)	160
Mini Blueberry	3 (1.2 oz)	150
Mini Chocolate Chip	3 (1.2 oz)	160
Mini Cinnamon Apple	3 (1.2 oz)	160
Mini Cinnamon Bites	3 (1.1 oz)	130
Mini Rocky Road	3 (1.2 oz)	160
Muffin Loaf Apple Spice	1 (3.7 oz)	430
Muffin Loaf Banana Nut	1 (3.8 oz)	460
Muffin Loaf Blueberry	1 (3.8 oz)	440
Muffin Loaf Chocolate Chocolate Chip	1 (3.8 oz)	400
Muffin Loaf Raspberry	1 (3.8 oz)	440
Oat Bran	1 (1.5 oz)	160
Otis Spunkmeyer		
Mayport Almond Poppy Seed	½ muffin (2 oz)	210
Mayport Apple Cinnamon	1 (2.25 oz)	240
Mayport Banana Nut	1 (2.25 oz)	270
Mayport Cheese Streusel	½ muffin (2 oz)	220
Mayport Chocolate Chocolate Chip	1 (2.25 oz)	260
Mayport Chocolate Chip	½ muffin (2 oz)	240
Mayport Cinnamon Spice	½ muffin (2 oz)	230
Mayport Corn	½ muffin (2 oz)	230
Mayport Harvest Bran	1 (2.25 oz)	240
Mayport Lemon	½ muffin (2 oz)	230
Mayport Orange	½ muffin (2 oz)	230
Mayport Pineapple	½ muffin (2 oz)	210

FOOD	PORTION	CALS.

Otis Spunkmeyer (CONT.)

Mayport Wild Blueberry	1 (2.25 oz)	230
Mayport Low Fat Apple Cinnamon	1 (4 oz)	380
Mayport Low Fat Banana Nut	1 (4 oz)	350
Mayport Low Fat Chocolate Chocolate Chip	1 (4 oz)	370
Mayport Low Fat Wild Blueberry	1 (4 oz)	350

Weight Watchers

Fat Free Apple Crisp	1 (2.5 oz)	160
Fat Free Cranberry Orange	1 (2.5 oz)	160
Fat Free Double Chocolate	1 (2.5 oz)	180
Fat Free Wild Blueberry	1 (2.5 oz)	160
Low Fat Apple Cinnamon	1 (2.5 oz)	170
Low Fat Blueberry	1 (2.5 oz)	180
Low Fat Carrot	1 (2.5 oz)	160
Low Fat Chocolate Chip	1 (2.5 oz)	180
Low Fat Cranberry Orange	1 (2.5 oz)	180
Low Fat Lemon Poppy	1 (2.5 oz)	190

MULBERRIES

fresh	1 cup	61

MULLET

striped cooked	3 oz	127

MUNG BEANS
DRIED

cooked	1 cup	213

SPROUTS

canned	½ cup	8
cooked	½ cup	13
raw	½ cup	16
stir fried	½ cup	31

MUNGO BEANS

dried cooked	1 cup	190

MUSHROOMS
CANNED

straw	1 cup (6.4 oz)	58

BinB

Pieces & Stems	1 can (4.2 oz)	30
Sliced	1 can (4.2 oz)	30
Sliced With Garlic	1 can (4.2 oz)	35
Whole	1 can (4.2 oz)	30

Green Giant

Pieces & Stems	½ cup (4.2 oz)	30

FOOD	PORTION	CALS.
Green Giant (CONT.)		
Sliced	½ cup (4.2 oz)	30
Whole	½ cup (4.2 oz)	30
Seneca		
Mushrooms	½ cup	25
DRIED		
cloud ear	1 (5 g)	13
cloud ears	1 cup (1 oz)	80
shiitake	4 (0.5 oz)	44
straw	1 piece (6 g)	2
FRESH		
enoki raw	1 (4 in)	2
morel	3.5 oz	9
oyster raw	1 sm (0.5 oz)	6
oyster raw	1 lg (5.2 oz)	55
portabella sliced	1 serv (2 oz)	4
raw	1 (0.5 oz)	5
raw sliced	½ cup	9
shitake cooked	4 (2.5 oz)	40
sliced cooked	½ cup	21
whole cooked	1 (0.4 oz)	3
Mother Earth		
Organic	4 oz	35
FROZEN		
Empire		
Breaded	7 (2.8 oz)	90
Fresh Like		
Mushrooms	3.5 oz	28
MUSKRAT		
roasted	3 oz	199
MUSSELS		
blue raw	1 cup	129
fresh blue cooked	3 oz	147
MUSTARD		
dry mustard seed yellow	1 tsp	15
yellow ready-to-use	1 tsp	5
Blanchard & Blanchard		
Mustard	1 tsp (5 g)	0
Boar's Head		
Delicatessen Style	1 tsp (5 g)	0
Honey	1 tsp (5 g)	10
Grey Poupon		
Country Dijon	1 tsp	6

FOOD	PORTION	CALS.
Grey Poupon (CONT.)		
Dijon	1 tsp	6
Parisian	1 tsp	6
Hain		
Stone Ground	1 tbsp	14
Stone Ground No Salt Added	1 tbsp	14
Kosciuszko		
Spicy Brown	1 tsp	5
Kraft		
Horseradish Mustard	1 tsp (5 g)	0
Mustard	1 tsp (5 g)	0
McIlhenny		
Coarse Ground	1 tsp (0.2 oz)	4
Spicy	1 tsp (0.2 oz)	6
Plochman		
Dijon	1 tsp (5 g)	7
Spoonable Salad	1 tsp (5 g)	4
Squeeze Salad	1 tsp (5 g)	4
Stone Ground	1 tsp (5 g)	6
Russer		
Deli	1 tsp (5 g)	4
Tree Of Life		
Dijon	1 tsp (5 g)	0
Dijon Imported	1 tsp (5 g)	5
Low Sodium	1 tsp (5 g)	3
Stone Ground	1 tsp (5 g)	0
Yellow	1 tsp (5 g)	0
Watkins		
Country Mill	1 tsp (7 g)	15
Dusseldorf	1 tsp (7 g)	10
Horseradish	1 tsp (7 g)	10
Jalapeno	1 tsp (7 g)	10
Onion	1 tsp (7 g)	10
Parisienne	1 tsp (7 g)	10

MUSTARD GREENS

FOOD	PORTION	CALS.
fresh chopped cooked	½ cup	11
fresh raw chopped	½ cup	7
Allen		
Mustard Greens	½ cup (4.1 oz)	30
Birds Eye		
Chopped	1 cup (3 oz)	30
Sunshine		
Mustard Greens	½ cup (4.1 oz)	30

FOOD	PORTION	CALS.

NATTO
| natto | ½ cup | 187 |

NAVY BEANS
CANNED
Allen
| Navy Beans | ½ cup (4.5 oz) | 110 |
Eden
| Organic | ½ cup (4.3 oz) | 100 |
| Organic | ½ cup (4.6 oz) | 110 |
Trappey
| With Bacon | ½ cup (4.5 oz) | 110 |
| With Bacon & Jalapeno | ½ cup (4.5 oz) | 110 |
DRIED
Hurst
| HamBeens w/ Ham | 3 tbsp (1.2 oz) | 120 |
SPROUTS
| cooked | 3.5 oz | 78 |
| raw | ½ cup | 35 |

NECTARINE
| fresh | 1 | 67 |
Dole
| Nectarine | 1 | 70 |

NEUFCHATEL
Philadelphia
| Neufchatel | 1 oz | 70 |
WisPride
| Garden Vegetable Cup | 2 tbsp (1.1 oz) | 60 |
| Garlic & Herb Cup | 2 tbsp (1.1 oz) | 60 |

NON-DAIRY CREAMERS
(*see* COFFEE WHITENERS)

NON-DAIRY WHIPPED TOPPINGS
(*see* WHIPPED TOPPINGS)

NOODLE DISHES
(*see also* NOODLES, PASTA DINNERS)
CANNED
Van Camp's
| Noodlee Weenee | 1 can (8 oz) | 230 |
FROZEN
Luigino's
| Stroganoff | 1 pkg (8 oz) | 310 |
MIX
Kraft
| Noodle Classics Cheddar Cheese as prep | 1 cup (7.4 oz) | 400 |

FOOD	PORTION	CALS.
Kraft (CONT.)		
Noodle Classics Savory Chicken as prep	1 cup (8.5 oz)	340
Lipton		
Noodles & Sauce Alfredo Broccoli as prep	1 cup (2.2 oz)	340
Noodles & Sauce Alfredo as prep	1 cup (2.2 oz)	330
Noodles & Sauce Beef as prep	1 cup (2.1 oz)	280
Noodles & Sauce Butter as prep	1 cup (2.2 oz)	310
Noodles & Sauce Butter & Herb as prep	1 cup (2.2 oz)	300
Noodles & Sauce Chicken Broccoli as prep	1 cup (2.1 oz)	310
Noodles & Sauce Chicken Tetrazzini as prep	1 cup (2 oz)	300
Noodles & Sauce Chicken as prep	1 cup (2.1 oz)	290
Noodles & Sauce Creamy Chicken as prep	1 cup (2.1 oz)	320
Noodles & Sauce Parmesan as prep	1 cup (2.1 oz)	330
Noodles & Sauce Sour Cream & Chives as prep	1 cup (2.2 oz)	310
Noodles & Sauce Stroganoff as prep	1 cup (2 oz)	300
Noodles By Leonardo		
Macaroni & Cheese as prep	1 cup (2.5 oz)	250
Ultra Slim-Fast		
Noodles & Alfredo Sauce	2.3 oz	240
Noodles & Beef	2.3 oz	230
Noodles & Cheese	2.3 oz	230
Noodles & Chicken Sauce	2.3 oz	220
Noodles & Tomato Herb Sauce	2.3 oz	220
SHELF-STABLE		
Hormel		
Microcup Meals Noodles & Chicken	1 cup (7.5 oz)	200

NOODLES

cellophane	1 cup	492
chow mein	1 cup (1.6 oz)	237
egg cooked	1 cup (5.6 oz)	213
japanese soba cooked	1 cup (4 oz)	113
japanese somen cooked	1 cup (6.2 oz)	231
rice cooked	1 cup (6.2 oz)	192
spinach/egg cooked	1 cup (5.6 oz)	211
Creamette		
Egg	2 oz	220
Herb's		
Egg Fine	2 oz	220
Egg Medium	2 oz	220
Kluski Medium	2 oz	220
Kluski Wide	2 oz	220

FOOD	PORTION	CALS.
Hodgson Mill		
Veggie Egg	2 oz	200
Whole Wheat Egg	2 oz	190
Whole Wheat Spinach Egg	2 oz	190
Noodles By Leonardo		
Egg Fine	2 oz	210
Egg Medium	2 oz	210
Egg Wide	2 oz	210
San Giorgio		
Egg	2 oz	210
Shofar		
No Yolks	2 oz	210

NOPALES

cooked	1 cup (5.2 oz)	23
raw sliced	1 cup (3 oz)	14
raw sliced	½ cup (1.5 oz)	7

NUTMEG

ground	1 tsp	12
Watkins		
Ground	¼ tsp (0.5 g)	0

NUTRITION SUPPLEMENTS

(*see also* BREAKFAST BAR, BREAKFAST DRINKS, CEREAL BARS, SPORTS DRINKS)

BeneFit		
Chocolate	1 serv	120
Nutrition Bar	1 (2 oz)	240
Vanilla	1 serv	120
Boost		
Chocolate	1 can (8 oz)	240
Vanilla	8 oz	240
Breakthru		
Organic Chocolate Fudge	1 bar (2.1 oz)	230
Organic Cinnamon Crunch	1 bar (2.1 oz)	220
Organic Honey Graham	1 bar (2.1 oz)	220
Organic Mocha Fudge	1 bar (2.1 oz)	230
California Joe		
All Natural Protein Drink Mix as prep	1 serv (8 oz)	165
Calorie Shed		
Shake Fat Free No Sugar Caramel Ripple	½ cup (4 fl oz)	70
Shake Fat Free No Sugar Chocolate	½ cup (4 fl oz)	70
Shake Fat Free No Sugar Marshmellow Nougat	½ cup (4 fl oz)	70

FOOD	PORTION	CALS.
Dynatrim		
Dutch Chocolate as prep w/ 1% milk	8 oz	220
Strawberry Royale as prep w/ 1% milk	8 oz	220
Vanilla as prep w/ 1% milk	8 oz	220
Ensure		
Honey Graham Crunch	1 bar (2.2 oz)	130
Essential		
Protein Powder	1 serv (0.6 oz)	70
Fat Burner		
Diet Fruit Punch	8 fl oz	0
Fi-Bar		
Apple	1 (1 oz)	90
Cocoa Almond	1	130
Cocoa Peanut	1	130
Cranberry & Wild Berries	1 (1 oz)	100
Lemon	1 (1 oz)	90
Mandarin Orange	1 (1 oz)	99
Nuggets Almond Cappuccino Crunch	1 pkg	136
Nuggets Almond Butter Crunch	1 pkg	163
Nuggets Coconut Almond Crunch	1 pkg	136
Nuggets Peanut Butter Crunch	1 pkg	160
Raspberry	1 (1 oz)	100
Strawberry	1 (1 oz)	100
Treat Yourself Right Almond	1	152
Treat Yourself Right Peanutty Butter	1	152
Vanilla Almond	1	130
Vanilla Peanut	1	130
Gatorade		
GatorBar	1 (1.17 oz)	110
GatorLode	1 can (11.6 fl oz)	280
GatorPro	1 can (11 fl oz)	360
ReLode	1 pkt (0.75 oz)	80
GeniSoy		
Soy Protein Powder	1 scoop (0.6 oz)	60
Soy Protein Shake Chocolate	1 scoop (1.2 oz)	120
Soy Protein Shake Vanilla	1 scoop (1.2 oz)	130
Soy Protein Bar Chocolate	1 bar (2.2 oz)	210
Soy Protein Bar Chocolate Coated	1 bar (2.2 oz)	220
Healthy Pleasures		
Chocolate Irish Cream	1 bottle (10.5 oz)	260
Nancy Grey's		
Shake Hi-Protein Black Raspberry	1 cup (8 fl oz)	340
Shake Hi-Protein Chocolate	1 cup (8 fl oz)	340
Shake Hi-Protein Vanilla	1 cup (8 fl oz)	340

FOOD	PORTION	CALS.
NiteBite		
Chocolate Fudge	1 bar (0.9 oz)	100
Peanut Butter	1 bar (0.9 oz)	100
Nutra/Balance		
EggPro	4 oz	200
Frozen Pudding Butterscotch	4 oz	225
Frozen Pudding Chocolate	4 oz	225
Frozen Pudding Tapioca	4 oz	225
Frozen Pudding Vanilla	4 oz	225
NutraShake		
Chocolate	4 oz	200
Strawberry	4 oz	200
Vanilla	4 oz	200
With Fiber Strawberry	6 oz	300
With Fiber Vanilla	6 oz	300
Pounds Off		
All Flavors	1 bar (2.1 oz)	210
Dark Chocolate Ectasy	1 can (11 oz)	200
French Vanilla	1 can (11 oz)	220
Power Bar		
Malt-Nut	1 bar (2.3 oz)	230
Resource		
Fructose Sweetened	1 pkg (8 oz)	250
Fruit Beverage	1 pkg (8 oz)	180
Liquid Food	1 pkg (8 oz)	250
Plus Liquid Food	1 pkg (8 oz)	355
Sego		
Lite Chocolate	10 fl oz	150
Lite Dutch Chocolate	10 fl oz	150
Lite French Vanilla	10 fl oz	150
Lite Strawberry	10 fl oz	150
Lite Vanilla	10 fl oz	150
Very Chocolate	10 fl oz	225
Very Chocolate Malt	10 fl oz	225
Very Strawberry	10 fl oz	225
Very Vanilla	10 fl oz	225
Slim-Fast		
Powder Chocolate as prep w/ skim milk	8 oz	190
Powder Chocolate Malt as prep w/ skim milk	8 oz	190
Powder Strawberry as prep w/ skim milk	8 oz	190
Powder Vanilla as prep w/ skim milk	8 oz	190
Sobe		
Jing Essentials	1 bottle (14 oz)	140

FOOD	PORTION	CALS.
Sobe (CONT.)		
Qi Essentials	1 bottle (14 oz)	140
Shen Essentials	1 bottle (14 oz)	140
Sustacal		
Vanilla	8 oz	240
Sweet Success		
Chewy Bar Chocolate Brownie	1 (1.6 oz)	120
Chewy Bar Chocolate Peanut Butter	1 (1.6 oz)	120
Chewy Bar Chocolate Raspberry	1 (1.6 oz)	120
Chewy Bar Chocolate Chip	1 (1.6 oz)	120
Chewy Bar Oatmeal Raisin	1 (1.6 oz)	120
Chocolate Raspberry Truffle	1 can (10 fl oz)	200
Chocolate Raspberry as prep w/ skim milk	9 fl oz	180
Chocolate Mocha Supreme	1 can (10 fl oz)	200
Chocolate Mocha Supreme as prep w/ skim milk	9 fl oz	180
Classic Chocolate Chip as prep w/ skim milk	9 fl oz	180
Creamy Milk Chocolate	1 carton (12 fl oz)	220
Creamy Milk Chocolate	1 can (10 fl oz)	200
Creamy Milk Chocolate as prep w/ skim milk	9 fl oz	180
Creamy Vanilla Delight as prep w/ skim milk	9 fl oz	180
Dark Chocolate Fudge	1 can (10 fl oz)	200
Dark Chocolate Fudge	1 carton (12 fl oz)	220
Dark Chocolate Fudge as prep w/ skim milk	9 fl oz	180
Rich Chocolate Almond	1 carton (12 fl oz)	220
Rich Chocolate Almond	1 can (10 fl oz)	200
Rich Chocolate Almond as prep w/ skim milk	9 fl oz	180
Smooth Vanilla Creme	1 can (10 fl oz)	200
The Pumper		
Body Building MilkShake Chocolate	1 serv (13.5 oz)	390
Body Building Milkeshake Banana	1 serv (13.5 oz)	390
Think!		
Apple Spice	1 bar (2 oz)	205
Chocolate Almond Coconut Raisin	1 bar (2 oz)	243
Chocolate Fruit Harvest	1 bar (2 oz)	217
Ultra Slim-Fast		
Cafe Mocha as prep w/ skim milk	8 oz	200
Chocolate Royale as prep w/ skim milk	8 oz	200
Crunch Bar Cocoa Almond	1	110

FOOD	PORTION	CALS.
Ultra Slim-Fast (CONT.)		
Crunch Bar Cocoa Raspberry	1	100
Crunch Bar Vanilla Almond	1	110
Dutch Chocolate as prep w/ water	8 oz	220
French Vanilla as prep w/ skim milk	8 oz	190
French Vanilla as prep w/ water	8 oz	220
Fruit Juice Mix as prep w/ fruit juice	8 oz	200
Nutrition Bar Dutch Chocolate	1	130
Nutrition Bar Peanut Butter	1	140
Pina Colada as prep w/ skim milk	8 oz	180
Ready-To-Drink Chocolate Royale	12 oz	250
Ready-To-Drink Chocolate Royale	11 oz	230
Ready-To-Drink French Vanilla	12 oz	220
Ready-To-Drink French Vanilla	11 oz	230
Ready-To-Drink Strawberry Supreme	12 oz	220
Strawberry Supreme as prep w/ water	8 oz	220
Strawberry as prep w/ skim milk	8 oz	190
Vita-J		
Apple Juice	11.5 fl oz	8
Fruit Punch	11.5 fl oz	8
Grapefruit Cocktail w/ Raspberry	11.5 fl oz	8
Orange Juice	11.5 fl oz	8

NUTS MIXED
(*see also individual names*)

FOOD	PORTION	CALS.
Estee		
Fruit & Nut Mix	¼ cup	210
Fisher		
Mixed Deluxe Lightly Salted	1 oz	180
Mixed Deluxe Salted	1 oz	180
Mixed Oil Roasted 25% More Cashews Lightly Salted	1 oz	180
Mixed Oil Roasted 25% More Cashews Salted	1 oz	180
Nut & Fruit Pina Colada	1 oz	150
Nut & Fruit Raisin Cranberry	1 oz	150
Nut & Fruit Tropical Fruit	1 oz	140
Nut Toppings Oil Roasted With Peanuts	1 oz	190
Peanuts Cashews	1 oz	170
Guy's		
Mixed With Peanuts	1 oz	180
Tasty Mix	1 oz	130
Planters		
Cashews & Peanuts Honey Roasted	1 oz	150

FOOD	PORTION	CALS.
Planters (CONT.)		
Deluxe Oil Roasted	1 oz	170
Dry Roasted	1 oz	170
Honey Roasted	1 oz	140
Lightly Salted Oil Roasted	1 oz	170
No Brazils Lightly Salted Oil Roasted	1 oz	170
No Brazils Oil Roasted	1 oz	170
Oil Roasted	1 oz	170
Select Mix Cashews Almonds & Macadamias Oil Roasted	1 oz	170
Select Mix Cashews Almonds & Pecans Oil Roasted	1 oz	170
Unsalted Oil Roasted	1 oz	170

OCTOPUS

FOOD	PORTION	CALS.
fresh steamed	3 oz	140

OHELOBERRIES

FOOD	PORTION	CALS.
fresh	1 cup	39

OIL
(*see also* FAT)

FOOD	PORTION	CALS.
almond	1 tbsp	120
apricot kernel	1 tbsp	120
butter oil	1 tbsp	112
canola	1 tbsp	124
corn	1 tbsp	120
cottonseed	1 tbsp	120
cupu assu	1 tbsp	120
grapeseed	1 tbsp	120
hazelnut	1 tbsp	120
mustard	1 tbsp	124
olive	1 tbsp	119
palm	1 tbsp	120
peanut	1 tbsp	119
poppyseed	1 tbsp	120
rice bran	1 tbsp	120
safflower	1 tbsp	120
sesame	1 tbsp	120
sheanut	1 tbsp	120
soybean	1 tbsp	120
sunflower	1 tbsp	120
teaseed	1 tbsp	120
tomatoseed	1 tbsp	120
walnut	1 tbsp	120

FOOD	PORTION	CALS.
wheat germ	1 tbsp	120
Arrowhead		
Flax Seed	1 tbsp (0.5 fl oz)	120
Hazelnut	1 tbsp (0.5 fl oz)	120
Crisco		
Corn Canola	1 tbsp (0.5 fl oz)	120
Oil	1 tbsp (0.5 fl oz)	120
Puritan Canola	1 tbsp (0.5 fl oz)	120
Eden		
Hot Pepper Sesame	1 tbsp (0.5 oz)	130
Safflower	1 tbsp (0.5 oz)	120
Sesame	1 tbsp (0.5 oz)	140
Toasted Sesame	1 tbsp (0.5 oz)	130
Hain		
All Blend	1 tbsp	120
Almond	1 tbsp	120
Apricot Kernel	1 tbsp	120
Avocado	1 tbsp	120
Canola	1 tbsp	120
Canola Organic	1 tbsp	120
Coconut	1 tbsp	120
Corn	1 tbsp	120
Garlic & Oil	1 tbsp	120
Olive	1 tbsp	120
Peanut	1 tbsp	120
Rice Bran	1 tbsp	120
Safflower	1 tbsp	120
Safflower Hi-Oleic	1 tbsp	120
Safflower Organic	1 tbsp	120
Sesame	1 tbsp	120
Soy	1 tbsp	120
Sunflower	1 tbsp	120
Sunflower Organic	1 tbsp	120
Walnut	1 tbsp	120
Hollywood		
Canola	1 tbsp	120
Peanut	1 tbsp	120
Safflower	1 tbsp	120
Soy	1 tbsp	120
Sunflower	1 tbsp	120
House Of Tsang		
Hot Chili Sesame	1 tsp (5 g)	45
Mongolian Fire	1 tsp (5 g)	45
Pure Sesame	1 tsp (5 g)	45

FOOD	PORTION	CALS.
House Of Tsang (CONT.)		
Singapore Curry	1 tsp (5 g)	45
Wok Oil	1 tbsp (0.5 oz)	130
Orville Redenbacher's		
Oil	1 tbsp	120
Pam		
Butter	⅓ sec spray (0.3 g)	0
Cooking Spray	⅓ sec spray (0.3 g)	0
Olive Oil	⅓ sec spray (0.3 g)	0
Planters		
Peanut	1 tbsp (0.5 oz)	120
Popcorn	1 tbsp (0.5 oz)	120
Progresso		
Olive Extra Light	1 tbsp	119
Olive Extra Mild	1 tbsp (0.5 oz)	120
Olive Extra Virgin	1 tbsp (0.5 oz)	120
Olive Riviera Blend	1 tbsp (0.5 oz)	120
Smart Beat		
Canola	1 tbsp	120
Oil	1 tbsp	120
Tree Of Life		
Almond	1 tbsp (0.5 g)	130
Apricot Kernel	1 tbsp (0.5 g)	130
Avocado	1 tbsp (0.5 g)	130
Macadamia Nut	1 tbsp (0.5 g)	130
Olive Extra Virgin Organic	1 tbsp (0.5 g)	130
Sesame	1 tbsp (0.5 g)	130
Toasted Sesame	1 tbsp (0.5 oz)	130
Weight Watchers		
Butter Spray	⅓ sec spray	0
Cooking Spray	⅓ sec spray	0
Wesson		
Canola	1 tbsp	120
Cooking Spray Lite	0.5 sec spray	0
Corn	1 tbsp	120
Olive	1 tbsp	120
Sunflower	1 tbsp	120
Vegetable	1 tbsp	120
FISH OIL		
cod liver	1 tbsp	123
herring	1 tbsp	123
menhaden	1 tbsp	123
salmon	1 tbsp	123
sardine	1 tbsp	123

FOOD	PORTION	CALS.
shark	3.5 oz	945
whale	3.5 oz	945
Hain		
Cod Liver	1 tbsp	120
Cod Liver Cherry	1 tbsp	120
Cod Liver Mint	1 tbsp	120

OKRA
CANNED
Allen

Cut	½ cup (4.4 oz)	25
McIlhenny		
Pickled	2 pieces (1 oz)	7
Trappey		
Cocktail Hot	2 pieces (1 oz)	8
Cocktail Mild	1 piece (1 oz)	9
Creole Gumbo	½ cup (4.2 oz)	35
Cut	½ cup (4.4 oz)	25
FRESH		
sliced cooked	½ cup	25
sliced cooked	8 pods	27
FROZEN		
Birds Eye		
Cut	¾ cup (2.9 oz)	25
Whole	9 pods (3 oz)	25
Fresh Like		
Cut	3.5 oz	26
Whole	3.5 oz	32

OLIVES

green	3 extra lg	15
green	4 med	15
ripe	1 sm	4
ripe	1 lg	5
ripe	1 jumbo	7
spanish stuffed	5 (0.5 oz)	15
Italia In Tavola		
Black Olives Paste	1 tbsp (0.5 oz)	20
Progresso		
Oil Cured	6 (0.5 oz)	80
Olive Salad (drained)	2 tbsp (0.8 oz)	25

ONION
CANNED

chopped	½ cup	21
whole	1 (2.2 oz)	12

FOOD	PORTION	CALS.
Boar's Head		
Sweet Vidalia In Sauce	1 tbsp	10
Vlasic		
Lightly Spiced Cocktail Onions	1 oz	4
Watkins		
Liquid Spice	1 tbsp (0.5 oz)	120
DRIED		
flakes	1 tbsp	16
powder	1 tsp	7
Watkins		
Flakes	¼ tsp (1 g)	0
FRESH		
chopped cooked	½ cup	47
raw chopped	1 tbsp	4
raw chopped	½ cup	30
scallions raw chopped	1 tbsp	2
welsh raw	3.5 oz	34
Antioch Farms		
Vidalia	1 med	60
Dole		
Green Chopped	1 tbsp	2
Medium	1	60
FROZEN		
chopped cooked	½ cup	30
Birds Eye		
Diced	⅔ cup (3 oz)	30
Pearl Onions In Cream Sauce	½ cup (4.4 oz)	60
Fresh Like		
Diced	3.5 oz	29
Whole	3.5 oz	37
Kineret		
Rings	6 (3 oz)	200
Ore Ida		
Chopped	¾ cup (3 oz)	25
Onion Ringers	6 pieces (3 oz)	240
TAKE-OUT		
fried	½ cup (7.5 oz)	176
rings breaded & fried	8 to 9	275
OPOSSUM		
roasted	3 oz	188
ORANGE		
CANNED		
Del Monte		
Mandarin In Heavy Syrup	½ cup (4.4 oz)	80

FOOD	PORTION	CALS.
Dole		
Mandarin Segments	½ cup	70
Pineapple Mandarin Segments	½ cup	80
FRESH		
california navel	1	65
california valencia	1	59
florida	1	69
peel	1 tbsp	6
sections	1 cup	85
Dole		
Orange	1	50

ORANGE EXTRACT

FOOD	PORTION	CALS.
Virginia Dare	1 tsp	22

ORANGE JUICE

FOOD	PORTION	CALS.
fresh	1 cup	111
After The Fall		
Juice	1 bottle (10 oz)	110
Bright & Early		
Chilled	8 fl oz	120
Frozen	8 fl oz	120
Capri Sun		
Drink	1 pkg (7 oz)	100
Del Monte		
Juice	8 fl oz	110
Everfresh		
Juice	1 can (8 oz)	100
Ruby Red Orange Drink	1 can (8 oz)	130
Fresh Samantha		
Juice	1 cup (8 oz)	109
Hi-C		
Box	8.45 fl oz	130
Drink	8 fl oz	130
Drink	1 can (11.5 fl oz)	180
Hood		
From Concentrate	1 cup (8 oz)	120
Select	1 cup (8 oz)	120
With Calcium	1 cup (8 oz)	120
Kool-Aid		
Drink Mix Orange as prep	1 serv (8 oz)	60
Orange Drink as prep w/ sugar	1 serv (8 oz)	100
Libby		
Juice	6 fl oz	80

FOOD	PORTION	CALS.
Minute Maid		
Box	8.45 fl oz	120
Calcium Rich Chilled	8 fl oz	120
Calcium Rich frzn	8 fl oz	120
Chilled	8 fl oz	110
Country Style Chilled	8 fl oz	110
Country Style frzn	8 fl oz	110
Juices To Go	1 can (11.5 fl oz)	160
Juices To Go	1 bottle (16 fl oz)	110
Juices To Go	1 bottle (10 fl oz)	140
Orange Punch Box	8.45 fl oz	130
Premium Choice Chilled	8 fl oz	110
Pulp Free Chilled	8 fl oz	110
Pulp Free frzn	8 fl oz	110
Reduced Acid frzn	8 fl oz	110
Mott's		
From Concentrate	10 fl oz	130
Ocean Spray		
100% Juice	8 fl oz	120
Odwalla		
Juice	8 fl oz	110
Shasta Plus		
Orange Drink	1 can (11.5 oz)	160
Sippin' Pak		
100% Pure	8.45 fl oz	110
Snapple		
Juice	10 fl oz	130
Orangeade	8 fl oz	120
Tang		
Orange Drink as prep	1 serv (8 oz)	90
Sugar Free Orange as prep	1 serv (8 oz)	5
Tree Of Life		
Juice	8 fl oz	110
Tropicana		
& Calcium	8 fl oz	110
Double Vitamin C	8 fl oz	110
Juice	8 oz	110
Ruby Red	8 oz	110
Season's Best	8 oz	110
Season's Best Homestyle	8 fl oz	110
Tropical	8 oz	110
W/ Calcium	8 fl oz	110
Veryfine		
100% Juice	1 bottle (10 oz)	150

FOOD	PORTION	CALS.
Veryfine (CONT.)		
Chillers Artric Orange	8 fl oz	130
Juice Blend	1 can (11.5 oz)	160
Orange Drink	1 bottle (10 oz)	160

OREGANO
ground	1 tsp	5
Watkins		
Liquid Spice	1 tbsp (0.5 oz)	120

ORGAN MEATS
(*see* BRAINS, GIBLETS, GIZZARD, HEART, KIDNEY, LIVER, SWEETBREADS)

ORIENTAL FOOD
(*see* ASIAN FOOD, EGG ROLLS, DINNER, NOODLES, RICE, SUSHI)

OSTRICH
ostrich	3 oz	127

OYSTERS
CANNED
eastern	1 cup	170
Bumble Bee		
Whole	½ cup (3.5 oz)	100

FRESH
eastern cooked	6 med	58
eastern raw	6 med	58
pacific raw	1 med	41
steamed	1 med	41

TAKE-OUT
battered & fried	6 (4.9 oz)	368
breaded & fried	6 (4.9 oz)	368
eastern breaded & fried	6 med (88 g)	173
oysters rockefeller	3 oysters	66

PANCAKE/WAFFLE SYRUP
(*see also* SYRUP)
maple	1 cup (11.1 oz)	824
maple	1 tbsp (0.8 oz)	52
pancake syrup	1 tbsp (0.7 oz)	57
pancake syrup	1 cup (11 oz)	903
pancake syrup light	1 oz	46
pancake syrup w/ butter	1 tbsp (0.7 oz)	59
pancake syrup w/ butter	1 cup (11 oz)	933
Aunt Jemima		
Butter Rich	¼ cup (2.8 oz)	210
Butterlite	¼ cup (2.5 oz)	100

FOOD	PORTION	CALS.
Aunt Jemima (CONT.)		
Lite	¼ cup (2.5 oz)	100
Syrup	¼ cup (2.8 oz)	210
Brer Rabbit		
Dark	2 tbsp	120
Light	2 tbsp	120
Estee		
Maple	¼ cup	80
Log Cabin		
Country Kitchen	1 oz	103
Lite	1 oz	49
Mrs. Butter-worth's		
Original	¼ cup (2 oz)	230
Mrs.Richardson's		
Lite	¼ cup (2.5 oz)	100
Original Recipe	¼ cup (2.8 oz)	210
Red Wing		
Lite	¼ cup (2 oz)	100
Syrup	¼ cup (2 oz)	210
Tree Of Life		
Maple	¼ cup (2.1 oz)	200

PANCAKES
FROZEN

FOOD	PORTION	CALS.
plain	1 4 in diam (1.3 oz)	83
Aunt Jemima		
Blueberry	3 (3.4 oz)	210
Buttermilk	3 (3 oz)	180
Lowfat	3 (3.4 oz)	130
Original	3 (3.4 oz)	200
Downyflake		
Blueberry	3	290
Buttermilk	3	280
Pancakes And Sausages	1 pkg (5.5 oz)	430
Regular	3	280
Eggo		
Buttermilk	3 (4.1 oz)	270
Jimmy Dean		
Flapstick	1 (2.5 oz)	240
Flapstick Blueberry	1 (2.5 oz)	260
Quaker		
Lite Pancakes & Lite Links	1 pkg (6 oz)	310
Lite Pancakes & Lite Syrup	1 pkg (6 oz)	260
Pancakes & Sausages	1 pkg (6 oz)	420

FOOD	PORTION	CALS.
HOME RECIPE		
plain	1 (4 in diam)	86
MIX		
buckwheat	1 (4 in diam)	62
buttermilk	1 (4 in diam) 1.3 oz	74
plain	1 (4 in diam)	74
sugar free low sodium	1 (3 in diam)	44
whole wheat	1 (4 in diam)	92
Arrowhead		
Multigrain Pancake & Waffle Mix	¼ cup (1.2 oz)	120
Aunt Jemima		
Buckwheat Pancake & Waffle Mix	¼ cup (1.4 oz)	120
Buttermilk Pancake & Waffle Mix	⅓ cup (1.9 oz)	190
Original Pancake & Waffle Mix	⅓ cup (1.6 oz)	150
Pancake & Waffle Mix Regular	⅓ cup (1.9 oz)	190
Pancake & Waffle Mix Whole Wheat	¼ cup (1.4 oz)	130
Bisquick		
Shake 'N Pour Blueberry as prep	3	210
Shake 'N Pour as prep	3	200
Shake 'N Pour as prep	3	210
Estee		
Pancake Mix as prep	4 (4 in diam)	180
Fast Shake		
Blueberry	1 serv (2.5 oz)	251
Buttermilk	1 serv (2.5 oz)	258
Original	1 serv (2.5 oz)	266
Hodgson Mill		
Buckwheat	⅓ cup (1.8 oz)	160
Hungry Jack		
Potato as prep	3 (3 in diam)	90
Robin Hood		
Buttermilk as prep	3	230
Stone-Buhr		
Buckwheat	¼ cup (1.4 oz)	130
Oat Bran	¼ cup (1.4 oz)	130
Whole Wheat	¼ cup (1.4 oz)	120
Wanda's		
Blue Corn	⅓ cup mix per serv (1.7 oz)	170
TAKE-OUT		
blueberry	1 (4 in diam)	84
w/ butter & syrup	2 (8.1 oz)	520

FOOD	PORTION	CALS.
PANCREAS		
(see SWEETBREADS)		
PAPAYA		
fresh	1	117
fresh cubed	1 cup	54
Sonoma		
Dried Pieces	2 pieces (2 oz)	200
PAPAYA JUICE		
nectar	1 cup	142
Everfresh		
Premium Drink	1 can (8 oz)	140
Goya		
Nectar	6 oz	110
Kern's		
Nectar	6 fl oz	110
Libby		
Nectar	1 can (11.5 fl oz)	210
PAPRIKA		
paprika	1 tsp	6
Watkins		
Ground	¼ tsp (0.5 oz)	0
PARSLEY		
dry	1 tsp	1
dry	1 tbsp	1
fresh chopped	½ cup	11
Dole		
Chopped	1 tbsp	10
PARSNIPS		
fresh cooked	1 (5.6 oz)	130
fresh sliced cooked	½ cup	63
PASSION FRUIT		
purple fresh	1	18
PASSION FRUIT JUICE		
purple	1 cup	126
yellow	1 cup	149
Snapple		
Passion Supreme	10 fl oz	160
PASTA		
(see also NOODLES, PASTA DINNERS, PASTA SALAD)		
DRY		
corn cooked	1 cup (4.9 oz)	176

FOOD	PORTION	CALS.
elbows cooked	1 cup (4.9 oz)	197
shells small cooked	1 cup (4 oz)	162
shells small protein fortified cooked	1 cup (4 oz)	189
spaghetti cooked	1 cup (4.9 oz)	197
spaghetti protein fortified cooked	1 cup (4.9 oz)	230
spinach spaghetti cooked	1 cup (4.9 oz)	182
spirals cooked	1 cup (4.7 oz)	189
vegetable cooked	1 cup (4.7 oz)	172
whole wheat cooked	1 cup (4.9 oz)	174
whole wheat spaghetti cooked	1 cup (4.9 oz)	174
Anthony		
Pasta	2 oz	210
Barilla		
Conchiglie Rigate	1 cup (2 oz)	200
Gemelli as prep	1 cup (2 oz)	200
Pennette Rigate	1⅓ cups (2 oz)	200
Bella Via		
Angel Hair	2 oz	200
Artichoke Angel Hair as prep	⅝ cup	200
Artichoke Spaghetti as prep	⅝ cup	200
Elbows	2 oz	200
Fettucini as prep	⅝ cup	200
Linguini	2 oz	200
Penne as prep	⅝ cup	200
Rotelli	2 oz	200
Shells	2 oz	200
Spaghetti	2 oz	200
Ziti	2 oz	200
Classico		
Gnocchi Di Toscana	1 cup (2 oz)	210
Creamette		
Elbow Macaroni not prep	2 oz	210
Cuore		
Capellini cooked	1⅓ cup (2 oz)	190
Fusilli cooked	1⅓ cup (2 oz)	190
Tortiglioni cooked	1⅓ cup (2 oz)	190
De Bole's		
Whole Wheat Organic Elbows	2 oz	210
DeCecco		
Whole Wheat Linguine cooked	2 oz	180
DeFino		
Lasagna No Boil	1 oz	102
Ribbons No Boil	2 oz	204

FOOD	PORTION	CALS.
Delverde		
Spaghetti Whole Wheat	2 oz	206
Eden		
Elbows Whole Wheat Organic	2 oz	210
Elbows Whole Wheat Vegetable Organic	2 oz	210
Kudzu And Sweet Potato Pasta	2 oz	190
Kudzu Kiri Pasta	2 oz	190
Mung Bean Pasta Harusame	2 oz	190
Organic Endless Tubes	½ cup (1.9 oz)	210
Ribbons Durum Wheat Curry Organic	2 oz	220
Ribbons Durum Wheat Organic	2 oz	220
Ribbons Durum Wheat Paella Organic	2 oz	220
Ribbons Durum Wheat Parsley Garlic Organic	2 oz	220
Ribbons Durum Wheat Pesto Organic	2 oz	220
Ribbons Whole Wheat Spinach Organic	2 oz	200
Rice Pasta Bifun	2 oz	200
Shells Durum Wheat Vegetable Organic	2 oz	210
Soba	2 oz	200
Soba 100% Buckwheat	2 oz	200
Soba Lotus Root	2 oz	190
Soba Mugwort	2 oz	190
Soba Wild Yam Jinenjo	2 oz	190
Somen	2 oz	200
Spaghetti Durum Wheat Organic	2 oz	210
Spaghetti Kamut Organic	2 oz	210
Spaghetti Parsley Garlic Organic	2 oz	210
Spaghetti Whole Wheat Organic	2 oz	210
Spirals Durum Wheat Vegetable Organic	2 oz	210
Spirals Kamut Organic	2 oz	210
Spirals Sesame Rice Organic	2 oz	200
Spirals Whole Wheat Vegetable Organic	2 oz	210
Udon	2 oz	200
Udon Brown Rice	2 oz	200
Gioia		
Pasta	2 oz	210
Hodgson Mill		
Spaghetti Whole Wheat Spinach not prep	2 oz	190
Veggie Bows not prep	2 oz	200
Veggie Rotini not prep	2 oz	200
Veggie Wagon Wheels not prep	2 oz	200
Whole Wheat Spirals not prep	2 oz	190
La Molisana		
Radiatori	2 oz	230

FOOD	PORTION	CALS.
Lupini		
Elbow uncooked	½ cup (2 oz)	190
Spaghetti Light uncooked	½ cup (2 oz)	190
Spaghetti With Triticale	⅐ pkg (2 oz)	190
Luxury		
Pasta	2 oz	210
Merlino's		
Pasta	2 oz	210
Noodles By Leonardo		
Capellini	2 oz	200
Elbows not prep	½ cup (2 oz)	200
Fettucini	2 oz	200
Linguine not prep	½ cup (2 oz)	200
Rigatoni	2 oz	200
Rotini	2 oz	200
Shells not prep	½ cup (2 oz)	200
Spaghetti not prep	½ cup (2 oz)	200
Spaghettini	2 oz	200
Vermicelli not prep	½ cup (2 oz)	200
Penn Dutch		
Pasta	2 oz	210
Pomi		
Capellini	2 oz	210
Prince		
Egg	2 oz	221
Pasta	2 oz	210
Rainbow	2 oz	210
Spinach Egg	2 oz	220
Pritikin		
Spaghetti Whole Wheat	⅛ box (2 oz)	190
Spiral	⅔ cup (2 oz)	190
Red Cross		
Pasta	2 oz	210
Ronco		
Pasta	2 oz	210
Ronzoni		
Elbows	¾ cup (2 oz)	210
Fettucini	¾ cup (2 oz)	210
Fusilli	¾ cup (2 oz)	210
Lasagne	¾ cup (2 oz)	210
Manicotti	¾ cup (2 oz)	210
Mostaccioli	¾ cup (2 oz)	210
Rigatoni	¾ cup (2 oz)	210
Rotelle uncooked	¾ cup (2 oz)	210

FOOD	PORTION	CALS.
Ronzoni (cont.)		
Rotini uncooked	¾ cup (2 oz)	210
Shells uncooked	¾ cup (2 oz)	210
Shells Jumbo	¾ cup (2 oz)	210
Spaghetti not prep	¾ cup (2 oz)	210
Tubettini	¾ cup (2 oz)	210
San Giorgio		
Bowties Egg	2 oz	210
Capellini	2 oz	210
Elbow Macaroni	2 oz	210
Fettuccine Egg	2 oz	210
Fettuccini Florentine	2 oz	210
Lasagne	2 oz	210
Linguini	2 oz	210
Manicotti	2 oz	210
Rigatoni	2 oz	210
Rotini	2 oz	210
Shells	2 oz	210
Spaghetti	2 oz	210
Spaghetti Thin	2 oz	210
Vermicelli	2 oz	210
Ziti Cut	2 oz	210
Tree Of Life		
Cajun as prep	⅝ cup (4.9 oz)	200
Confetti as prep	⅝ cup (4.9 oz)	200
Garlic & Parsley as prep	⅝ cup (4.9 oz)	200
Jamaican Spice as prep	⅝ cup (4.9 oz)	200
Lemon Pepper as prep	⅝ cup (4.9 oz)	200
Spinach as prep	⅝ cup (4.9 oz)	200
Tex Mex as prep	⅝ cup (4.9 oz)	200
Thai as prep	⅝ cup (4.9 oz)	200
Tomato Basil as prep	⅝ cup (4.9 oz)	200
Vimco		
Pasta	2 oz	210
FRESH		
cooked	2 oz	75
spinach cooked	2 oz	74
Contadina		
Angel's Hair	1¼ cup (2.8 oz)	240
Fettuccine	1¼ cup (2.9 oz)	250
Fettuccine Cholesterol Free	1 cup (2.9 oz)	240
Light Ravioli Cheese	1 cup (3.1 oz)	240
Light Ravioli Garden Vegetable	1¼ cup (3.8 oz)	290
Light Tortellini Garlic & Cheese	1 cup (3.6 oz)	280

FOOD	PORTION	CALS.
Contadina (CONT.)		
Linguine	1¼ cup (3 oz)	260
Linguine Cholesterol Free	1¼ cup (3.1 oz)	250
Ravioli Beef And Garlic	1¼ cup (4 oz)	350
Ravioli Cheese	1 cup (3.1 oz)	280
Ravioli Chicken And Rosemary	1¼ cup (4 oz)	330
Tagliatelli Spinach	1¼ cup (3.1 oz)	270
Tortellini Spianch Three Cheese	¾ cup (3.1 oz)	280
Tortelloni Cheese	¾ cup (3 oz)	260
Tortelloni Cheese And Basil	1 cup (4 oz)	360
Tortelloni Chicken And Prosciutto	1 cup (3.8 oz)	360
Tortelloni Chicken And Vegetable	¾ cup (2.9 oz)	260
Tortelloni Spicy Italian Sausage And Bell Pepper	1 cup (3.6 oz)	330
Di Giorno		
Angel's Hair	1 cup	160
Beef & Roasted Garlic Tortellini	1 cup	340
Fettuccine	1 cup	200
Four Cheese Raviolo	1 cup	350
Herb Linguine	1 cup	200
Italian Sausage Ravioli In Green Bell Pepper Pasta	1¼ cup	350
Lemon Chicken Tortellini In Cracked Black Pepper Pasta	1 cup	270
Light Cheese Ravioli	1 cup	280
Linguine	1 cup	200
Mozzarella Garlic Tortelloni	1 cup	300
Pesto Tortelloni	1 cup	320
Portabello Mushroom Tortelloni	1 cup	310
Red Bell Pepper Fettuccine	1 cup	200
Spinach Fettuccine	1 cup	190
Sun-Dried Tomato Ravioli	1⅓ cup	380
Three Cheese Tortellini	¾ cup	250
Herb's		
Fettucine Bell Pepper Basil	2 oz	220
Fettucine Parsley Garlic	2 oz	220
Fettucine Spinach	2 oz	220
Ribbons Vegetable	2 oz	220
Ribbons Whole Wheat	2 oz	200
Rotini Mixed Vegetable	2 oz	210
Shells Mixed Vegetable	2 oz	210
Trios		
Ravioli Cracked Pepper Garlic Cheese	1 cup (4.3 oz)	340

FOOD	PORTION	CALS.
HOME RECIPE		
made w/o egg cooked	2 oz	71
plain made w/ egg cooked	2 oz	74
PASTA DINNERS		
(see also DINNER, PASTA SALAD*)*		
CANNED		
Chef Boyardee		
ABC's & 1,2,3's In Cheese Flavor Sauce	7.5 oz	180
ABC's & 1,2,3's w/ Mini Meatballs	7.5 oz	260
Beef Ravioli	7.5 oz	190
Beef Ravioli 99% Fat Free	1 cup (8.6 oz)	210
Beefaroni	7.5 oz	220
Cheese Ravioli In Meat Sauce	7.5 oz	200
Dinosaurs In Cheese Flavor Sauce	7.5 oz	180
Dinosaurs w/ Meatballs	7.5 oz	240
Elbows In Beef Sauce	7.5 oz	210
Lasagna	7.5 oz	230
Lasagna In Garden Vegetable Sauce	7.5 oz	170
Macaroni & Cheese	7.5 oz	180
Pasta Rings & Meatballs	7.5 oz	220
Rigatoni	7.5 oz	210
Rings & Franks	7.5 oz	190
Shells In Meat Sauce	7.5 oz	210
Shells In Mushroom Sauce	7.5 oz	170
Spaghetti & Meat Balls	7.5 oz	230
Tic Tac Toes In Cheese Flavor Sauce	7.5 oz	170
Tic Tac Toes w/ Mini Meatballs	7.5 oz	250
Turtles In Sauce	7.5 oz	160
Turtles w/ Meatballs	7.5 oz	210
Franco-American		
Beef RavioliO's In Meat Sauce	½ can (7.5 oz)	250
CircusO's Pasta In Tomato & Cheese Sauce	½ can (7.4 oz)	170
CircusO's Pasta With Meatballs In Tomato Sauce	½ can (7.4 oz)	210
Macaroni & Cheese	½ can (7.4 oz)	170
Spaghetti In Tomato Sauce w/ Cheese	½ can (7.4 oz)	180
Spaghetti w/ Meatballs In Tomato Sauce	½ can (7.4 oz)	220
SpaghettiO's With Meatballs	½ can (7.4 oz)	220
SpaghettiO's With Sliced Franks	½ can (7.4 oz)	220
SpaghettiO's In Tomato & Cheese Sauce	½ can (7.4 oz)	170
SportyO's In Tomato & Cheese Sauce	½ can (7.5 oz)	170
SportyO's Pasta With Meatballs In Tomato Sauce	½ can (7.4 oz)	210

FOOD	PORTION	CALS.
Franco-American (CONT.)		
TeddyO's In Tomato & Cheese Sauce	½ can (7.5 oz)	170
TeddyO's Pasta With Meatballs	½ can (7.4 oz)	210
Hormel		
Spaghetti & Meatballs	1 can (7.5 oz)	210
Kid's Kitchen		
Microwave Meals Cheezy Mac & Beef	1 cup (7.5 oz)	260
Microwave Meals Noodle Rings & Chicken	1 cup (7.5 oz)	150
Microwave Meals Spaghetti Rings & Franks	1 cup (7.5 oz)	240
Progresso		
Beef Ravioli	1 cup (9.1 oz)	260
Cheese Ravioli	1 cup (9.1 oz)	220
Van Camp's		
Spaghetti Weenee	1 can (8 oz)	230
FROZEN		
Amy's Organic		
Macaroni & Cheese	1 pkg (9 oz)	390
Macaroni & Soy Cheese	1 pkg (9 oz)	360
Pasta Primavera	1 pkg (9.5 oz)	320
Ravioli w/ Sauce	1 pkg (9.5 oz)	340
Tofu Vegetable Lasagna	1 pkg (9.5 oz)	300
Vegetable Lasagna	1 pkg (9.5 oz)	300
Whole Meals Cannelloni	1 pkg (9 oz)	260
Banquet		
Family Entree Lasagna w/ Meat Sauce	1 serv (8 oz)	240
Family Entree Macaroni & Beef	1 serv (8 oz)	230
Family Entree Macaroni & Cheese	1 serv (8 oz)	300
Family Entree Noodles & Chicken	1 serv (8 oz)	210
Family Entree Noodles & Beef	1 serv (7.5 oz)	140
Birds Eye		
Easy Recipe Meal Starter Cheesy Cheese	1 serv	280
Easy Recipe Meal Starter Chicken Primavera as prep	1 serv	280
Easy Recipe Meal Starter Chicken Alfredo as prep	1 serv	280
Pasta Secrets Creamy Peppercorn	2⅓ cups (6.6 oz)	300
Pasta Secrets Italian Pesto	2⅓ cups (6.4 oz)	240
Pasta Secrets Primavera	2⅓ cups (6.6 oz)	230
Pasta Secrets Three Cheese	2 cups (6.1 oz)	230
Pasta Secrets White Cheddar	2 cups (6.3 oz)	240
Pasta Secrets Zesty Garlic	2 cups (5.9 oz)	240
Budget Gourmet		
Cheese Ravioli	1 meal (9.5 oz)	290

FOOD	PORTION	CALS.
Budget Gourmet (CONT.)		
Lasagna Italian Sausage	1 meal (10 oz)	430
Lasagna Vegetable	1 meal (10.5 oz)	390
Lasagne Three Cheese	1 meal (10 oz)	390
Lasagne With Meat Sauce	1 meal (9.4 oz)	290
Linguini With Shrimp & Clams	1 meal (9.5 oz)	280
Linguini With Shrimp And Clams	1 meal (10 oz)	270
Macaroni & Cheese	1 meal (5.75 oz)	230
Macaroni & Cheese With Cheddar & Parmesan	1 meal (10.5 oz)	330
Mainicotti Cheese	1 meal (10 oz)	440
Pasta Alfredo With Broccoli	1 meal (5.5 oz)	210
Penne Pasta With Chunky Tomato Sauce & Italian Sausage	1 meal (10 oz)	320
Rigatoni In Cream Sauce With Broccoli & Chicken	1 meal (10.8 oz)	290
Spaghetti With Chunky Tomato & Meat Sauce	1 meal (10 oz)	300
Tortellini Cheese	1 meal (5.5 oz)	200
Ziti In Marinara Sauce	1 meal (6.25 oz)	200
Dining Light		
Cheese Cannelloni	9 oz	310
Formagg		
Penne Pasta Alfredo	⅔ cup (5 oz)	190
Penne Pasta Primavera	⅔ cup (5 oz)	190
Vegetable Pasta & Caesar Italian Garden	⅔ cup (5 oz)	190
Green Giant		
Create A Meal Creamy Alfredo as prep	1¼ cups (10 oz)	380
Create A Meal Creamy Cheddar as prep	1½ cups (10 oz)	290
Create A Meal Creamy Chicken Noodle as prep	1¼ cups (10 oz)	350
Pasta Accents Alfredo	2 cups (5.6 oz)	210
Pasta Accents Creamy Cheddar	2⅓ cups (6.7 oz)	250
Pasta Accents Florentine	2 cups (7.3 oz)	310
Pasta Accents Garden Herb Seasoning	2 cups (6.8 oz)	230
Pasta Accents Garlic Seasoning	2 cups (6.6 oz)	260
Pasta Accents Primavera	2¼ cups (7 oz)	320
Pasta Accents White Cheddar Sauce	1¾ cups (5.6 oz)	300
Healthy Choice		
Beef Macaroni Casserole	1 meal (8.5 oz)	200
Cheese Ravioli Parmigiana	1 meal (9 oz)	250
Chicken Broccoli Alfredo	1 meal (12.1 oz)	370
Chicken Fettucini Alfredo	1 meal (8.5 oz)	250
Classics Pasta Shells Marinara	1 meal (12 oz)	360

FOOD	PORTION	CALS.
Healthy Choice (CONT.)		
Classics Turkey Fettuccine Alla Crema	1 meal (12.5 oz)	350
Fettucini Alfredo	1 meal (8 oz)	240
Lasagna Roma	1 meal (13.5 oz)	390
Macaroni & Cheese	1 meal (9 oz)	290
Spaghetti Bolognese	1 meal (10 oz)	260
Three Cheese Manicotti	1 meal (11 oz)	310
Vegetable Pasta Italiano	1 meal (10 oz)	220
Zucchini Lasagna	1 meal (14 oz)	330
Kid Cuisine		
Macaroni & Cheese	1 pkg (10.6 oz)	420
Mini Cheese Ravioli	1 pkg (9.82 oz)	320
Le Menu		
Entree LightStyle Garden Vegetables Lasagna	10.5 oz	260
Entree LightStyle Lasagna With Meat Sauce	10 oz	290
Entree LightStyle Meat Sauce & Cheese Tortellini	8 oz	250
Entree LightStyle Spaghetti With Beef Sauce And Mushrooms	9 oz	280
LightStyle 3-Cheese Stuffed Shells	10 oz	280
LightStyle Cheese Tortellini	10 oz	230
Manicotto With Three Cheeses	11.75 oz	390
Lean Cuisine		
Alfredo Pasta Primavera	1 pkg (10 oz)	290
Angel Hair Pasta	1 pkg (10 oz)	220
Bow Tie Pasta & Creamy Tomato Sauce	1 pkg (9.5 oz)	260
Cafe Classics Bow Tie Pasta & Chicken	1 pkg (9.5 oz)	250
Cafe Classics Cheese Lasagna w/ Chicken Scaloppini	1 pkg (10 oz)	290
Cheddar Bake With Pasta	1 pkg (9 oz)	220
Cheese Cannelloni	1 pkg (9.1 oz)	230
Cheese Lasagna Casserole	1 pkg (10 oz)	270
Cheese Ravioli	1 pkg (8.5 oz)	270
Cheese Stuffed Shells	1 serv (8.9 oz)	230
Chicken Fettucini	1 pkg (9.25 oz)	280
Chicken Lasagna	1 pkg (10 oz)	270
Classic Cheese Lasagna	1 pkg (11.5 oz)	270
Fettucini Alfredo	1 pkg (9 oz)	300
Fettucini Primavera	1 pkg (10 oz)	270
Five Cheese Lasagna	1 serv (8 oz)	210
Lasagne With Meat Sauce	1 pkg (10.5 oz)	290
Macaroni & Beef	1 pkg (10 oz)	270

FOOD	PORTION	CALS.
Lean Cuisine (CONT.)		
Macaroni & Cheese	1 pkg (10 oz)	290
Penne Pasta Bolognese	1 pkg (9.5 oz)	270
Penne Pasta w/ Tomato Basil Sauce	1 pkg (10 oz)	270
Spaghetti w/ Meat Sauce	1 pkg (11.5 oz)	290
Spaghetti w/ Meatballs	1 pkg (9.5 oz)	280
Vegetable Lasagna	1 pkg (10.5 oz)	260
Life Choice		
Linguini Roma	1 meal (13.2 oz)	230
Sun Dried Tomato Manicotti	1 meal (11.65 oz)	220
Vegetable Lasagna Primavera	1 meal (11.2 oz)	170
Luigino's		
& Pomodoro Sauc With Meatballs	1 pkg (9 oz)	320
& Pomodoro Sauce With Meatballs	1 cup (6.3 oz)	270
Cheese Ravioli & Alfredo With Broccoli Sauce	1 pkg (8.5 oz)	420
Cheese Tortellini & Alfredo Sauce With Broccoli	1 pkg (8 oz)	390
Fettuccine Alfredo	1 cup (7.5 oz)	330
Fettuccine Alfredo	1 pkg (9.4 oz)	390
Fettuccine Alfredo With Broccoli	1 pkg (9.2 oz)	360
Fettuccine Carbonara	1 pkg (9 oz)	360
Lasagna Alfredo	1 pkg (9 oz)	360
Lasagna Alfredo	1 cup (6.3 oz)	300
Lasagna Pollo	1 pkg (9 oz)	320
Lasagna With Meat Sauce	1 pkg (9 oz)	290
Lasagna With Meat Sauce	1 cup (7.2 oz)	240
Lasagna With Vegetables	1 pkg (9 oz)	290
Linguini With Clams & Sauce	1 pkg (9 oz)	270
Linguini With Red Sauce	1 pkg (9 oz)	260
Linguini With Seafood	1 pkg (9 oz)	290
Macaroni & Cheese	1 pkg (9 oz)	370
Macaroni & Cheese	1 cup (7.2 oz)	310
Marinara Sauce Penne Pasta Italian Sausage & Peppers	1 pkg (9 oz)	350
Marinara Sauce Penne Pasta Italian Sausage & Peppers	1 cup (7.4 oz)	290
Meat Ravioli & Pomodoro Sauce	1 pkg (8.5 oz)	320
Minestrone With Penne Pasta	1 cup (6.3 oz)	180
Penne Pollo	1 pkg (9 oz)	330
Penne Primavera	1 pkg (9 oz)	350
Rigatoni Pomodoro Italiano	1 pkg (9 oz)	290
Shells & Cheese With Jalapenos	1 pkg (8.5 oz)	360
Spaghetti Bolognese	1 pkg (9 oz)	270

FOOD	PORTION	CALS.
Luigino's (CONT.)		
Spaghetti Marinara	1 pkg (10 oz)	250
Spinach Ravioli & Primavera Sauce	1 pkg (8.5 oz)	360
Morton		
Macaroni & Cheese	1 serv (8 oz)	220
Palmazone		
Macaroni 'n Cheese	½ pkg (6 oz)	260
Pasta Favorites		
Chicken Pasta Primavera	1 pkg (10.5 oz)	330
Fettuccini Alfredo	1 pkg (10.5 oz)	370
Italian Sausage & Peppers	1 pkg (10.5 oz)	340
Lasagna	1 pkg (10.5 oz)	290
Macaroni & Cheese	1 pkg (10.5 oz)	350
Pasta Primavera	1 pkg (10.5 oz)	320
Spaghetti w/ Meatballs	1 pkg (10.5 oz)	370
Vegetable Lasagna	1 pkg (10.5 oz)	260
White Cheddar & Rotini	1 pkg (10.5 oz)	350
Senor Felix's		
Lasagna Southwestern	1 serv (6 oz)	160
Stouffer's		
Cheddar Pasta w/ Beef & Tomatoes	1 pkg (11 oz)	450
Cheese Manicotti	1 pkg (9 oz)	380
Cheese Ravioli	1 pkg (10.6 oz)	380
Chicken Lasagna	1 serv (7.8 oz)	320
Fettucini Alfredo	1 pkg (10 oz)	520
Fettucini Primavera	1 pkg (10 oz)	430
Five Cheese Lasagna	1 pkg (10.75 oz)	360
Grilled Chicken & Angel Hair Pasta	1 pkg (10.9 oz)	380
Homestyle Chicken Fettucini	1 pkg (10.5 oz)	390
Homestyle Chicken Parmigiana w/ Spaghetti	1 pkg (12 oz)	460
Homestyle Veal Parmigiana w/ Spaghetti	1 pkg (11.9 oz)	430
Lasagna Bake	1 pkg (10.25 oz)	370
Lasagna w/ Meat Sauce	1 pkg (10.5 oz)	370
Macaroni & Cheese	1 cup (6 oz)	320
Macaroni & Cheese w/ Broccoli	1 pkg (10.5 oz)	360
Macaroni & Beef	1 pkg (11.5 oz)	420
Noodles Romanoff	1 pkg (12 oz)	490
Pasta Shells w/ American Cheese	1 cup (6 oz)	260
Salisbury Steak w/ Macaroni & Cheese	1 serv (11.3 oz)	410
Spaghetti w/ Meat Sauce	1 pkg (10 oz)	350
Spaghetti w/ Meatballs	1 pkg (12.6 oz)	440
Tuna Noodle Casserole	1 pkg (10 oz)	320
Turkey Tettrazini	1 pkg (10 oz)	360

FOOD	PORTION	CALS.
Stouffer's (CONT.)		
Vegetable Lasagna	1 pkg (10.5 oz)	440
Swanson		
Homestyle Lasagne With Meat Sauce	10.5 oz	400
Homestyle Macaroni & Cheese	10 oz	390
Homestyle Spaghetti With Italian Style Meatballs	13 oz	490
Macaroni & Cheese	12.25 oz	370
Macaroni & Cheese	7 oz	200
Spaghetti & Meatballs	12.5 oz	390
Tabatchnick		
Macaroni & Cheese	7.5 oz	280
Tyson		
Parmigiana	1 pkg (11.25 oz)	380
Ultra Slim-Fast		
Pasta Primavera	12 oz	340
Spaghetti With Beef & Mushroom Sauce	12 oz	370
Weight Watchers		
Garden Lasagna	1 pkg (11 oz)	270
Homestyle Macaroni & Cheese	1 pkg (9 oz)	290
Smart Ones Angel Hair Pasta	1 pkg (9 oz)	180
Smart Ones Bowtie Pasta & Mushrooms Marsala	1 pkg (9.65 oz)	270
Smart Ones Chicken Fettucini	1 pkg (10 oz)	300
Smart Ones Creamy Rigatoni w/ Broccoli & Chicken	1 pkg (9 oz)	230
Smart Ones Fettucini Alfredo w/ Broccoli	1 pkg (8.5 oz)	230
Smart Ones Lasagna Florentine	1 pkg (10 oz)	200
Smart Ones Lasagna Alfredo	1 pkg (9 oz)	300
Smart Ones Lasagna w/ Meat Sauce	1 pkg (9 oz)	240
Smart Ones Lasagna w/ Meat Sauce	1 pkg (10.25 oz)	270
Smart Ones Macaroni & Cheese	1 pkg (9 oz)	220
Smart Ones Pasta & Spinach Romano	1 pkg (10.4 oz)	260
Smart Ones Pasta w/ Tomato Basil Sauce	1 pkg (9.6 oz)	260
Smart Ones Penne Pasta w/ Sun-Dried Tomatoes	1 pkg (10 oz)	280
Smart Ones Penne Pollo	1 pkg (10 oz)	290
Smart Ones Ravioli Florentine	1 pkg (8.5 oz)	220
Smart Ones Spaghetti Marinara	1 pkg (9 oz)	280
Smart Ones Spaghetti w/ Meat Sauce	1 pkg (10 oz)	280
Smart Ones Spicy Penne & Ricotta	1 pkg (10.2 oz)	280
Smart Ones Tuna Noodle Casserole	1 pkg (9.5 oz)	270
Smart Ones Zita Mozzarella	1 pkg (9 oz)	290

FOOD	PORTION	CALS.
HOME RECIPE		
spaghetti w/ meatballs & tomato sauce	1 cup	330
MIX		
Casbah		
Pasta Fasul	1 pkg (1.6 oz)	150
Hain		
Pasta & Sauce Creamy Parmesan	¼ pkg	150
Pasta & Sauce Creamy Swiss	¼ pkg	170
Pasta & Sauce Fettuccine Alfredo	¼ pkg	180
Pasta & Sauce Italian Herb	¼ pkg	110
Pasta & Sauce Primavera	¼ pkg	140
Pasta & Sauce Tangy Cheddar	¼ pkg	180
Hamburger Helper		
Ravioli as prep	1 cup	280
Ravioli w/ White Cheese Topping as prep	1 cup	310
Kraft		
Deluxe Macaroni & Cheese Four Cheese Blend as prep	1 cup (6.2 oz)	320
Deluxe Macaroni & Cheese Original as prep	1 cup (6.1 oz)	320
Light Deluxe Macaroni & Cheese as prep	1 cup (6.5 oz)	290
Macaroni & Cheese All Shapes as prep	1 cup (6.9 oz)	410
Macaroni & Cheese Original as prep	1 cup (6.9 oz)	410
Macaroni & Cheese Original as prep light recipe	1 cup (6.4 oz)	290
Premium Macaroni & Cheese Cheesy Alfredo as prep	1 cup (6.9 oz)	410
Premium Macaroni & Cheese Mild White Cheddar as prep	1 cup (6.8 oz)	410
Premium Macaroni & Cheese Thick 'N Creamy as prep	1 cup (7.6 oz)	420
Premium Macaroni & Cheese Three Cheese as prep	1 cup (6.9 oz)	410
Spaghetti Classics Mild Italian as prep	1 cup (9.1 oz)	240
Spaghetti Classics Tangy Italian as prep	1 cup (8.9 oz)	240
Spaghetti Classics Zesty Cheese as prep	1 cup (8.6 oz)	240
Spaghetti Classics w/ Meat Sauce as prep	1 cup (8.2 oz)	330
Lipton		
Pasta & Sauce Angel Hair Chicken Broccoli as prep	1 cup	260
Pasta & Sauce Angel Hair Parmesan as prep	1 cup	280
Pasta & Sauce Bow Tie Chicken Primavera as prep	1 cup	290

FOOD	PORTION	CALS.
Lipton (CONT.)		
Pasta & Sauce Bow Tie Italian Cheese as prep	1 cup	300
Pasta & Sauce Butter & Herbs as prep	1 cup	270
Pasta & Sauce Cheddar Broccoli as prep	1 cup	340
Pasta & Sauce Chicken Herb Parmesan as prep	1 cup	80
Pasta & Sauce Chicken Stir-Fry as prep	1 cup	270
Pasta & Sauce Creamy Garlic as prep	1 cup	350
Pasta & Sauce Creamy Mushroom as prep	1 cup	320
Pasta & Sauce Garlic & Butter Linguine as prep	1 cup	260
Pasta & Sauce Mild Cheddar Cheese as prep	1 cup	290
Pasta & Sauce Roasted Garlic Chicken as prep	1 cup	290
Pasta & Sauce Roasted Garlic & Olive Oil w/ Tomato as prep	1 cup	270
Pasta & Sauce Rotini Primavera as prep	1 cup	320
Pasta & Sauce Savory Herb w/ Garlic as prep	1 cup	280
Pasta & Sauce Three Cheese Rotini as prep	1 cup	320
Melting Pot		
Terrazza Black Beans & Penne	1 cup	180
Terrazza Florentine Red Beans & Fusilli	1 cup	220
Terrazza Red Lentils & Bow Ties	1 cup	240
Terrazza Tuscan White Beans & Gemelli	1 cup	220
Nile Spice		
Pasta'n Sauce Mediterranean	1 pkg	210
Pasta'n Sauce Parmesan	1 pkg	200
Pasta'n Sauce Primavera	1 pkg	200
Ultra Slim-Fast		
Macaroni & Cheese	2.3 oz	230
Uncle Ben		
Country Inn Pasta & Sauce Angel Hair Parmesan	1 serv (2.2 oz)	245
Country Inn Pasta & Sauce Broccoli & White Cheddar	1 serv (2.2 oz)	240
Country Inn Pasta & Sauce Butter & Herb	1 serv (2 oz)	230
Country Inn Pasta & Sauce Creamy Garlic	1 serv (2.4 oz)	261
Country Inn Pasta & Sauce Fettuccine Alfredo	1 serv (2.2 oz)	310
Country Inn Pasta & Sauce Herb Linguine	1 serv (2.2 oz)	240

FOOD	PORTION	CALS.
Uncle Ben (CONT.)		
Country Inn Pasta & Sauce Mushroom Fettuccine	1 serv (2.2 oz)	250
Country Inn Pasta & Sauce Vegetable Alfredo	1 serv (2.2 oz)	240
Velveeta		
Rotini & Cheese w/ Broccoli as prep	1 cup (7.2 oz)	400
Shells & Cheese Bacon as prep	1 cup (6.8 oz)	360
Shells & Cheese Original as prep	1 cup (6.6 oz)	360
Shells & Cheese Salsa as prep	1 cup (7.5 oz)	380
SHELF-STABLE		
Chef Boyardee		
Microwave Main Meal Beans & Pasta	10.5 oz	200
Microwave Main Meal Beef Ravioli Suprema	10.5 oz	290
Microwave Main Meal Cheese Ravioli Suprema	10.5 oz	290
Microwave Main Meal Fettuccine	10.5 oz	290
Microwave Main Meal Lasagna	10.5 oz	290
Microwave Main Meal Meat Tortellini	10.5 oz	220
Microwave Main Meal Noodles w/ Chicken	10.5 oz	170
Microwave Main Meal Peas & Pasta	10.5 oz	190
Microwave Main Meal Spaghetti Suprema	10.5 oz	200
Microwave Main Meal Zesty Macaroni	10.5 oz	290
Microwave Main Meal Ziti In Sauce	10.5 oz	210
Hormel		
Microcup Meals Lasagna	1 cup (7.5 oz)	250
Microcup Meals Macaroni & Cheese	1 cup (7.5 oz)	260
Microcup Meals Ravioli w/ Tomato Sauce	1 cup (7.5 oz)	220
Microcup Meals Spaghetti & Meatballs	1 cup (7.5 oz)	220
Kid's Kitchen		
Microwave Meals Beefy Macaroni	1 cup (7.5 oz)	190
Microwave Meals Macaroni & Cheese	1 cup (7.5 oz)	260
Microwave Meals Mini Ravioli	1 cup (7.5 oz)	240
Microwave Meals Spaghetti & Meatballs	1 cup (7.5 oz)	220
Microwave Meals Spaghetti Ring & Meatballs	1 cup (7.5 oz)	250
Lunch Bucket		
Elbows In Tomato Sauce	1 pkg (7.5 oz)	190
Lasagna With Meatsauce	1 pkg (7.5 oz)	220
Light'n Healthy Italian Style Pasta	1 pkg (7.5 oz)	130
Light'n Healthy Pasta In Wine Sauce	1 pkg (7.5 oz)	130
Light'n Healthy Pasta'n Garden Vegetables	1 pkg (7.5 oz)	150
Macaroni'n Cheese	1 pkg (7.5 oz)	210

FOOD	PORTION	CALS.
Lunch Bucket (CONT.)		
Pasta'n Chicken	1 pkg (7.5 oz)	180
Spaghetti'n Meatsauce	1 pkg (7.5 oz)	240
My Own Meal		
Cheese Tortellini	1 pkg (10 oz)	340

PASTA MACHINE MIX
Wanda's

Dried Tomato	⅓ cup mix per serv (1.9 oz)	202
Durum & Semolina	⅓ cup mix per serv (1.9 oz)	199
Semolina Blend	⅓ cup mix per serv (1.9 oz)	202
Spinach	⅓ cup mix per serv (1.9 oz)	202
Whole Wheat & Semolina	⅓ cup mix per serv (1.9 oz)	198

PASTA SALAD
MIX
Kraft

Herb & Garlic as prep	¾ cup (4.9 oz)	280
Pasta Salad Classic Ranch w/ Bacon as prep	¾ cup (4.7 oz)	350
Pasta Salad Creamy Ceasar as prep	¾ cup (4.8 oz)	340
Pasta Salad Garden Primavera as prep	¾ cup (5 oz)	240
Pasta Salad Italian 97% Fat Free as prep	¾ cup (4.9 oz)	190
Pasta Salad Parmesan Peppercorn as prep	¾ cup (4.9 oz)	360
Suddenly Salad		
Classic Pasta	¾ cup	250
Classic Pasta Reduced Fat Recipe	¾ cup	210
Garden Italian 98% Fat Free	¾ cup	140
TAKE-OUT		
elbow macaroni salad	3.5 oz	160
italian style pasta salad	3.5 oz	140
mustard macaroni salad	3.5 oz	190
pasta salad w/ vegetables	3.5 oz	140

PASTRY
(*see* BROWNIE, CAKE, DANISH PASTRY)

PATE

antipasto pate	1 can (2.25 oz)	110
duck pate	1 oz	96
fish pate	1 oz	76

FOOD	PORTION	CALS.
goose liver smoked canned	1 tbsp (13 g)	60
liver canned	1 tbsp (13 g)	41
mushroom anchovy pate	1 can (2.25 oz)	130
pate foie gras	1 oz	127
pork pate	1 oz	107
pork pate en croute	1 oz	91
rabbit pate	1 oz	66
salmon pate	1 can (2.25 oz)	140
shrimp	1 can (2.25 oz)	140
smoked turkey	1 can (2.25 oz)	170
Sells		
Liver	2.08 oz	190

PEACH
CANNED
Del Monte

FOOD	PORTION	CALS.
Halves Cling In Heavy Syrup	½ cup (4.5 oz)	100
Halves Cling Lite	½ cup (4.4 oz)	60
Halves Cling Melba In Heavy Syrup	½ cup (4.5 oz)	100
Halves Freestone In Heavy Syrup	½ cup (4.5 oz)	100
Sliced Cling Fruit Naturals	½ cup (4.4 oz)	60
Sliced Cling In Heavy Syrup	½ cup (4.5 oz)	100
Sliced Cling Lite	½ cup (4.4 oz)	60
Sliced Freestone In Heavy Syrup	½ cup (4.5 oz)	100
Sliced Freestone Lite	½ cup (4.4 oz)	60
Snack Cups Diced Fruit Naturals	1 serv (4.5 oz)	60
Snack Cups Diced Fruit Naturals EZ-Open Lid	1 serv (4.2 oz)	60
Snack Cups Diced In Heavy Syrup	1 serv (4.5 oz)	100
Snack Cups Diced In Heavy Syrup EZ-Open Lid	1 serv (4.2 oz)	90
Snack Cups Diced Lite	1 serv (4.5 oz)	60
Snack Cups Diced Lite EZ-Open Lid	1 serv (4.2 oz)	60
Whole Cling In Heavy Syrup	½ cup (4.2 oz)	100
Hunt's		
Halves	½ cup (4.5 oz)	100
Slices	½ cup (4.5 oz)	100
Libby		
Halves Yellow Cling Lite	½ cup (4.4 oz)	60
Sliced Yellow Cling Lite	½ cup (4.4 oz)	60
DRIED		
halves	10	311
Del Monte		
Sun Dried	⅓ cup (1.4 oz)	90

FOOD	PORTION	CALS.
Sonoma		
Pieces	3-5 pieces (1.4 oz)	120
FRESH		
peach	1	37
sliced	1 cup	73
Dole		
Peach	2	70
FROZEN		
Big Valley		
Freestone	⅔ cup (4.9 oz)	50

PEACH JUICE

Goya		
Nectar	6 oz	110
Kern's		
Nectar	6 fl oz	110
Libby		
Nectar	1 can (11.5 fl oz)	210
Mott's		
Fruit Basket Orchard Peach Juice Cocktail as prep	8 fl oz	130
Snapple		
Dixie Peach	10 fl oz	140

PEANUT BUTTER

chunky	2 tbsp	188
chunky	1 cup	1520
smooth	2 tbsp	188
smooth	1 cup	1517
Arrowhead		
Creamy	2 tbsp (1.1 oz)	200
Crunchy	2 tbsp (1.1 oz)	200
BAMA		
Creamy	2 tbsp	200
Crunchy	2 tbsp	200
Jelly & Peanut Butter	2 tbsp	150
Crazy Richard's		
Natural Creamy	2 tbsp (1.1 oz)	190
Estee		
Creamy Low Sodium	2 tbsp (1 oz)	190
Hollywood		
Creamy	1 tbsp	35
Crunchy	1 tbsp	35
Unsalted	1 tbsp	35

FOOD	PORTION	CALS.
Jif		
Creamy	2 tbsp (1.1 oz)	190
Extra Crunchy	2 tbsp (1.1 oz)	190
Reduced Fat	2 tbsp (1.3 oz)	190
Simply Creamy	2 tbsp (1.1 oz)	190
Simply Extra Crunchy	2 tbsp (1.1 oz)	190
Peter Pan		
Creamy	2 tbsp	190
Creamy Salt Free	2 tbsp	190
Crunchy	2 tbsp	190
Crunchy Salt Free	2 tbsp	190
Red Wing		
Creamy	2 tbsp (1.1 oz)	200
Crunchy	2 tbsp (1.1 oz)	200
Skippy		
Reduced Fat Creamy	2 tbsp	190
Tree Of Life		
Creamy	2 tbsp (1 oz)	190
Creamy No Salt	2 tbsp (1 oz)	190
Creamy Organic	2 tbsp (1 oz)	190
Creamy Organic No Salt	2 tbsp (1 oz)	190
Crunchy	2 tbsp (1 oz)	190
Crunchy No Salt	2 tbsp (1 oz)	190
Crunchy Organic	2 tbsp (1 oz)	190
Crunchy Organic No Salt	2 tbsp (1 oz)	190
Peanut Wonder 78% Less Fat	2 tbsp (1 oz)	100
PEANUTS		
chocolate coated	10 (1.4 oz)	208
chocolate coated	1 cup (5.2 oz)	773
Beer Nuts		
Peanuts	1 pkg (1 oz)	180
Estee		
Candy Coated	¼ cup	200
Fisher		
Salted-In-Shell shelled	1 oz	170
Spanish Roasted	1 oz	180
Frito Lay		
Honey Roasted	1 serv (1.5 oz)	270
Hot	1 serv (1.1 oz)	190
Salted	1 oz	200
Guy's		
Dry Roasted	1 oz	170
Spanish Salted	1 oz	170

FOOD	PORTION	CALS.
Little Debbie		
Salted	1 pkg (1.2 oz)	230
Pennant		
Oil Roasted	1 oz	170
Planters		
Cocktail Lightly Salted Oil Roasted	1 oz	170
Cocktail Oil Roasted	1 oz	170
Cocktail Unsalted Oil Roasted	1 oz	170
Dry Roasted	1 oz	160
Fun Size! Oil Roasted	2 pkg (1 oz)	170
Heat Hot Spicy Oil Roasted	1 pkg (1.7 oz)	290
Heat Hot Spicy Oil Roasted	1 oz	160
Heat Hot Spicy Oil Roasted	1 pkg (2 oz)	330
Heat Mild Spicy Oil Roasted	1 oz	160
Honey Roasted	1 oz	160
Honey Roasted Dry Roasted	1 pkg (1.7 oz)	260
Lightly Salted Dry Roasted	1 oz	160
Lightly Salted Dry Roasted	1 pkg (1.75 oz)	290
Lightly Salted Oil Roasted	1 pkg (1.8 oz)	300
Munch'N Go Singles Heat Hot Spicy Oil Roasted	1 pkg (2.5 oz)	410
Reduced Fat Honey Roasted	⅓ cup (1 oz)	130
Salted Oil Roasted	1 pkg (1 oz)	170
Spanish Oil Roasted	1 oz	170
Spanish Raw	1 oz	150
Sweet N Crunchy	1 oz	140
Unsalted Dry Roasted	1 oz	160
Weight Watchers		
Honey Roasted	1 pkg (0.7 oz)	100

PEAR
CANNED
Del Monte

Halves Fruit Naturals	½ cup (4.4 oz)	60
Halves In Heavy Syrup	½ cup (4.5 oz)	100
Halves Lite	½ cup (4.4 oz)	60
Sliced In Heavy Syrup	½ cup (4.5 oz)	100
Sliced Lite	½ cup (4.4 oz)	60
Snack Cups Diced In Heavy Syrup	1 serv (4.5 oz)	100
Snack Cups Diced In Heavy Syrup EZ-Open Lid	1 serv (4.2 oz)	90
Snack Cups Diced Lite	1 serv (4.5 oz)	60
Snack Cups Diced Lite EZ-Open Lid	1 serv (4.2 oz)	60
Libby		
Halves Lite	½ cup (4.3 oz)	60

FOOD	PORTION	CALS.
Libby (CONT.)		
Sliced Lite	½ cup (4.3 oz)	60
DRIED		
Sonoma		
Pieces	3-4 pieces (1.4 oz)	120
FRESH		
asian	1 (4.3 oz)	51
pear	1	98
sliced w/ skin	1 cup	97
Dole		
Pear	1	100

PEAR JUICE

Goya		
Nectar	6 oz	120
Kern's		
Nectar	6 fl oz	120
Libby		
Nectar	1 can (11.5 fl oz)	220

PEAS
CANNED

Allen		
Crowder	½ cup (4.5 oz)	110
Purple Hull	½ cup (4.4 oz)	120
Crest Top		
Early June	½ cup (4.5 oz)	100
Del Monte		
Sweet	½ cup (4.4 oz)	60
Sweet 50% Less Salt	½ cup (4.4 oz)	60
Sweet No Salt Added	½ cup (4.4 oz)	60
Sweet Very Young	½ cup (4.4 oz)	60
East Texas Fair		
Cream Peas	½ cup (4.4 oz)	120
Crowder	½ cup (4.5 oz)	110
Lady Peas With Snaps	½ cup (4.3 oz)	100
Peas 'n Pork	½ cup (4.5 oz)	110
Pepper Peas	½ cup (4.5 oz)	120
Purple Hull	½ cup (4.4 oz)	120
White Acre	½ cup (4.3 oz)	100
Green Giant		
Sweet	½ cup (4.3 oz)	60
Sweet 50% Less Sodium	½ cup (4.3 oz)	60
Homefolks		
Crowder	½ cup (4.5 oz)	110

FOOD	PORTION	CALS.
Homefolks (CONT.)		
Purple Hull	½ cup (4.4 oz)	120
LeSueur		
Early Peas	½ cup (4.2 oz)	60
Early Peas 50% Less Sodium	½ cup (4.2 oz)	60
Sweet	½ cup (4.2 oz)	60
Sweet 50% Less Sodium	½ cup (4.2 oz)	60
Seneca		
Natural Pack	½ cup	60
Peas	½ cup	50
Sunshine		
Field Peas	½ cup (4.4 oz)	120
Lady Peas	½ cup (4.3 oz)	100
Trappey		
Field Peas With Bacon	½ cup (4.5 oz)	90
Field Peas With Snaps And Bacon	½ cup (4.5 oz)	110
DRIED		
Bascom's		
Yellow Split as prep	½ cup	110
Hurst		
HamBeens Green Split Peas w/ Ham	1 serv	120
FRESH		
green cooked	½ cup	67
green raw	½ cup	58
snap peas cooked	½ cup	34
snap peas raw	½ cup	30
Dole		
Sugar Peas	½ cup	30
FROZEN		
snap peas cooked	½ cup	42
Birds Eye		
Baby Pea Blend	¾ cup (2.6 oz)	40
Baby Sweet	⅔ cup (3.1 oz)	70
Field Peas w/ Snaps	⅔ cup (3.4 oz)	130
Purple Hull Peas	½ cup (2.8 oz)	110
Chun King		
Snow Pea Pods	½ pkg (3 oz)	35
Fresh Like		
Green	3.5 oz	85
Tiny Green	3.5 oz	63
Green Giant		
Butter Sauce	¾ cup (4 oz)	100
Butter Sauce LeSueur Baby Peas	¾ cup (4 oz)	100
Harvest Fresh LeSueur Baby	⅔ cup (3.2 oz)	70

FOOD	PORTION	CALS.
Green Giant (CONT.)		
Harvest Fresh Sugar Snap	⅔ cup (3.2 oz)	50
Harvest Fresh Sweet	⅔ cup (3.3 oz)	60
LaSueur Baby Sweet	⅔ cup (2.8 oz)	60
LaSueur Early June	⅔ cup (2.8 oz)	80
LaSueur Early June w/ Mushrooms	¾ cup (3 oz)	60
Select Sugar Snap	¾ cup (2.8 oz)	35
Sweet	⅔ cup (3.1 oz)	70
Tree Of Life		
Peas	⅔ cup (3.1 oz)	70
SPROUTS		
raw	½ cup	77
PECANS		
dry roasted	1 oz	187
dry roasted salted	1 oz	187
oil roasted	1 oz	195
oil roasted salted	1 oz	195
Planters		
Chips	1 pkg (2 oz)	390
Gold Measure Halves	1 pkg (2 oz)	390
Halves	1 oz	190
Honey Roasted	1 oz	180
Pieces	1 oz	190
Pieces	1 pkg (2 oz)	390
PECTIN		
powder	1 pkg (1.75 oz)	163
powder	¼ pkg (0.4 oz)	39
Slim Set		
Packet	1 pkg	208
Powder	1 tbsp	3
Sure Jell		
For Lower Sugar Recipes	¼ tsp (0.7 g)	5
Pectin	¼ tsp (0.9 g)	5
PEPEAO		
pepeao dried	½ cup	36
PEPPER		
black	1 tsp	5
cayenne	1 tsp	6
red	1 tsp	6
white	1 tsp	7
Ac'cent		
Lemon	½ tsp	0

FOOD	PORTION	CALS.
Ac'cent (CONT.)		
Seasoned	½ tsp	0
Lawry's		
Lemon	1 tsp	6
Watkins		
Black	¼ tbsp (0.5 g)	0
Cajun	¼ tbsp (0.5 g)	0
Cracked Black	¼ tbsp (0.5 g)	0
Dijon	¼ tbsp (0.5 g)	0
Garlic Peppercorn Blend	¼ tbsp (1 g)	0
Herb	¼ tbsp (0.5 g)	0
Italian	¼ tbsp (0.5 g)	0
Lemon	¼ tbsp (1 g)	0
Mexican	¼ tbsp (0.5 g)	0
Red Pepper Flakes	¼ tsp (0.5 oz)	0
Royal Pepper Blend	¼ tbsp (0.5 g)	0

PEPPERS
CANNED

FOOD	PORTION	CALS.
chili green	1 cup (5.5 oz)	29
Chi-Chi's		
Chilies Diced Green	2 tbsp (1.2 oz)	10
Chilies Green Whole	¾ pepper (1 oz)	10
Del Monte		
Chipotle In Spice Sauce	2 tbsp (1.1 oz)	20
Hot Chili	4 (1 oz)	10
Jalapeno Nacho Pickled Sliced	2 tbsp (1 oz)	5
Jalapeno Pickled Sliced	2 tbsp (1.1 oz)	5
Jalapeno Pickled Whole	2 tbsp (1.1 oz)	5
Jalapeno Whole	1 (0.7 oz)	3
Hebrew National		
Filet	¼ pepper (1 oz)	9
Hot Cherry	⅓ pepper (1 oz)	11
Red Filet	¼ pepper (1 oz)	9
McIlhenny		
Jalapeno Nacho Slices	12 slices (1.1 oz)	7
Old El Paso		
Green Chilies Chopped	2 tbsp (1 oz)	5
Green Chilies Whole	1 (1.2 oz)	10
Jalapenos Peeled	3 (1 oz)	10
Jalapenos Pickled	2 (0.9 oz)	5
Jalapenos Slices	2 tbsp (1.1 oz)	15
Progresso		
Cherry (drained)	2 tbsp (0.9 oz)	30

FOOD	PORTION	CALS.
Progresso (CONT.)		
Fried (drained)	2 tbsp (0.9 oz)	60
Hot Cherry	1 (1 oz)	15
Pepper Salad (drained)	2 tbsp (0.9 oz)	25
Roasted	½ piece (1 oz)	10
Tuscan (drained)	3 (1 oz)	10
Rosoff's		
Sweet	¼ pepper (1 oz)	9
Schorr's		
Filet Peppers	1 oz	9
Trappey		
Banana Mild	3 peppers (1 oz)	6
Banana Sliced Rings	21 slices (1 oz)	6
Cherry Hot	2 peppers (1 oz)	7
Cherry Mild	2 peppers (1 oz)	10
Dulcito Italian Pepperoncini	4 peppers (1 oz)	8
In Vinegar Hot	15 peppers (1 oz)	9
Jalapeno Hot Sliced	21 slices (1 oz)	4
Jalapeno Whole	2 peppers (1 oz)	11
Serano	7 peppers (1 oz)	7
Tempero Golden Greek Pepperoncini	4 peppers (1 oz)	7
Torrido Santa Fe Grande	3 peppers (1 oz)	10
Vlasic		
Hot Banana Pepper Rings	1 oz	4
Hot Cherry	1 oz	10
Jalapeno Mexican Hot	1 oz	8
Mexican Tiny Hot	1 oz	6
Mild Cherry	1 oz	8
Mild Greek Pepperoncini Salad Peppers	1 oz	4
DRIED		
ancho	1 (0.6 oz)	48
pasilla	1 (7 g)	24
FRESH		
banana raw	1 cup (4.4 oz)	33
banana raw	1 (4 in) (1.2 oz)	9
green chopped cooked	½ cup	19
green cooked	1 (2.6 oz)	20
green raw	1 (2.6 oz)	20
green raw chopped	½ cup	13
hungarian raw	1 (0.9 oz)	8
jalapeno raw	1 (0.5 oz)	4
jalapeno raw sliced	1 cup (3.2 oz)	27
red chopped cooked	½ cup	19
red cooked	1 (2.6 oz)	20

FOOD	PORTION	CALS.
red raw	1 (2.6 oz)	20
red raw chopped	½ cup	13
serrano raw	1 (6 g)	2
serrano raw chopped	1 cup (3.7 oz)	34
yellow raw	1 (6.5 oz)	50
yellow raw	10 strips	14
Dole		
Medium	1	25
FROZEN		
Birds Eye		
Diced Green	¾ cup (2.9 oz)	20

PERCH
FRESH

cooked	3 oz	99
ocean perch atlantic cooked	3 oz	103
FROZEN		
Gorton's		
Fishmarket Fresh Ocean Perch	5 oz	140
Van De Kamp's		
Battered Fillets	2 (4 oz)	300

PERSIMMONS

dried japanese	1	93
fresh	1	32
Sonoma		
Dried	6-8 pieces (1.4 oz)	140

PHEASANT

roasted	3.5 oz	215

PHYLLO DOUGH

phyllo dough	1 oz	85
sheet	1	57
Ekizian		
Sheets	½ lb	865

PICANTE
(*see* SALSA)

PICKLES
Del Monte

Dill Halves	¼ pickle (1 oz)	5
Dill Hamburger Chips	5 pieces (1 oz)	5
Dill Sweet Chips	5 pieces (1 oz)	40
Dill Sweet Gherkin	2 pickles (1 oz)	40
Dill Sweet Midgets	3 pickles (1 oz)	40

FOOD	PORTION	CALS.
Del Monte (CONT.)		
Dill Sweet Whole	2 pickles (1 oz)	40
Dill Tiny Kosher	1½ pickle (1 oz)	5
Dill Whole Pickles	1½ pickle (1 oz)	5
Hebrew National		
Half Sour	½ pickle (1 oz)	4
Kosher	⅓ pickle (1 oz)	4
Kosher Barrel Cured Dill	1 pkg	23
Kosher Barrel Cured Hot Dill	1 pkg	23
Kosher Chips	3 slices (1 oz)	4
Kosher Halves	⅓ pickle (1 oz)	4
Kosher Large	⅕ pickle (1 oz)	4
Kosher Spears	½ spear (1 oz)	4
Sour Garlic	⅓ pickle (1 oz)	3
McIlhenny		
Hot N' Sweet	4 (1 oz)	42
Rosoff's		
Half Sour	⅓ pickle (1 oz)	4
Half Sour Spears	½ spear (1 oz)	4
Kosher	⅓ pickle (1 oz)	4
Kosher Halves	⅓ pickle (1 oz)	4
Schorr's		
Garlic	⅓ pickle (1 oz)	3
Half Sour	½ spear (1 oz)	4
Half Sour	⅓ pickle (1 oz)	4
Kosher Deli	½ pickle (1 oz)	4
Kosher Halves	⅓ pickle (1 oz)	4
Kosher Spears	½ spear (1 oz)	4
Kosher Whole	⅓ pickle (1 oz)	4
Vlasic		
Bread & Butter Chips	1 oz	30
Bread & Butter Chunks	1 oz	25
Bread & Butter Stixs	1 oz	18
Deli Bread & Butter	1 oz	25
Deli Dill Halves	1 oz	4
Half-The-Salt Hamburger Dill Chips	1 oz	2
Half-The-Salt Kosher Crunchy Dills	1 oz	4
Half-The-Salt Kosher Dill Spears	1 oz	4
Half-The-Salt Sweet Butter Chips	1 oz	30
Hot & Spicy Garden Mix	1 oz	4
Kosher Baby Dills	1 oz	4
Kosher Crunchy Dills	1 oz	4
Kosher Dill Gherkins	1 oz	4
Kosher Dill Spears	1 oz	4

FOOD	PORTION	CALS.
Vlasic (CONT.)		
Kosher Snack Chunks	1 oz	4
No Garlic Dill Spears	1 oz	4
Original Dills	1 oz	2
Polish Snack Chunk Dills	1 oz	4
Zesty Crunchy Dills	1 oz	4
Zesty Dill Snack Chunks	1 oz	4
Zesty Dill Spears	1 oz	4

PIE
(*see also* PIE CRUST)

FILLING

apple	⅛ can (2.6 oz)	74
apple	1 can (21 oz)	599
cherry	⅛ can (2.6 oz)	85
cherry	1 can (21 oz)	683
pumpkin pie mix	1 cup	282
Comstock		
MoreFruit Light Cherry	⅓ cup (2.9 oz)	60
Libby		
Pumpkin Pie Mix	½ cup	100
None Such		
Mincemeat Condensed	¼ pkg	220
Mincemeat Ready-to-Use	⅓ cup	200
Mincemeat Ready-to-Use With Brandy & Rum	⅓ cup	220

FROZEN

apple	⅛ of 9 in pie (4.4 oz)	297
blueberry	⅛ of 9 in pie (4.4 oz)	289
cherry	⅛ of 9 in pie (4.4 oz)	325
chocolate creme	⅙ of 8 in pie (4 oz)	344
coconut creme	⅙ of 7 in pie (2.2 oz)	191
lemon meringue	⅙ of 8 in pie (4.5 oz)	303
peach	⅙ of 8 in pie (4.1 oz)	261
Amy's Organic		
Apple	1 serv (8 oz)	280
Banquet		
Apple	⅕ pie (4 oz)	300
Banana Cream	⅓ pie (4.7 oz)	350
Cherry	⅕ pie (4 oz)	290
Chocolate Cream	⅓ pie (4.7 oz)	360
Coconut Cream	⅓ pie (4.7 oz)	350
Lemon Cream	⅓ pie (4.7 oz)	360
Mincemeat	⅕ pie (4 oz)	310

FOOD	PORTION	CALS.
Banquet (CONT.)		
Peach	⅕ pie (4 oz)	260
Pumpkin	⅙ pie (4 oz)	250
Kineret		
Apple Homestyle	⅙ pie (4 oz)	313
McMillin's		
Apple	4 oz	430
Berry	4 oz	430
Cherry	4 oz	430
Chocolate Pudding	4 oz	420
Coconut Pudding	4 oz	450
Lemon	4 oz	450
Peach	4 oz	430
Strawberry	4 oz	400
Mrs. Smith's		
Apple	⅙ of 8 in pie (4.3 oz)	270
Apple	⅛ of 9 in pie (4.6 oz)	370
Apple	⅒ of 10 in pie (4.6 oz)	280
Apple Cranberry	⅙ of 8 in pie (4.3 oz)	280
Apple Lattice Ready To Serve	⅕ of 8 in pie (4.6 oz)	310
Banana Cream	¼ of 8 in pie (3.4 oz)	250
Berry	⅙ of 8 in pie (4.3 oz)	280
Blackberry	⅙ of 8 in pie (4.3 oz)	280
Blueberry	⅙ of 8 in pie	260
Boston Cream	⅛ of 8 in pie (2.4 oz)	170
Cherry	⅙ of 8 in pie	270
Cherry	⅛ of 9 in pie (4.6 oz)	320
Cherry Lattice Ready To Serve	⅕ of 8 in pie (4.6 oz)	320
Chocolate Cream	¼ of 8 in pie (3.4 oz)	290
Coconut Cream	¼ of 8 in pie (3.4 oz)	280
Coconut Custard	⅕ of 8 in pie (5 oz)	280
Dutch Apple	⅒ of 10 in pie (4.6 oz)	320
Dutch Apple	⅙ of 8 in pie	310
Dutch Apple	⅑ of 9 in pie (4.5 oz)	300
French Silk Cream	⅕ of 8 in pie (4.8 oz)	410
Hearty Pumpkin	⅕ of 8 in pie (5.2 oz)	280
Lemon Cream	¼ of 8 in pie (3.4 oz)	270
Lemon Meringue	⅕ of 8 in pie (4.8 oz)	300
Mince	⅙ of 8 in pie (4.3 oz)	300
Peach	⅙ of 8 in pie	260
Peach	⅛ of 9 in pie (4.6 oz)	310
Pecan	⅛ of 10 in pie (4.5 oz)	500
Pumpkin	⅑ of 10 in pie (5.1 oz)	250
Pumpkin	⅕ of 8 in pie (5.2 oz)	270

FOOD	PORTION	CALS.
Mrs. Smith's (CONT.)		
Red Raspberry	1/6 of 8 in pie (4.3 oz)	280
Strawberry Rhubarb	1/5 of 8 in pie (4.8 oz)	520
Strawberry Rhubarb	1/6 of 8 in pie (4.3 oz)	280
Pet-Ritz		
Apple	1/6 pie (4.33 oz)	330
Banana Cream	1/6 pie (2.33 oz)	170
Blueberry	1/6 pie (4.33 oz)	370
Cherry	1/6 pie (4.33 oz)	300
Chocolate Cream	1/6 pie (2.33 oz)	190
Coconut Cream	1/6 pie (2.33 oz)	190
Egg Custard	1/6 pie (4.0 oz)	200
Lemon Cream	1/6 pie (2.33 oz)	190
Mince	1/6 pie (4.33 oz)	280
Neapolitan Cream	1/6 pie (2.33 oz)	180
Peach	1/6 pie (4.33 oz)	320
Pumpkin Custard	1/6 pie (4.33 oz)	250
Strawberry Cream	1/6 pie (2.33 oz)	170
Sweet Potato	1/6 pie (3.33 oz)	150
Sara Lee		
Chocolate Silk	1/5 pie (4.8 oz)	500
Coconut Cream	1/5 pie (4.8 oz)	480
Fruit's Of The Forest	1/8 pie (4.6 oz)	340
Homestyle Apple	1/8 pie (4.6 oz)	340
Homestyle Blueberry	1/8 pie (4.6 oz)	360
Homestyle Cherry	1/8 pie (4.6 oz)	330
Homestyle Dutch Apple	1/8 pie (4.6 oz)	350
Homestyle Mince	1/8 pie (4.6 oz)	390
Homestyle Peach	1/8 pie (4.6 oz)	330
Homestyle Pecan	1/8 pie (4.2 oz)	520
Homestyle Pumpkin	1/8 pie (4.6 oz)	260
Homestyle Raspberry	1/8 pie (4.6 oz)	380
Lemon Meringue	1/6 pie (5 oz)	350
Slice Lemon Icebox	1 (3.5 oz)	260
Slice Southern Pecan	1 (4 oz)	470
Weight Watchers		
Mississippi Mud	1 piece (2.45 oz)	160
HOME RECIPE		
pecan	1/8 of 9 in pie (4.3 oz)	502
pumpkin	1/8 of 9 in pie (5.4 oz)	316
MIX		
banana cream no-bake	1/8 of 9 in pie (3.2 oz)	231
chocolate mousse no-bake	1/8 of 9 in pie (3.3 oz)	247
coconut creme no-bake	1/8 of 9 in pie (3.3 oz)	259

FOOD	PORTION	CALS.
Jell-O		
No Bake Chocolate Silk as prep	⅙ pie (4.4 oz)	320
Royal		
Key Lime Pie Filling	mix for 1 serv	50
Lemon Pie Filling	mix for 1 serv	50
Lemon Meringue No-Bake	⅛ pie	210
READY-TO-EAT		
Entenmann's		
Apple Homestyle	1 serv (2.1 oz)	140
Coconut Custard	1 serv (1.8 oz)	140
SNACK		
apple fried	1 (6.4 oz)	404
blueberry fried	1 (6.4 oz)	404
cherry fried	1 (6.4 oz)	404
lemon fried	1 (6.4 oz)	404
peach fried	1 (6.4 oz)	404
strawberry fried	1 (6.4 oz)	404
Dolly Madison		
Apple	1 (4.5 oz)	480
Blueberry	1 (4.5 oz)	480
Cherry	1 (4.5 oz)	470
Chocolate Pudding	1 (4.5 oz)	530
Peach	1 (4.5 oz)	480
Pecan	1 (3 oz)	360
Pecan Fried	1 (4.5 oz)	530
Pineapple	1 (4.5 oz)	460
Hostess		
Apple	1 (4.5 oz)	480
Blackberry	1 (4.5 oz)	520
Blueberry	1 (4.5 oz)	480
Cherry	1 (4.5 oz)	470
French Apple	1 (4.5 oz)	480
Lemon	1 (4.5 oz)	500
Peach	1 (4.5 oz)	480
Pineapple	1 (4.5 oz)	460
Strawberry	1 (4.5 oz)	510
Little Debbie		
Marshmallow Banana	1 pkg (1.4 oz)	160
Marshmallow Banana	1 pkg (2.7 oz)	320
Marshmallow Banana	1 pkg (2 oz)	240
Marshmallow Chocolate	1 pkg (1.4 oz)	160
Marshmallow Chocolate	1 pkg (2 oz)	240
Marshmallow Chocolate	1 pkg (2.7 oz)	320
Oatmeal Creme	1 pkg (1.3 oz)	170

FOOD	PORTION	CALS.
Little Debbie (CONT.)		
Oatmeal Creme	1 pkg (3 oz)	360
Oatmeal Creme	1 pkg (2.5 oz)	300
Raisin Creme	1 pkg (1.2 oz)	140
Raisin Creme	1 pkg (2.5 oz)	290
Pepperidge Farm		
Lemon	1 (4.5 oz)	500
Tastykake		
Apple	1 (4 oz)	270
Blueberry	1 (4 oz)	300
Cherry	1 (4 oz)	290
Coconut Creme	1 (4 oz)	370
French Apple	1 (4.2 oz)	310
Lemon	1 (4 oz)	300
Peach	1 (4 oz)	280
Pineapple	1 (4 oz)	290
Pineapple Cheese	1 (4 oz)	320
Pumpkin	1 (4 oz)	340
Strawberry	1 (3.5 oz)	320
Tastyklair	1 (4 oz)	400
TAKE-OUT		
apple	1/8 of 9 in pie (5.4 oz)	411
banana cream	1/8 of 9 in pie (5.2 oz)	398
blueberry	1/8 of 9 in pie (5.2 oz)	360
butterscotch	1/8 of 9 in pie (4.5 oz)	355
cherry	1/8 of 9 in pie (6.3 oz)	486
coconut creme	1/8 of 9 in pie (4.7 oz)	396
coconut custard	1/6 of 8 in pie (3.6 oz)	271
custard	1/8 of 9 in pie (4.5 oz)	262
lemon meringue	1/8 of 9 in pie (4.5 oz)	362
mince	1/8 of 9 in pie (5.8 oz)	477
pecan	1/6 of 8 in pie (4 oz)	452
pumpkin	1/6 of 8 in pie (3.8 oz)	229
vanilla cream	1/8 of 9 in pie (4.4 oz)	350

PIE CRUST
(*see also* PIE)

FROZEN

baked	1/8 of 9 in pie (0.6 oz)	82
baked	9 in shell (4.4 oz)	647
puff pastry baked	1 shell (1.4 oz)	223
Oronoque		
Deep Dish	1/6 pie (1.41 oz)	200
Pie Crust	1/6 pie (1.23 oz)	170

FOOD	PORTION	CALS.
Pepperidge Farm		
Puff Pastry Sheets	⅛ sheet (1.4 oz)	170
Puff Pastry Shell	1 (1.6 oz)	190
Puff Pastry Squares	1 sq (2 oz)	240
Pet-Ritz		
Deep Dish	⅛ pie (0.7 oz)	90
Regular	⅛ pie (0.6 oz)	80
Tart Shells	1 (1 oz)	130
HOME RECIPE		
baked	9 in shell (6.3 oz)	949
baked	⅛ of 9 in crust (0.8 oz)	119
MIX		
as prep	9 in crust (5.6 oz)	801
as prep	⅛ of 9 in pie (0.7 oz)	100
Flako		
Mix	¼ cup (0.9 oz)	130
Jiffy		
As prep	⅐ crust	180
READY-TO-EAT		
chocolate cookie crumb baked	⅛ of 9 in pie (1 oz)	139
chocolate cookie crumb baked	9 in crust (7.7 oz)	1130
chocolate cookie crumb chilled	9 in crust (7.8 oz)	1127
chocolate cookie crumb chilled	⅛ of 9 in pie (1 oz)	142
graham cracker baked	⅛ of 9 in pie (1 oz)	148
graham cracker baked	9 in crust (8.4 oz)	1181
graham cracker chilled	⅛ of 9 in pie (1 oz)	150
graham cracker chilled	9 in crust (8.6 oz)	1182
vanilla wafer cracker crumbs baked	9 in crust (6.1 oz)	937
vanilla wafer cracker crumbs baked	⅛ of 9 in pie (0.8 oz)	119
vanilla wafer cracker crumbs chilled	⅛ of 9 in pie (0.8 oz)	117
vanilla wafer cracker crumbs chilled	9 in crust (6.2 oz)	934
Generic Label		
Graham	⅛ pie (0.7 oz)	110
Honey Maid		
Graham	⅙ crust (1 oz)	140
Nabisco		
Nilla	⅙ crust (1 oz)	140
Oreo		
Crumb Crust	⅙ crust (1 oz)	140
REFRIGERATED		
All Ready		
Crust	⅛ pie (0.9 oz)	120
PIEROGI		
Empire		
Potato Cheese	3 (4.6 oz)	260

FOOD	PORTION	CALS.
Empire (CONT.)		
Potato Onion	3 (4.6 oz)	250
Golden		
Potato Cheese	3 (4 oz)	250
Potato Onion	3 (4 oz)	210
Mrs. T's		
Potato And Cheddar Cheese	1 (1.3 oz)	60
Potato And Onion	1 (1.3 oz)	50
PIG'S EARS AND FEET		
ear simmered	1	184
feet pickled	1 oz	58
feet pickled	1 lb	921
feet simmered	3 oz	165
Hormel		
Pickled Feet	2 oz	80
Pickled Hocks	2 oz	110
PIGEON		
w/ skin & bone	3.5 oz	169
PIGEON PEAS		
dried cooked	½ cup	102
PIGNOLIA		
(*see* PINE NUTS)		
PIKE		
northern cooked	3 oz	96
roe raw	3½ oz	130
walleye baked	3 oz	101
PIMIENTOS		
canned	1 tbsp	3
PINE NUTS		
Progresso		
Pignoli	1 jar (1 oz)	170
PINEAPPLE		
CANNED		
Del Monte		
Chunks In Heavy Syrup	½ cup (4.3 oz)	90
Chunks In Its Own Juice	½ cup (4.4 oz)	70
Crushed In Heavy Syrup	½ cup (4.4 oz)	90
Crushed In Its Own Juice	½ cup (4.3 oz)	70
Sliced In Heavy Syrup	½ cup (4.1 oz)	90
Sliced In Its Own Juice	½ cup (4 oz)	60

FOOD	PORTION	CALS.
Del Monte (CONT.)		
Snack Cups Tidbits In Juice	1 serv (4.5 oz)	70
Snack Cups Tidbits In Juice EZ-Open Lid	1 serv (4.2 oz)	60
Spears In Its Own Juice	½ cup (4.3 oz)	70
Tidbits In Its Own Juice	½ cup (4.3 oz)	70
Wedges In Its Own Juice	½ cup (4.3 oz)	70
Dole		
All Cuts Juice Pack	½ cup	70
All Cuts Syrup Pack	½ cup	90
Libby		
Crushed	1 cup with juice	140
Sliced In Unsweetened Juice	1 cup with juice	140
DRIED		
Sonoma		
Pieces	2 pieces (1.4 oz)	140
FRESH		
diced	1 cup	77
slice	1 slice	42
Dole		
Pineapple	2 slices	90

PINEAPPLE JUICE
After The Fall		
Mandarin Pineapple	1 can (12 oz)	150
Bright & Early		
Frozen	8 fl oz	120
Del Monte		
Juice	1 serv (11.5 oz)	190
Juice	6 fl oz	80
Juice	8 fl oz	110
Dole		
Chilled	8 oz	130
Minute Maid		
Box	8.45 fl oz	130
Frozen	8 fl oz	110

PINK BEANS
CANNED
Goya		
Spanish Style	7.5 oz	140

PINTO BEANS
CANNED
Allen		
Pinto Beans	½ cup (4.5 oz)	110

FOOD	PORTION	CALS.
Brown Beauty		
Pinto Beans	½ cup (4.5 oz)	110
Chi-Chi's		
Pinto Beans	½ cup (4.3 oz)	100
East Texas Fair		
Pinto Beans	½ cup (4.5 oz)	110
Eden		
Organic	½ cup (4.6 oz)	100
Organic Spicy w/ Jalapeno & Red Peppers	½ cup (4.6 oz)	125
Goya		
Spanish Style	7.5 oz	140
Green Giant		
Pinto Beans	½ cup (4.4 oz)	110
Old El Paso		
Pinto Beans	½ cup (4.6 oz)	110
Progresso		
Pinto Beans	½ cup (4.6 oz)	110
Trappey		
Jalapinto With Bacon	½ cup (4.5 oz)	120
With Bacon	½ cup (4.5 oz)	120
DRIED		
Arrowhead		
Dried	¼ cup (1.5 oz)	150
Bean Cuisine		
Dried	½ cup	115
Hurst		
HamBeens w/ Ham	3 tbsp (1.2 oz)	120
SPROUTS		
cooked	3½ oz	22
raw	3½ oz	62

PINYON
(*see* PINE NUTS)

PISTACHIOS

FOOD	PORTION	CALS.
Dole		
Shelled	1 oz	163
Shells On	1 oz	90
Fisher		
Red Tint	1 oz	170
Planters		
Munch'N Go Singles Shelled Dry Roasted	1 pkg (2 oz)	330
Red Salted Dry Roasted	1 pkg	160
Uncolored Dry Roasted	½ cup	160

FOOD	PORTION	CALS.

Sonoma
| Salted Shelled | ¼ cup (1 oz) | 190 |

PITANGA
| fresh | 1 cup | 57 |
| fresh | 1 | 2 |

PIZZA
DOUGH
Boboli
| Shell + Sauce | ⅛ lg shell (2.6 oz) | 170 |
| Shell + Sauce | ⅙ sm shell (2.6 oz) | 170 |

House of Pasta
| Frozen | ⅛ of 14 in pie (1.9 oz) | 140 |

Jiffy
| As prep | ¼ crust | 180 |

Pillsbury
| Crust | ⅕ crust (2 oz) | 150 |

Robin Hood
| Crust | ¼ crust | 160 |

Sassafras
| Cornmeal Pizza Crust | 1 slice (1.4 oz) | 140 |
| Italian Pizza Crust Mix | 1 slice (1.4 oz) | 140 |

Wanda's
| Crust Mix Oregano & Basil | ⅒ pie (1.4 oz) | 149 |
| Crust Mix Oregano & Basil Whole Wheat | ⅒ pie (1.4 oz) | 141 |

Watkins
| Crust Mix | ⅛ pkg (1.8 oz) | 180 |

FROZEN
Amy's Organic
Cheese	1 (13 oz)	310
Pocket Sandwich Cheese Pizza	1 (4.5 oz)	290
Pocket Sandwich Veggie Pepperoni Pizza	1 (4.5 oz)	220
Roasted Vegetable	1 (12 oz)	270
Spinach	1 (14 oz)	320

Celeste
Italian Bread Deluxe	1 (5.1 oz)	290
Italian Bread Garlic & Herb Zesty Chicken	1 (5 oz)	260
Italian Bread Pepperoni	1 (5 oz)	320
Italian Bread Zesty Four Cheese	1 (4.6 oz)	300
Large Cheese	¼ pie (4.4 oz)	320
Large Deluxe	¼ pie (5.5 oz)	350
Large Pepperoni	¼ pie (4.7 oz)	350
Large Suprema With Meat	⅕ pie (4.6 oz)	290
Large Zesty Four Cheese	¼ pie (4.4 oz)	330

FOOD	PORTION	CALS.
Celeste (CONT.)		
Small Cheese	1 (7.5 oz)	540
Small Deluxe	1 (8.2 oz)	540
Small Hot & Zesty Four Cheese	1 (7 oz)	530
Small Original Four Cheese	1 (7 oz)	540
Small Pepperoni	1 (6.7 oz)	520
Small Sausage	1 (7.5 oz)	530
Small Suprema Vegetable	1 (7.5 oz)	480
Small Suprema With Meat	1 (9 oz)	580
Small Zesty Four Cheese	1 (7 oz)	530
Croissant Pocket		
Stuffed Sandwich Pepperoni Pizza	1 piece (4.5 oz)	350
Di Giorno		
Rising Crust 12 inch Four Cheese	⅙ pie (4.9 oz)	320
Rising Crust 12 inch Italian Sausage	⅙ pie (5.3 oz)	360
Rising Crust 12 inch Pepperoni	⅙ pie (5.2 oz)	370
Rising Crust 12 inch Supreme	⅙ pie (5.8 oz)	380
Rising Crust 12 inch Three Meat	⅙ pie (5.4 oz)	380
Rising Crust 12 inch Vegetable	⅙ pie (5.6 oz)	310
Rising Crust 8 inch Chicken Supreme	⅓ pie (4.8 oz)	270
Rising Crust 8 inch Four Cheese	⅓ pie (4 oz)	260
Rising Crust 8 inch Italian Sausage	⅓ pie (4.4 oz)	300
Rising Crust 8 inch Pepperoni	⅓ pie (4.2 oz)	300
Rising Crust 8 inch Spinach	⅓ pie (4.3 oz)	250
Rising Crust 8 inch Supreme	⅓ pie (4.7 oz)	310
Rising Crust 8 inch Three Meat	⅓ pie (4.4 oz)	310
Rising Crust 8 inch Vegetable	⅓ pie (4.6 oz)	250
Empire		
3 Pack	1 (3 oz)	210
Bagel	1 (2 oz)	150
English Muffin	1 (2 oz)	130
Pizza	½ pie (5 oz)	340
Healthy Choice		
French Bread Cheese	1 (5.6 oz)	310
French Bread Pepperoni	1 (6 oz)	360
French Bread Sausage	1 (6 oz)	330
French Bread Supreme	1 (6.35 oz)	340
Hot Pocket		
Stuffed Sandwich Pepperoni & Sausage Pizza	1 (4.5 oz)	340
Stuffed Sandwich Pepperoni Pizza	1 (4.5 oz)	350
Jack's		
Great Combinations 12 inch Bacon Cheeseburger	¼ pie (4.7 oz)	360

FOOD	PORTION	CALS.
Jack's (CONT.)		
Great Combinations 12 inch Double Cheese	¼ pie (4.9 oz)	380
Great Combinations 12 inch Pepperoni	¼ pie (5.2 oz)	410
Great Combinations 12 inch Pepperoni & Mushrooms	¼ pie (4.8 oz)	340
Great Combinations 12 inch Sausage	¼ pie (5.4 oz)	390
Great Combinations 12 inch Sausage & Mushroom	¼ pie (4.9 oz)	310
Great Combinations 12 inch Sausage & Pepperoni	¼ pie (4.8 oz)	350
Great Combinations 12 inch Supreme	¼ pie (5.2 oz)	350
Great Combinations 9 inch Double Cheese	½ pie (5.5 oz)	430
Great Combinations 9 inch Pepperoni & Sausage	½ pie (5.1 oz)	380
Naturally Rising 12 inch Bacon Cheeseburger	⅙ pie (5 oz)	350
Naturally Rising 12 inch Canadian Bacon	⅙ pie (4.9 oz)	280
Naturally Rising 12 inch Cheese	⅙ pie (4.5 oz)	290
Naturally Rising 12 inch Combination w/ Sausage & Pepperoni	⅙ pie (5.2 oz)	360
Naturally Rising 12 inch Pepperoni	⅙ pie (4.9 oz)	350
Naturally Rising 12 inch Pepperoni Supreme	⅙ pie (5.1 oz)	340
Naturally Rising 12 inch Sausage	⅙ pie (5.1 oz)	340
Naturally Rising 12 inch Spicy Italian Sausage	⅙ pie (5.1 oz)	330
Naturally Rising 12 inch The Works	⅙ pie (5.3 oz)	330
Naturally Rising 9 inch Cheese	⅓ pie (4.7 oz)	300
Naturally Rising 9 inch Combination w/ Sausage & Pepperoni	¼ pie (4.2 oz)	300
Naturally Rising 9 inch Pepperoni	⅓ pie (5.2 oz)	360
Naturally Rising 9 inch Sausage	⅓ pie (5.4 oz)	360
Naturally Rising 9 inch The Works	¼ pie (4.5 oz)	280
Original 12 inch Canadian Bacon	¼ pie (4.4 oz)	280
Original 12 inch Cheese	⅓ pie (5 oz)	360
Original 12 inch Hamburger	¼ pie (4.4 oz)	300
Original 12 inch Pepperoni	¼ pie (4.3 oz)	330
Original 12 inch Sausage	¼ pie (4.3 oz)	300
Original 12 inch Spicy Italian Sausage	¼ pie (4.3 oz)	290
Original 9 inch Pepperoni	½ pie (5 oz)	380
Original 9 inch Sausage	½ pie (5.1 oz)	360
Pizza Bursts Combination Sausage & Pepperoni	6 pieces (3 oz)	250

FOOD	PORTION	CALS.
Jack's (CONT.)		
Pizza Bursts Pepperoni	6 pieces (3 oz)	260
Pizza Bursts Sausage	6 pieces (3 oz)	250
Pizza Bursts Supercheese	6 pieces (3 oz)	250
Pizza Bursts Supreme	6 pieces (3 oz)	250
Kid Cuisine		
Cheese	1 (8 oz)	430
Hamburger	1 (8.30 oz)	400
Kineret		
Bagel Pizza	2 (4 oz)	300
Slice	1 (4.9 oz)	490
Lean Cuisine		
French Bread Cheese	1 pkg (6 oz)	300
French Bread Deluxe	1 pkg (6.1 oz)	300
French Bread Pepperoni	1 pkg (5.25 oz)	310
Lean Pockets		
Stuffed Sandwich Pizza Deluxe	1 (4.5 oz)	270
Old El Paso		
Pizza Burrito Cheese	1 (3.5 oz)	320
Pizza Burrito Pepperoni	1 (3.5 oz)	260
Pizza Burrito Sausage	1 (3.5 oz)	260
Pepperidge Farm		
Gourmet Crust Cheese	1 (4.4 oz)	390
Gourmet Crust Pepperoni	1 (4.5 oz)	420
Small World		
Four Cheese	1 (4 oz)	240
Special Delivery		
Organic	⅓ pizza (5.3 oz)	320
Organic Soy Kaas	⅓ pizza (5.3 oz)	320
Stouffer's		
French Bread Bacon Cheddar	1 piece (5.7 oz)	430
French Bread Cheese	1 piece (5.2 oz)	370
French Bread Cheeseburger	1 piece (6 oz)	420
French Bread Deluxe	1 piece (6.2 oz)	430
French Bread Double Cheese	1 piece (5.9 oz)	400
French Bread Pepperoni	1 piece (5.6 oz)	430
French Bread Pepperoni & Mushroom	1 piece (6.1 oz)	440
French Bread Sausage	1 piece (6 oz)	420
French Bread Sausage & Pepperoni	1 piece (6.25 oz)	470
French Bread Three Meat	1 piece (6.25 oz)	460
French Bread Vegetable Deluxe	1 piece (6.4 oz)	380
French Bread White Pizza	1 piece (5.1 oz)	460
Tombstone		
Double Top Pepperoni	⅙ pie (4.5 oz)	340

FOOD	PORTION	CALS.
Tombstone (CONT.)		
Double Top Sausage	⅙ pie (4.6 oz)	320
Double Top Sausage & Pepperoni	⅙ pie (4.6 oz)	340
Double Top Supreme	⅙ pie (4.7 oz)	330
Double Top Two Cheese	⅙ pie (5.2 oz)	380
For One ½ Less Fat Cheese	1 pie (6.5 oz)	460
For One ½ Less Fat Vegetable	1 pie (7.2 oz)	360
For One Extra Cheese	1 pie (6.9 oz)	520
For One Pepperoni	1 pie (6.9 oz)	550
For One Supreme	1 pie (7.5 oz)	550
Light Supreme	⅕ pie (4.8 oz)	270
Light Vegetable	⅕ pie (4.6 oz)	240
Original 12 inch Canadian Bacon	¼ pie (5.5 oz)	350
Original 12 inch Deluxe	⅕ pie (4.8 oz)	310
Original 12 inch Extra Cheese	¼ pie (5.1 oz)	350
Original 12 inch Hamburger	⅕ pie (4.4 oz)	310
Original 12 inch Pepperoni	¼ pie (5.3 oz)	400
Original 12 inch Sausage	⅕ pie (4.4 oz)	300
Original 12 inch Sausage & Mushroom	⅕ pie (4.6 oz)	300
Original 12 inch Sausage & Pepperoni	⅕ pie (4.4 oz)	320
Original 12 inch Supreme	⅕ pie (5.1 oz)	320
Original 9 inch Deluxe	⅓ pie (4.4 oz)	280
Original 9 inch Extra Cheese	½ pie (5.6 oz)	380
Original 9 inch Hamburger	⅓ pie (4 oz)	280
Original 9 inch Pepperoni	⅓ pie (4 oz)	300
Original 9 inch Pepperoni & Sausage	⅓ pie (4.1 oz)	300
Original 9 inch Sausage	⅓ pie (4 oz)	280
Original 9 inch Supreme	⅓ pie (4.4 oz)	310
Oven Rising Italian Sausage	⅙ pie (5.1 oz)	320
Oven Rising Pepperoni	⅙ pie (4.9 oz)	340
Oven Rising Supreme	⅙ pie (5.1 oz)	320
Oven Rising Three Cheese	⅙ pie (4.8 oz)	320
Oven Rising Three Meat	⅙ pie (5.1 oz)	340
Thin Crust Four Meat Combo	¼ pie (5 oz)	380
Thin Crust Italian Sausage	¼ pie (5 oz)	370
Thin Crust Pepperoni	¼ pie (4.8 oz)	400
Thin Crust Supreme	¼ pie (5 oz)	380
Thin Crust Supreme Taco	¼ pie (5.1 oz)	370
Thin Crust Three Cheese	¼ pie (4.7 oz)	360
Weight Watchers		
Smart Ones Deluxe Combo	1 (6.57 oz)	380
Smart Ones Pepperoni	1 (5.56 oz)	390
SAUCE		
Boboli		
Sauce	¼ cup (2.5 oz)	40

·OOD	PORTION	CALS.
Boboli (CONT.)		
Sauce	1 pkg (1.2 oz)	20
Contadina		
Flavored With Pepperoni	¼ cup	40
Pizza Sauce	¼ cup	35
Squeeze	¼ cup	35
With Italian Cheeses	¼ cup	40
Eden		
Pizza Pasta Sauce	½ cup (4.4 oz)	80
Muir Glen		
Organic	¼ cup (2.2 oz)	40
Progresso		
Pizza Sauce	¼ cup (2.2 oz)	35
Ragu		
Quick Traditional	3 tbsp (1.7 oz)	35
Tree Of Life		
Sauce	¼ cup (1.9 oz)	30
TAKE-OUT		
cheese	12 in pie	1121
cheese	⅛ of 12 in pie	140
cheese deep dish individual	1 (5.5 oz)	460
cheese meat & vegetables	12 in pie	1472
cheese meat & vegetables	⅛ of 12 in pie	184
pepperoni	⅛ of 12 in pie	181
pepperoni	12 in pie	1445
PLANTAINS		
fresh uncooked	1 (6.3 oz)	218
sliced cooked	½ cup	89
Chifles		
Plantain Chips	1 pkg (2 oz)	170
PLUMS		
FRESH		
Dole		
Plums	2	70
POI		
poi	½ cup	134
POKEBERRY SHOOTS		
cooked	½ cup	16
Allen		
Pokeberry Shoots	½ cup (4.1 oz)	35
POLENTA		
(*see* CORNMEAL)		
POLLACK		
atlantic baked	3 oz	100

FOOD	PORTION	CALS.
POMEGRANATES		
pomegranate	1	104
POMPANO		
florida cooked	3 oz	179
POPCORN		
(see also CHIPS, POPCORN CAKES, PRETZELS, SNACKS)		
air-popped	1 cup (0.3 oz)	31
air-popped	1 oz	108
caramel coated	1 oz	122
caramel coated	1 cup (1.2 oz)	152
carmel coated w/ peanuts	⅔ cup (1 oz)	114
cheese	1 cup (0.4 oz)	58
cheese	1 oz	149
oil popped	1 oz	142
oil popped	1 cup (0.4 oz)	55
Barrel O' Fun		
Baked Curl	1 oz	150
Caramel Corn	1 oz	115
Corn Pop	1 oz	190
Popcorn	1 oz	160
White Cheddar Pops	1 oz	170
Chester's		
Butter	3 cups	160
Caramel Craze	¾ cup	130
Cheddar Cheese	3 cups	190
Microwave Butter	5 cups	200
Cracker Jack		
Fat Free Butter Toffee	¾ cup	110
Fat Free Caramel	¾ cup	110
Original	½ cup	120
Estee		
Caramel	1 cup	120
Greenfield		
Caramel	1 cup (1 oz)	120
Herr's		
Regular	3 cups (1 oz)	140
Jiffy Pop		
Bag Butter	3 cups	90
Bag Lite	3 cups	70
Bag Regular	3 cups	100
Glazed Popcorn Clusters	1 oz	120
Microwave Butter	4 cup	140
Microwave Regular	4 cup	140

FOOD	PORTION	CALS.
Jiffy Pop (CONT.)		
Pan Butter	4 cup	130
Pan Regular	4 cup	130
Louise's		
Fat-Free Apple Cinnamon	1 oz	100
Fat-Free Buttery Toffee	1 oz	100
Fat-Free Caramel	1 oz	100
Newman's Own		
Microwave Butter Flavor	3½ cups	170
Microwave Light Butter	3½ cups	110
Microwave Light Natural	3½ cups	110
Microwave Natural	3½ cups	170
Popcorn unpopped	3 tbsp	110
Orville Redenbacher's		
Gourmet Hot Air	3 cups	40
Gourmet Original	3 cups	80
Gourmet White	3 cups	80
Microwave Gourmet	3 cups	100
Microwave Gourmet Butter	3 cups	100
Microwave Gourmet Butter Toffee	2½ cups	210
Microwave Gourmet Caramel	2½ cups	240
Microwave Gourmet Cheddar Cheese	3 cups	130
Microwave Gourmet Frozen	3 cups	100
Microwave Gourmet Frozen Butter	3 cups	100
Microwave Gourmet Light	3 cups	70
Microwave Gourmet Light Butter	3 cups	70
Microwave Gourmet Salt Free	3 cups	100
Microwave Gourmet Salt Free Butter	3 cups	100
Microwave Gourmet Sour Cream 'n Onion	3 cups	160
Planters		
Fiddle Faddle Caramel Fat Free	1 cup (1 oz)	110
Pop Secret		
94% Fat Free Butter	1 cup (5 g)	20
94% Fat Free Natural	1 cup (5 g)	20
Butter	1 cup (7 g)	35
Cheddar Cheese	1 cup (6 g)	30
Jumbo Pop Butter	1 cup (7 g)	40
Jumbo Pop Movie Theater Butter	1 cup (7 g)	40
Light Butter	1 cup (5 g)	20
Light Movie Theater Butter	1 cup (5 g)	25
Light Natural	1 cup (5 g)	25
Movie Theater Butter	1 cup (7 g)	40
Nacho Cheese	1 cup (6 g)	30
Natural	1 cup (7 g)	35

FOOD	PORTION	CALS.
Pop Secret (CONT.)		
Pop Chips	1½ cups (1 oz)	130
Real Butter	1 cup (7 g)	35
Smartfood		
Butter	3 cups	150
Low Fat Toffee Crunch	¾ cup	110
Reduced Fat Golden Butter	3⅓ cups	130
Reduced Fat White Cheddar	3 cups	140
White Cheddar	2 cups	190
Snyder's		
Butter	1 oz	140
Ultra Slim-Fast		
Lite N' Tasty	½ oz	60
Utz		
Au Natural	3 cups (1 oz)	120
Butter	2 cups (1 oz)	170
Cheese	2 cups (1 oz)	150
Hulless Puff'N Corn	2 cups (1 oz)	180
Hulless Puff'N Corn Hot Cheese	1 pkg (1.75 oz)	290
Hulless Pull'N Corn Cheese	2 cups (1 oz)	170
White Cheddar	2 cups (1 oz)	150
Weight Watchers		
Butter	1 pkg (0.66 oz)	90
Butter Toffee	1 pkg (0.9 oz)	110
Caramel	1 pkg (0.9 oz)	100
Microwave	1 pkg (1 oz)	100
White Cheddar Cheese	1 pkg (0.66 oz)	90
Wise		
Tender Eating	0.5 oz	70
With Real Premium White Cheddar Cheese	0.5 oz	70

POPCORN CAKES

FOOD	PORTION	CALS.
popcorn cake	1 (0.3 oz)	38
Lundberg		
Organic Lightly Salted	1	60
Organic Unsalted	1	60
Rye With Caraway Lightly Salted	1	59
Mother's		
Butter Flavor	1 (0.3 oz)	35
Unsalted	1 (0.3 oz)	35
Orville Redenbacher's		
Chocolate Peanut Crunch Mini	6 pieces (0.5 oz)	60
Peanut Caramel Crunch	6 (0.5 oz)	60
Quaker		
Blueberry Crunch	1 (0.5 oz)	50

FOOD	PORTION	CALS.
Quaker (CONT.)		
Butter Mini	6 (0.5 oz)	50
Butter Popped	1 (0.3 oz)	35
Caramel	1 (0.5 oz)	50
Caramel Mini	5 (0.5 oz)	50
Cheddar Cheese Mini	6 (0.5 oz)	50
Lightly Salted Mini	7 (0.5 oz)	50
Monterey Jack	1 (0.4 oz)	40
Strawberry Crunch	1 (0.5 oz)	50
White Cheddar	1 (0.4 oz)	40

POPOVER

home recipe as prep w/ 2% milk	1 (1.4 oz)	87
home recipe as prep w/ whole milk	1 (1.4 oz)	90
mix as prep	1 (1.2 oz)	67

POPPY SEEDS

poppy seeds	1 tsp	15

PORK

(*see also* BACON, BACON SUBSTITUTES, CANADIAN BACON, DELI MEATS/
COLD CUTS, HAM, PORK DISHES, SAUSAGE)

CANNED
Hormel

Pickled Tidbits	2 oz	100

FRESH

boston blade roast lean & fat cooked	3 oz	229
boston blade steak lean & fat cooked	3 oz	220
center loin roast lean bone in cooked	3 oz	169
center loin chop lean bone in cooked	3 oz	172
center rib chop lean & fat bone in cooked	3 oz	213
center rib roast lean & fat bone in cooked	3 oz	217
fresh ham rump lean roasted	3 oz	175
fresh ham rump lean & fat roasted	3 oz	214
fresh ham shank lean roasted	3 oz	183
fresh ham shank lean & fat roasted	3 oz	246
fresh ham whole lean roasted	3 oz	179
fresh ham whole lean roasted diced	1 cup	285
fresh ham whole lean & fat roasted	3 oz	232
fresh ham whole lean & fat roasted diced	1 cup	369
ground cooked	3 oz	252
leg loin & shoulder lean only roasted	3 oz	198
loin chop lean bone in braised	3 oz	191
loin chop lean bone in broiled	3 oz	199
loin roast lean bone in roasted	3 oz	210

FOOD	PORTION	CALS.
loin whole lean & fat braised	3 oz	203
loin whole lean & fat broiled	3 oz	206
loin whole lean & fat roasted	3 oz	211
lungs braised	3 oz	84
pancreas cooked	3 oz	186
ribs country style lean & fat braised	3 oz	252
shoulder arm picnic lean & fat roasted	3 oz	269
shoulder whole lean & fat roasted	3 oz	248
shoulder whole lean & fat roasted diced	1 cup	394
shoulder whole lean roasted	3 oz	196
shoulder whole lean roasted diced	1 cup	311
sirloin chop lean & fat bone in braised	3 oz	208
sirloin roast lean & fat bone in cooked	3 oz	222
spareribs braised	3 oz	338
spleen braised	3 oz	127
tail simmered	3 oz	336
tenderloin lean roasted	3 oz	139
top loin chop boneless lean & fat cooked	3 oz	198
top loin roast boness lean & fat cooked	3 oz	192
Oscar Mayer		
Sweet Morsel Smoked Boneless Pork Shoulder Butt	3 oz	180

PORK DISHES

Jimmy Dean

BBQ Pork Rib Sandwich	1 (5.4 oz)	440

TAKE-OUT

pork roast	2 oz	70
tourtiere	1 piece (4.9 oz)	451[1]

POSOLE

(*see* HOMINY)

POT PIE

Amy's Organic

Broccoli	1 (7.5 oz)	430
Country Vegetable	1 (7.5 oz)	370
Shepard's	1 (8 oz)	160
Vegetable	1 (7.5 oz)	360
Vegetable Non-Dairy	1 (7.5 oz)	320

Award Brand

Beef	1 (7 oz)	350
Chicken	1 (7 oz)	350

Banquet

Family Entree Chicken Pie	1 serv (8 oz)	450

FOOD	PORTION	CALS.
Banquet (CONT.)		
Macaroni & Cheese	1 pkg (6.5 oz)	200
Vegetable & Cheese	1 (7 oz)	390
Vegetable Pie w/ Beef	1 (7 oz)	330
Vegetable Pie w/ Chicken	1 (7 oz)	350
Vegetable Pie w/ Turkey	1 (7 oz)	370
Empire		
Chicken	1 (8.1 oz)	440
Turkey	1 (8.1 oz)	470
Great Value		
Beef	1 (7 oz)	390
Chicken	1 (7 oz)	380
Turkey	1 (7 oz)	400
Lean Cuisine		
Chicken Pie	1 pkg (9.5 oz)	290
Turkey & Country Vegetable	1 pkg (9.5 oz)	320
Morton		
Beef	1 (7 oz)	310
Chicken	1 (7 oz)	320
Macaroni & Cheese	1 (6 oz)	160
Turkey	1 (7 oz)	300
Mrs. Paterson's		
Aussie Pie Chicken	1 (5.5 oz)	460
Aussie Pie Philly Steak	1 (5.5 oz)	420
Ozark Valley		
Chicken	1 (7 oz)	330
Macaroni & Cheese	1 (6.5 oz)	160
Turkey	1 (7 oz)	280
Stouffer's		
Beef Pie	1 pkg (10 oz)	450
Chicken Pie	1 pkg (10 oz)	540
Turkey	1 pkg (10 oz)	530
Swanson		
Beef	7 oz	370
Beef Hungry Man	16 oz	610
Chicken	7 oz	380
Chicken Homestyle	8 oz	410
Hungry Man Chicken	16 oz	630
Hungry Man Turkey	16 oz	650
Turkey	7 oz	380
TAKE-OUT		
beef	1/3 of 9 in pie (7.4 oz)	515
chicken	1/3 of 9 in pie (8.1 oz)	545

FOOD	PORTION	CALS.

POTATO
(*see also* CHIPS, KNISH, PANCAKES)
CANNED
Allen

Refried Potatoes	½ cup (4.5 oz)	150
Butterfield		
Diced	⅔ cup (5.7 oz)	100
Sliced	½ cup (5.7 oz)	100
Whole	2½ pieces (5.6 oz)	90
Del Monte		
New Sliced	⅔ cup (5.4 oz)	60
New Whole	⅔ cup (5.5 oz)	60
Hormel		
Au Gratin & Bacon	1 can (7.5 oz)	250
Seneca		
Potatoes	½ cup	80
Sunshine		
Whole	2½ pieces (5.6 oz)	90
FRESH		
baked w/ skin	1 (6.5 oz)	220
boiled	½ cup	68
microwaved	1 (7 oz)	212
Purely Idaho		
Oven Roasts	1 serv (3 oz)	70
Yukon Gold		
Fresh	1 (5.3 oz)	110
FROZEN		
Birds Eye		
Whole	3 (2.6 oz)	50
Budget Gourmet		
Baked With Broccoli And Cheese	1 pkg (10.5 oz)	300
Cheddared Potatoes	1 pkg (5.5 oz)	260
Cheddared Potatoes With Broccoli	1 pkg (5 oz)	150
Three Cheese Potatoes	1 pkg (5.75 oz)	220
Empire		
Crinkle Cut French Fries	½ cup (3 oz)	90
Latkes Potato Pancakes	1 (2 oz)	80
Latkes Mini Potato Pancakes	2 (2 oz)	90
Golden		
Potato Pancakes	1 (1.3 oz)	71
Healthy Choice		
Cheddar Broccoli Potatoes	1 meal (10.5 oz)	310
Garden Potato Casserole	1 meal (9.25 oz)	200

FOOD	PORTION	CALS.
Kineret		
Crinkle Cut	18 pieces (3 oz)	120
Kugel	1 piece (2.5 oz)	150
Latkes	1 (1.5 oz)	90
Latkes Mini	10 (3 oz)	160
Lean Cuisine		
Deluxe Cheddar	1 pkg (10.4 oz)	270
Roasted Potatoes w/ Broccoli & Cheddar Cheese Sauce	1 pkg (10.25 oz)	260
MicroMagic		
French Fries Low Fat	1 pkg (3 oz)	130
Oh Boy!		
Stuffed With Cheddar Cheese	1 (6 oz)	130
Stuffed With Real Bacon	1 (6 oz)	120
Ore Ida		
Cheddar Browns	1 patty (3 oz)	90
Cottage Fries	14 pieces (3 oz)	130
Crispers!	17 pieces (3 oz)	220
Crispers! Nacho	10 pieces (3 oz)	170
Crispers! Texas	3 oz	170
Crispy Crowns!	12 pieces (3 oz)	100
Crispy Crunchies	12 pieces (3 oz)	160
Deep Fries Crinkle Cuts	18 pieces (3 oz)	160
Deep Fries French Fries	22 pieces (3 oz)	160
Dinner Fries Country Style	8 pieces (3 oz)	110
Fast Fries	23 pieces (3 oz)	140
Fast Fries Ranch	22 pieces (3 oz)	150
Golden Crinkles	16 pieces (3 oz)	120
Golden Fries	16 pieces (3 oz)	120
Golden Patties	1 (2.5 oz)	140
Golden Twirls	28 pieces (3 oz)	160
Hash Browns Country Style	1 cup (2.6 oz)	60
Hash Browns Shredded	1 patty (3 oz)	70
Hash Browns Southern Style	¾ cup (3 oz)	70
Hot Tots	9 pieces (3 oz)	150
Mashed Natural Butter	½ cup (2.1 oz)	80
Microwave Crinkle Cuts	1 pkg (3.5 oz)	180
Microwave Hash Browns	1 patty (2 oz)	110
Microwave Tater Tots	1 pkg (3.75 oz)	190
O'Brien Potatoes	¾ cup (3 oz)	60
Pixie Crinkles	33 pieces (3 oz)	140
Shoestrings	38 pieces (3 oz)	150
Snackin' Fries	1 pkg (5 oz)	180
Snackin' Fries Extra Zesty	1 pkg (5 oz)	180

FOOD	PORTION	CALS.
Ore Ida (CONT.)		
Tater ABC's	10 pieces (3 oz)	190
Tater Tots	9 pieces (3 oz)	160
Tater Tots Bacon	9 pieces (3 oz)	150
Tater Tots Onion	9 pieces (3 oz)	150
Toaster Hash Browns	2 patties (3.5 oz)	190
Topped Broccoli & Cheese	½ (6 oz)	150
Topped Salsa & Cheese	½ (5.5 oz)	160
Topped Vegetable Primavera	1 (6.1 oz)	160
Twice Baked Butter	1 (5 oz)	200
Twice Baked Cheddar Cheese	1 (5 oz)	190
Twice Baked Ranch	1 (5 oz)	180
Twice Bakes Sour Cream & Chives	1 (5 oz)	180
Waffle Fries	15 pieces (3 oz)	140
Wedges With Skin	9 pieces (3 oz)	110
Zesties!	12 pieces (3 oz)	160
Stouffer's		
Au Gratin	½ cup (5.75 oz)	130
Scalloped	1 serv (5 oz)	140
Scalloped	½ cup (5.75 oz)	140
Weight Watchers		
Smart Ones Baked Broccoli & Cheese	1 pkg (10 oz)	250
MIX		
Barbara's		
Mashed not prep	⅓ cup (0.8 oz)	70
Country Store		
Mashed not prep	⅓ cup	70
Hungry Jack		
Au Gratin as prep	½ cup	150
Cheddar & Bacon as prep	½ cup	150
Chessy Scalloped as prep	½ cup	150
Creamy Scalloped as prep	½ cup	150
Mashed Butter Flavored as prep	½ cup	150
Mashed Flakes as prep	½ cup	160
Mashed Garlic Flavored as prep	½ cup	150
Mashed Parsley Butter as prep	½ cup	150
Mashed Sour Cream 'n Chives as prep	½ cup	150
Sour Cream & Chives as prep	½ cup	160
Idaho		
Mashed Potato Flakes as prep	½ cup	150
Mashed Potato Granules as prep	½ cup	160
Shake 'N Bake		
Perfect Potatoes Crispy Cheddar	⅙ pkg (7 g)	30
Perfect Potatoes Herb & Garlic	⅙ pkg (7 g)	20

FOOD	PORTION	CALS.
Shake 'N Bake (CONT.)		
Perfect Potatoes Home Fries	⅙ pkg (7 g)	20
Perfect Potatoes Parmesan Peppercorn	⅙ pkg (7 g)	25
Perfect Potatoes Savory Onion	⅙ pkg (7 g)	20
REFRIGERATED		
Simply Potatoes		
Au Gratin	¼ pkg (3 oz)	130
Hash Browns	⅕ pkg (4 oz)	100
Hash Browns Onion	⅕ pkg (4 oz)	120
Hash Browns Southwest Style	⅕ pkg (4 oz)	100
Mashed	⅕ pkg (4 oz)	90
Scalloped	¼ pkg (3 oz)	100
SHELF-STABLE		
Lunch Bucket		
Scalloped	1 pkg (7.5 oz)	160
Micro Cup Meals		
Microcup Meals Scalloped Potatoes w/ Ham	1 cup (7.5 oz)	240
TAKE-OUT		
baked topped w/ cheese sauce	1	475
baked topped w/ cheese sauce & bacon	1	451
baked topped w/ cheese sauce & broccoli	1	402
baked topped w/ cheese sauce & chili	1	481
baked topped w/ sour cream & chives	1	394
hash brown	½ cup (2.5 oz)	151
indian yogurt potatoes	1 serv	315
mashed	½ cup	111
mustard potato salad	3.5 oz	120
o'brien	1 cup	157
potato pancakes	1 (1.3 oz)	101
potato salad	½ cup	179
potato salad w/ vegetables	3.5 oz	120

POUT
ocean fillet baked	4.8 oz	139

PRESERVE
(*see* JAM/JELLY/PRESERVE)

PRETZELS
(*see also* CHIPS, POPCORN, SNACKS)

chocolate covered	1 (0.4 oz)	50
chocolate covered	1 oz	130
dutch twist	4 (2.1 oz)	229
pretzels	1 oz	108

FOOD	PORTION	CALS.
rods	4 (2 oz)	229
sticks	120 (2 oz)	229
twists	10 (2.1 oz)	229
whole wheat	2 sm (1 oz)	103
whole wheat	2 med (2 oz)	205
Barrel O' Fun		
Mini	1 oz	110
Sticks	1 oz	110
Twists	1 oz	110
Estee		
Chocolate Covered	7	130
Dutch	2 (1.1 oz)	130
Unsalted	23 (1 oz)	120
Formagg		
Pretzel Nuts	1 oz	120
Gardetto's		
Mustard	1 pkg (0.5 oz)	50
Herr's		
Hard Sourdough	1 (1 oz)	100
Manischewitz		
Bagel Pretzels Original	4 (1 oz)	110
Mister Salty		
Chips	16 (1 oz)	110
Dutch	2 (1.1 oz)	120
Fat Free Chips	16 (1 oz)	100
Mini	22 (1 oz)	110
Sticks Fat Free	47 (1 oz)	110
Twist Fat Free	9 (1 oz)	110
Mr. Phipps		
Chips Lower Sodium	16 (1 oz)	120
Chips Original	16 (1 oz)	120
Chips Original Fat Free	16 (1 oz)	100
Nabisco		
Air Crisps Fat Free	23 pieces (1 oz)	110
Nestle		
Flipz Milk Chocolate Covered	9 pieces (1 oz)	130
Flipz White Fudge Covered	9 pieces (1 oz)	130
Newman's Own		
Salted Rounds Organic	1 pkg (1.4 oz)	150
Planters		
Twists	1 oz	100
Twists	1 pkg (1.5 oz)	160
Quinlan		
Beers	1 oz	110

FOOD	PORTION	CALS.
Quinlan (CONT.)		
Hard Sourdough	1 oz	110
Logs	1 oz	110
Nuggets	1 oz	110
Rods	1 oz	110
Sticks	1 oz	110
Thins	1 oz	110
Rold Gold		
Crispy's Thins	4 (1 oz)	110
Fat Free Cheddar Cheese	17 (1 oz)	110
Fat Free Honey Mustard	17 (1 oz)	110
Fat Free Sticks	48 (1 oz)	110
Fat Free Thins	12 pieces (1 oz)	110
Fat Free Tiny Twists	18 pieces (1 oz)	110
Rods	3 (1 oz)	110
Sour Dough Nuggets	11 (1 oz)	110
Seyfart's		
Butter Rods	1 oz	110
Snyder's		
Dips White Fudge	1 oz	130
Logs	1 oz	310
Minis	1 oz	310
Minis Unsalted	1 oz	310
Nibblers	1 oz	310
Oat Bran	1 oz	120
Old Fashioned Hard	1 oz	111
Old Fashioned Hard Unsalted	1 oz	100
Old Tyme	1 oz	310
Old Tyme Unsalted	1 oz	110
Rods	1 oz	310
Snaps	24 (1 oz)	120
Sourdough Hard Buttermilk Ranch	1 oz	130
Sourdough Hard Cheddar Cheese	1 oz	160
Sourdough Hard Honey Mustard & Onion	1 oz	130
Stix	1 oz	310
Very Thins	1 oz	310
Sunshine		
California Pretzels	1 oz	110
Ultra Slim-Fast		
Lite N' Tasty	1 oz	100
Utz		
Country Store Stix	5 (1 oz)	110
Fat Free Hard	1 (0.8 oz)	90
Fat Free Hard No Salt Added	1 (0.8 oz)	90

FOOD	PORTION	CALS.
Utz (CONT.)		
Fat Free Sour Dough Nuggets	10 (1 oz)	100
Fat Free Stix	14 (1 oz)	100
Fat Free Thin	10 (1 oz)	100
Honey Mustard & Onion	⅓ cup (1 oz)	130
Rods	3 (1 oz)	120
Specials	5 (1 oz)	110
Specials Extra Dark	5 (1 oz)	110
Specials Unsalted	5 (1 oz)	110
Wheels	20 (1 oz)	100
Weight Watchers		
Oat Bran Nuggets	1 pkg (1.5 oz)	170

PRICKLYPEAR

fresh	1	42

PRUNE JUICE

canned	1 cup	181
Del Monte		
Juice	8 fl oz	170
Ocean Spray		
100% Juice	8 fl oz	180

PRUNES
DRIED

dried	10	201
Del Monte		
Pitted	¼ cup (1.4 oz)	120
Unpitted	⅓ cup (1.4 oz)	110
Sonoma		
Pitted	¼ cup (1.4 oz)	120
Sunsweet		
Orange Essence Pitted Prunes	6 (1.4 oz)	100

PUDDING

(*see also* CUSTARD, PUDDING POPS)

HOME RECIPE

bread pudding	1 recipe 6 serv (26.4 oz)	1266
chocolate as prep w/ whole milk	½ cup (5.5 oz)	221
corn	⅔ cup	181
cornstarch	½ cup (4.4 oz)	137
rice	½ cup (5.3 oz)	217

MIX

banana as prep w/ 2% milk	½ cup (4.9 oz)	142
banana as prep w/ whole milk	½ cup (4.9 oz)	157
chocolate as prep w/ 2% milk	½ cup (5 oz)	150

FOOD	PORTION	CALS.
chocolate as prep w/ whole milk	½ cup (5 oz)	158
coconut cream as prep w/ 2% milk	½ cup (4.9 oz)	148
coconut cream as prep w/ whole milk	½ cup (4.9 oz)	160
instant banana as prep w/ 2% milk	½ cup (5.2 oz)	152
instant banana as prep w/ whole milk	½ cup (5.2 oz)	167
instant chocolate as prep w/ whole milk	½ cup (5.2 oz)	164
instant coconut cream as prep w/ 2% milk	½ cup (5.2 oz)	157
instant coconut cream as prep w/ whole milk	½ cup (5.2 oz)	172
instant lemon as prep w/ 2% milk	½ cup (5.2 oz)	155
instant lemon as prep w/ whole milk	½ cup (5.2 oz)	169
instant vanilla as prep w/ 2% milk	½ cup (5 oz)	147
instant vanilla as prep w/ whole milk	½ cup (5 oz)	181
Instant chocolate as prep w/ 2% milk	½ cup (5.2 oz)	149
lemon	½ cup (5.1 oz)	163
rice as prep w/ 2% milk	½ cup (5.1 oz)	161
rice as prep w/ whole milk	½ cup (5.1 oz)	175
tapioca as prep w/ 2% milk	½ cup (5 oz)	147
tapioca as prep w/ whole milk	½ cup (5 oz)	161
vanilla as prep w/ 2% milk	½ cup (4.9 oz)	141
vanilla as prep w/ whole milk	½ cup (4.9 oz)	155
Emes		
Dietetic as prep w/ skim milk	½ cup (4 fl oz)	71
Jell-O		
Americana Rice as prep w/ skim milk	½ cup (5.2 oz)	140
Americana Tapioca as prep w/ skim milk	½ cup (5.1 oz)	130
Banana Cream as prep w/ 2% milk	½ cup (5.1 oz)	140
Butterscotch as prep w/ 2% milk	½ cup (5.2 oz)	160
Chocolate as prep w/ 2% milk	½ cup (5.2 oz)	150
Chocolate Fudge as prep w/ 2% milk	½ cup (5.2 oz)	150
Coconut Cream as prep w/ 2% milk	½ cup (5.1 oz)	150
Fat Free Chocolate as prep w/ skim milk	½ cup (5.2 oz)	130
Fat Free Vanilla as prep w/ skim milk	½ cup (5.1 oz)	130
Instant Banana Cream as prep w/ 2% milk	½ cup (5.2 oz)	150
Instant Butterscotch as prep w/ 2% milk	½ cup (5.2 oz)	150
Instant Chocolate as prep w/ 2% milk	½ cup (5.2 oz)	160
Instant Chocolate Fudge as prep w/ 2% milk	½ cup (4.2 oz)	160
Instant Coconut Cream as prep w/ 2% milk	½ cup (4.2 oz)	160
Instant French Vanilla as prep w/ 2% milk	½ cup (4.2 oz)	150
Instant Lemon as prep w/ 2% milk	½ cup (4.2 oz)	150
Instant Pistachio as prep w/ 2% milk	½ cup (4.2 oz)	160
Instant Vanilla as prep w/ 2% milk	½ cup (4.2 oz)	150
Instant Fat Free Chocolate as prep w/ skim milk	½ cup (5.3 oz)	140

FOOD	PORTION	CALS.
Jell-O (CONT.)		
Instant Fat Free Devil's Food as prep w/ skim milk	½ cup (5.3 oz)	140
Instant Fat Free Sugar Free Banana as prep w/ skim milk	½ cup (4.6 oz)	70
Instant Fat Free Sugar Free Butterscotch as prep w/ skim milk	½ cup (4.6 oz)	70
Instant Fat Free Sugar Free Chocolate Fudge as prep w/ skim milk	½ cup (4.7 oz)	80
Instant Fat Free Sugar Free Chocolate as prep w/ skim milk	½ cup (4.6 oz)	80
Instant Fat Free Sugar Free Vanilla as prep w/ skim milk	½ cup (4.6 oz)	70
Instant Fat Free Sugar Free White Chocolate as prep w/ skim milk	½ cup (4.6 oz)	70
Instant Fat Free Vanilla as prep w/ skim milk	½ cup (5.2 oz)	140
Instant Fat Free White Chocolate as prep w/ skim milk	½ cup (5.2 oz)	140
Lemon as prep	½ cup (4.4 oz)	140
Milk Chocolate as prep w/ 2% milk	½ cup (5.2 oz)	150
Sugar Free Chocolate as prep w/ 2% milk	½ cup (4.6 oz)	90
Sugar Free Vanilla as prep w/ 2% milk	½ cup (4.5 oz)	80
Vanilla as prep w/ 2% milk	½ cup (5.1 oz)	140
Louisiana Purchase		
Bread	1 serv (1.3 oz)	150
My*T*Fine		
Butterscotch	mix for 1 serv	90
Chocolate	mix for 1 serv	100
Chocolate Almond	mix for 1 serv	100
Chocolate Fudge	mix for 1 serv	100
Lemon	mix for 1 serv	90
Vanilla	mix for 1 serv	90
Vanilla Tapioca	mix for 1 serv	80
Royal		
Banana Cream	mix for 1 serv	80
Banana Cream Instant	mix for 1 serv	90
Butterscotch	mix for 1 serv	90
Butterscotch Instant	mix for 1 serv	90
Cherry Vanilla Instant	mix for 1 serv	90
Chocolate	mix for 1 serv	90
Chocolate Almond Instant	mix for 1 serv	120
Chocolate Chocolate Chip Instant	mix for 1 serv	110
Chocolate Instant	mix for 1 serv	110

FOOD	PORTION	CALS.
Royal (CONT.)		
Chocolate Peanut Butter Instant	mix for 1 serv	110
Chocolate Sugar Free Instant	mix for 1 serv	50
Dark 'n Sweet Chocolate	mix for 1 serv	90
Dark'N Sweet Instant	mix for 1 serv	110
Lemon Instant	mix for 1 serv	90
Pistachio Instant	mix for 1 serv	90
Strawberry Instant	mix for 1 serv	100
Toasted Coconut Instant	mix for 1 serv	100
Vanilla	mix for 1 serv	80
Vanilla Chocolate Chip Instant	mix for 1 serv	90
Vanilla Instant	mix for 1 serv	90
READY-TO-EAT		
banana	1 pkg (5 oz)	180
chocolate	1 pkg (5 oz)	189
lemon	1 pkg (5 oz)	177
rice	1 pkg (5 oz)	231
tapioca	1 pkg (5 oz)	169
vanilla	1 pkg (4 oz)	146
Del Monte		
Snack Cups Banana	1 serv (4 oz)	140
Snack Cups Butterscotch	1 serv (4 oz)	140
Snack Cups Chocolate	1 serv (4 oz)	160
Snack Cups Chocolate Fudge	1 serv (4 oz)	150
Snack Cups Chocolate Peanut Butter	1 serv (4 oz)	160
Snack Cups Lite Chocolate	1 serv (4 oz)	100
Snack Cups Lite Vanilla	1 serv (4 oz)	90
Snack Cups Tapioca	1 serv (4 oz)	140
Snack Cups Vanilla	1 serv (4 oz)	150
Handi-Snacks		
Banana	1 serv (3.5 oz)	120
Butterscotch	1 serv (3.5 oz)	120
Chocolate	1 serv (3.5 oz)	130
Chocolate Fudge	1 serv (3.5 oz)	130
Fat Free Chocolate	1 serv (3.5 oz)	90
Fat Free Vanilla	1 serv (3.5 oz)	90
Tapioca	1 serv (3.5 oz)	120
Vanilla	1 serv (3.5 oz)	120
Hunt's		
Snack Pack Banana	1 (4 oz)	158
Snack Pack Butterscotch	1 (4 oz)	153
Snack Pack Chocolate	1 (4 oz)	167
Snack Pack Chocolate Fudge	1 (4 oz)	167
Snack Pack Chocolate Marshmallow	1 (4 oz)	155

FOOD	PORTION	CALS.
Hunt's (CONT.)		
Snack Pack Fat Free Chocolate	1 (4 oz)	96
Snack Pack Fat Free Tapioca	1 (4 oz)	95
Snack Pack Fat Free Vanilla	1 (4 oz)	93
Snack Pack Lemon	1 (4 oz)	162
Snack Pack Swirl Chocolate Caramel	1 (4 oz)	168
Snack Pack Swirl Chocolate Peanut Butter	1 (4 oz)	166
Snack Pack Swirl Milk Chocolate	1 (4 oz)	164
Snack Pack Swirl Smores	1 (4 oz)	154
Snack Pack Tapioca	1 (4 oz)	151
Snack Pack Vanilla	1 (4 oz)	163
Imagine Foods		
Lemon Dream	1 (4 oz)	120
Jell-O		
Chocolate	1 serv (4 oz)	160
Chocolate Marshmallow	1 serv (4 oz)	160
Chocolate Vanilla Swirls	1 serv (4 oz)	160
Free Chocolate	1 serv (4 oz)	100
Free Chocolate Vanilla Swirl	1 serv (4 oz)	100
Free Devil's Food	1 serv (4 oz)	100
Free Rocky Road	1 serv (4 oz)	100
Free Vanilla	1 serv (4 oz)	100
Tapioca	1 serv (4 oz)	140
Tapioca	1 serv (4 oz)	100
Vanilla	1 serv (4 oz)	160
Kozy Shack		
Banana	1 pkg (4 oz)	130
Chocolate	1 pkg (4 oz)	140
Light Chocolate	1 pkg (4 oz)	110
Light Vanilla	1 pkg (4 oz)	110
Rice	1 pkg (4 oz)	130
Tapioca	1 pkg (4 oz)	140
Vanilla	1 pkg (4 oz)	130
Snack Pack		
Banana	4.25 oz	145
Butterscotch	4.25 oz	170
Chocolate	4.25 oz	170
Chocolate Marshmallow	4.25 oz	165
Chocolate Fudge	4.25 oz	165
Lemon	4.25 oz	150
Light Chocolate	4.25 oz	100
Light Tapioca	4.25 oz	100
Tapioca	4.25 oz	150
Vanilla	4.25 oz	170

FOOD	PORTION	CALS.
Swiss Miss		
Butterscotch	4 oz	180
Chocolate	4 oz	180
Chocolate Fudge	4 oz	220
Chocolate Sundae	4 oz	220
Light Chocolate	4 oz	100
Light Chocolate Fudge	4 oz	100
Light Vanilla	4 oz	100
Light Vanilla Chocolate Parfait	4 oz	100
Tapioca	4 oz	160
Vanilla	4 oz	190
Vanilla Parfait	4 oz	180
Vanilla Sundae	4 oz	200
Ultra Slim-Fast		
Butterscotch	4 oz	100
Chocolate	4 oz	100
Vanilla	4 oz	100
TAKE-OUT		
bread pudding	½ cup (4.4 oz)	212
chocolate	½ cup (5.5 oz)	206
tapioca	½ cup (5.3 oz)	189
vanilla	½ cup (4.3 oz)	130

PUDDING POPS

(*see also* ICE CREAM AND FROZEN DESSERTS, YOGURT FROZEN)

chocolate	1 (1.6 oz)	72
vanilla	1 (1.6 oz)	75

PUMMELO

fresh	1	228
sections	1 cup	71

PUMPKIN
CANNED
Libby

Solid Pack	½ cup	60
FRESH		
flowers cooked	½ cup	10
leaves cooked	½ cup	7
SEEDS		
dried	1 oz	154
roasted	1 cup	1184
salted & roasted	1 oz	148
whole roasted	1 oz	127
whole salted roasted	1 cup	285

FOOD	PORTION	CALS.
PURSLANE		
cooked	1 cup	21
QUAHOGS		
(*see* CLAM)		
QUAIL		
breast w/o skin raw	1 (2 oz)	69
w/ skin raw	1 quail (3.8 oz)	210
QUICHE		
TAKE-OUT		
lorraine	⅛ of 8 in pie	600
QUINCE		
fresh	1	53
QUINOA		
Arrowhead		
Quinoa	¼ cup (1.4 oz)	140
Eden		
Not Prep	¼ cup (1.6 oz)	170
RABBIT		
domestic w/o bone roasted	3 oz	167
wild w/o bone stewed	3 oz	147
RACCOON		
roasted	3 oz	217
RADICCHIO		
leaf	3.5 oz	18
raw shredded	½ cup	5
RADISHES		
DRIED		
chinese	½ cup	157
daikon	½ cup	157
FRESH		
chinese raw	1 (12 oz)	62
chinese raw sliced	½ cup	8
chinese sliced cooked	½ cup	13
daikon raw	1 (12 oz)	62
daikon raw sliced	½ cup	8
daikon sliced cooked	½ cup	13
red raw	10	7
red sliced	½ cup	10
white icicle raw	1 (0.5 oz)	2
white icicle raw sliced	½ cup	7

FOOD	PORTION	CALS.
Dole		
Radishes	7	20
SPROUTS		
raw	½ cup	8
RAISINS		
chocolate coated	10 (0.4 oz)	39
chocolate coated	1 cup (6.7 oz)	741
golden seedless	1 cup	437
seedless	1 cup	434
seedless	1 tbsp	27
Del Monte		
Golden	¼ cup (1.4 oz)	130
Raisins	1 box (1.5 oz)	140
Raisins	1 box (1 oz)	90
Raisins	1 box (0.5 oz)	45
Raisins	¼ cup (1.4 oz)	130
Yogurt Raisins Strawberry	1 pkg (0.9 oz)	110
Yogurt Raisins Vanilla	1 pkg (0.9 oz)	110
Yogurt Raisins Vanilla	1 pkg (1 oz)	120
Yogurt Raisins Vanilla	3 tbsp (1 oz)	130
Dole		
CinnaRaisins	1 pkg (1 oz)	95
Golden	½ cup	250
Seedless	½ cup	250
Estee		
Chocolate Covered	¼ cup	180
Sonoma		
Monukka Thompson	¼ cup (1.4 oz)	130
Tree Of Life		
Organic	¼ cup (1.4 oz)	130
RASPBERRIES		
CANNED		
in heavy syrup	½ cup	117
FRESH		
raspberries	1 cup	61
Dole		
Raspberries	1 cup	45
FROZEN		
sweetened	1 cup	256
Big Valley		
Raspberries	⅔ cup (4.9 oz)	80

FOOD	PORTION	CALS.
Birds Eye		
Red	½ cup (4.4 oz)	90

RASPBERRY JUICE
Crystal Geyser
Juice Squeeze Mountain Raspberry	1 bottle (12 fl oz)	135
Crystal Light		
Raspberry Ice Drink	1 serv (8 oz)	5
Raspberry Ice Drink Mix as prep	1 serv (8 oz)	5
Dole		
Country Raspberry	8 fl oz	140
Fresh Samantha		
Raspberry Dream	1 cup (8 oz)	120
Kool-Aid		
Drink Mix as prep	1 serv (8 oz)	60
Raspberry Drink as prep w/ sugar	1 serv (8 oz)	100
Splash Blue Raspberry Drink	1 serv (8 oz)	120

RED BEANS
CANNED
Allen
Red Beans	½ cup (4.5 oz)	160
Green Giant		
Red Beans	½ cup (4.5 oz)	100
Hunt's		
Small	½ cup (4.5 oz)	89
Van Camp's		
Red Beans	½ cup (4.6 oz)	90
DRIED
Bean Cuisine
| Dried | ½ cup | 115 |
MIX
Bean Cuisine
Pasta & Beans Barcelona Red With Radiatore	½ cup	170
Mahatma		
Red Beans & Rice	1 cup	190

RED KIDNEY BEANS
DRIED
Hurst
| HamBeens w/ Ham | 1 serv | 120 |

RELISH
| cranberry orange | ½ cup | 246 |
| hamburger | 1 tbsp | 19 |

FOOD	PORTION	CALS.
hot dog	1 tbsp	14
sweet	1 tbsp	19
Del Monte		
Hamburger	1 tbsp (0.5 oz)	20
Hot Dog	1 tbsp (0.5 oz)	15
Sweet Pickle	1 tbsp (0.5 oz)	20
Green Giant		
Corn	1 tbsp (0.6 oz)	20
Old El Paso		
Jalapeno	1 tbsp (0.5 oz)	5
Vlasic		
Dill	1 oz	2
Hamburger	1 oz	40
Hot Dog	1 oz	40
Hot Piccalilli	1 oz	35
India	1 oz	30
Sweet	1 oz	30

RENNIN
tablet	1 (0.9 g)	1

RHUBARB
fresh	½ cup	13
frzn as prep w/ sugar	½ cup	139

RICE
(*see also* BRAN, CEREAL, FLOUR, RICE CAKES, WILD RICE)

FOOD	PORTION	CALS.
brown long grain cooked	1 cup (6.8 oz)	216
brown medium grain cooked	1 cup (6.8 oz)	218
glutinous cooked	1 cup (6.1 oz)	169
white long grain cooked	1 cup (5.5 oz)	205
white long grain instant cooked	1 cup (5.8 oz)	162
white medium grain cooked	1 cup (6.5 oz)	242
white short grain cooked	1 cup (6.5 oz)	242
Arrowhead		
Basmati Brown	¼ cup (1.5 oz)	150
Basmati White	¼ cup (1.5 oz)	150
Brown Quick Regular	⅓ cup (1.5 oz)	150
Brown Quick Spanish Style	¼ pkg (1.4 oz)	150
Brown Quick Vegetable Herb	¼ pkg (1.4 oz)	150
Brown Quick Wild Rice & Herb	¼ pkg (1.3 oz)	140
Birds Eye		
Rice & Broccoli In Cheese Sauce	1 pkg (10 oz)	290
White & Wild	1 cup (6.6 oz)	180
Budget Gourmet		
Oriental Rice With Vegetables	1 pkg (5.75 oz)	230

FOOD	PORTION	CALS.
Budget Gourmet (CONT.)		
Rice Pilaf With Green Beans	1 pkg (5.5 oz)	230
Carolina		
Red Beans & Rice as prep	¼ pkg	190
Casbah		
Basmati as prep	1 cup	158
Jambalaya	1 pkg (1.4 oz)	130
La Fiesta	1 pkg (1.6 oz)	170
Nutted Pilaf as prep	1 cup	220
Pilaf as prep	1 cup	200
Spanish Pilaf as prep	1 cup	200
Thai Yum	1 pkg (1.7 oz)	180
Chun King		
Fried Rice	1 pkg (8 oz)	290
Fried Rice With Chicken	1 pkg (8 oz)	270
Goodman's		
Rice & Vermicelli For Beef	¾ cup	160
Rice & Vermicelli For Chicken	¾ cup	160
Goya		
Arroz Amarillo	¼ cup (1.6 oz)	170
Green Giant		
Rice & Broccoli	1 pkg (10 oz)	320
Rice Medley	1 pkg (10 oz)	240
Rice Pilaf	1 pkg (10 oz)	230
White & Wild	1 pkg (10 oz)	250
Hain		
Almondine	½ cup	130
Oriental 3-Grain Goodness	½ cup	120
Kitchen Del Sol		
Mediterranean Paella Costa Brave as prep	½ cup (1.2 oz)	130
Mediterranean Sunny Lemon Pilaf as prep	½ cup (1.2 oz)	110
Mediterranean Tomato & Basil With Pine Nuts	½ cup (1 oz)	110
Lipton		
Golden Saute Onion Mushroom	½ cup (2.1 oz)	240
Oriental Stir Fry as prep	1 cup	270
Rice & Sauce Alfredo Broccoli as prep	1 cup	320
Rice & Sauce Beef as prep	1 cup	270
Rice & Sauce Cajun Style as prep	1 cup	270
Rice & Sauce Cajun Style w/ Beans as prep	1 cup	310
Rice & Sauce Cheddar Broccoli as prep	1 cup	280
Rice & Sauce Chicken & Parmesan Risotto as prep	1 cup	270

FOOD	PORTION	CALS.
Lipton (CONT.)		
Rice & Sauce Chicken Broccoli as prep	1 cup	280
Rice & Sauce Chicken Flavor as prep	1 cup	280
Rice & Sauce Creamy Chicken as prep	1 cup	290
Rice & Sauce Herb & Butter as prep	1 cup	280
Rice & Sauce Medley as prep	1 cup	270
Rice & Sauce Mushroom as prep	1 cup	270
Rice & Sauce Mushroom & Herb as prep	1 cup	290
Rice & Sauce Oriental as prep	1 cup	280
Rice & Sauce Pilaf as prep	1 cup	260
Rice & Sauce Scampi Style as prep	1 cup	270
Rice & Sauce Spanish as prep	1 cup	270
Rice & Sauce Teriyaki as prep	1 cup	270
Roasted Chicken as prep	1 cup	260
Salsa Style as prep	1 cup	220
Southwestern Chicken Flavor as prep	1 cup	260
Luigino's		
Fried Rice Chicken	1 pkg (8 oz)	250
Fried Rice Pork	1 pkg (8 oz)	250
Fried Rice Pork & Shrimp	1 pkg (8 oz)	250
Fried Rice Shrimp	1 pkg (8 oz)	220
Risotto Parmesano	1 pkg (8 oz)	360
Mahatma		
Broccoli & Cheese	1 cup	200
Jambalaya	1 cup (2 oz)	190
Long Grain & Wild	1 cup (2 oz)	190
Pilaf	1 cup (2 oz)	190
Spanish	1 cup (2 oz)	180
Yellow Rice Mix	1 cup	190
Melting Pot		
Risotto Melanese w/ Saffron	1 cup	210
Risotto Primavera	1 cup	200
Risotto Sun-Dried Tomatoes & Peas	1 cup	200
Risotto Three Cheese	1 cup	200
Risotto Wild Mushroom	1 cup	200
Minute		
Boil-In-Bag White as prep	1 cup (5.7 oz)	190
Instant Brown as prep	1 cup (5.2 oz)	170
Instant White as prep	1 cup (5.7 oz)	160
Long Grain & Wild Seasoned w/ Herbs as prep	1 cup (7.8 oz)	230
Near East		
Barley Pilaf as prep	1 cup	220
Beef Pilaf as prep	1 cup	220

FOOD	PORTION	CALS.
Near East (CONT.)		
Curry Rice as prep	1 cup	220
Lentil Pilaf as prep	1 cup	210
Long Grain & Wild as prep	1 cup	220
Pilaf Brown Rice as prep	1 cup	220
Pilaf Chicken as prep	1 cup	220
Pilaf Kosher as prep	1 cup	220
Spanish Pilaf as prep	1 cup	230
Old El Paso		
Mexican	½ cup (4 oz)	410
Spanish	1 cup (8.6 oz)	130
Pritikin		
Mexican	⅓ cup (2 oz)	200
Oriental	⅓ cup (2 oz)	190
Success		
Beef Oriental	½ cup	190
Broccoli & Cheese	½ cup	200
Brown & Wild	½ cup	190
Classic Chicken	½ cup	150
Long Grain & Wild	½ cup	190
Pilaf	½ cup	200
Spanish	½ cup	190
Ultra Slim-Fast		
Oriental Style	2.3 oz	240
Rice & Chicken Sauce	2.3 oz	240
Uncle Ben		
Boil-In-Bag	1 serv (0.9 oz)	94
Brown	1 serv (1.6 oz)	158
Brown & Wild Fast Cooking	1 serv (1.3 oz)	120
Country Inn Broccoli Almondine	1 serv (1.2 oz)	124
Country Inn Broccoli & White Cheddar	1 serv (1.2 oz)	131
Country Inn Broccoli Au Gratin	1 serv (1.1 oz)	116
Country Inn Chicken Stock	1 serv (1.2 oz)	123
Country Inn Chicken With Wild Rice	1 serv (1.1 oz)	108
Country Inn Creamy Chicken & Mushroom	1 serv (1.3 oz)	138
Country Inn Creamy Chicken & Wild Rice	1 serv (1.3 oz)	135
Country Inn Green Bean Almondine	1 serv (1.2 oz)	128
Country Inn Herbed Au Gratin	1 serv (1.2 oz)	119
Country Inn Homestyle Chicken & Vegetables	1 serv (1.3 oz)	139
Country Inn Rice Florentine	1 serv (1.2 oz)	212
Country Inn Vegetable Pilaf	1 serv (1.2 oz)	115
In An Instant	1 serv (1.1 oz)	111
Long Grain & Wild Chicken Stock Sauce	1 serv (1.3 oz)	133

FOOD	PORTION	CALS.
Uncle Ben (CONT.)		
Long Grain & Wild Fast Cooking	1 serv (1 oz)	101
Long Grain & Wild Garden Vegetable Blend	1 serv (1.3 oz)	128
Long Grain & Wild Original	1 serv (1 oz)	96
White Converted	1 serv (1.2 oz)	123
Van Camp's		
Spanish	1 cup (9 oz)	180
Watkins		
Brown & Wild	¼ cup (1.6 oz)	160
Calico Medley	¼ cup (1.6 oz)	160
East/West Medley	¼ cup (1.6 oz)	160
Heartland Medley	¼ cup (1.6 oz)	160
Minnesota Medley	¼ cup (1.6 oz)	160
White & Wild	¼ cup (1.6 oz)	160
TAKE-OUT		
nasi goreng indonesian rice & vegetables	1 cup (4.9 oz)	130
paella	1 serv (7 oz)	308

RICE CAKES

(*see also* POPCORN CAKES)

FOOD	PORTION	CALS.
brown rice	1 (0.3 oz)	35
brown rice & buckwheat	1 (0.3 oz)	34
brown rice & buckwheat unsalted	1 (0.3 oz)	34
brown rice & corn	1 (0.3 oz)	35
brown rice & rye	1 (0.3 oz)	35
brown rice & sesame seed	1 (0.3 oz)	35
brown rice multigrain	1 (0.3 oz)	35
brown rice multigrain unsalted	1 (0.3 oz)	35
brown rice unsalted	1 (0.3 oz)	35
Estee		
Banana Nut	5	60
Cinnamon Spice	5	60
Granny Smith Apple	5	60
Mixed Berry	5	60
Peanut Butter Crunch	5	60
Hain		
5-Grain	1	40
Mini Apple Cinnamon	0.5 oz	60
Mini Barbeque	0.5 oz	70
Mini Cheese	0.5 oz	60
Mini Honey Nut	0.5 oz	60
Mini Nacho Cheese	0.5 oz	70
Mini Plain	0.5 oz	60

FOOD	PORTION	CALS.
Hain (CONT.)		
Mini Plain No Salt Added	0.5 oz	60
Mini Ranch	0.5 oz	70
Mini Teriyaki	½ oz	50
Plain	1	40
Plain No Salt Added	1	40
Sesame	1	40
Sesame No Salt	1	40
Lundberg		
Organic Lightly Salted	1	60
Organic Unsalted	1	60
Premium Lightly Salted	1	60
Premium Unsalted	1	60
Sesame Lightly Salted	1	59
Mother's		
Mini Apple	5 (0.5 oz)	50
Mini Caramel	5 (0.5 oz)	50
Mini Cinnamon	5 (0.5 oz)	50
Mini Plain Unsalted	7 (0.5 oz)	60
Multigrain Lightly Salted	1 (0.3 oz)	35
Rye Unsalted	1 (0.3 oz)	35
Wheat Unsalted	1 (0.3 oz)	35
Pritikin		
Mini Apple Crisp	5 (0.5 oz)	50
Multigrain	1 (0.3 oz)	35
Multigrain Unsalted	1 (0.3 oz)	35
Plain	1 (0.3 oz)	35
Plain Unsalted	1 (0.3 oz)	35
Sesame Low Sodium	1 (0.3 oz)	35
Sesame Unsalted	1 (0.3 oz)	35
Quaker		
Apple Cinnamon	1 (0.5 oz)	50
Banana Crunch	1 (0.5 oz)	50
Cinnamon Crunch	1 (0.5 oz)	50
Mini Apple Cinnamon	5 (0.5 oz)	50
Mini Banana Nut	5 (0.5 oz)	50
Mini Butter Popped Corn	6 (0.5 oz)	50
Mini Caramel Corn	5 (0.5 oz)	50
Mini Chocolate Crunch	5 (0.5 oz)	50
Mini Cinnamon Crunch	5 (0.5 oz)	50
Mini Honey Nut	5 (0.5 oz)	50
Mini Monterey Jack	6 (0.5 oz)	50
Mini White Cheddar	6 (0.5 oz)	50
Salt-Free	1 (0.3 oz)	35

FOOD	PORTION	CALS.
Quaker (CONT.)		
Salted	1 (0.3 oz)	35
Tree Of Life		
Fat Free Mini Apple Cinnamon	15	60
Fat Free Mini Caramel	15	60
Fat Free Mini Honey Nut	15	60
Fat Free Mini Jalapeno	15	60
Fat Free Mini Plain	15	50
Weight Watchers		
Apple Cinnamon	1 oz	110
Butter	1 oz	110
Caramel	1 oz	110
White Cheddar	1 oz	100

ROCKFISH

pacific cooked	3 oz	103

ROE

(*see also individual fish names*)

fish	3.5 oz	39
fresh baked	1 oz	58

ROLL

(*see also* BISCUIT, CROISSANT, ENGLISH MUFFIN, MUFFIN, POPOVER, SCONE)

FROZEN

New York		
Garlic	1 (2 oz)	210
Sara Lee		
Deluxe Cinnamon Rolls w/ Icing	1 (2.7 oz)	370
Deluxe Cinnamon Rolls w/o Icing	1 (2.7 oz)	320

HOME RECIPE

dinner as prep w/ 2% milk	1 (2½ in)	111
dinner as prep w/ whole milk	1 (2½ in)	112
raisin & nut	1 (2 oz)	196

MIX

Natural Ovens		
German Hard	1 (2.1 oz)	138
Gourmet Dinner	1 (1 oz)	50
Hearty Sandwich	1 (1.8 oz)	110

READY-TO-EAT

brioche sweet roll	1 (3.5 oz)	410
brown & serve	1 (1 oz)	85
cheese	1 (2.3 oz)	238
cinnamon raisin	1 (2¾ in)	223

FOOD	PORTION	CALS.
dinner	1 (1 oz)	85
egg	1 (2½ in)	107
french	1 (1.3 oz)	105
hamburger	1 (1.5 oz)	123
hamburger multi-grain	1 (1.5 oz)	113
hamburger reduced calorie	1 (1.5 oz)	84
hard	1 (3½ in)	167
hotdog	1 (1.5 oz)	123
hotdog multi-grain	1 (1.5 oz)	113
hotdog reduced calorie	1 (1.5 oz)	84
kaiser	1 (3½ in)	167
oat bran	1 (1.2 oz)	78
rye	1 (1 oz)	81
wheat	1 (1 oz)	77
whole wheat	1 (1 oz)	75
Alvarado St. Bakery		
Burger Buns	1 (2.2 oz)	140
Hot Dog Buns	1 (2.2 oz)	140
Arnold		
8-inch Francisco	1 (2.5 oz)	210
Augusto Pan Cubano	1	230
Bakery Light	1 (1.5 oz)	80
Bran'nola Buns	1 (1.5 oz)	100
Deli Kaiser	1	170
Deli Onion	1	170
Dinner Plain	1 (0.7 oz)	50
Dinner Sesame	1 (0.7 oz)	50
Dutch Egg	1	130
French Francisco	1 (2.5 oz)	210
French Mini Francisco	1	130
Hamburger	1	120
Hot Dog	1 (1.5 oz)	110
Hot Dog Bran'nola	1 (1.5 oz)	110
Hot Dog New England Style	1	110
Italian 8-inch Savoni	1	210
Kaiser Francisco	1 (2 oz)	180
Onion Premium	1 (2.6 oz)	180
Onion Soft	1	140
Party Petite	2	70
Potato	1	140
Sandwich Soft Sesame	1	130
Sourdough Brown N' Serve	1 (1 oz)	100
Sourdough Francisco	1 (1 oz)	100
Wheat Old Fashioned	2	80

FOOD	PORTION	CALS.
August Bros.		
Dinner	1	90
Kaiser	1	170
Onion	1	160
Sesame Cubano	1	170
Bread Du Jour		
Cracked Wheat	1 (1.2 oz)	100
Italian	1 (1.2 oz)	90
Sourdough	1 (1.2 oz)	90
Dicarlo's		
Extra Sourdough	1 (1.6 oz)	100
French	1 (1 oz)	70
Freihofer's		
Brown 'N Serve	1 (1 oz)	80
Home Pride		
Dinner Wheat	1 (1.9 oz)	160
Hamburger Potato Bun	1 (1.9 oz)	130
Hot Dog Potato Bun	1 (1.9 oz)	130
Sandwich Roll Wheat	1 (1.9 oz)	160
White	2 (1.6 oz)	130
Levy		
Sub Old Country	1	180
Martin's		
Big Marty Poppy	1	170
Big Marty Sesame	1	170
Hoagie	1	240
Hoagie Sesame	1	240
Potato Dinner	1	100
Potato Long	1	140
Potato Party	1	50
Potato Sandwich	1	140
Sandwich Whole Wheat 100% Stoneground	1	160
Pepperidge Farm		
Brown & Serve Club	1 (1.6 oz)	120
Roman Meal		
Brown & Serve	2 (2 oz)	140
Dinner	2 (2 oz)	136
Hamburger	1 (1.6 oz)	111
Hotdog	1 (1.5 oz)	103
Sandwich	1 (2.7 oz)	181
Sandwich	1 (2.7 oz)	181
San Francisco		
Sourdough	1 (1.8 oz)	180

FOOD	PORTION	CALS.
The Baker		
Honey Cinnamon Raisin	1 (2 oz)	150
Wonder		
Brown & Serve	1 (1 oz)	80
Brown & Serve Sourdough	1 (1 oz)	70
Brown & Serve Wheat	1 (1 oz)	80
Bun	1 (3 oz)	220
Club French	1 (1.6 oz)	120
Club Grain	1 (1.6 oz)	120
Club Sourdough	1 (1.6 oz)	120
Dinner	2 (1.6 oz)	130
Dinner Honey Rich	1 (1.3 oz)	100
Dinner Wheat	2 (1.6 oz)	140
Hamburger	1 (2.5 oz)	190
Hamburger	1 (2 oz)	150
Hamburger	1 (2.5 oz)	180
Hamburger	1 (1.5 oz)	110
Hamburger Wheat	1 (1.9 oz)	140
Hamburger Wheat	1 (1.5 oz)	120
Hoagie French	1 (3 oz)	220
Hoagie Grain	1 (3 oz)	220
Hoagie Sourdough	1 (3 oz)	220
Hot Dog	1 (2 oz)	160
Kaiser	1 (2.2 oz)	180
Kaiser Hoagie	1 (3 oz)	220
Multigrain	1 (1.8 oz)	140
Potato Bun	1 (1.5 oz)	110
Steak	1 (2.5 oz)	190
REFRIGERATED		
cinnamon w/ frosting	1	109
crescent	1 (1 oz)	98
Pillsbury		
Apple Cinnamon	1 (1.5 oz)	150
Caramel	1 (1.7 oz)	170
Cinnamon w/ Icing	1 (1.5 oz)	150
Cinnamon Raisin w/ Icing	1 (1.7 oz)	170
Cornbread Twists	1 (1.4 oz)	140
Crecents Reduced Fat	1 (1 oz)	100
Crescent	1 (1 oz)	110
Dinner	1 (1.4 oz)	110
Dinner Wheat	1 (1.4 oz)	110
Orange Sweet Roll w/ Icing	1 (1.7 oz)	150
ROSELLE		
fresh	1 cup	28

FOOD	PORTION	CALS.
ROSEMARY		
dried	1 tsp	4
RUTABAGA		
CANNED		
Sunshine		
Diced	½ cup (4.2 oz)	30
FRESH		
cooked mashed	½ cup	41
SABLEFISH		
baked	3 oz	213
smoked	1 oz	72
SAFFLOWER		
seeds dried	1 oz	147
SAFFRON		
saffron	1 tsp	2
SAGE		
ground	1 tsp	2
Watkins		
Sage	¼ tsp (0.5 g)	0
SALAD		
(*see also* LETTUCE, PASTA SALAD)		
MIX		
Dole		
Caesar Salad	⅓ pkg (3.5 oz)	170
Classic Blend	3.5 oz	25
Coleslaw Blend	3.5 oz	30
French Blend	3.5 oz	25
Italian Blend	3.5 oz	25
Salad-In-A- Minute Oriental	3.5 oz	110
Salad-In-A- Minute Spinach	3.5 oz	180
Fresh Express		
American Salad	1½ cups (3 oz)	20
Caesar Salad	1½ cups (3 oz)	140
European Salad	1½ cups (3 oz)	20
Garden Salad	1½ cups (3 oz)	20
Italian Salad	1½ cups (3 oz)	20
Oriental Salad	1½ cups (3 oz)	120
Riviera Salad	1½ cups (3 oz)	10
Spinach Salad	1½ cups (3 oz)	130
Suddenly Salad		
Caesar	¾ cup	220

FOOD	PORTION	CALS.
Suddenly Salad (CONT.)		
Caesar Low Fat Recipe	¾ cup	170
Italian Pepperoni	1 cup	190
Italian Pepperoni Low Fat Recipe	1 cup	180
Ranch & Bacon	¾ cup	330
Ranch & Bacon Low Fat Recipe	¾ cup	180
Weight Watchers		
Caesar Salad	1 serv (3.5 oz)	60
Caesar Salad w/ Cookies	1 pkg (4.3 oz)	160
European Salad	1 serv (3.5 oz)	60
European Salad w/ Cookies	1 pkg (4.3 oz)	160
Garden Salad	1 serv (3.5 oz)	60
Garden Salad w/ Cookies	1 pkg (4 oz)	120
TAKE-OUT		
caesar	2 cups (5 oz)	235
tossed w/o dressing	1½ cups	32
tossed w/o dressing	¾ cup	16
tossed w/o dressing w/ cheese & egg	1½ cups	102
tossed w/o dressing w/ chicken	1½ cups	105
tossed w/o dressing w/ pasta & seafood	1½ cups (14.6 oz)	380
tossed w/o dressing w/ shrimp	1½ cups	107

SALAD DRESSING
MIX

FOOD	PORTION	CALS.
Et Tu		
Caesar Salad Kit	1 serv	140
Good Seasons		
Cheese Garlic as prep	2 tbsp (1 oz)	140
Fat Free Honey Mustard as prep	2 tbsp (1.2 oz)	20
Fat Free Italian as prep	2 tbsp (1.1 oz)	10
Fat Free Ranch as prep	2 tbsp (1.2 oz)	20
Fat Free Zesty Herb as prep	2 tbsp (1.1 oz)	10
Garlic & Herbs as prep	2 tbsp (1 oz)	140
Gourmet Caesar as prep	2 tbsp (1.1 oz)	150
Gourmet Parmesan Italian as prep	2 tbsp (1.1 oz)	150
Honey French as prep	2 tbsp (1.2 oz)	160
Honey Mustard as prep	2 tbsp (1.1 oz)	150
Italian as prep	2 tbsp (1 oz)	140
Mexican Spice as prep	2 tbsp (1.1 oz)	140
Mild Italian as prep	2 tbsp (1.1 oz)	150
Oriental Sesame as prep	2 tbsp (1.1 oz)	150
Reduced Calorie Italian as prep	2 tbsp (1 oz)	50
Reduced Calorie Zesty Italian as prep	2 tbsp (1 oz)	50
Roasted Garlic as prep	2 tbsp (1.1 oz)	150

FOOD	PORTION	CALS.
Good Seasons (CONT.)		
Zesty Italian as prep	2 tbsp (1 oz)	140
Hain		
No Oil 1000 Island	1 tbsp	12
No Oil Bleu Cheese	1 tbsp	14
No Oil Buttermilk	1 tbsp	11
No Oil Caesar	1 tbsp	6
No Oil French	1 tbsp	12
No Oil Garlic & Cheese	1 tbsp	6
No Oil Herb	1 tbsp	2
No Oil Italian	1 tbsp	2
READY-TO-EAT		
Estee		
Creamy French	2 tbsp (1 oz)	10
Italian	2 tbsp	5
Hain		
1000 Island	1 tbsp	50
Canola Garden Tomato	1 tbsp	60
Canola Italian	1 tbsp	50
Canola Spicy French Mustard	1 tbsp	50
Canola Tangy Citrus	1 tbsp	50
Creamy Caesar	1 tbsp	60
Creamy Caesar Low Salt	1 tbsp	60
Creamy French	1 tbsp	60
Creamy Italian	1 tbsp	80
Creamy Italian No Salt Added	1 tbsp	80
Cucumber Dill	1 tbsp	80
Dijon Vinaigrette	1 tbsp	50
Garlic & Sour Cream	1 tbsp	70
Honey & Sesame	1 tbsp	60
Italian Cheese Vinaigrette	1 tbsp	55
Old Fashioned Buttermilk	1 tbsp	70
Poppyseed Rancher's	1 tbsp	60
Savory Herb No Salt Added	1 tbsp	90
Swiss Cheese Vinaigrette	1 tbsp	60
Traditional Italian	1 tbsp	80
Traditional Italian No Salt Added	1 tbsp	60
Hollywood		
Caesar	1 tbsp	70
Creamy French	1 tbsp	70
Creamy Italian	1 tbsp	90
Dijon Vinaigrette	1 tbsp	60
Italian	1 tbsp	90
Italian Cheese	1 tbsp	80

FOOD	PORTION	CALS.
Hollywood (CONT.)		
Old Fashion Buttermilk	1 tbsp	75
Poppy Seed Rancher's	1 tbsp	75
Thousand Island	1 tbsp	60
Kraft		
⅓ Less Fat Catalina	2 tbsp (1.2 oz)	80
⅓ Less Fat Cucumber Ranch	2 tbsp (1.1 oz)	60
⅓ Less Fat Italian	2 tbsp (1.1 oz)	70
⅓ Less Fat Ranch	2 tbsp (1.1)	110
⅓ Less Fat Thousand Island	2 tbsp (1.2 oz)	70
Bacon & Tomato	2 tbsp (1.1 oz)	140
Buttermilk Ranch	2 tbsp (1.1 oz)	150
Caesar Italian	2 tbsp (1.1 oz)	100
Caesar Ranch	2 tbsp (1.1 oz)	110
Catalina	2 tbsp (1.1 oz)	120
Catalina With Honey	2 tbsp (1.1 oz)	130
Classic Caesar	2 tbsp (1.1 oz)	110
Coleslaw	2 tbsp (1.1 oz)	130
Creamy French	2 tbsp (1.1 oz)	160
Creamy Garlic	2 tbsp (1.1 oz)	110
Creamy Italian	2 tbsp (1.1 oz)	110
Cucumber Ranch	2 tbsp (1.1 oz)	140
Free Blue Cheese	2 tbsp (1.2 oz)	45
Free Caesar Italian	2 tbsp (1.2 oz)	25
Free Catalina	2 tbsp (1.2 oz)	35
Free Classic Caesar	2 tbsp (1.2 oz)	45
Free Creamy Italian	2 tbsp (1.2 oz)	50
Free French	2 tbsp (1.2 oz)	45
Free Garlic Ranch	2 tbsp (1.2 oz)	45
Free Honey Dijon	2 tbsp (1.2 oz)	45
Free Italian	2 tbsp (1.2 oz)	20
Free Peppercorn Ranch	2 tbsp (1.2 oz)	45
Free Ranch	1 tbsp (1.2 oz)	50
Free Red Wine Vinegar	2 tbsp (1.1 oz)	15
Free Thousand Island	2 tbsp (1.2 oz)	40
Garlic Ranch	2 tbsp (1.1 oz)	180
Herb Vinaigrette	2 tbsp (1.1 oz)	140
Honey Dijon	2 tbsp (1.1 oz)	110
Honey Mustard	2 tbsp (1.1 oz)	110
House Italian w/ Olive Oil Blend	2 tbsp (1.1 oz)	120
Peppercorn Ranch	2 tbsp (1 oz)	170
Pesto Italian	2 tbsp (1.1 oz)	90
Ranch	2 tbsp (1 oz)	170
Roka Blue Cheese	2 tbsp (1.1 oz)	130

FOOD	PORTION	CALS.
Kraft (CONT.)		
Russian	2 tbsp (1.2 oz)	130
Sour Cream & Onion Ranch	2 tbsp (1 oz)	170
Thousand Island	2 tbsp (1.1 oz)	110
Thousand Island With Bacon	2 tbsp (1.1 oz)	130
Tomato & Herb Italian	2 tbsp (1.1 oz)	100
Zesty Italian	2 tbsp (1.1 oz)	110
Marzetti		
Bacon Spinach Salad	2 tbsp	80
Blue Cheese	2 tbsp	160
Buttermilk & Herb	2 tbsp	180
Buttermilk Bacon Ranch	2 tbsp	180
Buttermilk Blue Cheese	2 tbsp	160
Buttermilk Parmesan Pepper	2 tbsp	170
Buttermilk Parmesan Ranch	2 tbsp	160
Buttermilk Ranch	2 tbsp	180
Buttermilk Veggie Dip	2 tbsp	170
Caesar	2 tbsp	150
Caesar Ranch	2 tbsp	190
California French	2 tbsp	160
Celery Seed	2 tbsp	160
Chunky Blue Cheese	2 tbsp	150
Classic Caesar Ranch	2 tbsp	190
Country French	2 tbsp	150
Cracked Peppercorn	2 tbsp	140
Creamy Garlic Italian	2 tbsp	160
Creamy Italian	2 tbsp	150
Crispy Celery Seed	2 tbsp	160
Dijon Honey Mustard	2 tbsp	140
Dijon Ranch	2 tbsp	170
Dutch Sweet'N Sour	2 tbsp	160
Fat Free California French	2 tbsp	45
Fat Free Honey Dijon	2 tbsp	60
Fat Free Honey French	2 tbsp	45
Fat Free Italian	2 tbsp	15
Fat Free Peppercorn Ranch	2 tbsp	30
Fat Free Ranch	2 tbsp	30
Fat Free Raspberry	2 tbsp	70
Fat Free Slaw	2 tbsp	45
Fat Free Sweet & Sour	2 tbsp	45
Fat Free Thousand Island	2 tbsp	35
Garden Ranch	2 tbsp	180
Gusto Italian	2 tbsp	120
Honey Dijon	2 tbsp	140

FOOD	PORTION	CALS.
Marzetti (CONT.)		
Honey Dijon Ranch	2 tbsp	150
Honey French	2 tbsp	160
Honey French Blue Cheese	2 tbsp	160
House Caesar	2 tbsp	150
Italian With Olive Oil	2 tbsp	120
Light Blue Cheese	2 tbsp	60
Light Buttermilk Ranch	2 tbsp	90
Light California French	2 tbsp	80
Light Chunky Blue Cheese	2 tbsp	80
Light French	2 tbsp	40
Light French	2 tbsp	40
Light Honey French	2 tbsp	80
Light Italian	2 tbsp	60
Light Ranch	2 tbsp	90
Light Red Wine Vinegar & Oil	2 tbsp	20
Light Slaw	2 tbsp	60
Light Sweet & Sour	2 tbsp	100
Light Thousand Island	2 tbsp	70
Old Fashioned Poppyseed	2 tbsp	140
Olde Venice Italain	2 tbsp	130
Olde World Caesar	2 tbsp	150
Parmesan Pepper	2 tbsp	160
Peppercorn Ranch	2 tbsp	180
Poppyseed	2 tbsp	160
Potato Salad Dressing	2 tbsp	120
Ranch	2 tbsp	180
Red Wine Vinegar & Oil	2 tbsp	130
Romano Cheese Caesar	2 tbsp	150
Romano Italian	2 tbsp	160
Savory Italian	2 tbsp	110
Slaw	2 tbsp	170
Southern Slaw	2 tbsp	100
Sweet & Saucy	2 tbsp	140
Sweet & Sour	2 tbsp	160
Thousand Island	2 tbsp	150
Vintage Champagne	2 tbsp	150
Wilde Raspberry	2 tbsp	150
Nasoya		
Creamy Dill	2 tbsp (1 oz)	63
Creamy Italian	2 tbsp (1 oz)	60
Garden Herb	2 tbsp (1 oz)	61
Sesame Garlic	2 tbsp (1 oz)	63
Thousand Island	2 tbsp (1 oz)	62

FOOD	PORTION	CALS.
Newman's Own		
Balsamic Vinaigrette	2 tbsp (1.1 oz)	90
Caesar	2 tbsp (1.1 oz)	150
Light Italian	2 tbsp (1.1 oz)	20
Olive Oil & Vinegar	2 tbsp (1 oz)	150
Ranch	2 tbsp (1 oz)	180
Pfeiffer		
1000 Island	2 tbsp	140
California French	2 tbsp	140
French	2 tbsp	150
Honey Dijon	2 tbsp	140
Lite Italian	2 tbsp	50
Ranch	2 tbsp	180
Savory Italian	2 tbsp	110
Pritikin		
Dijon Balsamic Vinaigrette	2 tbsp (1 oz)	3
French	2 tbsp (1 oz)	35
Honey Dijon	2 tbsp (1 oz)	45
Honey French	2 tbsp (1 oz)	40
Italian	2 tbsp (1 oz)	20
Raspberry Vinaigrette	2 tbsp (1 oz)	45
Red Wing		
"K" Dressing	1 tbsp (0.5 oz)	70
Chunky Blue Cheese	2 tbsp (1 oz)	130
Creamy Ranch	2 tbsp (1 oz)	150
French Traditional	2 tbsp (1 oz)	130
Italian Traditional	2 tbsp (1 oz)	100
Spicy Sweet French	2 tbsp (1 oz)	130
Thousand Island Thick & Rich	2 tbsp (1 oz)	110
Seven Seas		
1/3 Less Fat Creamy Italian	2 tbsp (1.1 oz)	60
1/3 Less Fat Italian w/ Olive Oil Blend	2 tbsp (1.1 oz)	45
1/3 Less Fat Ranch	2 tbsp (1.1 oz)	100
1/3 Less Fat Red Wine Vinegar & Oil	2 tbsp (1.1 oz)	45
1/3 Less Fat Viva Italian	2 tbsp (1.1 oz)	45
2 Cheese Italian	2 tbsp (1.1 oz)	70
Chunky Blue Cheese	2 tbsp (1.1 oz)	130
Classic Caesar	2 tbsp (1.1 oz)	100
Creamy Italian	2 tbsp (1.1 oz)	120
Free Ranch	2 tbsp (1.2 oz)	45
Free Red Wine Vinegar	2 tbsp (1.1 oz)	15
Free Sour Cream & Onion Ranch	2 tbsp (1.2 oz)	50
Free Viva Italian	2 tbsp (1.1 oz)	10
Green Goddess	2 tbsp (1.1 oz)	130

FOOD	PORTION	CALS.
Seven Seas (CONT.)		
Herbs & Spices	2 tbsp (1.1 oz)	90
Ranch	2 tbsp (1.1 oz)	160
Red Wine Vinegar & Oil	2 tbsp (1.1 oz)	90
Viva Italian	2 tbsp (1.1 oz)	90
Viva Russian	2 tbsp (1.1 oz)	150
Tree Of Life		
Cafe Venice	2 tbsp (1 oz)	100
Fat Free Blue Cheese	2 tbsp (1 oz)	15
Fat Free Honey French	2 tbsp (1 oz)	35
Fat Free Italian Garlic	2 tbsp (1 oz)	20
Fat Free Oriental Ginger	2 tbsp (1 oz)	15
Frisco's Raspberry	2 tbsp (1 oz)	120
Maison Caesar	2 tbsp (1 oz)	70
Shanghai Palace	2 tbsp (1 oz)	80
Ultra Slim-Fast		
French	1 tbsp	20
Italian	1 tbsp	6
W.J. Clark		
Ginger Orange Vinaigrette	1 tbsp	73
Herbs & Romano	1 tbsp	67
Lemon Peppercorn	1 tbsp	72
Lime Cilantro Vinaigrette	1 tbsp	73
Poppy Seed	1 tbsp	75
Sweet Pepper Basil	1 tbsp	69
Tarragon Honey Mustard	1 tbsp	66
Walden Farms		
Fat Free Balsamic Vinaigrette	2 tbsp (1 oz)	15
Fat Free Bleu Cheese	2 tbsp (1 oz)	25
Fat Free Caesar	2 tbsp (1 oz)	25
Fat Free Creamy Italian With Parmesan	1 tbsp (1 oz)	25
Fat Free French Style	2 tbsp (1 oz)	25
Fat Free Honey Dijon	2 tbsp (1 oz)	25
Fat Free Italian	2 tbsp (1 oz)	10
Fat Free Ranch	2 tbsp (1 oz)	25
Fat Free Raspberry Vinaigrette	2 tbsp (1 oz)	20
Fat Free Russian	2 tbsp (1 oz)	30
Fat Free Sodium Free Italian	2 tbsp (1 oz)	10
Fat Free Sugar Free Italian	2 tbsp (1 oz)	0
Fat Free Thousand Island	2 tbsp (1 oz)	35
Italian With Sun Dried Tomato	2 tbsp (1 oz)	15
Ranch With Sun Dried Tomato	2 tbsp (1 oz)	25
Weight Watchers		
Fat Free Caesar	1 pkg (0.75 oz)	5

FOOD	PORTION	CALS.
Weight Watchers (CONT.)		
Fat Free Caesar	2 tbsp	10
Fat Free Creamy Italian	2 tbsp	30
Fat Free French Style	2 tbsp	40
Fat Free Honey Dijon	2 tbsp	45
Fat Free Italian	2 tbsp	10
Fat Free Ranch	2 tbsp	35
Fat Free Ranch	1 pkg (0.75 oz)	25
Wishbone		
Caesar	2 tbsp (1 oz)	90
Chunky Blue Cheese	2 tbsp (1 oz)	150
Classic House Italian	2 tbsp (1 oz)	140
Classic Olive Oil Italian	2 tbsp (1 oz)	60
Creamy Caesar	2 tbsp (1 oz)	180
Creamy Italian	2 tbsp (1 oz)	110
Creamy Roasted Garlic	2 tbsp (1 oz)	110
Deluxe French	2 tbsp (1 oz)	120
Fat Free Chunky Blue Cheese	2 tbsp (1 oz)	35
Fat Free Chunky Blue Cheese	2 tbsp	35
Fat Free Creamy Italian	2 tbsp (1 oz)	35
Fat Free Creamy Roasted Garlic	2 tbsp (1 oz)	40
Fat Free Deluxe French	2 tbsp (1 oz)	30
Fat Free Honey Dijon	2 tbsp (1 oz)	45
Fat Free Italian	2 tbsp (1 oz)	10
Fat Free Parmesan & Onion	2 tbsp (1 oz)	45
Fat Free Ranch	2 tbsp (1 oz)	40
Fat Free Red Wine Vinaigrette	2 tbsp (1 oz)	35
Fat Free Sweet N' Spicy French	2 tbsp (1 oz)	30
Fat Free Thousand Island	2 tbsp (1 oz)	35
Italian	2 tbsp (1 oz)	80
Lite French	2 tbsp (1 oz)	50
Lite Italian	2 tbsp (1 oz)	15
Lite Ranch	2 tbsp (1 oz)	100
Olive Oil Vinaigrette	2 tbsp (1 oz)	60
Oriental	2 tbsp (1 oz)	70
Parmesan & Onion	2 tbsp (1 oz)	110
Ranch	2 tbsp (1 oz)	160
Red Wine Vinaigrette	2 tbsp (1 oz)	80
Robusto Italian	2 tbsp (1 oz)	90
Russian	2 tbsp (1 oz)	110
Sweet N' Spicy French	2 tbsp (1 oz)	140
Thousand Island	2 tbsp (1 oz)	140

SALMON
CANNED

Bumble Bee

Keta	3.5 oz	160

FOOD	PORTION	CALS.
Bumble Bee (CONT.)		
Pink	3.5 oz	160
Pink Skinless & Boneless	3.25 oz	120
Red	3.5 oz	180
Red Skinless & Boneless	3.25 oz	130
FRESH		
atlantic baked	3 oz	155
chinook baked	3 oz	196
chum baked	3 oz	131
coho cooked	3 oz	157
roe raw	3.5 oz	207
sockeye cooked	3 oz	183
SMOKED		
chinook	1 oz	33
Nathan's		
Nova	2 oz	80
TAKE-OUT		
roulette w/ spinach stuffing	1 serv (4 oz)	160

SALSA

(*see also* KETCHUP, SAUCE, SPANISH FOOD)

FOOD	PORTION	CALS.
Chi-Chi's		
Con Queso	2 tbsp (1.1 oz)	90
Hot	2 tbsp (1 oz)	10
Medium	2 tbsp (1 oz)	10
Mild	2 tbsp (1 oz)	10
Picante Hot	2 tbsp (1 oz)	10
Picante Medium	2 tbsp (1 oz)	10
Picante Mild	2 tbsp (1 oz)	10
Verde Medium	2 tbsp (1.2 oz)	15
Verde Mild	2 tbsp (1.2 oz)	15
Del Monte		
Mexicana	2 tbsp (1.1 oz)	5
Taquera	2 tbsp (1.1 oz)	5
Verde	2 tbsp (1.1 oz)	10
Guiltless Gourmet		
Picante Hot	1 oz	6
Picante Medium	1 oz	6
Hain		
Hot	¼ cup	22
Mild	¼ cup	20
Heluva Good Cheese		
Cheese & Salsa	2 tbsp (1.1 oz)	80
Thick & Chunky Hot	2 tbsp (1.2 oz)	10

FOOD	PORTION	CALS.
Heluva Good Cheese (CONT.)		
Thick & Chunky Mild	2 tbsp (1.2 oz)	10
Hot Cha Cha		
Medium	2 tbsp (1 oz)	5
Hunt's		
Alfresco Medium	2 tbsp (1.1 oz)	10
Alfresco Mild	2 tbsp (1.1 oz)	10
Hot	2 tbsp (1.1 oz)	27
Medium	2 tbsp (1.1 oz)	27
Mild	2 tbsp (1.1 oz)	27
Picante Medium	2 tbsp (1.1 oz)	11
Picante Mild	2 tbsp (1.1 oz)	11
Louise's		
Fat Free BBQ Black Bean	1 oz	10
Fat Free Black Bean	1 oz	10
Fat Free Medium	1 oz	10
Fat Free Mild	1 oz	10
Fat Free Nacho Queso	1 oz	15
Muir Glen		
Organic Fat Free Hot	2 tbsp (1.1 oz)	10
Organic Fat Free Medium	2 tbsp (1.1 oz)	10
Organic Fat Free Mild	2 tbsp (1.1 oz)	10
Newman's Own		
Bandito Hot	2 tbsp (1.1 oz)	10
Bandito Medium	2 tbsp (1.1 oz)	10
Bandito Mild	2 tbsp (1.1 oz)	10
Peach	2 tbsp (1.1 oz)	25
Pineapple	2 tbsp (1.1 oz)	15
Roasted Garlic	2 tbsp (1.1 oz)	10
Old El Paso		
Green Chili Medium	2 tbsp (1 oz)	10
Homestyle	2 tbsp (1 oz)	5
Homestyle Mild	2 tbsp (1 oz)	5
Picante Hot	2 tbsp (1 oz)	10
Picante Medium	2 tbsp (1 oz)	10
Picante Mild	2 tbsp (1 oz)	10
Picante Thick'n Chunky Hot	2 tbsp (1 oz)	10
Picante Thick'n Chunky Medium	2 tbsp (1 oz)	10
Picante Thick'n Chunky Mild	2 tbsp (1 oz)	10
Pico De Gallo Hot	2 tbsp (1 oz)	5
Pico De Gallo Medium	1 tbsp (1 oz)	5
Salsa Verde	2 tbsp (1 oz)	10
Thick'n Chunky Hot	2 tbsp (1 oz)	10
Thick'n Chunky Medium	2 tbsp (1 oz)	10

FOOD	PORTION	CALS.
Old El Paso (CONT.)		
Thick'n Chunky Mild	2 tbsp (1 oz)	10
Ortega		
Hot Green Chili	1 tbsp	6
Medium Green Chili	1 tbsp	6
Mild Green Chili	1 tbsp	8
Pace		
Picante	2 tbsp (1 fl oz)	7
Thick & Chunky	2 tbsp (1 fl oz)	12
Progresso		
Italian Hot	2 tbsp (1 oz)	30
Italian Medium	2 tbsp (1 oz)	10
Italian Mild	2 tbsp (1 oz)	10
Tabasco		
Picante	2 tbsp (1.5 oz)	17
Taco Bell		
Smooth 'N Zesty Picante Medium	2 tbsp (1.1 oz)	15
Smooth 'N Zesty Picante Mild	2 tbsp (1.1 oz)	15
Thick 'N Chunky Salsa Hot	2 tbsp (1.1 oz)	15
Thick 'N Chunky Salsa Medium	2 tbsp (1.1 oz)	15
Thick 'N Chunky Salsa Mild	2 tbsp (1.1 oz)	15
Tostitos		
Con Queso	2.3 oz	80
Hot	2.3 oz	30
Low Fat Con Queso	2.5 oz	80
Medium	2.3 oz	30
Mild	2.3 oz	30
Restaurant Style	2.2 oz	30
Ultimate Garden	2.4 oz	30
Tree Of Life		
Hot	2 tbsp (1 oz)	10
Medium	2 tbsp (1 oz)	10
Mild	2 tbsp (1 oz)	10
No Salt	2 tbsp (1 oz)	10
Utz		
Chunky	2 tbsp (1 fl oz)	60
Watkins		
Salsa Seasoning Blend	⅛ tsp (0.5 g)	0
Tropical	2 tbsp (1 oz)	60
Wise		
Picante	2 tbsp	12

SALSIFY

FOOD	PORTION	CALS.
fresh sliced cooked	½ cup	46
raw sliced	½ cup	55

FOOD	PORTION	CALS.

SALT/SEASONED SALT
   (*see also* SALT SUBSTITUTES)

salt	1 tbsp (18 g)	0
salt	1 tsp (6 g)	0
Hain		
Sea Salt	1 tsp	0
Sea Salt Iodized	1 tsp	0
Watkins		
Bacon Cheese Salt	¼ tbsp (1 g)	0
Butter Salt	¼ tbsp (1 g)	0
Cheese Salt	¼ tbsp (1 g)	0
Garlic Salt	¼ tsp (1 g)	0
Salt & Vinegar Seasoning	¼ tsp (1 g)	0
Seasoning Salt	¼ tsp (1 g)	0
Sour Cream & Onion Salt	¼ tbsp (1 g)	0

SALT SUBSTITUTES
Cardia

Salt Alternative	1 pkg (0.6 g)	0
Estee		
Salt-It	¼ tsp	0
Mrs. Dash		
Onion & Herb	⅛ tsp (0.02 oz)	2
NoSalt		
Salt Alternative	1 pkg (0.75 g)	0
Papa Dash		
Lite Salt	½ tsp (1 g)	0

SANDWICH
TAKE-OUT

chicken fillet plain	1	515
chicken fillet w/ cheese lettuce mayonnaise & tomato	1	632
fish fillet w/ tartar sauce	1	431
fish fillet w/ tartar sauce & cheese	1	524
fried egg w/ cheese	1	340
fried egg w/ cheese & ham	1	348
ham w/ cheese	1	353
roast beef submarine sandwich w/ tomato lettuce & mayonnaise	1	411
roast beef w/ cheese	1	402
roast beef plain	1	346
steak w/ tomato lettuce salt & mayonnaise	1	459
submarine w/ salami ham cheese lettuce tomato onion & oil	1	456

FOOD	PORTION	CALS.
tuna salad submarine sandwich w/ lettuce & oil	1	584

SAPODILLA
fresh	1	140
fresh cut up	1 cup	199

SAPOTES
fresh	1	301

SARDINES
CANNED
Del Monte

In Tomato Sauce	1 fish (1.4 oz)	50

Port Clyde

In Louisiana Hot Sauce	1 can (3.75 oz)	170
In Mustard Sauce	1 can (3.75 oz)	150
In Soybean Oil Select Small	1 can (3.3 oz)	220
In Soybean Oil With Hot Chilies	1 can (3.3 oz)	155
In Soybean Oil drained	1 can (3.3 oz)	220
In Spring Water	1 can (3.3 oz)	170
In Tomato Sauce	1 can (3.75 oz)	150

Underwood

Brisling In Olive Oil	3.75 oz	260
In Mustard Sauce	3.75 oz	220
In Sild Oil drained	3.75 oz	460
In Soya Oil drained	3 oz	230
In Tomato Sauce	3.75 oz	220
With Tabasco Pepper Sauce drained	3 oz	220

Viking's Delight

Brisling In Olive Oil	1 can (3.75 oz)	460
Brisling In Olive Oil drained	1 can (3.75 oz)	260

SAUCE
(*see also* BARBECUE SAUCE, GRAVY, PIZZA SAUCE, SALSA, SPAGHETTI SAUCE, TOMATO)

JARRED
Boar's Head

Ham Glaze Brown Sugar & Spice	2 tbsp (1.4 oz)	120

Cheez Whiz

Cheese	2 tbsp (1.2 oz)	90
Cheese Jalapeno Pepper	2 tbsp (1.2 oz)	90
Cheese Mild Salsa	2 tbsp (1.2 oz)	100

Chi-Chi's

Enchilada	¼ cup (2.1 oz)	30
Taco	1 tbsp (0.5 oz)	10

FOOD	PORTION	CALS.
Contadina		
Sweet 'n Sour	2 tbsp	40
Del Monte		
Cocktail	¼ cup (2.7 oz)	100
Sloppy Joe Hickory Flavor	¼ cup (2.4 oz)	70
Sloppy Joe Italian Style	¼ cup (2.4 oz)	70
Sloppy Joe Original	¼ cup (2.4 oz)	70
El Molino		
Taco Red Mild	2 tbsp	10
Escoffier		
Diable	1 tbsp	20
Fritos		
Texas-Style Chili Hearty Topping	2.3 oz	50
Utimate Taco Hearty Topping	2.3 oz	50
Green Giant		
Sloppy Joe	¼ cup (2.6 oz)	50
Sloppy Joe as prep w/ meat	1 serv (4.4 oz)	200
Heluva Good Cheese		
Cocktail	¼ cup (1.6 oz)	40
Hormel		
Not-So-Sloppy-Joe Sauce	¼ cup (2.2 oz)	70
House Of Tsang		
Bangkok Padang	1 tbsp (0.6 oz)	45
Hoisin	1 tsp (6 g)	15
Mandarin Marinade	1 tbsp (0.6 oz)	25
Saigon Sizzle	1 tbsp (0.6 oz)	40
Spicy Brown Bean	1 tsp (6 g)	15
Stir Fry Classic	1 tbsp (0.6 oz)	25
Stir Fry Sweet & Sour	1 tbsp (0.6 oz)	30
Stir Fry Szechuan Spicy	1 tbsp (0.6 oz)	20
Sweet & Sour Concentrate	1 tsp (6 g)	10
Teriyaki Korean	1 tbsp (0.6 oz)	30
Hunt's		
Chicken Sensations Barbecue Flavor	1 tbsp (0.5 oz)	35
Chicken Sensations Italian Garlic	1 tbsp (0.5 oz)	30
Chicken Sensations Lemon Herb	1 tbsp (0.5 oz)	31
Chicken Sensations South Westren	1 tbsp (0.5 oz)	27
Pepper Sauce Original	1 tsp (5.2 g)	1
Steak	1 tbsp (0.6 oz)	10
Just Rite		
Hot Dog	2 oz	60
Kraft		
Cocktail	¼ cup (2.3 oz)	60
Fat Free Tartar Sauce	2 tbsp (1.1 oz)	25

FOOD	PORTION	CALS.
Kraft (CONT.)		
Lemon & Herb Tartar Sauce	2 tbsp (1 oz)	150
Reduced Fat Sandwich Spread	1 tbsp (0.5 oz)	35
Sandwich Spread	1 tbsp (0.5 oz)	50
Sweet'n Sour	2 tbsp (1.2 oz)	60
Tartar	2 tbsp (1.1 oz)	90
Lawry's		
Marinade Lemon Pepper	1 tbsp (0.5 oz)	10
Teriyaki Marinade	2 tbsp	72
Lea & Perrins		
Steak	1 oz	40
Manwich		
Bold	¼ cup (2.2 oz)	62
Burrito	¼ cup (2.2 oz)	25
Mexican	¼ cup (2.2 oz)	27
Original	¼ cup (2.2 oz)	32
Taco	¼ cup (2.2 oz)	31
Thick & Chunky	¼ cup (2.3 oz)	44
Marzetti		
Teriyaki Stir-Fry	2 tbsp	80
McIlhenny		
Tabasco	1 tsp	1
Mrs. Dash		
Steak	1 tbsp (0.4 oz)	17
Newman's Own		
Spicy Simmer Sauce Diavolo	½ cup (4.4 oz)	70
Old El Paso		
Enchilada Hot	¼ cup (2 oz)	30
Enchilada Mild	¼ cup (2 oz)	25
Green Chili Enchilada Sauce	¼ cup (2.1 oz)	30
Taco Hot	1 tbsp (0.5 oz)	5
Taco Medium	1 tbsp (0.5 oz)	5
Taco Mild	1 tbsp (0.5 oz)	5
Taco Sauce	1 tbsp (0.5 oz)	5
Taco Sauce Extra Chunky Medium	1 tbsp (0.5 oz)	5
Taco Sauce Extra Chunky Mild	1 tbsp (0.5 oz)	5
Ortega		
Taco Thick & Smooth Hot	1 tbsp	8
Taco Thick & Smooth Mild	1 tbsp	8
Progresso		
Alfredo	½ cup (4.4 oz)	310
Red Wing		
Chili Sauce	1 tbsp (0.6 oz)	20
Seafood Cocktail	¼ cup (2 oz)	90

FOOD	PORTION	CALS.
Sauce Arturo		
Original	¼ cup (2.2 fl oz)	50
Simmer Chef		
Golden Honey Mustard	½ cup (4 fl oz)	150
Hearty Onion & Mushroom	½ cup (4 fl oz)	50
Snow's		
Newburg With Sherry	⅓ cup	120
Welsh Rarebit Cheese	½ cup	170
Tabasco		
Caribbean Steak Sauce	1 tbsp (0.6 oz)	15
Garlic Basting Sauce	1 tbsp (0.6 oz)	20
Habanero Sauce	1 tsp (0.2 oz)	5
Hot Sauce w/ Garlic	1 tsp (0.2 oz)	0
Jalepeno Pepper Sauce	1 tbsp	15
New Orleans Steak Sauce	1 tbsp (0.6 oz)	15
Pepper Sauce	1 tsp (0.2 oz)	0
Taco Bell		
Taco Sauce Medium	2 tbsp (1.1 oz)	15
Taco Sauce Mild	2 tbsp (1.1 oz)	15
The Restaurant Hot Sauce	1 tsp (5 g)	0
Tostitos		
Beef Fiesta Nacho	2.4 oz	120
Chicken Quesadilla Topping	2.5 oz	90
Watkins		
Inferno Hot Pepper Sauce	2 tbsp (1 oz)	35
Steak Sauce	1 tbsp (0.5 oz)	20
MIX		
Cajun King		
Etoufee Seasoning Mix	3.5 oz	383
Jambalaya Seasoning Mix	3.5 oz	375
Durkee		
A La King as prep	1 cup	60
Cheese as prep	¼ cup	25
Hollandaise as prep	2 tbsp	10
Nacho Cheese as prep	2 tbsp	25
White as prep	¼ cup	20
French's		
Cheese as prep	¼ cup	25
Hollandaise as prep	2 tbsp	10
Watkins		
Beef Marinade	¼ tbsp (2 g)	5
Calypso Hot Pepper Sauce	1 tsp (5 g)	10
Caribbean Red Pepper Sauce	1 tsp (5 g)	10
Chicken & Pork Marinade	¼ tbsp (2 g)	5

FOOD	PORTION	CALS.
Watkins (CONT.)		
Fish & Seafood Marinade	¼ tbsp (2 g)	10
Meat Magic	1 tsp (6 g)	10
SHELF-STABLE		
Cheez Whiz		
Cheese Sqeezable	2 tbsp (1.2 oz)	100
Fresh Gourmet		
Stir 'n Sauce Italian	1 tbsp (0.5 oz)	30
TAKE-OUT		
bearnaise	1 oz	177

SAUERKRAUT

FOOD	PORTION	CALS.
Boar's Head		
Sauerkraut	2 tbsp (1 oz)	5
Del Monte		
Canned	½ cup (4.2 oz)	15
Hebrew National		
Gallon Kraut	½ cup	25
New Kraut	½ cup (3.1 oz)	50
Rosoff's		
Sauerkraut	½ cup (3.2 oz)	50
Schorr's		
New Kraut	½ cup (3.2 oz)	50
Seneca		
Canned	2 tbsp	5
Vlasic		
Old Fashioned	1 oz	4

SAUSAGE

(*see also* HOT DOG, SAUSAGE SUBSTITUTES)

FOOD	PORTION	CALS.
bierschinken	3.5 oz	174
bierwurst	3.5 oz	258
bockwurst	3.5 oz	276
bratwurst pork cooked	1 link (3 oz)	256
brotwurst pork	1 oz	92
brotwurst pork & beef	1 link (2.5 oz)	226
chipolata	3.5 oz	342
chorizo	3.5 oz	499
fleischwurst	3.5 oz	305
jagdwurst	3.5 oz	211
zungenwurst (tongue)	3.5 oz	285
Aidells		
Andouille Cajun Cooked	1 (3.5 oz)	220
Burmese Curry Cooked	1 (3.5 oz)	220
Chicken & Apple Fresh	1 (1.9 oz)	110

FOOD	PORTION	CALS.
Aidells (CONT.)		
Chicken & Apple Smoked	1 (3.5 oz)	220
Chicken & Turkey New Mexico Smoked	1 (3.5 oz)	220
Chicken & Turkey Thai Fresh	1 (3.5 oz)	200
Chicken & Turkey Thai Smoked	1 (3.5 oz)	220
Chicken & Turkey With Sun-Dried Tomatoes & Basil Fresh	1 (3.5 oz)	200
Chicken & Turkey With Sun-Dried Tomatoes & Basil Smoked	1 (3.5 oz)	200
Creole Hot Cooked	1 (3.5 oz)	220
Duck & Turkey Smoked	1 (3.5 oz)	220
Hunter's Cooked	1 (3.5 oz)	240
Italian Hot Fresh	1 (3.5 oz)	230
Italian Mild Fresh	1 (3.5 oz)	230
Lamb & Beef With Rosemary Fresh	1 (3.5 oz)	220
Lemon Chicken Cooked	1 (3.5 oz)	220
Mexican Chorizo Beef Fresh	1 (3.5 oz)	400
Whiskey Fennel Cooked	1 (3.5 oz)	230
Banner		
Sausage Tripe	2 oz	90
Bilinski's		
Chicken & Vegetable	1 (3 oz)	80
Chicken Italian With Peppers & Onions	1 (3 oz)	120
Boar's Head		
Bratwurst	1 (4 oz)	300
Hot Smoked	1 (3.2 oz)	280
Kielbasa	2 oz	120
Knockwurst	1 (4 oz)	310
Golden Brown		
Beef	1	80
Mild	1	100
Spicy	1	100
Healthy Choice		
Low Fat Smoked	2 oz	70
Low Fat Smoked Polska Kielbasa	2 oz	70
Hebrew National		
Beef Knocks	1 (3 oz)	260
Polish Beef	1 link	240
Hillshire		
Beer Bratwurst	1 (2 oz)	190
Bratwurst Fresh	1 (2 oz)	190
Bratwurst Light Fresh	1 (2 oz)	150
Bratwurst Spicy	1 (2 oz)	180
Flavorseal Kielbasa Polska	2 oz	190

FOOD	PORTION	CALS.
Hillshire (CONT.)		
Flavorseal Kielbasa Polska Beef	2 oz	190
Flavorseal Kielbasa Polska Lite	2 oz	130
Flavorseal Kielbasa Polska Mild	2 oz	190
Flavorseal Kielbasa Polska Turkey	2 oz	90
Flavorseal Smoked	2 oz	190
Flavorseal Smoked Beef	2 oz	180
Flavorseal Smoked Beef & Cheddar	2 oz	190
Flavorseal Smoked Country Recipe	2 oz	180
Flavorseal Smoked Hot	2 oz	180
Flavorseal Smoked Lite	2 oz	130
Flavorseal Smoked Turkey	2 oz	90
Flavorseal Smoked w/ Italian Seasoning	2 oz	200
Italian Mild	1 (2 oz)	190
Italian Mild Light	1 (2 oz)	150
Italian Hot	1 (2 oz)	180
Italian Hot Light	1 (2 oz)	150
Kielbasa Fresh Polska	1 (2 oz)	190
Kielbasa Fresh Polska Lower Fat	1 (2 oz)	150
Links 80% Fat Free Cheddar Hots	2 oz	150
Links 80% Fat Free Kielbasa	2 oz	130
Links 80% Fat Free Smokies	2 oz	130
Links Brats Fully Cooked	2 oz	170
Links Bratwurst Smoked	2 oz	190
Links Bun Size Cheddarwurst	2 oz	200
Links Bun Size Kielbasa	2 oz	180
Links Bun Size Smoked	2 oz	180
Links Bun Size Smoked Beef	2 oz	180
Links Cheddarwurst	2 oz	190
Links Cheddarwurst Lite	1 link (2.7 oz)	190
Links Hot	2 oz	190
Links Hot Beef	2 oz	190
Links Hot Lite	1 link (2.7 oz)	190
Links Keilbasa Polska	2 oz	190
Links Keilbasa Polska Lite	1 link (2.7 oz)	190
Links Knockwurst Lite	2 oz	180
Links Lit'l Polskas	2 oz	180
Links Lit'l Smokies	2 oz	180
Links Lit'l Smokies Beef	2 oz	180
Links Lit'l Smokies Cheddar	2 oz	180
Links Lit'l Smokies Light	2 oz	120
Links Polish	2 oz	190
Links Smoked	2 oz	190
Mexican Style	1 (2 oz)	190

FOOD	PORTION	CALS.
Hillshire (CONT.)		
Mexican Style Lower Fat	1 (2 oz)	150
Hormel		
Kielbasa	2 oz	150
Light & Lean 97 Dinner Smoked	2 oz	60
Pickled Hot	6 (2 oz)	140
Pickled Smoked	6 (2 oz)	140
Smoked Summer	2 oz	200
Vienna	2 oz	140
Vienna Chicken	2 oz	110
Jimmy Dean		
Brick Sausage	2.5 oz	270
Bulk	2.5 oz	300
Hickory Smoked Dinner Sausage	2 oz	170
Pattie Pre-Cooked	1 (1.9 oz)	230
Polska Kielbaska	2 oz	170
Sage Pattie	1 (2 oz)	200
Sausage Pattie Raw	1 (2 oz)	200
Skinless Link	2 (2 oz)	200
Skinless Link	4 (2 oz)	200
Little Sizzlers		
Brown & Serve	3 links (2.1 oz)	190
Brown & Serve	2 patties (1.8 oz)	190
Cooked	2 patties (1.8 oz)	230
Cooked	3 links (1.8 oz)	230
Heat & Serve Pork cooked	3 links (1.8 oz)	230
Louis Rich		
Polska Kielbasa	2 oz	90
Turkey Hot	2.5 oz	120
Turkey Original	2.5 oz	120
Turkey Smoked	2 oz	90
Mr. Turkey		
Breakfast	2.5 oz	130
Hearty Blend Polish Kielbasa	1 oz	70
Hearty Blend Smoked	1 oz	70
Hot Smoked	1 oz	45
Italian Smoked	1 oz	45
Polish Kielbasa	1 oz	45
Smoked	1 oz	45
Old Smokehouse		
Summer Sausage	2 oz	200
Oscar Mayer		
Pork cooked	2 links (1.7 oz)	170
Smokies Beef	1 (1.5 oz)	120

FOOD	PORTION	CALS.
Oscar Mayer (CONT.)		
Smokies Cheese	1 (1.5 oz)	130
Smokies Link	1 (1.5 oz)	130
Smokies Little	6 (2 oz)	170
Smokies Little Cheese	6 (2 oz)	180
Perdue		
Breakfast Links Turkey Cooked	2 links (2 oz)	100
Hot Italian Turkey Cooked	1 link (2.4 oz)	110
Sweet Italian Turkey Cooked	1 link (2.4 oz)	110
Rudy's Farm		
Italian Hot	2.5 oz	240
Italian Mild	2.5 oz	240
Italian Mild Natural Casing	1 (2 oz)	190
Morning Right Link	3 (2.9 oz)	150
Morning Right Pattie	2 (2.9 oz)	150
Pattie Pre-Cooked	1 (1.4 oz)	100
Smoked	4 (2.1 oz)	200
Sweet Link	1 (3.9 oz)	380
Shady Brook		
Turkey Breakfast	2 oz	80
Turkey Hot Italian	2 oz	100
Turkey Old World Style	4 oz	190
Turkey Sweet Italian	2 oz	100
Shofar		
Knockwurst Beef	1 (3 oz)	260
Turkey Store		
Breakfast	2 links (2 oz)	140
Tyson		
Country Pork	3.5 oz	320
Wampler Longacre		
Breakfast Links	1 (2.8 oz)	170
Italian Links	1 (2.8 oz)	170
Tinderlings Garlic & Pepper	1 (3.5 oz)	143
Turkey	1 link (1 oz)	60
Turkey	1 pattie (2 oz)	120
TAKE-OUT		
pork	1 patty (1 oz)	100
pork	1 link (0.5 oz)	48

SAUSAGE DISHES

Jimmy Dean		
Italian Sausage & Mozzarella Sandwich	1 (4.5 oz)	380

SAUSAGE SUBSTITUTES

GardenSausage		
Patty	1 (2.5 oz)	140

FOOD	PORTION	CALS.
Knox Mountain Farm		
No-So-Sausage	1 serv (1/10 pkg)	120
Lightlife		
Lean Links Breakfast	1.25 oz	69
Lean Links Italian	1.5 oz	83
Loma Linda		
Linketts	1 (1.2 oz)	70
Little Links	2 (1.6 oz)	90
Morningstar Farms		
Breakfast Links	2 (1.6 oz)	60
Breakfast Patties	1 (1.3 oz)	70
Grillers	1 patty (2.2 oz)	140
Sausage Style Recipe Crumbles	2/3 cup (1.9 oz)	90
Natural Touch		
Vegan Sausage Crumbles	1/2 cup (1.9 oz)	60
White Wave		
Meatless Healthy Links	2 (1.6 oz)	140
Worthington		
Leanies	1 link (1.4 oz)	110
Prosage Links	2 (1.6 oz)	60
Saucettes	1 link (1.3 oz)	90
Super Links	1 (1.7 oz)	110
Veja Links	1 (1.1 oz)	50
SAVORY		
ground	1 tsp	4
SCALLOP		
HOME RECIPE		
breaded & fried	2 lg	67
TAKE-OUT		
breaded & fried	6 (5 oz)	386
SCONE		
apricot scone	1	232
Finnegan's		
Cranberry	1 (2.7 oz)	90
Irish Raisin	1 (2.7 oz)	90
Health Valley		
Apple Kiwi	1	180
Cinnamon Raisin	1	180
Cranberry Orange	1	180
Mountain Blueberry	1	180
Pineapple Banana	1	180
TAKE-OUT		
orange poppy	1 (3 oz)	260
raisin	1 (3 oz)	270

FOOD	PORTION	CALS.

SCROD
Gorton's
Microwave Entree Baked | 1 pkg | 320

SCUP
fresh baked | 3 oz | 115

SEA BASS
(*see* BASS)

SEA TROUT
(*see* TROUT)

SEAWEED
Eden

Agar Agar Bars	1 tbsp (2.5 oz)	10
Agar Agar Flakes	1 tbsp (2.5 oz)	10
Arame	½ cup (0.3 oz)	30
Hiziki	½ cup (0.3 oz)	30
Kombu	3.5 in piece (3.3 g)	10
Nori	1 sheet (2.5 g)	10
Sushi Nori	1 sheet (2.5 g)	10
Wakame	½ cup (0.3 oz)	25
Wakame Flakes	½ cup (0.3 oz)	25

Maine Coast

Alaria	⅓ cup (7 g)	18
Dulse	⅓ cup (7 g)	18
Dulse Flakes	1 oz	75
Kelp	⅓ cup (7 g)	17
Kelp Crunch	1 bar (1 oz)	129
Kelp Crunch Peanut-Raisin	1 bar (1 oz)	129
Laver	⅓ cup (7 g)	22
Sea Seasoning Dulse	1 g	3
Sea Seasoning Dulse With Celery	1 g	3
Sea Seasoning Dulse With Garlic	1 g	3
Sea Seasoning Dulse With Sesame	1 g	3
Sea Seasoning Kelp	1 g	3
Sea Seasoning Kelp With Cayenne	1 g	3
Sea Seasoning Nori	1 g	3
Sea Seasoning Nori With Ginger	1 g	3

SEITAN
(*see* WHEAT)

SEMOLINA
dry | 1 cup (5.9 oz) | 601

FOOD	PORTION	CALS.
SESAME		
sesame butter	1 tbsp	95
sesame crunch candy	20 pieces (1.2 oz)	181
sesame crunch candy	1 oz	146
sesame sticks	1 oz	153
sesame sticks unsalted	1 oz	153
Arrowhead		
Sesame Tahini	1 oz	170
Casbah		
Tahini Sauce Mix as prep	¼ cup	160
Eden		
Sesame Shake	½ tsp (1.5 g)	10
Sesame Shake Garlic	½ tsp (1.5 g)	10
Sesame Shake Organic Seaweed	½ tsp (1.5 g)	10
Joyva		
Tahini	2 tbsp (1 oz)	200
Planters		
Nut Mix	1 oz	150
Stone-Buhr		
Seeds Raw	4 tsp (1 oz)	180
SESBANIA		
flower	1	1
flowers cooked	1 cup	23
SHAD		
american baked	3 oz	214
roe baked w/ butter & lemon	3.5 oz	126
roe raw	3.5 oz	130
SHALLOTS		
dried	1 tbsp	3
raw chopped	1 tbsp	7
SHARK		
batter-dipped & fried	3 oz	194
SHEEPSHEAD FISH		
cooked	3 oz	107
SHELLFISH		
(*see individual names,* SHELLFISH SUBSTITUTES)		
SHELLFISH SUBSTITUTES		
Louis Kemp		
Crab Delights Chunk Style	2 oz	54
Lobster Delights	2 oz	60

FOOD	PORTION	CALS.
Louis Kemp (CONT.)		
Maryland Style Cakes	2.5 oz	154
Ocean Magic		
Imitation King Crab	3 oz	80

SHERBET
(*see also* ICES AND ICE POPS)

	PORTION	CALS.
orange	½ cup (4 fl oz)	132
orange	1 bar (2.75 fl oz)	91
Borden		
Orange	½ cup	110
Breyers		
Fat Free Orange	½ cup (3 oz)	110
Fat Free Rainbow	½ cup (3 oz)	110
Fat Free Raspberry	½ cup (3 oz)	120
Fat Free Tropical	½ cup (3 oz)	110
Orange	½ cup (3 oz)	120
Rainbow	½ cup (3 oz)	120
Raspberry	½ cup (3 oz)	120
Tropical	½ cup (3 oz)	120
Hood		
Lime Orange Lemon	½ cup (3.1 oz)	120
Orange	½ cup (3.1 oz)	120
Rainbow Swirl	½ cup (3.1 oz)	120
Raspberry Orange Lime	½ cup (3.1 oz)	120
Sealtest		
Lime	½ cup (3 oz)	130
Orange	½ cup (3 oz)	130
Rainbow Orange Red Raspberry Lime	½ cup (3 oz)	130
Red Raspberry	½ cup (3 oz)	130

SHRIMP
FRESH

	PORTION	CALS.
cooked	4 large	22
FROZEN		
Cajun Cookin'		
Shrimp Creole	12 oz	390
Shrimp Etouffee	17 oz	360
Shrimp Jambalaya	12 oz	450
Gorton's		
Butterfly Shrimp	4 oz	160
Microwave Crunchy Shrimp	5 oz	380
Microwave Entree Shrimp Scampi	1 pkg	390
Shrimp Crisps	4 oz	280

FOOD	PORTION	CALS.
Van De Kamp's		
Breaded Butterfly	7 (4 oz)	280
Breaded Popcorn	20 (4 oz)	270
Breaded Whole	7 (4 oz)	240
TAKE-OUT		
breaded & fried	6 to 8 (6 oz)	454
SMELT		
rainbow cooked	3 oz	106
SNACKS		
(*see also* CHIPS, FRUIT SNACKS, NUTS MIXED, POPCORN, POPCORN CAKES, PRETZELS, RICE CAKES)		
oriental mix	1 oz	155
pork skins	1 oz	154
pork skins barbecue	1 oz	152
trail mix	1 oz	131
trail mix	1 cup (5.3 oz)	693
trail mix tropical	1 oz	115
trail mix w/ chocolate chips	1 oz	137
trail mix w/ chocolate chips	1 cup (5.1 oz)	707
Baken-ets		
BBQ	9 (0.5 oz)	70
Hot N'Spicy	7 (0.5 oz)	70
Hot N'Spicy Cracklins	8 (0.5 oz)	80
Regular	9 (0.5 oz)	80
Regular Cracklins	8 (0.5 oz)	40
Barbara's		
Cheese Puffs Bakes	1½ cups (1 oz)	160
Cheese Puffs Jalapeno	¾ cup (1 oz)	150
Cheese Puffs Original	¾ cup (1 oz)	150
Big Dipper		
Bagel Chips Lowfat Barbeque	12 (1 oz)	110
Bagel Chips Lowfat Garlic	12 (1 oz)	120
Bagel Chips Lowfat Original	12 (1 oz)	110
Bugles		
Baked Cheddar Cheese	1½ cups (1 oz)	130
Baked Original	1 pkg (1.4 oz)	170
Baked Original	1½ cups (1 oz)	130
Nacho	1⅓ cups (1 oz)	160
Nacho	1 pkg (0.9 oz)	130
Original	1 pkg (1.5 oz)	230
Original	1⅓ cups (1 oz)	160
Ranch	1⅓ cups (1 oz)	160
Smokin BBQ	1⅓ cups (1 oz)	150

FOOD	PORTION	CALS.
Bugles (CONT.)		
Sour Cream & Onion	1⅓ cups (1 oz)	160
Cheetos		
Crunchy	21 pieces (1 oz)	160
Curls	15 pieces (1 oz)	150
Curls	15 pieces (1 oz)	150
Flamin' Hot	21 pieces (1 oz)	160
Nacho Cheese	23 pieces (1 oz)	160
Puffed Balls	38 pieces (1 oz)	150
Puffs	29 pieces (1 oz)	160
Zig Zags	17 pieces (1 oz)	170
Cheez Doodles		
Crunchy	1 oz	160
Puffed	1 oz	150
Cheez Waffies		
Snacks	1 oz	140
Chex Mix		
Bold'n Zesty	1 pkg (1.7 oz)	230
Cheddar Cheese	1 pkg (1.7 oz)	220
Hot'n Spicy	⅔ cup (1 oz)	130
Hot'n Spicy	1 pkg (1.7 oz)	210
Traditional	1 pkg (1.7 oz)	210
Combos		
Cheddar Cheese Cracker	1 pkg (1.7 oz)	250
Cheddar Cheese Cracker	1 oz	140
Cheddar Cheese Pretzel	1 oz	130
Cheddar Cheese Pretzel	1 pkg (1.8 oz)	240
Chili Cheese w/ Corn Shell	1 oz	140
Chili Cheese w/ Corn Shell	1 pkg (1.7 oz)	230
Mustard Pretzel	1 pkg (1.8 oz)	230
Mustard Pretzel	1 oz	130
Nacho Cheese Pretzel	1 pkg (1.7 oz)	230
Nacho Cheese Pretzel	1 oz	130
Nacho Cheese w/ Tortilla Shell	1 oz	140
Nacho Cheese w/ Tortilla Shell	1 pkg (1.7 oz)	230
Peanut Butter Cracker	1 oz	140
Pepperoni & Cheese Pizza	1 oz	140
Pepperoni & Cheese Pizza	1 pkg (1.7 oz)	240
Pizzeria Pretzel	1 pkg (1.8 oz)	230
Pizzeria Pretzel	1 oz	130
Tortilla Ranch	1 bag (1.7 oz)	240
Tortilla Ranch	1 oz	140
Cornnuts		
Barbecue	1 oz	120

FOOD	PORTION	CALS.
Cornnuts (CONT.)		
Nacho Cheese	1 oz	120
Original	1 oz	120
Original	1 pkg (2 oz)	260
Picante	1 oz	120
Ranch	1 oz	120
Doo Dads		
Snacks	1 oz	130
Energy Food Factory		
Poprice Cheddar Cheese	0.5 oz	60
Poprice Herb & Garlic	0.5 oz	50
Poprice Lite	0.5 oz	50
Poprice Original No Salt	0.5 oz	45
Frito Lay		
Funyuns	13 (1 oz)	140
Munchos	16 (1 oz)	160
Munchos BBQ	14 (1 oz)	160
Hapi		
Chili Bits	½ cup (1 oz)	110
Health Valley		
Cheddar Lites Green Onion	1¾ cups	120
Cheddar Lites Original	1¾ cups	120
Corn Puffs Caramel	2 cups	120
Low Fat Potato Puffs Cheddar Cheese	1½ cups	110
Low Fat Potato Puffs Garlic w/ Cheese	1½ cups	260
Low Fat Potato Puffs Zesty Ranch	1½ cups	110
Innovative Foods		
Roasted Sweet Corn	1 pkg (0.8 oz)	76
Mr. Peanut		
Peanut Butter Crisps Graham	12 pieces (1.1 oz)	150
Pita Puffs		
Barbeque	35 (1 oz)	120
Lowfat Garlic	35 (1 oz)	110
Lowfat Original	35 (1 oz)	110
Lowfat Salsa	35 (1 oz)	110
Pizza	35 (1 oz)	120
Ranch	35 (1 oz)	120
Planters		
Cheez Balls	1 oz	150
Cheez Balls	1 pkg (1 oz)	150
Cheez Curls	1 pkg (1.2 oz)	190
Cheez Curls	1 oz	150
Heat Snack Mix	1 oz	140

FOOD	PORTION	CALS.
Snyder's		
Cheddar Cheese Twists	1 oz	150
Kruncheez	1 oz	160
Onion Toasters	1 oz	150
Snack Mix	1 oz	170
Sopaipillas Apple & Cinnamon	1 oz	150
Splurge		
Snack Mix Fat Free Original	⅔ cup (1 oz)	100
Ultra Slim-Fast		
Lite N' Tasty Cheese Curls	1 oz	110
Utz		
Caramel Corn Clusters	1⅛ cups (1 oz)	120
Cheese Balls	50 (1 oz)	150
Cheese Curls	18 (1 oz)	150
Cheese Curls Crunchy	30 (1 oz)	160
Cheese Curls Reduced Fat	32 (1 oz)	140
Onion Rings	41 (1 oz)	140
Party Mix	¾ cup (1 oz)	140
Pork Cracklins	0.5 oz	90
Pork Cracklins Hot & Spicy	0.5 oz	80
Pork Rinds	0.5 oz	80
Pork Rinds BBQ	0.5 oz	80
Weight Watchers		
Cheese Curls	1 pkg (0.5 oz)	70

SNAIL
cooked	3 oz	233

SNAPPER
cooked	3 oz	109

SODA
(*see also* DRINK MIXERS, SPORTS DRINKS, WATER)

7 Up		
Cherry	1 oz	13
Cherry Diet	1 oz	tr
Diet	1 oz	tr
Gold	1 oz	13
Gold Diet	1 oz	tr
Original	1 oz	12
After The Fall		
Raspberry Ginger Ale	1 can (12 oz)	150
Barrelhead		
Root Beer	8 fl oz	110
Burst		
Cola Strawberry	8 fl oz	11

FOOD	PORTION	CALS.
Canada Dry		
Birch Beer Brown	8 fl oz	110
Birch Beer Clear	8 fl oz	110
Black Cherry Wishniak	8 fl oz	130
Cactus Cooler	8 fl oz	110
California Strawberry	8 fl oz	110
Club	8 fl oz	0
Club Sodium Free	8 fl oz	0
Concord Grape	8 fl oz	120
Diet Ginger Ale	8 fl oz	0
Diet Ginger Ale Cherry	8 fl oz	0
Diet Ginger Ale Cranberry	8 fl oz	0
Diet Ginger Ale Lemon	8 fl oz	5
Diet Tonic Water	8 fl oz	0
Diet Tonic Water Twist Of Lime	8 fl oz	0
Ginger Ale	8 fl oz	100
Ginger Ale Cherry	8 fl oz	110
Ginger Ale Cranberry	8 fl oz	100
Ginger Ale Golden	8 fl oz	100
Ginger Ale Lemon	8 fl oz	100
Half & Half	8 fl oz	110
Hi-Spot	8 fl oz	110
Island Lime	8 fl oz	140
Jamaica Cola	8 fl oz	110
Lemon Sour	8 fl oz	100
Peach	8 fl oz	120
Pina Pineapple	8 fl oz	110
Seltzer	8 fl oz	0
Seltzer Cherry	8 fl oz	0
Seltzer Cranberry Lime	8 fl oz	0
Seltzer Grapefruit	8 fl oz	0
Seltzer Lemon Lime	8 fl oz	0
Seltzer Mandarin Orange	8 fl oz	0
Seltzer Peach	8 fl oz	0
Seltzer Raspberry	8 fl oz	0
Seltzer Strawberry	8 fl oz	0
Seltzer Tropical	8 fl oz	0
Sunripe Orange	8 fl oz	140
Tahitian Treat	8 fl oz	150
Tonic Water	8 fl oz	100
Tonic Water Twist Of Lime	8 fl oz	100
Vanilla Cream	8 fl oz	120
Vichy Water	8 fl oz	0
Wild Cherry	8 fl oz	110

FOOD	PORTION	CALS.
Clearly 2		
Black Cherry	8 fl oz	2
Key Lime	8 fl oz	2
Clearly Canadian		
Alpine Fruit & Berries	8 fl oz	90
Boysenberry Mist	8 fl oz	2
Coastal Cranberry	8 fl oz	90
Country Raspberry	8 fl oz	80
Green Apple	8 fl oz	80
Mountain Blackberry	8 fl oz	100
Orchard Peach Strawberry	8 fl oz	90
Soda	8 fl oz	0
Summer Strawberry	8 fl oz	80
Western Longanberry	8 fl oz	80
Wild Cherry	8 fl oz	90
Coca-Cola		
Cherry	8 fl oz	104
Classic	8 fl oz	97
Classic Caffeine-Free	8 fl oz	97
Coke II	8 fl oz	105
Diet	8 fl oz	1
Diet Cherry	8 fl oz	1
Diet Coke Caffeine-free	8 fl oz	1
Cott		
Cola	8 fl oz	110
Ginger Ale	8 fl oz	90
Grape	8 fl oz	130
Orange	8 fl oz	140
Pineapple	8 fl oz	130
Punch	8 fl oz	130
Seltzer	8 fl oz	0
Crush		
Cherry	8 fl oz	140
Grape	8 fl oz	110
Orange	8 fl oz	140
Orange Diet	8 fl oz	0
Pineapple	8 fl oz	140
Strawberry	8 fl oz	130
Tropical Fruit Punch	1 bottle (10 fl oz)	180
Diet Rite		
Black Cherry Salt/Sodium Free	8 fl oz	2
Cola	8 fl oz	1
Cola Caffeine/Sugar Free	8 fl oz	1
Cola Salt/Sodium Free	8 fl oz	1

FOOD	PORTION	CALS.
Diet Rite (CONT.)		
Fruit Punch Salt/Sodium Free	8 fl oz	2
Golden Peach Salt/Sodium Free	8 fl oz	2
Key Lime Salt/Sodium Free	8 fl oz	7
Pink Grapefruit Salt/Sodium Free	8 fl oz	2
Red Raspberry Salt/Sodium Free	8 fl oz	3
Tangerine Salt/Sodium Free	8 fl oz	2
White Grape Salt/Sodium Free	8 fl oz	1
Dr Pepper		
Diet	1 oz	tr
Free	1 oz	12
Free Diet	1 oz	tr
Original	1 oz	13
Dr. Nehi		
Soda	8 fl oz	100
Fanta		
Ginger Ale	8 fl oz	86
Grape	8 fl oz	117
Orange	8 fl oz	118
Root Beer	8 fl oz	111
Fresca		
Soda	8 fl oz	3
Health Valley		
Ginger Ale	1 bottle	160
Rootbeer Old Fashioned	1 bottle	160
Sarsaparilla Rootbeer	1 bottle	160
Hires		
Cream	8 fl oz	130
Cream Soda Diet	8 fl oz	0
Original Mocha	8 fl oz	100
Original Mocha Diet	8 fl oz	5
Root Beer	8 fl oz	130
Root Beer Diet	8 fl oz	0
IBC		
Root Beer	8 oz	110
Kick		
Soda	8 fl oz	120
Mello Yellow		
Diet	8 fl oz	4
Soda	8 fl oz	119
Minute Maid		
Berry	8 fl oz	111
Diet Orange	8 fl oz	2
Fruit Punch	8 fl oz	117

FOOD	PORTION	CALS.
Minute Maid (CONT.)		
Grape	8 fl oz	121
Grapefruit	8 fl oz	108
Orange	8 fl oz	118
Peach	8 fl oz	110
Pineapple	8 fl oz	109
Raspberry	8 fl oz	111
Soda	8 fl oz	110
Strawberry	8 fl oz	122
Mountain Dew		
Diet	8 fl oz	2
Soda	8 fl oz	118
Mr. PiBB		
Diet	8 fl oz	1
Soda	6 oz	97
Mug		
Cream	8 fl oz	122
Diet Cream	8 fl oz	2
Diet Root Beer	8 fl oz	1
Root Beer	8 fl oz	141
Nehi		
Cream	8 fl oz	120
Fruit Punch	8 fl oz	120
Ginger Ale	8 fl oz	90
Grape	8 fl oz	120
Orange	8 fl oz	130
Peach	8 fl oz	130
Pineapple	8 fl oz	130
Quinine Water	8 fl oz	90
Root Beer	8 fl oz	120
Strawberry	8 fl oz	120
Wild Red	8 fl oz	120
Old Colony		
Grape	8 fl oz	140
Orangina		
Sparkling Citrus	6 fl oz	80
Pepsi		
Caffeine Free	8 fl oz	105
Diet	8 fl oz	1
Diet Caffeine Free	8 fl oz	1
Regular	8 fl oz	105
Ramblin' Root Beer		
Ramblin' Root Beer	8 fl oz	120

FOOD	PORTION	CALS.
Razing Razberry		
Cola	8 fl oz	117
Royal Crown		
Caffeine Free Cola	8 fl oz	110
Cherry	8 fl oz	110
Cola	8 fl oz	100
Diet	8 fl oz	1
Diet Caffeine Free	8 fl oz	1
Diet Cranberry Apple Salt/Sodium Free	8 fl oz	2
Diet Cranberry Salt/Sodium Free	8 fl oz	2
Royal Mistic		
'N Juice Black Cherry	12 fl oz	146
'N Juice Peach Vanilla	12 fl oz	146
'N Juice Tangerine Orange	12 fl oz	146
'N Juice Tropical Supreme	12 fl oz	152
'N Juice Wild Berry	12 fl oz	156
Caribbean Fruit Punch	16 fl oz	230
Grape Strawberry	16 fl oz	230
Sparkling Diet With Lime Kiwi	11.1 fl oz	0
Sparkling Diet With Raspberry Boysenberry	11.1 fl oz	0
Sparkling Diet With Royal Peach	11.1 fl oz	0
Sparkling Diet With Wild Cherry	11.1 fl oz	0
Sparkling With Lime Kiwi	11.1 fl oz	112
Sparkling With Mandarin Orange Pineappple	11.1 fl oz	120
Sparkling With Mango Passion	11.1 fl oz	112
Sparkling With Raspberry Boysenberry	11.1 fl oz	112
Sparkling With Royal Peach	11.1 fl oz	112
Sparkling With Wild Cherry	11.1 fl oz	112
Schweppes		
Bitter Lemon	8 fl oz	110
Club	8 fl oz	0
Club Sodium Free	8 fl oz	0
Diet Ginger Ale	8 fl oz	0
Diet Ginger Ale Dry Grape	8 fl oz	2
Diet Ginger Ale Raspberry	8 fl oz	0
Ginger Ale	8 fl oz	90
Ginger Ale Dry Grape	8 fl oz	100
Ginger Ale Raspberry	8 fl oz	100
Ginger Beer	8 fl oz	100
Grape	8 fl oz	130
Grapefruit	8 fl oz	110
Lemon Sour	8 fl oz	110

FOOD	PORTION	CALS
Schweppes (CONT.)		
Lemon-Lime	8 fl oz	100
Seltzer Black Berry	8 fl oz	0
Seltzer Lemon	8 fl oz	0
Seltzer Lemon Lime	8 fl oz	0
Seltzer Lime	8 fl oz	0
Seltzer Orange	8 fl oz	0
Seltzer Peaches & Cream	8 fl oz	0
Seltzer Raspberry	8 fl oz	0
Tonic Citrus	8 fl oz	90
Tonic Cranberry	8 fl oz	90
Tonic Raspberry	8 fl oz	90
Tonic Water Diet	8 fl oz	0
Shasta		
Black Cherry	1 can (12 oz)	170
Caffeine Free Cola	1 can (12 oz)	160
Cherry Cola	1 can (12 oz)	160
Club Soda	1 can (12 oz)	0
Cola	1 can (12 oz)	170
Creme	1 can (12 oz)	190
Diet Black Cherry	1 can (12 oz)	0
Diet Caffeine Free Cola	1 can (12 oz)	0
Diet Cherry Cola	1 can (12 oz)	0
Diet Cola	1 can (12 oz)	0
Diet Creme	1 can (12 oz)	0
Diet Doc Shasta	1 can (12 oz)	0
Diet Ginger Ale	1 can (12 oz)	0
Diet Grape	1 can (12 oz)	0
Diet Grapefruit	1 can (12 oz)	0
Diet Grapefruit	1 can (12 oz)	0
Diet Kiwi-Strawberry	1 can (12 oz)	0
Diet Lemon-Lime Twist	1 can (12 oz)	0
Diet Orange	1 can (12 oz)	0
Diet Pineapple-Orange	1 can (12 oz)	0
Diet Raspberry Creme	1 can (12 oz)	0
Diet Red Pop	1 can (12 oz)	0
Diet Root Beer	1 can (12 oz)	0
Diet Strawberry	1 can (12 oz)	0
Diet Strawberry-Peach	1 can (12 oz)	0
Doc Shasta	1 can (12 oz)	160
Fruit Punch	1 can (12 oz)	200
Ginger Ale	1 can (12 oz)	130
Grape	1 can (12 oz)	190
Kiwi-Strawberry	1 can (12 oz)	170

FOOD	PORTION	CALS.
Shasta (CONT.)		
Lemon-Lime Twist	1 can (12 oz)	150
Moon Mist	1 can (12 oz)	180
Orange	1 can (12 oz)	200
Peach	1 can (12 oz)	170
Pineapple	1 can (12 oz)	200
Pineapple-Orange	1 can (12 oz)	180
Quinine/Tonic	1 can (12 oz)	130
Raspberry Creme	1 can (12 oz)	170
Red Pop	1 can (12 oz)	170
Root Beer	1 can (12 oz)	170
Strawberry	1 can (12 oz)	190
Strawberry-Peach	1 can (12 oz)	170
Slice		
Diet Lemon Lime	8 fl oz	5
Diet Mandarin	8 fl oz	5
Lemon Lime	8 fl oz	100
Mandarin Orange	8 fl oz	128
Red	8 fl oz	128
Snapple		
Amazin' Grape	8 fl oz	120
Cherry Lime Ricky	8 fl oz	110
Creme D'Vanilla	8 fl oz	130
French Cherry	8 fl oz	120
Kiwi Peach	8 fl oz	120
Kiwi Strawberry	8 fl oz	130
Mango Madness	8 fl oz	130
Passion Supreme	8 fl oz	120
Peach Melba	8 fl oz	120
Raspberry	8 fl oz	120
Seltzer Black Cherry	8 fl oz	0
Seltzer Lemon Lime	8 fl oz	0
Seltzer Original	8 fl oz	0
Seltzer Tangerine	8 fl oz	0
Tru Root Beer	8 fl oz	110
Sprite		
Diet	8 fl oz	3
Soda	8 fl oz	100
Sundrop		
Cherry	8 fl oz	130
Diet	8 fl oz	5
Soda	8 fl oz	140
Sunkist		
Cactus Cooler	8 fl oz	110

FOOD	PORTION	CALS.
Sunkist (CONT.)		
Cherry	8 fl oz	140
Diet Citrus	8 fl oz	0
Diet Orange	8 fl oz	5
Fruit Punch	8 fl oz	130
Orange	8 fl oz	140
Peach	8 fl oz	120
Pineapple	8 fl oz	140
Strawberry	8 fl oz	140
TAB		
Soda	8 fl oz	1
Tropical Chill		
Cola	8 fl oz	117
Diet	8 fl oz	1
Upper 10		
Diet	8 fl oz	3
Diet Salt/Sodium Free	8 fl oz	3
Salt Free	8 fl oz	100
Soda	8 fl oz	100
Wink		
Diet	8 fl oz	5
Soda	8 fl oz	130
Yoo-Hoo		
Original	9 fl oz	150

SOLDIER BEANS
Bean Cuisine
Dried	½ cup	115

SOLE
FRESH
cooked	3 oz	99

FROZEN
Gorton's
Fishmarket Fresh	5 oz	110
Microwave Entree In Lemon Butter	1 pkg	380
Microwave Entree In Wine Sauce	1 pkg	180
Van De Kamp's		
Lightly Breaded Fillets	1 (4 oz)	220
Natural Fillets	1 (4 oz)	110

TAKE-OUT
battered & fried	3.2 oz	211
breaded & fried	3.2 oz	211

FOOD	PORTION	CALS.
SORBET		
(*see* ICES AND ICE POPS)		
SORGHUM		
sorghum	1 cup (6.7 oz)	651
SOUFFLE		
spinach	1 cup	218
SOUP		
CANNED		
College Inn		
Beef Broth	½ can (7 oz)	16
Chicken Broth	½ can (7 oz)	35
Chicken Broth Lower Salt	½ can (7 oz)	20
Gorton's		
New England Clam Chowder as prep w/ whole milk	¼ can	140
Goya		
Black Bean	7.5 oz	160
Hain		
Chicken Broth	8.75 fl oz	70
Chicken Broth No Salt Added	8.75 fl oz	60
Chicken Noodle	9.5 fl oz	120
Chicken Noodle No Salt Added	9.5 fl oz	120
Creamy Mushroom	9.25 fl oz	110
Italian Vegetable Pasta	9.5 fl oz	160
Italian Vegetable Pasta Low Sodium	9.5 fl oz	140
Minestrone	9.5 fl oz	170
Minestrone No Salt Added	9.5 fl oz	160
Mushroom Barley	9.5 fl oz	100
New England Clam Chowder	9.5 fl oz	180
Split Pea	9.5 fl oz	170
Split Pea No Salt Added	9.5 fl oz	170
Turkey Rice	9.5 fl oz	100
Turkey Rice No Salt Added	9.5 fl oz	120
Vegetable Chicken	9.5 fl oz	120
Vegetable Chicken No Salt Added	9.5 fl oz	130
Vegetable Broth	9.5 fl oz	45
Vegetable Broth Low Sodium	9.5 fl oz	40
Vegetable Split Pea	9.5 fl oz	170
Vegetable Split Pea No Salt Added	9.5 fl oz	170
Vegetarian Lentil	9.5 fl oz	160
Vegetarian Lentil No Salt Added	9.5 fl oz	160
Vegetarian Vegetable	9.5 fl oz	140

FOOD	PORTION	CALS.
Hain (CONT.)		
Vegetarian Vegetable No Salt Added	9.5 fl oz	150
Health Valley		
5 Bean Vegetable	1 cup	250
Beef Broth Fat Free	1 cup	20
Beef Broth Fat Free No Salt	1 cup	20
Black Bean & Vegetable	1 cup	110
Chicken Broth	1 cup	45
Chicken Broth Fat Free	1 cup	30
Chicken Broth No Salt	1 cup	45
Country Corn & Vegetable	1 cup	70
Garden Vegetable	1 cup	80
Italian Plus Carotene	1 cup	80
Lentil & Carrot	1 cup	100
Organic Black Bean	1 cup	110
Organic Lentil No Salt	1 cup	90
Organic Minestrone	1 cup	100
Organic Mushroom Barley No Salt	1 cup	60
Organic Potato Leek	1 cup	70
Organic Potato Leek No Salt	1 cup	70
Organic Split Pea	1 cup	110
Organic Split Pea No Salt	1 cup	110
Organic Tomato	1 cup	90
Organic Vegetable No Salt	1 cup	80
Pasta Bolognese	1 cup	100
Pasta Cacciatore	1 cup	100
Pasta Romano	1 cup	100
Real Italian Minestrone	1 cup	90
Rotini & Vegetable	1 cup	100
Split Pea & Carrots	1 cup	110
Super Broccoli Carotene	1 cup	70
Tomato Vegetable	1 cup	80
Vegetable Barley	1 cup	90
Vegetable Power Carotene	1 cup	70
Healthy Choice		
Bean & Ham	1 cup (8.7 oz)	184
Beef & Potato	1 cup (8.5 oz)	119
Chicken Corn Chowder	1 cup (8.8 oz)	176
Chicken Pasta	1 cup (8.6 oz)	118
Chicken With Rice	1 cup (8.4 oz)	108
Chili Beef	1 cup (9.1 oz)	166
Clam Chowder	1 cup (8.8 oz)	123
Country Vegetable	1 cup (8.6 oz)	104
Cream Of Mushroom	1 cup (8.8 oz)	77

FOOD	PORTION	CALS.
Healthy Choice (CONT.)		
Cream Of Chicken With Mushrooms	1 cup (8.9 oz)	127
Cream Of Chicken With Vegetables	1 cup (8.9 oz)	127
Garden Vegetable	1 cup (8.6 oz)	118
Hearty Chicken	1 cup (8.7 oz)	132
Lentil	1 cup (8.7 oz)	146
Minestrone	1 cup (8.6 oz)	112
Old Fashion Chicken Noodle	1 cup (8.8 oz)	137
Split Pea & Ham	1 cup (8.8 oz)	155
Tomato Garden	1 cup (8.6 oz)	106
Turkey With Wild Rice	1 cup (8.4 oz)	92
Vegetable Beef	1 cup (8.8 oz)	130
Herb-Ox		
Beef Liquid	2 tsp (0.4 oz)	20
Chicken Liquid	2 tsp (0.4 oz)	15
Old El Paso		
Black Bean With Bacon	1 cup (8.6 oz)	160
Chicken Vegetable	1 cup (8.4 oz)	110
Chicken With Rice	1 cup (8.4 oz)	90
Garden Vegetable	1 cup (8.4 oz)	110
Hearty Beef	1 cup (8.4 oz)	120
Hearty Chicken Noodle	1 cup (8.4 oz)	110
Pritikin		
Chicken & Rice	1 cup (8.8 oz)	80
Chicken Broth	1 cup (8.5 oz)	15
Chicken Pasta	1 cup (8.6 oz)	100
Hearty Vegetable	1 cup (8.8 oz)	90
Lentil	1 cup (8.4 oz)	130
Minestrone	1 cup (8.8 oz)	90
Split Pea	1 cup (9.2 oz)	140
Three Bean Chili	½ cup (4.5 oz)	90
Vegetable Broth	1 cup (8.3 oz)	20
Vegetarian Vegetables	1 cup (9 oz)	100
Progresso		
Bean And Ham	1 cup (8.4 oz)	160
Beef	1 can (10.5 fl oz)	180
Beef Barley	1 cup (8.5 oz)	130
Beef Minestrone	1 cup (8.5 oz)	140
Beef Noodle	1 cup (8.5 oz)	140
Beef Vegetable & Rotini	1 cup (8 oz)	120
Broccoli & Shells	1 cup (8.5 oz)	70
Chickarina	1 cup (8.3 oz)	120
Chicken Minestrone	1 cup (8.4 oz)	120
Chicken Vegetables & Penne	1 cup (8.4 oz)	100

FOOD	PORTION	CALS.
Progresso (CONT.)		
Chicken & Wild Rice	1 cup (8.4 oz)	100
Chicken Barley	1 cup (8.5 oz)	110
Chicken Broth	1 cup ((8.2 oz)	20
Chicken Noodle	1 cup (8.4 oz)	80
Chicken Noodle	1 can (10.5 oz)	110
Chicken Rice Vegetable	1 cup (8.4 oz)	110
Chicken Rice Vegetable	1 can (10.5 oz)	130
Clam & Rotini Chowder	1 cup (8.8 oz)	200
Corn Chowder	1 cup (8.6 oz)	180
Cream Of Chicken	1 cup (8.4 oz)	170
Cream Of Mushroom	1 cup (8.4 oz)	140
Creamy Tortellini	1 cup (8.4 oz)	210
Escarole In Chicken Broth	1 cup (8.1 oz)	25
Green Split Pea	1 cup (8.6 oz)	170
Healthy Classics Beef Barley	1 cup (8.5 oz)	140
Healthy Classics Beef Vegetable	1 cup (8.5 oz)	150
Healthy Classics Chicken Noodle	1 cup (8.3 oz)	80
Healthy Classics Chicken Rice With Vegetables	1 cup (8.4 oz)	90
Healthy Classics Cream Of Broccoli	1 cup (8.6 oz)	90
Healthy Classics Garlic & Pasta	1 cup (8.5 oz)	100
Healthy Classics Lentil	1 cup (8.5 oz)	120
Healthy Classics Minestrone	1 cup (8.5 oz)	120
Healthy Classics New England Clam Chowder	1 cup (8.6 oz)	120
Healthy Classics Split Pea	1 cup (8.9 oz)	180
Healthy Classics Tomato Garden Vegetable	1 cup (8.6 oz)	100
Healthy Classics Vegetable	1 cup (8.4 oz)	80
Hearty Minestrone With Shells	1 cup (8.4 oz)	120
Hearty Black Bean	1 cup (8.5 oz)	170
Hearty Chicken	1 can (10.5 fl oz)	120
Hearty Chicken & Rotini	1 cup (8.4 oz)	90
Hearty Penne In Chicken Broth	1 cup (8.4 oz)	70
Hearty Tomato & Rotini	1 cup (8.4 oz)	90
Hearty Vegetable With Rotini	1 cup (8.4 oz)	110
Homestyle Chicken Vegetable	1 cup (8.4 oz)	100
Lentil	1 can (10.5 fl oz)	170
Lentil	1 cup (8.5 oz)	140
Lentil & Shells	1 cup (8.5 oz)	130
Lentil With Sausage	1 cup (8.5 oz)	170
Macaroni & Bean	1 cup (8.6 oz)	160
Manhattan Clam Chowder	1 cup (8.4 oz)	110
Meatballs & Pasta Pearls	1 cup (8.3 oz)	140

FOOD	PORTION	CALS.
Progresso (CONT.)		
Minestrone	1 cup (8.4 oz)	130
Minestrone	1 can (10.5 fl oz)	170
New England Clam Chowder	1 can (10.5 oz)	220
New England Clam Chowder	1 cup (8.4 oz)	180
Spicy Chicken & Penne	1 cup (8.5 oz)	120
Split Pea With Ham	1 cup (8.5 oz)	160
Tomato	1 cup (8.5 oz)	90
Tomato Tortellini	1 cup (8.4 oz)	120
Tomato Beef & Rotini	1 cup (8.5 oz)	140
Tortellini In Chicken Broth	1 cup (8.3 oz)	80
Vegetable	1 cup (8.4 oz)	90
Zesty Minestrone	1 cup (8.3 oz)	150
Snow's		
Manhattan Clam Chowder as prep w/ water	7.5 fl oz	70
New England Clam Chowder as prep w/ milk	7.5 fl oz	140
New England Corn Chowder as prep w/ milk	7.5 fl oz	150
New England Fish Chowder as prep w/ milk	7.5 fl oz	130
New England Seafood Chowder as prep w/ milk	7.5 fl oz	130
Swanson		
Beef Broth	7.25 oz	18
Chicken Broth	7.25 oz	30
Chicken Broth Seasoned w/ Italian Herbs	1 cup (8 oz)	25
Chicken Broth Seasoned w/ Italian Herbs	1 cup (8 oz)	25
Natural Goodness Clear Chicken Broth	7.25 oz	20
Vegetable Broth	7.25 fl oz	20
Weight Watchers		
Chicken & Rice	1 can (10.5 oz)	110
Chicken Noodle	1 can (10.5 oz)	150
Minestrone	1 can (10.5 oz)	130
Vegetable	1 can (10.5 oz)	130
FROZEN		
Tabatchnick		
Barley Mushroom	1 serv (7.5 oz)	70
Barley Mushroom No Salt Added	1 serv (7.5 oz)	70
Broccoli Cream Of	1 serv (7.5 oz)	90
Cabbage	1 serv (7.5 oz)	60
Chicken With Dumplings	1 serv (7.5 oz)	70
Corn Chowder	1 serv (7.5 oz)	150

FOOD	PORTION	CALS.
Tabatchnick (CONT.)		
Minestrone	1 serv (7.5 oz)	150
New England Potato	1 serv (7.5 oz)	150
New York Chicken	1 serv (7.5 oz)	35
Old Fashion Potato	1 serv (7.5 oz)	70
Pea	1 serv (7.5 oz)	180
Pea No Salt Added	1 serv (7.5 oz)	180
Spinach Cream Of	1 serv (7.5 oz)	90
Vegetable	1 serv (7.5 oz)	110
Vegetable No Salt Added	1 serv (7.5 oz)	110
Wisconsin Cheddar Vegetable	1 serv (7.5 oz)	140
Yankee Bean	1 serv (7.5 oz)	160
MIX		
Arrowhead		
Bean & Barley	¼ cup (1.9 oz)	170
Bean Cuisine		
Bean Bouillabaisse	1 cup (7.5 fl oz)	174
Island Black Bean	1 cup (8.7 fl oz)	210
Lots of Lentil	1 cup (7.7 oz)	166
Mesa Maize	1 cup (9.2 fl oz)	179
Rocky Mountain Red Bean	1 cup (8.6 oz)	202
Sante Fe Corn Chowder	1 cup (9.2 oz)	179
Thick As Fog Split Pea	1 cup (8.6 fl oz)	189
Ultima Pasta E Fagioli	1 cup (8.6 fl oz)	179
White Bean Provencal	1 cup (7.7 fl oz)	166
Casbah		
Black Bean	1 pkg (1.7 oz)	170
Split Pea	1 pkg (2.3 oz)	230
Sweet Corn Chowder	1 pkg (1.2 oz)	125
Vegetarian Chili	1 pkg (1.8 oz)	170
Cup-A-Ramen		
Beef With Vegetables Low Fat as prep	8 oz	220
Beef With Vegetables as prep	8 oz	270
Chicken With Vegetables Low Fat as prep	8 oz	220
Chicken With Vegetables as prep	8 oz	270
Oriental With Vegetables Low Fat as prep	8 oz	220
Oriental With Vegetables as prep	8 oz	270
Shrimp With Vegetables Low Fat as prep	8 oz	230
Shrimp With Vegetables as prep	8 oz	280
Cup-a-Soup		
Broccoli & Cheese as prep	1 serv (6 oz)	70
Chicken Vegetable as prep	1 serv (6 oz)	50
Chicken Broth as prep	1 serv (6 oz)	20
Chicken Broth w/ Pasta Fat Free as prep	1 serv (6 oz)	45

FOOD	PORTION	CALS.
Cup-a-Soup (CONT.)		
Chicken Noodle as prep	1 serv (6 oz)	50
Cream Of Chicken as prep	1 serv (6 oz)	70
Creamy Chicken Vegetable as prep	1 serv (6 oz)	80
Creamy Mushroom as prep	1 serv (6 oz)	60
Green Pea as prep	1 serv (6 oz)	80
Hearty Chicken Noodle as prep	1 serv (6 oz)	60
Ring Noodle as prep	1 serv (6 oz)	50
Spring Vegetable as prep	1 serv (6 oz)	45
Tomato as prep	1 serv (6 oz)	100
Emes		
Beef Base	1 tsp	18
Chicken Base	1 tsp	18
Fantastic		
Cha-Cha Chili Low Fat	1 pkg	220
Goodman's		
Cup Of Soup Beef	1 pkg (1½ cups)	180
Cup Of Soup Chicken Noodle	1 pkg (1½ cups)	180
Cup Of Soup Vegetable	1 pkg (1½ cups)	180
Matzo Ball & Soup	1 cup	40
Matzo Ball & Soup 50% Less Salt	1 serv	50
Noodleman	1 cup	45
Noodleman Low Sodium	1 cup	50
Onion	1 cup	30
Onion Low Sodium	1 cup	30
Hain		
Cheese & Broccoli	¾ cup	310
Cheese Savory	¾ cup	250
Savory Lentil	¾ cup	130
Savory Minestrone	¾ cup	110
Savory Mushroom	¾ cup	210
Savory Mushroom No Salt Added	¾ cup	250
Savory Onion	¾ cup	50
Savory Onion No Salt Added	¾ cup	50
Savory Potato Leek	¾ cup	260
Savory Split Pea	¾ cup	310
Savory Tomato	¾ cup	220
Savory Vegetable	¾ cup	80
Savory Vegetable No Salt Added	¾ cup	80
Health Valley		
Chicken Noodles w/ Vegetables	1 serv	110
Corn Chowder w/ Tomatoes	1 serv	100
Creamy Potatoe w/ Broccoli	1 serv	70
Garden Split Pea w/ Carrots	1 serv	130

FOOD	PORTION	CALS.
Health Valley (CONT.)		
Lentil w/ Couscous	1 serv	130
Pasta Italiano	1 serv	140
Pasta Marinara	1 serv	100
Pasta Parmesan	1 serv	100
Spicy Black Bean w/ Couscous	1 serv	130
Zesty Black Bean w/ Rice	1 serv	100
Herb-Ox		
Beef Bouillon	1 cube (3.5 g)	5
Beef Instant Bouillon Powder	1 tsp (4 g)	5
Beef Instant Broth & Seasoning Pack	1 pkg (4.5 g)	5
Beef Instant Broth & Seasoning Pack Low Sodium	1 pkg (4 g)	10
Chicken Bouillon	1 cube (4 g)	5
Chicken Instant Bouillon Powder	1 tsp (4 g)	5
Chicken Instant Broth & Seasoning Pack	1 pkg (4 g)	5
Chicken Instant Broth & Seasoning Pack Low Sodium	1 pkg (4 g)	10
Vegetable Bouillon	1 cube (4 g)	5
Hodgson Mill		
13 Bean not prep	1.5 oz	100
Hurst		
15 Bean Soup Beef	1 serv (6 oz)	120
15 Bean Soup Cajun	1 serv	120
15 Bean Soup Chicken	1 serv (6 oz)	120
15 Bean Soup Chili	1 serv (6 oz)	120
15 Bean Soup Ham	1 serv	120
HamBeens Great Northern Bean	1 serv	120
HamBeens Navy Bean	1 serv	120
Pasta Fagioli	1 serv	120
Spanish American Pinto Bean	1 serv	120
Spanish-American Black Bean	1 serv	120
Knorr		
Black Bean Cup-A-Soup as prep	1 pkg	200
Broccoli as prep	8 fl oz	160
Cauliflower as prep	8 fl oz	100
Chef's Series Wild Mushroom as prep	8 fl oz	100
Chick 'N Pasta as prep	8 fl oz	90
Chicken Bouillon as prep	8 fl oz	16
Chicken Flavored Noodle as prep	8 fl oz	100
Chicken Noodle Instant as prep	6 fl oz	25
Fine Herb as prep	8 fl oz	130
Fish Bouillon as prep	8 fl oz	10
French Onion as prep	8 fl oz	50

FOOD	PORTION	CALS.
Knorr (CONT.)		
Hearty Minestrone Cup-A-Soup as prep	1 pkg	150
Lentil Cup-A-Soup as prep	1 pkg	220
Mushroom as prep	8 fl oz	100
Navy Bean Cup-A-Soup as prep	1 pkg	140
Oriental Hot And Sour as prep	8 fl oz	50
Oxtail Hearty Beef as prep	8 fl oz	70
Potato Leek Cup-A-Soup as prep	1 pkg	120
Spinach as prep	8 fl oz	100
Spring Vegetable With Herbs as prep	8 fl oz	30
Tomato Basil as prep	8 fl oz	90
Tortellini In Brodo as prep	8 fl oz	60
Vegetable Cup-A-Soup as prep	1 pkg	100
Vegetable as prep	8 fl oz	35
Vegetarian Vegetable Bouillon as prep	8 fl oz	16
Kojel		
Hearty Potato With Vegetables Instant	1 serv (6 fl oz)	60
Noodle Soup Chicken Flavor Instant	1 serv (6 fl oz)	70
Split Pea Instant	1 serv (6 fl oz)	60
Tomato Instant	1 serv (6 fl oz)	50
Vegetable Chicken Couscous Instant	1 serv (6 fl oz)	80
Lipton		
Chicken Noodle w/ White Chicken Meat as prep	1 cup	80
Extra Noodle w/ Chicken Broth as prep	1 cup	90
Giggle Noodle w/ Chicken Broth as prep	1 cup	70
Recipe Secrets Beefy Mushroom	1½ tbsp (0.4 oz)	35
Recipe Secrets Beefy Onion	1 tbsp (0.3 oz)	25
Recipe Secrets Fiesta Herb w/ Red Pepper as prep	1 cup	30
Recipe Secrets Golden Herb w/ Lemon as prep	1 cup	35
Recipe Secrets Golden Onion	1⅔ tbsp (0.5 oz)	50
Recipe Secrets Italian Herb w/ Tomato as prep	1 cup	40
Recipe Secrets Onion as prep	1 cup	20
Recipe Secrets Onion Mushroom as prep	1 cup	30
Recipe Secrets Savory Herb With Garlic as prep	1 cup	30
Recipe Secrets Vegetable as prep	1 cup	30
Ring-O-Noodle w/ Chicken Broth as prep	1 cup	70
Soup Secrets Chicken 'N Onion as prep	1 cup	120
Soup Secrets Chicken w/ Pasta & Beans as prep	1 cup	110

FOOD	PORTION	CALS.
Lipton (CONT.)		
Soup Secrets Country Chicken w/ Pasta & Herbs as prep	1 cup	100
Soup Secrets Honestyle Lentil w/ Bow Tie Pasta as prep	1 cup	130
Soup Secrets Minestrone as prep	1 cup	110
Sprial Pasta w/ Chicken Broth as prep	1 cup	60
Lite Line		
Beef Bouillon Instant Low Sodium	1 tsp	12
Chicken Bouillon Instant Low Sodium	1 tsp	12
Maruchan		
Instant Lunch Oriental Noodles Beef	1 pkg (2.25 oz)	290
Instant Lunch Oriental Noodles Chicken	1 pkg (2.25 oz)	290
Instant Lunch Oriental Noodles Chicken Mushroom	1 pkg (2.25 oz)	280
Instant Lunch Oriental Noodles Mushroom	1 pkg (2.25 oz)	290
Instant Lunch Oriental Noodles Pork	1 pkg (2.25 oz)	290
Instant Lunch Oriental Noodles Shrimp	1 pkg (2.25 oz)	290
Instant Lunch Oriental Noodles Toast Onion	1 pkg (2.25 oz)	270
Instant Lunch Oriental Noodles Vegetable Beef	1 pkg (2.25 oz)	290
Instant Wonton Chicken	1 pkg (1.49 oz)	200
Instant Wonton Hot & Sour	1 pkg (1.49 oz)	200
Instant Wonton Oriental	1 pkg (1.49 oz)	190
Instant Wonton Pork	1 pkg (1.49 oz)	200
Instant Wonton Shrimp	1 pkg (1.49 oz)	200
Oriental Noodle Picante Style Beef	1 pkg (2.25 oz)	290
Oriental Noodle Picante Style Chicken	1 pkg (2.25 oz)	290
Oriental Noodle Picante Style Shrimp	1 pkg (2.25 oz)	300
Ramen Beef	½ pkg (1.5 oz)	190
Ramen Chicken	½ pkg (1.5 oz)	190
Ramen Chicken Mushroom	½ pkg (1.5 oz)	190
Ramen Chili	½ pkg (1.5 oz)	190
Ramen Mushroom	½ pkg (1.5 oz)	190
Ramen Oriental	½ pkg (1.5 oz)	190
Ramen Pork	½ pkg (1.5 oz)	190
Ramen Shrimp	½ pkg (1.5 oz)	190
Wonton Beef	⅓ pkg (0.68 oz)	90
Wonton Chicken	⅓ pkg (0.67 oz)	90
Wonton Pork	⅓ pkg (0.68 oz)	90
Wonton Vegetable	⅓ pkg (0.7 oz)	90
Morga		
Vegetable Bouillon No Salt Added	½ cube (5 g)	25

FOOD	PORTION	CALS.
Morga (CONT.)		
Vegetable Broth Fat Free	1 tsp (4 g)	10
Nile Spice		
Couscous Almondine	1 pkg	200
Couscous Garbanzo	1 pkg	220
Couscous Lentil Curry	1 pkg	200
Couscous Minestrone	1 pkg	180
Couscous Parmesan	1 pkg	200
Homestyle Black Bean	1 pkg	190
Homestyle Chicken Flavored Vegetable	1 pkg	120
Homestyle Lentil	1 pkg	180
Homestyle Minestrone	1 pkg	160
Homestyle Red Beans & Rice	1 pkg	190
Homestyle Split Pea	1 pkg	200
Homestyle Sweet Corn Chowder	1 pkg	120
Italian Tomato	1 pkg	140
Potato Leek	1 pkg	150
Potato Romano	1 pkg	140
Ramen Noodle		
Beef Low Fat as prep	8 oz	160
Beef as prep	8 oz	190
Chicken Low Fat as prep	8 oz	160
Chicken as prep	8 oz	190
Oriental Low Fat as prep	8 oz	150
Oriental as prep	8 oz	190
Pork Low Fat as prep	8 oz	150
Pork as prep	8 oz	200
Ultra Slim-Fast		
Beef Noodle	6 oz	45
Chicken Leek	6 oz	50
Chicken Noodle	6 oz	45
Creamy Broccoli	6 oz	75
Creamy Tomato	6 oz	60
Hearty Vegetable	6 oz	50
Onion	6 oz	45
Potato Leek	6 oz	80
Weight Watchers		
Instant Beef Broth	1 pkg (0.16 oz)	10
Instant Chicken Broth	1 pkg (0.16 oz)	10
Wyler's		
Beef Bouillon Instant	1 tsp	6
Beef Bouillon Instant Cube	1	6
Chicken Bouillon Instant	1 tsp	8
Chicken Bouillon Instant Cube	1	8

FOOD	PORTION	CALS.
Wyler's (CONT.)		
Onion Bouillon Instant	1 tsp	10
Vegetable Bouillon Instant	1 tsp	6
SHELF-STABLE		
Hormel		
Micro Cup Bean & Ham	1 cup (7.5 oz)	190
Micro Cup Beef Vegetable	1 cup (7.5 oz)	90
Micro Cup Broccoli Cheese w/ Ham	1 cup (7.5 oz)	170
Micro Cup Chicken & Rice	1 cup (7.5 oz)	110
Micro Cup Chicken Noodle	1 cup (7.5 oz)	110
Micro Cup New England Clam Chowder	1 cup (7.5 oz)	130
Micro Cup Potato Cheese w/ Ham	1 cup (7.5 oz)	190
Lunch Bucket		
Chicken Noodle	1 pkg (7.25 oz)	90
Country Vegetable	1 pkg (7.25 oz)	70
TAKE-OUT		
gazpacho	1 cup	46
hot & sour	1 serv (14 oz)	173
onion soup gratinee	1 serv	492

SOUR CREAM

(*see also* SOUR CREAM SUBSTITUTES)

FOOD	PORTION	CALS.
Breakstone's		
Free	2 tbsp (1.1 oz)	35
Reduced Fat	2 tbsp (1.1 oz)	45
Sour Cream	2 tbsp (1 oz)	60
Friendship		
Light	2 tbsp (1 oz)	35
Sour Cream	2 tbsp (1 oz)	60
Heluva Good Cheese		
Fat-Free	2 tbsp (1.1 oz)	20
Light	2 tbsp (1.1 oz)	40
Sour Cream	2 tbsp (1.1 oz)	60
Hood		
Fat Free	2 tbsp (1 oz)	20
Light	2 tbsp (1 oz)	40
Sour Cream	2 tbsp (1 oz)	60
Knudsen		
Free	2 tbsp (1.1 oz)	35
Hampshire	2 tbsp (1 oz)	60
Light	2 tbsp (1.1 oz)	50
Naturally Yours		
No Fat	2 tbsp (1 fl oz)	15

SOUR CREAM SUBSTITUTES

FOOD	PORTION	CALS.
Pet		
Imitation	1 tbsp	25

FOOD	PORTION	CALS.
Tofutti		
Better Than Sour Cream Sour Supreme	1 oz	50

SOURSOP
fresh	1	416
fresh cut up	1 cup	150

SOY
(*see also* CHEESE SUBSTITUTES, ICE CREAM AND FROZEN DESSERTS, MILK SUBSTITUTES, MISO, SOY SAUCE, SOYBEANS, TEMPEH, TOFU, YOGURT FROZEN)

lecithin	1 tbsp	104
Loma Linda		
Soyagen All Purpose	¼ cup (1 oz)	130
Soyagen Carob	¼ cup (1 oz)	130
Soyagen No Sucrose	¼ cup (1 oz)	130

SOY SAUCE
shoyu	1 tbsp	9
tamari	1 tbsp	11
Eden		
Shoyu Organic	1 tbsp (0.5 oz)	15
Shoyu Traditional	1 tbsp (0.5 oz)	15
Tamari Organic Domestic	1 tbsp (0.5 oz)	15
Tamari Organic Imported	1 tbsp (0.5 oz)	15
House Of Tsang		
Dark	1 tbsp (0.6 oz)	10
Ginger Flavored	1 tbsp (0.6 oz)	20
Light	1 tbsp (0.6 oz)	5
Low Sodium	1 tbsp (0.6 oz)	5
Low Sodium Ginger	1 tbsp (0.6 oz)	10
Low Sodium Mushroom	1 tbsp (0.6 oz)	10
Ka-Me		
Chinese Light	1 tbsp (0.5 fl oz)	5
Trappey		
Chef Magic	1 tbsp (0.5 oz)	23
Tree Of Life		
Shoyu	1 tbsp (0.5 oz)	15
Tamari Reduced Sodium	1 tbsp (0.5 oz)	20
Tamari Wheat Free	1 tbsp (0.5 oz)	15

SOYBEANS
(*see also* MILK SUBSTITUTES, MISO, SOY, SOY SAUCE, TEMPEH, TOFU)

dry-roasted	½ cup	387
green cooked	½ cup	127
honey toasted	¼ cup (1 oz)	130

FOOD	PORTION	CALS.
roasted	½ cup	405
sprouts raw	½ cup	43
sprouts steamed	½ cup	38
sprouts stir fried	1 cup	125

SPAGHETTI
(*see* PASTA, PASTA DINNERS, PASTA SALAD, SPAGHETTI SAUCE)

SPAGHETTI SAUCE
(*see also* PIZZA SAUCE, TOMATO)

JARRED

Classico

Beef & Pork	4 fl oz	80
Four Cheese	4 fl oz	70
Ripe Olives & Mushrooms	4 fl oz	50
Spicy Red Pepper	4 fl oz	50
Sweet Peppers & Onions	4 fl oz	50
Tomato & Basil	4 fl oz	60

Contadina

Italian	¼ cup	15
Sauce	¼ cup	20
Thick & Zesty	¼ cup	15

Del Monte

Traditional	½ cup (4.4 oz)	80
Traditional No Sugar Added	½ cup (4.4 oz)	60
With Garlic & Onion	½ cup (4.4 oz)	70
With Green Peppers & Mushrooms	½ cup (4.4 oz)	70
With Meat	½ cup (4.4 oz)	40
With Mushrooms	½ cup (4.4 oz)	80

Eden

Organic No Salt Added	½ cup (4.4 oz)	80

Enrico's

Fat Free Organic Basil	½ cup (4 oz)	50
Fat Free Organic Garlic	½ cup (4 oz)	50
Fat Free Organic Hot Pepper	½ cup (4 oz)	50
Fat Free Organic Mushroom	½ cup (4 oz)	60
Fat Free Organic Traditional	½ cup (4 oz)	45

Healthy Choice

Extra Chunky Garlic & Onion	½ cup (4.4 oz)	43
Extra Chunky Italian Vegetable	½ cup (4.4 oz)	39
Extra Chunky Mushroom	½ cup (4.4 oz)	41
Garlic & Herbs	½ cup (4.4 oz)	47
Super Chunky Mushroom & Sweet Peppers	½ cup (4.4 oz)	44
Super Chunky Tomato, Mushroom & Garlic	½ cup (4.4 oz)	46

FOOD	PORTION	CALS.
Healthy Choice (CONT.)		
Super Chunky Vegetable Primavera	½ cup (4.4 oz)	46
Traditional	½ cup (4.4 oz)	47
With Meat	½ cup (4.4 oz)	47
With Mushrooms	½ cup (4.4 oz)	47
Hunt's		
Chunky Marinara	½ cup (4.4 oz)	60
Chunky Tomato Garlic & Onion	½ cup (4.4 oz)	61
Chunky Vegetable	½ cup (4.4 oz)	63
Classic Garlic & Onion	½ cup (4.4 oz)	58
Classic Tomato & Basil	½ cup (4.4 oz)	48
Classic Italian With Parmesan	½ cup (4.4 oz)	50
Home Style With Meat	½ cup (4.4 oz)	56
Home Style With Mushrooms	½ cup (4.4 oz)	56
Homestyle Traditional	½ cup (4.4 oz)	56
Italian Cheese & Garlic	½ cup (4.5 oz)	65
Italian Sausage	½ cup (4.5 oz)	77
Old Country Garlic & Herbs	½ cup (4.4 oz)	63
Old Country Italian Style Vegetables	½ cup (4.4 oz)	64
Old Country Traditional	½ cup (4.4 oz)	53
Old Country With Meat	½ cup (4.4 oz)	56
Old Country With Mushrooms	½ cup (4.4 oz)	53
Original Traditional	½ cup (4.4 oz)	65
Original With Meat	½ cup (4.4 oz)	65
Original With Mushrooms	½ cup (4.4 oz)	65
Mama Rizzo's		
Mushroom Onion	½ cup (4.3 oz)	60
Pepper Mushroom Onion	½ cup (4.3 oz)	60
Pepper Primavera Vegetable	½ cup (4.2 oz)	50
Pepper Tomato Basil Garlic	½ cup (4.7 oz)	60
Primavera Vegetable	½ cup (4.2 oz)	50
Tomato Basil Garlic	½ cup (4.6 oz)	60
Muir Glen		
Organic Cabernet Marinara	½ cup (4.4 oz)	45
Organic Chunky Style	½ cup (4.5 oz)	80
Organic Fat Free Tomato Basil	½ cup (4.3 oz)	50
Organic Garlic Onion	½ cup (4.3 oz)	50
Organic Garlic Roasted Garlic	½ cup (4.4 oz)	45
Organic Green Pepper & Mushroom	½ cup (4.5 oz)	70
Organic Italian Herb	½ cup (4.5 oz)	60
Organic Romano Cheese	½ cup (4.5 oz)	90
Organic Sun Dried Tomato	½ cup (4.4 oz)	40
Organic Sweet Pepper Onion	½ cup (4.4 oz)	40
Organic Tomato Basil	½ cup (4.3 oz)	50

FOOD	PORTION	CALS.
Newman's Own		
Marinara Ventian	½ cup (4.4 oz)	60
Marinara Ventian w/ Mushrooms	½ cup (4.4 oz)	60
Pasta Sauce Bambolina	½ cup (4.5 oz)	100
Pasta Sauce Roasted Garlic & Red & Green Peppers	½ cup (4.7 oz)	70
Pasta Sauce Say Cheese	½ cup (4.4 oz)	90
Sockarooni	½ cup (4.4 oz)	60
Prego		
Chunky Sausage & Green Peppers	4 oz	160
Extra Chunky Garden Combination	4 oz	80
Extra Chunky Mushroom & Tomato	4 oz	110
Extra Chunky Mushroom & Green Pepper	4 oz	100
Extra Chunky Mushroom & Onion	4 oz	100
Extra Chunky Mushroom With Extra Spice	4 oz	100
Extra Chunky Tomato & Onion	4 oz	110
Marinara	4 oz	100
Meat Flavored	4 oz	140
Mushroom	4 oz	130
Onion & Garlic	4 oz	110
Regular	4 oz	130
Three Cheese	4 oz	100
Tomato & Basil	4 oz	100
Pritikin		
Chunky Garden	½ cup (4 oz)	50
Marinara	½ cup (4 oz)	60
Original	½ cup (4 oz)	60
Progresso		
Marinara	½ cup (4.3 oz)	90
Meat Flavored	½ cup (4.4 oz)	100
Mushroom	½ cup (4.4 oz)	100
Sauce	½ cup (4.4 oz)	100
Ragu		
Fino Italian Garden Medley	½ cup (4.5 oz)	90
Fino Italian Garlic & Basil	½ cup (4.5 oz)	90
Fino Italian Parmesan	½ cup (4.5 oz)	100
Fino Italian Sliced Mushroom	½ cup (4.5 oz)	90
Fino Italian Tomato & Herb	½ cup (4.5 oz)	90
Fino Italian Zesty Tomato	½ cup (4.5 oz)	90
Gardenstyle Chunky Garden Combination	½ cup (4.5 oz)	120
Gardenstyle Chunky Green & Red Pepper	½ cup (4.5 oz)	120
Gardenstyle Chunky Mushroom & Green Pepper	½ cup (4.5 oz)	120
Gardenstyle Chunky Mushroom & Onion	½ cup (4.5 oz)	120

FOOD	PORTION	CALS.
Ragu (CONT.)		
Gardenstyle Chunky Tomato Garlic & Onion	½ cup (4.5 oz)	120
Gardenstyle Super Mushroom	½ cup (4.5 oz)	120
Gardenstyle Super Vegetable Primavera	½ cup (4.5 oz)	110
Homestyle Mushroom	½ cup (4.5 oz)	120
Homestyle Tomato & Herb	½ cup (4.5 oz)	120
Homestyle With Meat	½ cup (4.5 oz)	130
Light Chunky Mushroom	½ cup (4.4 oz)	50
Light Garden Harvest	½ cup (4.4 oz)	50
Light No Sugar Added	½ cup (4.4 oz)	60
Light Tomato & Herb	½ cup (4.4 oz)	50
Old World Style Marinara	½ cup (4.4 oz)	90
Old World Style Mushrooms	½ cup (4.4 oz)	80
Old World Style Traditional	½ cup (4.4 oz)	80
Old World Style With Meat	½ cup (4.4 oz)	90
Sauce	4 fl oz	80
Thick & Hearty Mushroom	½ cup (4.5 oz)	120
Thick & Hearty Spaghetti Sauce	4 oz	100
Thick & Hearty Tomato & Herb	½ cup (4.5 oz)	120
Thick & Hearty With Meat	1.2 cup (4.5 oz)	130
Tree Of Life		
Pasta Sauce	½ cup (4 oz)	50
Pasta Sauce Calabrese	½ cup (3.9 oz)	60
Pasta Sauce Fat Free Classic	½ cup (3.9 oz)	40
Pasta Sauce Fat Free Mushroom & Basil	½ cup (3.9 oz)	30
Pasta Sauce Fat Free Onion & Garlic	½ cup (3.9 oz)	30
Pasta Sauce Fat Free Sweet Pepper	½ cup (3.9 oz)	30
Pasta Sauce No Salt	½ cup (3.9 oz)	50
MIX		
Durkee		
American Style as prep	½ cup	15
Family Style as prep	½ cup	20
Spaghetti Sauce as prep	½ cup	15
With Mushrooms as prep	½ cup	15
Zesty as prep	½ cup	20
French's		
All American as prep	½ cup	20
Italian as prep	½ cup	16
Mushroom as prep	½ cup	20
Thick as prep	½ cup	10
Zesty Pasta as prep	½ cup	20
REFRIGERATED		
Contadina		
Alfredo	½ cup (4.2 fl oz)	400

FOOD	PORTION	CALS.
Contadina (CONT.)		
Four Cheese Sauce With White Wine & Shallots	½ cup (4.2 fl oz)	320
Light Alfredo	½ cup (4.2 fl oz)	190
Light Chunky Tomato	½ cup (4.4 fl oz)	45
Light Garden Vegetable	½ cup (4.4 fl oz)	45
Marinara	½ cup (4.4 fl oz)	80
Pesto With Basil	¼ cup (2 oz)	310
Pesto With Sun Dried Tomatoes	¼ cup (2 oz)	250
Plum Tomato With Basil	½ cup (4.4 fl oz)	70
Spicy Italian Sausage & Bell Pepper	½ cup (4.4 fl oz)	100
Di Giorno		
Alfredo	¼ cup (2.2 oz)	180
Basil Pesto	¼ cup (2.2 oz)	320
Four Cheese	¼ cup (2.2 oz)	160
Garlic Pesto	¼ cup (2.1 oz)	340
Light Alfredo Sauce	¼ cup (2.4 oz)	140
Marinara	½ cup (4.5 oz)	70
Plum Tomato Cream Sauce	½ cup (4.4 oz)	160
Plum Tomato & Mushroom	½ cup (4.4 oz)	60
Roasted Red Bell Pepper Cream Sauce	¼ cup (2.3 oz)	140

SPANISH FOOD

(*see also* BEANS, CHIPS, CHILI, DINNER, PEPPERS, SALSA, SNACKS, SAUCE, TORTILLA)

CANNED

FOOD	PORTION	CALS.
Chi-Chi's		
Pico De Gallo	2 tbsp (1.2 oz)	10
Derby		
Tamales	2	160
El Molino		
Enchilada Sauce Hot	2 tbsp	16
Green Chili Sauce Mild	2 tbsp	10
Guiltless Gourmet		
Picante Mild	1 oz	6
Queso Mild Cheddar	1 oz	22
Hormel		
Tamales Beef	3 (7.5 oz)	280
Tamales Chicken	3 (7.5 oz)	210
Tamales Hot Spicy Beef	3 (7.5 oz)	280
Tamales Jumbo Beef	2 (6.9 oz)	270
Old El Paso		
Tamales	3 (7.2 oz)	330

FOOD	PORTION	CALS.
Van Camp's		
Tamales	2 (5.1 oz)	210
FROZEN		
Amy's Organic		
Black Bean Vegetable Enchilada	1 (4.75 oz)	130
Burritos Bean & Cheese	1 (6 oz)	280
Burritos Bean & Rice Non-Dairy	1 (6 oz)	250
Burritos Black Bean Vegetable	1 (6 oz)	320
Burritos Breakfast	1 (6 oz)	230
Cheese Enchilada	1 (4.7 oz)	210
Mexican Tamale Pie	1 (8 oz)	220
Pocket Sandwich Tamale	1 (4.5 oz)	250
Whole Meals Cheese Enchilada	1 pkg (9 oz)	330
Whole Meals Enchilada	1 pkg (10 oz)	250
Banquet		
Beef Enchilada	1 pkg (11 oz)	320
Chimichanga Meal	1 pkg (9.5 oz)	470
Enchilada Cheese	1 pkg (11 oz)	350
Enchilada Chicken	1 pkg (11 oz)	360
Family Entree Beef Enchilada w/ Cheese	1 serv (4.67 oz)	130
Chi-Chi's		
Burro Beef	1 pkg (15.9 oz)	590
Burro Chicken	1 pkg (15.9 oz)	540
Chimichanga Beef	1 pkg (15.9 oz)	630
Chimichanga Chicken	1 pkg (15.9 oz)	580
Enchilada Chicken Suprema	1 pkg (15.9 oz)	600
Enchilida Baja	1 pkg (15.9 oz)	590
Healthy Choice		
Beef Burrito Ranchero Medium	1 (5.4 oz)	290
Beef Burrito Ranchero Mild	1 (5.4 oz)	300
Beef Enchilada Rio Grande	1 meal (13.4 oz)	410
Burrito Chicken Con Queso	1 (5.4 oz)	280
Chicken Enchilada Supreme	1 meal (13.4 oz)	390
Enchiladas Suiza Chicken	1 meal (10 oz)	270
Fiesta Chicken Fajitas	1 meal (7 oz)	260
Jimmy Dean		
Burrito Breakfast Bacon	1 (4 oz)	260
Burrito Breakfast Sausage	1 (4 oz)	250
Le Menu		
Entree LightStyle Enchiladas Chicken	8 oz	280
Lean Cuisine		
Chicken Enchilada Suiza w/ Mexican Style Rice	1 pkg (9 oz)	280

FOOD	PORTION	CALS.
Life Choice		
Burrito Black Bean	1 meal (13.2 oz)	410
Vegetable Enchilada Sonora	1 meal (14 oz)	420
Lightlife		
Vegetarian Taco	2 oz	51
Old El Paso		
Burrito Bean & Cheese	1 (4.9 oz)	290
Burrito Beef & Bean Hot	1 (5 oz)	320
Burrito Beef & Bean Medium	1 (5 oz)	320
Burrito Beef & Bean Mild	1 (5 oz)	330
Chimichanga Beef	1 (4.5 oz)	370
Chimichanga Chicken	1 (4.5 oz)	350
Patio		
Burrito Bean & Cheese	1 (5 oz)	270
Burrito Chicken	1 (5 oz)	260
Burrito Red Chili	1 (5 oz)	270
Burritos Beef & Bean	1 (5 oz)	280
Burritos Beef & Bean Green Chili	1 (5 oz)	260
Burritos Beef & Bean Red Chili	1 (5 oz)	260
Enchilada Beef Dinner	1 meal (12 oz)	320
Enchilada Cheese Dinner	1 meal (12 oz)	330
Enchilada Chicken	1 pkg (12 oz)	380
Family Entree Beef Enchilada	2 (5.7 oz)	170
Family Entree Enchilada Beef	2 (5.3 oz)	250
Family Entree Enchilada Beef & Cheese	2 (5.3 oz)	250
Family Entree Enchilada Cheese	2 (5.7 oz)	170
Fiesta Dinner	1 meal (12 oz)	340
Mexican Dinner	1 meal (13.25 oz)	440
Salis Con Queso	1 pkg (11 oz)	390
Patio Britos		
Beef & Bean	10 (6 oz)	420
Nacho Beef	10 (6 oz)	410
Nacho Cheese	10 (6 oz)	360
Spicy Chicken	10 (6 oz)	400
Rudy's Farm		
Burrito Beef/Bean	1 (5 oz)	326
Burrito Hot Beef/Bean	1 (5 oz)	305
Senor Felix's		
Burrito Black Bean	1 (10 oz)	540
Burrito Black Bean Soy	1 (5 oz)	240
Burrito Chicken	1 (10 oz)	520
Burrito Hot Potato	1 (10 oz)	560
Burrito Soy Hot	1 (10 oz)	520
Burritos Charbroiled Chicken	1 + 4 tsp sauce (6.7 oz)	320

FOOD	PORTION	CALS.
Senor Felix's (CONT.)		
Burritos Sonora Style	1 + 4 tsp sauce (6.7 oz)	280
Burritos Yucatan Style	1 + 4 tsp sauce (6.7 oz)	310
Empanadas Chicken	1 (4.7 oz)	340
Empanadas Corn & Rice	1 (4.7 oz)	280
Empanadas Pumpkin & Mushroom	1 (4.7 oz)	260
Empanadas Spinach & Ricotta	1 (4.7 oz)	260
Enchilada Red Pepper	1 (10 oz)	420
Enchilada Soy Verda	1 (10 oz)	430
Enchilada Supreme Soy Cheese	1 (10 oz)	460
Enchilada Verde	1 (5 oz)	423
Tamales Blue Corn & Soy Cheese	2 + 4 tsp sauce (5.7 oz)	240
Tamales Chicken	2 + 4 tsp sauce (5.7 oz)	240
Tamales Gourmet Vegetarian	2 + 4 tsp sauce	240
Taquitos Blue Corn Soy	3 + 4 tsp sauce (5.2 oz)	230
Taquitos Chicken	2 + 4 tsp sauce (5.7 oz)	240
Stouffer's		
Chicken Enchilada	1 serv (4.8 oz)	230
Swanson		
Enchiladas Beef	13.75 oz	480
Mexican Style Combination	14.25 oz	490
Mexican Style Hungry Man	20.25 oz	820
Today's Tamales		
Cheese & Chili	1 pkg (7 oz)	390
Del Sol	1 pkg (6.5 oz)	310
Original Bean	1 pkg (7 oz)	330
Spicy Taco	1 pkg (7 oz)	310
Tyson		
Fajita Kit Beef	3.8 oz	160
Fajita Kit Chicken	4 oz	80
Weight Watchers		
Smart Ones Chicken Enchiladas Suiza	1 pkg (9 oz)	270
Smart Ones Santa Fe Style Rice & Beans	1 pkg (10 oz)	290
MIX		
Hain		
Taco Seasoning Mix	1/10 pkg	10
Old El Paso		
Burrito Seasoning Mix	2 tsp (6 g)	20
Dinner Kit Burrito as prep	1	280
Dinner Kit Soft Taco as prep	2	380
Dinner Kit Taco as prep	2	270
Enchilada Sauce Mix	2 tsp (4 g)	10
Taco Mix 40% Less Sodium	2 tsp (6 g)	20
Taco Seasoning Mix	2 tsp (6 g)	20

FOOD	PORTION	CALS.
Ortega		
Taco Meat Seasoning Mix Mild	1 filled taco	90
Taco Bell		
Home Originals Chicken Fajita Dinner as prep	2 (6.9 oz)	340
Home Originals Chicken Fajita Seasoning Mix	1 tbsp (8 g)	25
Home Originals Soft Taco Dinner as prep	2 (6.3 oz)	410
Home Originals Taco Dinner as prep	2 (4.4 oz)	280
Home Originals Taco Seasoning Mix	2 tsp (6 g)	20
Home Originals Ultimate Bean Burrito Dinner as prep	1 (4.4 oz)	200
Home Originals Ultimate Nachos as prep	12 pieces (4.6 oz)	240
READY-TO-EAT		
taco shell baked	1 med (0.5 oz)	61
taco shell baked w/o salt	1 med (0.5 oz)	61
Chi-Chi's		
Taco Shells White Corn	2 (1.2 oz)	170
Taco Shells Yellow Corn	2 shells (1.2 oz)	170
Old El Paso		
Taco Shells Mini	7 (1.1 oz)	160
Taco Shells Regular	3 (1.1 oz)	170
Taco Shells Super	2 (1.3 oz)	190
Taco Shells White Corn	3 (1.1 oz)	170
Tostaco Shells	1 (0.8 oz)	130
Tostada Shells	3 (1.1 oz)	160
Taco Bell		
Home Originals Taco Shells	3 (1.1 oz)	150
TAKE-OUT		
burrito w/ apple	1 lg (5.4 oz)	484
burrito w/ apple	1 sm (2.6 oz)	231
burrito w/ beans	2 (7.6 oz)	448
burrito w/ beans & cheese	2 (6.5 oz)	377
burrito w/ beans & chili peppers	2 (7.2 oz)	413
burrito w/ beans & meat	2 (8.1 oz)	508
burrito w/ beans cheese & beef	2 (7.1 oz)	331
burrito w/ beans cheese & chili peppers	2 (11.8 oz)	663
burrito w/ beef	2 (7.7 oz)	523
burrito w/ beef & chili peppers	2 (7.1 oz)	426
burrito w/ beef cheese & chili peppers	2 (10.7 oz)	634
burrito w/ cherry	1 lg (5.4 oz)	484
burrito w/ cherry	1 sm (2.6 oz)	231
chimichanga w/ beef	1 (6.1 oz)	425
chimichanga w/ beef & cheese	1 (6.4 oz)	443

FOOD	PORTION	CALS.
chimichanga w/ beef & red chili peppers	1 (6.7 oz)	424
chimichanga w/ beef cheese & red chili peppers	1 (6.3 oz)	364
enchilada eggplant	1	142
enchilada w/ cheese	1 (5.7 oz)	320
enchilada w/ cheese & beef	1 (6.7 oz)	324
enchirito w/ cheese beef & beans	1 (6.8 oz)	344
frijoles w/ cheese	1 cup (5.9 oz)	226
nachos w/ cheese	6 to 8 (4 oz)	345
nachos w/ cheese & jalapeno peppers	6 to 8 (7.2 oz)	607
nachos w/ cheese beans ground beef & peppers	6 to 8 (8.9 oz)	568
nachos w/ cinnamon & sugar	6 to 8 (3.8 oz)	592
taco	1 sm (6 oz)	370
taco salad	1½ cups	279
taco salad w/ chili con carne	1½ cups	288
tostada w/ beans & cheese	1 (5.1 oz)	223
tostada w/ beans beef & cheese	1 (7.9 oz)	334
tostada w/ beef & cheese	1 (5.7 oz)	315
tostada w/ guacamole	2 (9.2 oz)	360

SPARE RIBS
(*see* PORK)

SPELT
Arrowhead

Spelt	1 oz	83

SPICES
(*see individual names,* HERBS/SPICES)

SPINACH
CANNED
Del Monte

50% Less Salt	½ cup (4 oz)	30
Chopped	½ cup (4 oz)	30
No Salt Added	½ cup (4 oz)	30
Whole Leaf	½ cup (4 oz)	30
Popeye		
Chopped	½ cup (4.1 oz)	40
Leaf	½ cup (4.2 oz)	45
Low Sodium	½ cup (4.2 oz)	35
Sunshine		
Chopped	½ cup (4.1 oz)	40

FRESH

cooked	½ cup	21
malabar cooked	1 cup (1.5 oz)	10

FOOD	PORTION	CALS.
Dole		
Spinach	3 oz	9
Fresh Express		
Spinach	1½ cups (3 oz)	40
FROZEN		
Amy's Organic		
Pocket Sandwich Spinach Feta	1 (4.5 oz)	200
Birds Eye		
Creamed	½ cup (4.3 oz)	100
Whole Leaf	1 cup (2.8 oz)	20
Budget Gourmet		
Au Gratin	1 pkg (5.5 oz)	160
Fresh Like		
Cut Leaf	3.5 oz	21
Green Giant		
Butter Sauce	½ cup (3.4 oz)	40
Creamed	½ cup (3.8 oz)	80
Cut Leaf	¾ cup (2.6 oz)	25
Harvest Fresh	½ cup (3.5 oz)	25
Stouffer's		
Creamed	1 serv (4.5 oz)	160
Souffle	1 serv (4 oz)	150
Tabatchnick		
Creamed	7.5 oz	60
TAKE-OUT		
indian saag	1 serv	28
spanakopita spinach pie	1 cup (6 oz)	196

SPORTS DRINKS
(*see also* NUTRITION SUPPLEMENTS)

FOOD	PORTION	CALS.
Gatorade		
Citrus Cooler	1 cup (8 oz)	50
Fruit Punch	1 cup (8 oz)	50
Grape	1 cup (8 oz)	50
Iced Tea Cooler	1 cup (8 oz)	50
Lemon-Lime	1 cup (8 oz)	50
Lemonade	1 cup (8 oz)	50
Orange	1 cup (8 fl oz)	50
Tropical Fruit	1 cup (8 oz)	50
Powerade		
Fruit Punch	8 fl oz	72
Grape	8 fl oz	73
Lemon-Lime	8 fl oz	70
Orange	8 fl oz	72

FOOD	PORTION	CALS.
Slice		
All Sport Diet Lemon Lime	8 fl oz	1
All Sport Lemon Lime	8 fl oz	72
All Sport Orange	8 fl oz	74
All Sport Punch	8 fl oz	81
Snapple		
Sport Fruit	1 bottle	80
Sport Lemon	1 bottle	80
Sport Lemon Lime	1 bottle	80
Sport Orange	1 bottle	80
Ultra Fuel		
Lemon Lime	16 fl oz	400
SPOT		
baked	3 oz	134
SPROUTS		
Fresh Alternatives		
Deli Blend	½ cup (1 oz)	10
Salad Blend	½ cup (1 oz)	10
Sandwich Blend	½ cup (1 oz)	5
SQUAB		
boneless baked	3.5 oz	175
breast w/o skin raw	1 (3.5 oz)	135
w/o skin raw	1 squab (5.9 oz)	239
SQUASH		
(*see also* ZUCCHINI)		
CANNED		
Allen		
Yellow	½ cup (4.2 oz)	25
Sunshine		
Yellow	½ cup (4.2 oz)	25
FRESH		
acorn cooked mashed	½ cup	41
butternut baked	½ cup	41
crookneck raw sliced	½ cup	12
crookneck sliced cooked	½ cup	18
hubbard baked	½ cup	51
scallop sliced cooked	½ cup	14
spaghetti cooked	½ cup	23
Nature's Pasta		
Spaghetti Squash	1 cup (5.5 oz)	20
SEEDS		
salted & roasted	1 oz	148

FOOD	PORTION	CALS.

SQUID
fried	3 oz	149

SQUIRREL
roasted	3 oz	147

STAR FRUIT
fresh	1	42
Sonoma		
Dried	7-9 pieces (1.4 oz)	140

STRAWBERRIES
FRESH

Dole		
Strawberries	8	50

FROZEN

Big Valley		
Strawberries	⅔ cup (4.9 oz)	50
Birds Eye		
Halves	½ cup (4.7 oz)	120
Halves In Lite Syrup	½ cup (4.6 oz)	70
Whole	½ cup (4.5 oz)	100

STRAWBERRY JUICE
Capri Sun		
Strawberry Cooler Drink	1 pkg (7 oz)	90
Kern's		
Nectar	6 fl oz	110
Kool-Aid		
Drink as prep w/ sugar	1 serv (8 oz)	100
Drink Mix as prep	1 serv (8 oz)	60
Libby		
Nectar	1 can (11.5 fl oz)	210
Veryfine		
Juice-Ups	8 fl oz	140

STUFFING/DRESSING
MIX

bread dry as prep	½ cup	178
cornbread as prep	½ cup	179
Arnold		
All Purpose Seasoned	0.5 oz	50
Corn	0.5 oz	50
Herb Seasoned	0.5 oz	50
Sage & Onion	0.5 oz	50
Kellogg's		
Croutettes Mix	1 cup (1.2 oz)	120

FOOD	PORTION	CALS.
Pepperidge Farm		
Herb Seasoned	¾ cup (1.5 oz)	170
Italian Style Chicken Herb	½ cup (1.2 oz)	130
Italian Style Cornbread	½ cup (1.2 oz)	130
Stove Top		
Chicken as prep w/ margarine	½ cup (3.6 oz)	170
Cornbread as prep w/ margarine	½ cup (3.6 oz)	170
Flexible Serve Chicken as prep w/ margarine	½ cup (3.3 oz)	170
Flexible Serve Cornbread as prep w/ margarine	½ cup (3.3 oz)	160
Flexible Serve Homestyle Herb as prep w/ margarine	½ cup (3.3 oz)	170
For Beef as prep w/ margarine	½ cup (3.7 oz)	180
For Pork as prep w/ margarine	½ cup (3.6 oz)	170
For Turkey as prep w/ margarine	½ cup (3.6 oz)	170
Long Grain & Wild Rice as prep w/ margarine	½ cup (3.7 oz)	180
Lower Sodium Chicken as prep w/ margarine	½ cup (3.6 oz)	180
Microwave Chicken as prep w/ margarine	½ cup (3.5 oz)	160
Microwave Homestyle Cornbread as prep w/ margarine	½ cup (3 oz)	160
Mushroom & Onion as prep w/ margarine	½ cup (3.6 oz)	180
San Francisco Style as prep w/ margarine	½ cup (3.6 oz)	170
Savory Herb as prep w/ margarine	½ cup (3.6 oz)	170
Traditional Sage as prep w/ margarine	½ cup (3.6 oz)	180
TAKE-OUT		
bread	½ cup (3½ oz)	195
STURGEON		
cooked	3 oz	115
roe raw	3.5 oz	207
smoked	1 oz	48
SUCKER		
white baked	3 oz	101
SUGAR		
(*see also* FRUCTOSE, SUGAR SUBSTITUTES, SYRUP)		
brown packed	1 cup (7.7 oz)	828
brown unpacked	1 cup (5.1 oz)	546
maple	1 piece (1 oz)	100
powdered	1 tbsp (0.3 oz)	31
powdered unsifted	1 cup (4.2 oz)	467

FOOD	PORTION	CALS.
white	1 cup (7 oz)	773
white	1 packet (6 g)	25
white	1 tbsp	45
white	1 tsp (4 g)	15
C&H		
White	1 tsp	16
Domino		
White	1 tsp	16
Hain		
Turbinado	1 tbsp	50
Hollywood		
Turbinado	1 tbsp	50

SUGAR SUBSTITUTES
(*see also* FRUCTOSE)

Mrs. Bateman's		
Sugarlike	1 tsp (4 g)	4
NatraTaste		
Packet	1 pkg (1 g)	0
Sweet One		
Packet	1 pkg (1 g)	4
Sweet'N Low		
Granulated	1 pkg (1g)	4
Weight Watchers		
Sweetner	1 serv (1 g)	5

SUGAR-APPLE

fresh	1	146
fresh cut up	1 cup	236

SUNCHOKE

fresh raw sliced	½ cup	57

SUNDAE TOPPINGS
(*see* ICE CREAM TOPPINGS)

SUNFISH

pumpkinseed baked	3 oz	97

SUNFLOWER

Fisher		
Seeds Oil Roasted	1 oz	170
Seeds Salted In Shell shelled	1 oz	160
Seeds Salted In Shell unshelled	1 oz	170
Frito Lay		
Seeds	1 oz	180

FOOD	PORTION	CALS.
Planters		
Kernels	1 pkg (1.7 oz)	290
Kernels	1 pkg (2 oz)	340
Kernels Barbecue	1 pkg (1.7 oz)	290
Kernels Honey Roasted	1 pkg (1.7 oz)	280
Kernels Salted	1 oz	170
Munch'N Go Singles Dry Roasted	1 pkg	120
Nuts Dry Roasted	¼ cup (1.1 oz)	190
Original With Shell Dry Roasted	¾ cup	160
Stone-Buhr		
Seeds Raw	4 tsp (1 oz)	170

SUSHI
TAKE-OUT

california roll	1 piece (0.8 oz)	28
kim chi	⅓ cup (5.8 oz)	18
sashimi	1 serv (6 oz)	198
tuna roll	1 piece (0.7 oz)	23
vegetable roll	1 piece (1.2 oz)	27
vinegared ginger	⅓ cup (1.6 oz)	48
wasabi	2 tsp (0.3 oz)	5
yellowtail roll	1 piece (0.6 oz)	25

SWAMP CABBAGE

chopped cooked	½ cup	10

SWEET POTATO
(*see also* YAM)
CANNED

Princella		
Mashed	⅔ cup (5.1 oz)	120
Royal Prince		
Candied	½ cup (4.9 oz)	210
Halves	3 pieces (5.7 oz)	190
Orange Pineapple	½ cup (4.8 oz)	210
Sugary Sam		
Mashed	⅔ cup (5.1 oz)	120

FRESH

baked w/ skin	1 (3.5 oz)	118
leaves cooked	½ cup	11

TAKE-OUT

candied	3.5 oz	144

SWEETBREADS

beef braised	3 oz	230
lamb braised	3 oz	199
veal braised	3 oz	218

FOOD	PORTION	CALS.
SWISS CHARD		
cooked	½ cup	18
SWORDFISH		
cooked	3 oz	132
SYRUP		
(*see also* ICE CREAM TOPPINGS, PANCAKE/WAFFLE SYRUP)		
corn dark	1 tbsp (0.7 oz)	56
corn dark	1 cup (11.5 oz)	925
corn light	1 cup (11.5 oz)	925
corn light	1 tbsp (0.7 oz)	56
malt	1 tbsp (0.8 oz)	76
malt	1 cup (13 oz)	1222
maple	1 tbsp (0.8 oz)	52
maple	1 cup (11.1 oz)	824
rose hip	3.5 oz	33
sorghum	1 cup (11.6 oz)	957
sorghum	1 tbsp (0.7 oz)	61
Estee		
Blueberry	¼ cup	80
McIlhenny		
Cane	2 tbsp (1.4 oz)	130
Quik		
Strawberry	2 tbsp (1.5 oz)	110
Red Wing		
Strawberry	2 tbsp (1.4 oz)	110
Tree Of Life		
Maple	¼ cup (2.1 oz)	200
Rice Syrup	2 tbsp (1 oz)	120
Whistling Wings		
Blueberry	1 oz	45
Raspberry	1 oz	60
TACO		
(*see* SPANISH FOOD)		
TAHINI		
(*see* SESAME)		
TAMARIND		
fresh	1	5
fresh cut up	1 cup	287
TANGERINE		
CANNED		
in light syrup	½ cup	76
juice pack	½ cup	46

FOOD	PORTION	CALS.
FRESH		
sections	1 cup	86
tangerine	1	37
Dole		
Tangerine	2	70
TANGERINE JUICE		
fresh	1 cup	106
After The Fall		
Juice	1 can (12 oz)	170
Fresh Samantha		
Fresh Juice	1 cup (8 oz)	106
Minute Maid		
Frozen	8 fl oz	120
TAPIOCA		
pearl dry	½ cup (2.7 oz)	272
Minute		
Minute Tapioca	1½ tsp (6 g)	20
TARO		
chips	10 (0.8 oz)	115
chips	1 oz	141
leaves cooked	½ cup	18
shoots sliced cooked	½ cup	10
sliced cooked	½ cup (2.3 oz)	94
TARRAGON		
ground	1 tsp	5
TEA/HERBAL TEA		
(*see also* ICED TEA)		
HERBAL		
Bigelow		
Almond Orange	5 fl oz	tr
Apple Orchard	5 fl oz	5
Apple Spice	5 fl oz	tr
Chamomile	5 fl oz	tr
Chamomile Mint	5 fl oz	tr
Cinnamon Orange	5 fl oz	tr
Early Riser	5 fl oz	3
Feeling Free	5 fl oz	1
Fruit & Almond	5 fl oz	1
Hibiscus & Rose Hips	5 fl oz	1
I Love Lemon	5 fl oz	1
Lemon & C	5 fl oz	tr

FOOD	PORTION	CALS.
Bigelow (CONT.)		
Looking Good	5 fl oz	1
Mint Blend	5 fl oz	tr
Mint Medley	5 fl oz	1
Orange & C	5 fl oz	tr
Orange & Spice	5 fl oz	1
Peppermint	5 fl oz	tr
Roasted Grains & Carob	5 fl oz	3
Spearmint	5 fl oz	tr
Sweet Dreams	5 fl oz	1
Take-A-Break	5 fl oz	3
Celestial Seasonings		
Almond Sunset	8 fl oz	3
Bengal Spice	8 fl oz	5
Caffeine Free	8 fl oz	2
Chamomile	8 fl oz	2
Cinnamon Apple Spice	8 fl oz	<3
Cinnamon Rose	8 fl oz	<4
Country Peach Spice	8 fl oz	3
Cranberry Cove	8 fl oz	2
Emperor's Choice	8 fl oz	4
Ginseng Plus	8 fl oz	3
Grandma's Tummy Mint	8 fl oz	2
Lemon Mist	8 fl oz	3
Lemon Zinger	8 fl oz	4
Mama Bear's Cold Care	8 fl oz	6
Mandarin Orange Spice	8 fl oz	5
Mellow Mint	8 fl oz	2
Mint Magic	8 fl oz	1
Orange Zinger	8 fl oz	6
Peppermint	8 fl oz	2
Raspberry Patch	8 fl oz	4
Red Zinger	8 fl oz	4
Roastaroma	8 fl oz	10
Sleepytime	8 fl oz	4
Spearmint	8 fl oz	5
Strawberry Fields	8 fl oz	4
Sunburst C	8 fl oz	3
Tropical Escape	8 fl oz	1
Wild Forest Blackberry	8 fl oz	2
Lipton		
Bedtime Story	1 tea bag	0
Cinnamon Apple	1 tea bag	0
Country Cranberry	1 tea bag	0

FOOD	PORTION	CALS.
Lipton (CONT.)		
Gentle Orange	1 tea bag	0
Ginger Twist	1 tea bag	0
Golden Lemon Honey	1 tea bag	0
Lemon Soother	1 tea bag	0
Peppermint Breeze	1 tea bag	0
REGULAR		
Bigelow		
Chinese Fortune	5 fl oz	1
Cinnamon Stick	5 fl oz	1
Constant Comment	5 fl oz	1
Darjeeling Blend	5 fl oz	1
Earl Gray	5 fl oz	1
English Teatime	5 fl oz	1
Lemon Lift	5 fl oz	1
Orange Pekoe	5 fl oz	1
Peppermint Stick	5 fl oz	1
Plantation Mint	5 fl oz	1
Raspberry Royale	5 fl oz	1
Celestial Seasonings		
Cinnamon Vienna	8 fl oz	2
Earl Grey Extraordinary	8 fl oz	3
English Breakfast Classic	8 fl oz	3
Lemon	8 fl oz	7
Mint	8 fl oz	4
Morning Thunder	8 fl oz	3
Naturally Decaffeinated	8 fl oz	10
Orange Spice	8 fl oz	7
Orange Spice Decaff	8 fl oz	7
Organically Grown	8 fl oz	12
Raspberry	8 fl oz	7
General Foods		
International Instant Tea Decaffeinated English Breakfast Creme	1 serv (8 oz)	70
International Instant Tea Decaffeinated Viennese Cinnamon Creme	1 serv (8 oz)	70
International Instant Tea English Breakfast Creme as prep	1 serv (8 oz)	70
International Instant Tea English Raspberry Creme as prep	1 serv (8 oz)	70
International Instant Tea Island Orange Creme as prep	1 serv (8 oz)	70
International Instant Tea Viennese Cinnamon Creme as prep	1 serv (8 oz)	70

FOOD	PORTION	CALS.
Lipton		
Brisk Tea as prep	1 serv	0
Decaffeinated Brisk Tea as prep	1 serv	0
English Blend as prep	1 cup	0
Flavored Blackberry	1 tea bag	0
Flavored Decaffeinated Orange & Spice	1 tea bag	0
Flavored Honey & Lemon	1 tea bag	0
Flavored Mint	1 tea bag	0
Flavored Orange & Spice	1 tea bag	0
Flavored Raspberry	1 tea bag	0
Green Tea	1 tea bag	0
Green Tea Orange, Passionfruit & Jasmine	1 tea bag	0
Loose Tea	1 tsp (2 g)	0
Tetley		
Tea Bag as prep	1	0

TEFF
Arrowhead

Whole Grain	¼ cup (1.6 oz)	160

TEMPEH
Lightlife

Garden Vege	4 oz	142
Tempeh	4 oz	182
White Wave		
Burger	1 patty (3 oz)	110
Lemon Broil	1 patty (2 oz)	130
Organic Wild Rice	⅓ block (2.7 oz)	140
Teriyaki Burger	1 patty (3 oz)	110

THYME

ground	1 tsp	4
Watkins		
Thyme	¼ tsp (0.5 oz)	0

TILEFISH

cooked	3 oz	125

TOFU

fresh fried	1 piece (0.5 oz)	35
fuyu salted & fermented	1 block (⅓ oz)	13
koyadofu dried frozen	1 piece (½ oz)	82
okara	½ cup	47
regular	½ cup	94
Casbah		
Gyro as prep w/ tofu	1 patty (2 oz)	105

FOOD	PORTION	CALS.
Hinoichi		
Firm	1 inch slice (3 oz)	60
Long Life		
Tofu	3 oz	60
Mori-Nu		
Extra Firm	1 in slice (3 oz)	55
Firm	1 in slice (3 oz)	50
Lite Extra Firm	1 in slice (3 oz)	35
Lite Firm	1 in slice (3 oz)	35
Soft	1 in slice (3 oz)	45
Nasoya		
Chinise 5 Spice	¼ block (3 oz)	68
Extra Firm	⅕ block (3.2 oz)	92
Firm	⅕ block (3.2 oz)	76
French Country	⅕ block (3 oz)	68
Silken	⅕ block (3.2 oz)	48
Soft	⅕ block (3.2 oz)	63
Tree Of Life		
Baked	⅕ block (3.2 oz)	150
Firm	⅕ block (3.2 oz)	100
Raw Firm	⅕ block (3.2 oz)	100
Ready Ground Hot & Spicy	⅓ pkg (3 oz)	60
Ready Ground Original	⅓ pkg (3 oz)	60
Ready Ground Savory Garlic	⅓ pkg (3 oz)	60
Reduced Fat	⅕ block (3.2 oz)	90
Savory Baked	⅕ block (3.2 oz)	140
Smoked Hot'N Spicy	½ block (3 oz)	120
Smoked Original	½ block (3 oz)	120
White Wave		
Baked Tofus Teriyaki Oriental Style	¼ block (2 oz)	120
Hard	4 oz	120
International Baked Italian Garlic Herb	¼ pkg (2 oz)	120
International Baked Mexican Jalapeno	¼ pkg (2 oz)	120
International Baked Oriental Teriyaki	¼ pkg (2 oz)	120
International Baked Thai Sesame Peanut	¼ pkg (2 oz)	120
Soft	4 oz	120
YOGURT		
Stir Fruity		
Black Cherry	6 oz	141
Blueberry	6 oz	140
Lemon Chiffon	6 oz	152
Mixed Berry	6 oz	149
Orange	6 oz	143
Peach	6 oz.	160

FOOD	PORTION	CALS.
Stir Fruity (CONT.)		
Pina Colada	6 oz	162
Raspberry	6 oz	155
Spiced Apple	6 oz	167
Strawberry	6 oz	140
Tropical Fruit	6 oz	170

TOMATILLO
fresh	1 (1.2 oz)	11
fresh chopped	½ cup	21

TOMATO
(*see also* PIZZA, SPAGHETTI SAUCE)

CANNED

Amore		
Sun-Dried Tomato Paste	1 tsp (6 g)	15
Contadina		
Crushed	¼ cup	20
Italian Paste	2 tbsp	40
Italian Style Pear	½ cup	25
Italian Style Stewed	½ cup	40
Mexican Style Stewed	½ cup	40
Pasta Ready Primavera	½ cup	50
Pasta Ready Tomatoes	½ cup	50
Pasta Ready With Crushed Red Pepper	½ cup	60
Pasta Ready With Mushrooms	½ cup	50
Pasta Ready With Olives	½ cup	60
Pasta Ready With Three Cheeses	½ cup	70
Paste	2 tbsp	30
Peeled Whole	½ cup	25
Puree	¼ cup	20
Recipe Ready	½ cup	25
Stewed	½ cup	40
Del Monte		
Paste	2 tbsp (1.2 oz)	30
Peeled Diced	½ cup (4.4 oz)	25
Puree	¼ cup (2.2 oz)	30
Sauce	¼ cup (2.1 oz)	20
Sauce No Salt Added	¼ cup (2.1 oz)	20
Stewed Cajun Style	½ cup (4.4 oz)	35
Stewed Chunky Chili	½ cup (4.5 oz)	30
Stewed Chunky Pasta	½ cup (4.5 oz)	45
Stewed Chunky Pizza	½ cup (4.5 oz)	35
Stewed Chunky Salsa	½ cup (4.5 oz)	35
Stewed Italian Style	½ cup (4.4 oz)	30

FOOD	PORTION	CALS.
Del Monte (CONT.)		
Stewed Mexican Style	½ cup (4.4 oz)	35
Stewed Original	½ cup (4.4 oz)	35
Stewed Original No Salt Added	½ cup (4.4 oz)	35
Wedges	½ cup (4.4 oz)	35
Whole Peeled	½ cup (4.4 oz)	25
Eden		
Crushed Organic	¼ cup (2.1 oz)	20
Sauce Lightly Seasoned	¼ cup (2.1 oz)	25
Hebrew National		
Pickled	⅓ tomato (1 oz)	4
Hunt's		
Choice Cut	½ cup (4.2 oz)	22
Choice Cut Diced Tomatoes & Green Chiles	2 tbsp (0.4 oz)	1
Choice Cut Diced Tomatoes & Italian Herb	½ cup (4.2 oz)	24
Choice Cut Diced Tomatoes & Roasted Garlic	½ cup (4.2 oz)	24
Crushed	½ cup (4.2 oz)	29
Crushed Angela Mia	½ cup (4.2 oz)	27
Paste	2 tbsp (1.2 oz)	30
Paste Italian	2 tbsp (1.2 oz)	27
Paste No Salt Added	2 tbsp (1.2 oz)	30
Paste With Garlic	2 tbsp (1.2 oz)	28
Pear Shaped	½ cup (4.6 oz)	20
Puree	¼ cup (2.2 oz)	24
Ready Sauce Chunky Chili	¼ cup (2.2 oz)	22
Ready Sauce Chunky Italian	¼ cup (2.2 oz)	26
Ready Sauce Chunky Mexican	¼ cup (2.2 oz)	21
Ready Sauce Chunky Special	¼ cup (2.2 oz)	21
Ready Sauce Chunky Tomato	¼ cup (2.2 oz)	15
Ready Sauce Country Herb	¼ cup (2.2 oz)	33
Ready Sauce Garlic	¼ cup (2.2 oz)	29
Ready Sauce Garlic & Herb	¼ cup (2.2 oz)	26
Ready Sauce Meatloaf Fixins	¼ cup (2.2 oz)	23
Ready Sauce Original	¼ cup (2.2 oz)	30
Ready Sauce Salsa	¼ cup (2.2 oz)	18
Sauce	¼ cup (2.2 oz)	16
Sauce Italian	¼ cup (2.2 oz)	32
Sauce No Salt Added	¼ cup (2.2 oz)	16
Sauce With Herb	¼ cup (2.2 oz)	32
Stewed	½ cup (4.2 oz)	33
Stewed Italian	4 oz	40
Tomatoes	½ cup (4.2 oz)	33

FOOD	PORTION	CALS.
Hunt's (CONT.)		
Whole	2 (5.2 oz)	22
Muir Glen		
Organic Chunky Sauce	¼ cup (2.3 oz)	20
Organic Crushed With Basil	¼ cup (2.3 oz)	25
Organic Diced	½ cup (4.5 oz)	25
Organic Diced No Salt Added	½ cup (4.5 oz)	25
Organic Ground Peeled	¼ cup (2.3 oz)	10
Organic Italian Style Diced	½ cup (4.4 oz)	25
Organic Paste	2 tbsp (1.2 oz)	30
Organic Puree	¼ cup (2.2 oz)	20
Organic Sauce	¼ cup (2.2 oz)	20
Organic Sauce No Salt Added	¼ cup (2.2 oz)	20
Organic Stewed	½ cup (4.5 oz)	30
Organic Stewed Italian Style	½ cup (4.4 oz)	30
Organic Stewed Mexican Style	½ cup (4.4 oz)	30
Organic Whole Peeled	½ cup (4.6 oz)	30
Old El Paso		
Tomatoes & Jalapenos	¼ cup (2 oz)	15
Tomatoes & Green Chilies	¼ cup (2 oz)	10
Progresso		
Crushed	¼ cup (2.1 oz)	20
Paste	2 tbsp (1.2 oz)	30
Peeled Whole	½ cup (4.2 oz)	25
Peeled w/ Basil	½ cup (4.2 oz)	25
Puree	¼ cup (2.2 oz)	25
Puree Thick Style	¼ cup (2.2 oz)	30
Sauce	¼ cup (2.1 oz)	20
Ro-Tel		
Diced Tomatoes & Green Chilies	½ cup (4.4 oz)	20
Rosoff's		
Pickled	⅓ tomato (1 oz)	5
Schorr's		
Pickled	⅓ tomato (1 oz)	4
Sonoma		
Dried Spice Medley oil drained	1 tbsp (0.5 oz)	50
Pesto	¼ cup (2 oz)	110
Tapenade	1 tbsp (0.7 oz)	70
Tree Of Life		
Sauce	¼ cup (2 oz)	20
DRIED		
sun dried	1 piece	5
sun dried in oil	1 piece (3 g)	6

FOOD	PORTION	CALS.
Sonoma		
Bits	2-3 tsp (5 g)	15
Dried	2-3 halves (5 g)	15
Halves	2-3 halves (5 g)	15
Julienne	7-9 pieces (5 g)	15
Pasta Toss	½ cup (0.7 oz)	70
Season It	2-3 tsp (5 g)	20
FRESH		
green	1	30
red	1 (4.5 oz)	26
red chopped	1 cup	35
TAKE-OUT		
stewed	1 cup	80

TOMATO JUICE

Del Monte		
Snap-E-Tom	6 fl oz	40
Snap-E-Tom	8 fl oz	50
Snap-E-Tom	10 fl oz	60
Dole		
Juice	1 bottle (12 oz)	85
Hunt's		
Juice	8 fl oz	22
No Salt Added	8 fl oz	34
Mott's		
Beefamato	8 fl oz	80
Clamato	8 fl oz	100
Clamato Caesar	8 fl oz	100
Muir Glen		
Organic	8 oz	40

TONGUE

beef simmered	3 oz	241
lamb braised	3 oz	234
pork braised	3 oz	230

TOPPINGS

(*see* ICE CREAM TOPPINGS)

TORTILLA

(*see also* CHIPS TORTILLA, SPANISH FOOD)

corn	1 (6 in diam)	56
corn w/o salt	1 (6 in diam) 0.09 oz	56
flour w/o salt	1 (8 in diam) 1.2 oz	114
Alvarado St. Bakery		
Burrito Size	1 (2.2 oz)	170

FOOD	PORTION	CALS.
Alvarado St. Bakery (CONT.)		
Fajita Size	1 (1.6 oz)	130
Old El Paso		
Flour	1 (1.4 oz)	150
Soft Taco Tortilla	2 (1.8 oz)	180
Tyson		
Burrito Style Flour	1	170
Burrito Style Hand Stretched Small Flour	1	106
Burrito Style Heat Pressed Large Flour	1	182
Enchilada Style Corn	1	54
Fajito Style Flour	1	89
Soft Taco Flour	1	121
Whole Wheat	1	120
Zapata		
Tortilla	1 (1.2 oz)	100

TORTILLA CHIPS
(*see* CHIPS)

TREE FERN

chopped cooked	½ cup	28

TRITICALE

dry	1 cup (6.7 oz)	645

TROUT

baked	3 oz	162
seatrout baked	3 oz	113
Clear Springs		
Rainbow	3.5 oz	140

TUMERIC

ground	1 tsp	8

TUNA
(*see also* TUNA DISHES)

CANNED

Bumble Bee		
Chunk Light In Oil	2 oz	160
Chunk Light In Water	2 oz	60
Chunk White In Oil	2 oz	160
Chunk White In Water	2 oz	70
Chunk White In Water Diet	2 oz	60
Solid White In Oil	2 oz	130
Solid White In Water	2 oz	70
Progresso		
In Olive Oil	¼ cup (2 oz)	160

FOOD	PORTION	CALS.
Tree Of Life		
Tongol In Spring Water	2 oz	60
Tongol In Spring Water No Salt Water	2 oz	70
FRESH		
bluefin cooked	3 oz	157
skipjack baked	3 oz	112
yellowfin baked	3 oz	118

TUNA DISHES
MIX
Bumble Bee

FOOD	PORTION	CALS.
Tuna Mix-ins Classic Italian	⅓ pkg (0.17 oz)	25
Tuna Mix-ins Garden & Herb	⅓ pkg (0.17 oz)	25
Tuna Mix-ins Lemon Herb	⅓ pkg (0.17 oz)	25
Tuna Mix-ins Zesty Tomato	⅓ pkg (0.17 oz)	25
Tuna Helper		
AuGratin 50% Less Fat Recipe as prep	1 cup	240
AuGratin as prep	1 cup	300
Cheesy Broccoli 50% Less Fat Recipe as prep	1 cup	240
Cheesy Broccoli as prep	1 cup	290
Cheesy Pasta 50% Less Fat Recipe as prep	1 cup	230
Cheesy Pasta as prep	1 cup	280
Creamy Broccoli 50% Less Fat Recipe as prep	1 cup	240
Creamy Broccoli as prep	1 cup	310
Creamy Pasta 50% Less Fat Recipe as prep	1 cup	230
Creamy Pasta as prep	1 cup	300
Fettuccine Alfredo 50% Less Fat Recipe as prep	1 cup	240
Fettuccine Alfredo as prep	1 cup	310
Garden Cheddar 50% Less Fat Recipe as prep	1 cup	240
Garden Cheddar as prep	1 cup	290
Pasta Salad Low Fat Recipe as prep	⅔ cup	230
Pasta Salad as prep	⅔ cup	380
Tetrazzini 50% Less Fat Recipe as prep	1 cup	230
Tetrazzini as prep	1 cup	300
Tuna Melt Reduced Fat Recipe as prep	1 cup	240
Tuna Melt as prep	1 cup	300
Tuna Pot Pie as prep	1 cup	440
Tuna Romanoff 50% Less Fat Recipe as prep	1 cup	240

FOOD	PORTION	CALS.
Tuna Helper (cont.)		
Tuna Romanoff as prep	1 cup	280
TAKE-OUT		
tuna salad	1 cup	383
TURBOT		
european baked	3 oz	104

TURKEY

(*see also* DINNER, HOT DOG, TURKEY DISHES, TURKEY SUBSTITUTES)

CANNED

FOOD	PORTION	CALS.
Hormel		
Chunk Turkey Ham	2 oz	70
Swanson		
White	2.5 oz	80
Underwood		
Chunky Light	2 oz	75
FRESH		
back w/ skin roasted	½ back (9 oz)	637
breast w/ skin roasted	4 oz	212
dark meat w/ skin roasted	3.6 oz	230
dark meat w/o skin roasted	1 cup (5 oz)	262
dark meat w/o skin roasted	3 oz	170
ground cooked	3 oz	188
leg w/ skin roasted	1 (1.2 lbs)	1133
leg w/ skin roasted	2.5 oz	147
light meat w/ skin roasted	4.7 oz	268
light meat w/ skin roasted	from ½ turkey (2.3 lbs)	2069
light meat w/o skin roasted	4 oz	183
neck simmered	1 (5.3 oz)	274
skin roasted	from ½ turkey (9 oz)	1096
skin roasted	1 oz	141
w/ skin roasted	½ turkey (4 lbs)	3857
w/ skin roasted	8.4 oz	498
w/ skin neck & giblets roasted	½ turkey (8.8 lbs)	4123
w/o skin roasted	1 cup (5 oz)	238
w/o skin roasted	7.3 oz	354
wing w/ skin roasted	1 (6.5 oz)	426
Butterball		
Ground All White Meat	3 oz	100
Louis Rich		
Ground	4 oz	190
Patties White	1 (4 oz)	170
Mr. Turkey		
Ground 85% Fat Free	3.5 oz	210

FOOD	PORTION	CALS.
Mr. Turkey (CONT.)		
Ground 91% Fat Free	3.5 oz	170
Perdue		
Breast Tenderloins Cooked	3 oz	110
Breast Boneless Cooked	3 oz	110
Breast Cutlets Thin Sliced Cooked	1 (2.5 oz)	90
Breast Fillets Cooked	3 oz	110
Burger Cooked	1 (3 oz)	170
Cubed Steak Cooked	3 oz	120
Dark Cooked	3 oz	200
Drumsticks Roasted	3 oz	150
Drumsticks Cooked	3 oz	150
Ground Cooked	3 oz	170
Ground Breast Cooked	3 oz	110
Half Breast Cooked	3 oz	170
Thighs Cooked	3 oz	180
Tom Wings Cooked	3 oz	160
White Cooked	3 oz	170
Whole Breast Cooked	3 oz	170
Wings Roasted	1 (3 oz)	180
Wings Drummettes Roasted	1 (3.5 oz)	180
Shady Brook		
Cutlets	4 oz	130
Drumstick	4 oz	170
Ground Breast	4 oz	120
Ground Lean	4 oz	170
Ground Turkey 85%	4 oz	220
Mesquite Seasoned Tenderloin	4 oz	110
OnlyOne Boneless Breast Roast	4 oz	130
Split Breast	4 oz	190
Tenderloin	4 oz	130
Teriyaki Seasoned Tenderloin	4 oz	120
Thigh	4 oz	220
Turkey Burgers	4 oz	170
Turkey Meatloaf Lean	4 oz	150
Whole Breast	4 oz	190
Whole Turkey	4 oz	180
Wing	4 oz	220
Zesty Lemon Seasoned Tenderlion	4 oz	120
Swift-Eckrich		
Ground All White	3 oz	100
The Turkey Store		
Seasoned Cuts Turkey Breast Roast	4 oz	110

FOOD	PORTION	CALS.
Wampler Longacre		
Ground raw	1 oz	60
FROZEN		
Empire		
Patties	1 (3.1 oz)	200
READY-TO-EAT		
Alpine Lace		
Breast Fat Free	2 oz	50
Boar's Head		
Breast Cracked Pepper Smoked	2 oz	60
Breast Golden Skin On	2 oz	60
Breast Golden Skinless	2 oz	60
Breast Hickory Smoked	2 oz	70
Breast Low Sodium Skinless	2 oz	60
Breast Lower Sodium Skin On	2 oz	60
Breast Maple Glazed Honey Coat	2 oz	70
Breast Ovengold Skin On	2 oz	60
Breast Ovengold Skinless	2 oz	60
Breast Roasted Mesquite Smoked Skin On	2 oz	60
Breast Roasted Mesquite Smoked Skinless	2 oz	60
Breast Roasted Salsalito	2 oz	60
Pastrami Seasoned	2 oz	60
Carl Buddig		
Honey Turkey	1 oz	40
Turkey	1 oz	50
Turkey Ham	1 oz	40
Empire		
Barbecue Whole	5 oz	250
Bologna	3 slices (1.8 oz)	90
Oven Prepared Breast Slices	3 slices (1.8 oz)	50
Pastrami	3 slices (1.8 oz)	60
Salami	3 slices (1.8 oz)	70
Smoked Breast Slices	3 slices (1.8 oz)	40
Falls		
BBQ	3 oz	140
Gourmet Breast	3 oz	80
Premium Cooked Breast	3 oz	100
Healthy Choice		
Deli-Thin Roasted Breast	6 slices (2 oz)	60
Deli-Thin Smoked Breast	6 slices (2 oz)	60
Deli-Thin Turkey Ham	6 slices (2 oz)	60
Fresh-Trak Honey Roast & Smoked Breast	1 slice (1 oz)	35
Fresh-Trak Oven Roasted Breast	1 slice (1 oz)	35
Honey Roasted & Smoked	1 slice (1 oz)	35

FOOD	PORTION	CALS.
Healthy Choice (CONT.)		
Oven Roasted Breast	1 slice (1 oz)	35
Smoked Breast	1 slice (1 oz)	30
Variety Pack Regular	3 slices (2.2 oz)	70
Hebrew National		
Deli Thin Hickory Smoked	1.8 oz	55
Deli Thin Lemon Garlic	1.8 oz	50
Deli Thin Oven Roasted	1.8 oz	80
Hillshire		
Deli Select Honey Roasted Breast	1 slice	10
Deli Select Oven Roasted Breast	1 slice	10
Deli Select Smoked Breast	1 slice	10
Deli Select Turkey Ham	1 slice	10
Flavor Pack 90-99% Fat Free Honey Roasted Breast	1 slice (0.75 oz)	20
Flavor Pack 90-99% Fat Free Oven Roasted Breast	1 slice (0.75 oz)	20
Flavor Pack 90-99% Fat Free Smoked Breast	1 slice (0.75 oz)	20
Honey Cured Breast	1 oz	35
Lunch 'N Munch Smoked Turkey/ Cheddar	1 pkg (4.5 oz)	350
Lunch 'N Munch Smoked Turkey/ Cheddar/ Brownie	1 pkg (4.5 oz)	400
Lunch 'N Munch Turkey/Cheddar/ Brownie/Hi-C	1 pkg (4.5 oz + 6 fl oz)	500
Smoked Breast	1 oz	35
Hormel		
Light & Lean 97 Breast Sliced	1 slice (1 oz)	30
Light & Lean 97 Mesquite Smoked Breast	1 slice (1 oz)	30
turkey pepperoni	17 slices (1 oz)	80
Jordan's		
Healthy Trim Fat Free Oven Roasted Breast	1 slice (1 oz)	20
Healthy Trim Fat Free Oven Roasted Smoked Breast	1 slice (1 oz)	20
Louis Rich		
Bologna	1 slice (28 g)	50
Breaded Nuggets	4 (3.2 oz)	260
Breaded Patties	1 (3 oz)	220
Breaded Sticks	3 (3 oz)	230
Breast Skinless Hickory Smoked	2 oz	50
Breast Skinless Honey Roasted	2 oz	60
Breast Skinless Oven Roasted	2 oz	50
Breast Skinless Rotisserie	2 oz	50
Breast Slices Hickory Smoked	1 slice (2 oz)	50

FOOD	PORTION	CALS.
Louis Rich (CONT.)		
Breast Slices Honey Roasted	1 slice (2 oz)	60
Breast Slices Oven Roasted	1 slice (2 oz)	50
Breast Slices Rotisserie	1 slice (2 oz)	50
Carving Board Hickory Smoked	2 slices (1.6 oz)	40
Carving Board Oven Roasted Thin	6 slices (2.1 oz)	60
Carving Board Oven Roasted Traditional	2 slices (1.6 oz)	40
Carving Board Rotisserie	2 slices (1.6 oz)	40
Cotto Salami	1 slice (28 g)	40
Deli-Thin Oven Roasted	4 slices (1.8 oz)	50
Deli-Thin Smoked	4 slices (1.8 oz)	50
Fat Free Hickory Smoked Breast	1 slice (1 oz)	25
Fat Free Oven Roasted Breast	1 slice (1 oz)	25
Fat Free Oven Roasted Deli-Thin Breast	4 slices (1.8 oz)	45
Fat Free Turkey Ham Honey	2 slices (1.7 oz)	35
Fat Free Turkey Ham Smoked	2 slices (1.7 oz)	35
Hickory Smoked	1 slice (1 oz)	30
Oven Roasted	1 slice (1 oz)	30
Pastrami	1 slice (1 oz)	30
Salami	1 slice (28 g)	40
Smoked	1 slice (1 oz)	30
Turkey Ham	1 slice (1 oz)	30
Turkey Ham Chopped	1 slice (1 oz)	45
Turkey Ham Honey Cured	1 slice (1 oz)	30
Mr. Turkey		
Deli Cuts Hardwood Smoked Breast	3 slices	30
Deli Cuts Honey Roasted Breast	3 slices	30
Deli Cuts Oven Roasted Breast	3 slices	30
Deli Cuts Turkey Ham	3 slices	35
Deli Cuts Turkey Pastrami	3 slices	35
Hardwood Smoked Breast	1 slice	30
Hardwood Smoked Turkey Ham	1 slice	35
Honey Cured Turkey Ham	1 slice	30
Oven Roasted Breast	1 slice	30
Smoked Breakfast Turkey Ham	1 oz	30
Turkey Bologna	1 slice	70
Turkey Cotto Salami	1 slice	50
Turkey Ham	1 slice	35
Turkey Pastrami	1 slice	30
Oscar Mayer		
Free Oven Roasted Breast	4 slices (1.8 oz)	40
Free Smoked Breast	4 slices (1.8 oz)	40
Lunchables Fun Pack Turkey/Pacific Cooler	1 pkg (11.2 oz)	460

FOOD	PORTION	CALS.
Oscar Mayer (CONT.)		
Lunchables Fun Pack Turkey/Surger Cooler	1 pkg (11.2 oz)	440
Lunchables Turkey/Cheddar	1 pkg (4.5 oz)	360
Oven Roasted White	1 slice (1 oz)	30
Smoked White	1 slice (1 oz)	30
Perdue		
Nuggets Dinosaur	3 (3 oz)	200
Sara Lee		
Hardwood Smoked Breast Of Turkey	2 oz	60
Hardwood Smoked Turkey Ham	2 oz	60
Honey Roasted Breast Of Turkey	2 oz	60
Honey Roasted Turkey Ham	2 oz	70
Mesquite Smoked Breast Of Turkey	2 oz	60
Oven Roasted Breast Of Turkey	2 oz	60
Peppered Breast Of Turkey	2 oz	50
Seasoned Breast Of Turkey Pastrami	2 oz	60
Shady Brook		
Black Forest Turkey Ham	2 oz	70
Browned Homestyle Oven Roasted Breast	2 oz	60
Browned Slow Roasted Breast	2 oz	60
Carved Breast Italian Seasoned	2 oz	60
Carved Breast Natural Roast	2 oz	60
Carved Breast Peppered	2 oz	60
Hickory Smoked Breast	2 oz	50
Honey Roasted Breast	2 oz	60
Honey Roasted Breast Covered w/ Cracked Pepper	2 oz	60
Meatballs Italian Style	3 oz	130
Smoked Drumstick	3 oz	180
Smoked Neck	3 oz	150
Smoked Whole Turkey	3 oz	150
Smoked Wing	3 oz	200
Tyson		
Breast	1 slice	20
Ham	1 slice	23
Wampler Longacre		
Bologna	1 oz	60
Breast Chops	1 serv (4 oz)	120
Breast Sliced	1 slice (1 oz)	35
Breast Sliced Smoked	1 slice (0.75 oz)	20
Burger	1 (3 oz)	170
Burger	1 (4 oz)	230
Burger Barbecue	1 (4 oz)	240

FOOD	PORTION	CALS.
Wampler Longacre (CONT.)		
Chef Select Breast Skinless	1 oz	35
Chef Select Breast Smoked	1 oz	35
Chunk Dark Smoked Cured	1 oz	45
Chunk Ham 12% Water Smoked	1 oz	45
Chunk Ham 20% Water	1 oz	40
Chunk Pastrami	1 oz	35
Cook-In-The-Bag Breast	1 oz	30
Cook-In-The-Bag Breast Mini	1 oz	30
Cook-In-The-Bag Combo Roast	1 oz	35
Cook-In-The-Bag Thigh Roast	1 oz	40
Dark Smoked Cured	1 oz	45
Deli Chef Breast And White Meat No Skin	1 oz	40
Gourmet Breast	1 oz	35
Gourmet Breast Mini	1 oz	35
Gourmet Breast Mini Smoked	1 oz	35
Gourmet Breast Smoked	1 oz	30
Gourmet Brown & Glazed Breast	1 oz	35
Gourmet Brown & Roasted Breast	1 oz	35
Gourmet Honey Cured Breast	1 oz	30
Lean-Lite Breast Skinless	1 oz	35
Lean-Lite Deli Breast	1 oz	35
Lean-Lite Deli Breast Smoked	1 oz	35
Old Fashioned Brown & Roasted Breast	1 oz	35
Pastrami	1 oz	35
Premium Breast Skinless	1 oz	30
Premium Brown & Roasted Breast Skinless	1 oz	16
Roll Combo	1 oz	44
Roll Sliced Breast	1 slice (0.75 oz)	30
Roll White	1 oz	45
Salami	1 oz	50
Salt Watchers Breast Skinless	1 oz	35
Seasoned Roast	1 oz	40
Sliced Salami	1 slice (0.8 oz)	45
Tenderlings BBQ	1 serv (4 oz)	110
Tenderlings Cajun	1 serv (4 oz)	110
Tenderlings Garlic & Pepper	1 serv (4 oz)	110
Tenderlings Original	1 serv (4 oz)	110
Turkey Ham 12% Water Baked	1 oz	45
Turkey Ham 20% Water Baked	1 oz	40
Unseasoned Roast	1 oz	40

FOOD	PORTION	CALS.
Wampler Longacre (CONT.)		
Whole Browned & Roasted	1 oz	60

TURKEY DISHES
(*see also* DINNER, TURKEY SUBSTITUTES)
CANNED
Dinty Moore
| Stew | 1 cup (8.5 oz) | 140 |

FROZEN
Hot Pocket
| Stuffed Sandwich Turkey & Ham With Cheese | 1 (4.5 oz) | 320 |

Lean Pockets
| Stuffed Sandwich Turkey & Ham With Cheddar | 1 (4.5 oz) | 260 |
| Stuffed Sandwich Turkey Broccoli & Cheese | 1 (4.5 oz) | 260 |

Luigino's
| Gravy Dressing & Turkey | 1 pkg (8 oz) | 340 |

READY-TO-EAT
Shady Brook
| Meatloaf | 1 serv (16 oz) | 470 |

Wampler Longacre
Meatloaf Italian	1 serv (4 oz)	114
Meatloaf Mexican	1 serv (4 oz)	114
Meatloaf Original	1 serv (4 oz)	126
Salad	1 oz	60
Salad Turkey Ham	1 oz	50
Teriyaki	1 serv (4 oz)	112

SHELF-STABLE
Dinty Moore
| Microwave Cup Stew | 1 pkg (7.5 oz) | 130 |

TURKEY SUBSTITUTES
Harvest Direct
| TVP Poultry Chunks | 3.5 oz | 280 |
| TVP Poultry Ground | 3.5 oz | 280 |

Soy Is Us
| Turkey Not! | ½ cup (1.75 oz) | 140 |

White Wave
| Meatless Sandwich Slices | 2 slices (1.6 oz) | 80 |

Worthington
| Smoked Turkey Meatless | 3 slices (2 oz) | 140 |

FOOD	PORTION	CALS.
Worthington (CONT.)		
Turkee Slices	3 slices (3.3 oz)	130

TURNIPS
CANNED
Allen

Chopped Greens And Diced Turnip	½ cup (4.2 oz)	30
Greens	½ cup (4.2 oz)	25

Sunshine

Chopped Greens And Diced Turnip	½ cup (4.2 oz)	30
Greens	½ cup (4.2 oz)	25

FRESH

cooked mashed	½ cup (4.2 oz)	47
cubed cooked	½ cup (3 oz)	33
greens chopped cooked	½ cup	15
raw cubed	½ cup (2.4 oz)	25

FROZEN
Birds Eye

Chopped Greens	1 cup (3.1 oz)	30
Greens w/ Diced Root	1 cup (3 oz)	25

VANILLA
Virginia Dare

Vanilla Extract	1 tsp	10

VEAL
(*see also* DINNER, VEAL DISHES)

cutlet lean only braised	3 oz	172
cutlet lean only fried	3 oz	156
ground broiled	3 oz	146
loin chop w/ bone lean & fat braised	1 chop (2.8 oz)	227
loin chop w/ bone lean only braised	1 chop (2.4 oz)	155
shoulder w/ bone lean only braised	3 oz	169
sirloin w/ bone lean & fat roasted	3 oz	171
sirloin w/ bone lean only roasted	3 oz	143

VEGETABLE JUICE
Dole

Vegetable Blend	1 bottle (12 oz)	90
Mott's		
Vegetable Juice as prep	8 fl oz	60
Muir Glen		
Organic	8 oz	70
Organic Reduced Sodium	8 oz	70
Odwalla		
Vegetable Cocktail	8 fl oz	70

FOOD	PORTION	CALS.
V8		
No Salt Added	6 fl oz	35
Original	6 fl oz	35
Spicy Hot	6 fl oz	35
Splash Tropical Blend	8 fl oz	120

VEGETABLES MIXED
(*see also* VEGETABLE JUICE)

CANNED

FOOD	PORTION	CALS.
Allen		
Green Beans And Potatoes	½ cup (4.2 oz)	35
Okra & Tomatoes	½ cup (4 oz)	25
Okra Tomatoes & Corn	½ cup (4.1 oz)	30
Chi-Chi's		
Diced Tomatoes & Green Chilies	¼ cup (2.5 oz)	20
Del Monte		
Mixed	½ cup (4.4 oz)	40
Peas And Carrots	½ cup (4.5 oz)	60
Green Giant		
Garden Medley	½ cup (4.2 oz)	40
Mixed	½ cup (4.3 oz)	60
Sweet Peas & Carrots	½ cup (4.3 oz)	50
Sweet Peas & Tiny Pearl Onion	½ cup (4.4 oz)	60
House Of Tsang		
Vegetables & Sauce Cantonese Classic	½ cup (4.2 oz)	70
Vegetables & Sauce Hong Kong Sweet & Sour	½ cup (4.5 oz)	160
Vegetables & Sauce Szechuan Hot & Spicy	½ cup (4.2 oz)	70
Vegetables & Sauce Tokyo Teriyaki	½ cup (4.4 oz)	100
LeSueur		
Early Peas w/ Mushrooms & Pearl Onions	½ cup (4.3 oz)	60
Seneca		
Peas & Carrots	½ cup	60
Succotash	½ cup	90
Sunshine		
Green Beans And Potatoes	½ cup (4.2 oz)	35
Trappey		
Okra & Tomatoes	½ cup (4 oz)	25
Okra Tomatoes & Corn	½ cup (4.1 oz)	30

FROZEN

FOOD	PORTION	CALS.
Amy's Organic		
Pocket Sandwich Mediterranean Vegetables	1 (4.5 oz)	220
Pocket Sandwich Roasted Vegetables	1 (4.5 oz)	220

FOOD	PORTION	CALS.
Amy's Organic (CONT.)		
Pocket Sandwich Vegetable Pie	1 (5 oz)	230
Big Valley		
California Blend	¾ cup (3 oz)	25
Italian Blend	¾ cup (3 oz)	30
Oriental Blend	¾ cup (3 oz)	25
Stew Vegetables	⅔ cup (3 oz)	40
Winter Blend	¾ cup (3 oz)	25
Birds Eye		
Baby Bean & Carrot Blend	1 cup (2.9 oz)	30
Broccoli Cauliflower Carrots w/ Cheese	½ cup (3.9 oz)	70
Brussels Sprouts Cauliflower Carrots	½ cup (3.1 oz)	30
Chicken Viola Garlic	2 cups (6.2 oz)	260
Chicken Viola Pesto	2¼ cups (6.6 oz)	250
Chicken Viola Three Cheese	1¾ cups (6.2 oz)	240
Chicken Voila Teriyaki	2⅓ cups (6.1 oz)	230
Farm Fresh Broccoli Carrots Water Chestnuts	½ cup (3.3 oz)	30
Farm Fresh Broccoli Cauliflower	½ cup (3.2 oz)	20
Farm Fresh Broccoli Cauliflower Carrots	½ cup (3.2 oz)	25
Farm Fresh Broccoli Cauliflower Red Peppers	½ cup (3.3 oz)	20
Farm Fresh Broccoli Corn Red Peppers	½ cup (3.6 oz)	50
Farm Fresh Broccoli Red Peppers Onions Mushrooms	½ cup (3.5 oz)	25
Farm Fresh Brussels Sprouts Cauliflower Carrots	½ cup (3.1 oz)	30
Farm Fresh Cauliflower Carrots Snow Peas Pods	½ cup (3.2 oz)	30
For Soup	⅔ cup (3 oz)	45
For Stew	¾ cup (2.9 oz)	40
Gumbo Blend	¾ cup (3 oz)	40
International French Country Style	⅔ cup (4.4 oz)	110
International New England Style	1 pkg (9 oz)	260
International Oriental Style	½ cup (3 oz)	60
International Stir Fry Style	½ cup 3.6 oz)	60
Internationals Bavarian Style	1 cup (5.5 oz)	150
Internationals California Style	½ cup (3 oz)	100
Internationals Italian Style	1 cup (5.8 oz)	150
Peas & Carrots	⅔ cup (3 oz)	50
Peas & Pearl Onions	⅔ cup (4.2 oz)	90
Peas & Potatoes In Cream Sauce	½ cup (4.4 oz)	90
Seasoning Blend	¾ cup (2.9 oz)	20
Stir Fry Asparagus	2 cups (5.8 oz)	90

FOOD	PORTION	CALS.
Birds Eye (CONT.)		
Stir Fry Broccoli	1 cup (3.3 oz)	30
Stir Fry Pepper	1 cup (2.9 oz)	25
Stir Fry Sugar Snap	¾ cup (2.6 oz)	35
Stir Fry Whole Green Bean	1¾ cup (5.3 oz)	100
Budget Gourmet		
Mandarin Vegetables	1 pkg (5.25 oz)	160
New England Recipe Vegetables	1 pkg (5.5 oz)	230
Spring Vegetables In Cheese Sauce	1 pkg (5 oz)	130
Fresh Like		
California Blend	3.5 oz	31
Chuckwagon Blend	3.5 oz	71
Italian Blend	3.5 oz	33
Midwestern Blend	3.5 oz	42
Mixed	3.5 oz	69
Oriental Blend	3.5 oz	26
Peas & Carrots	3.5 oz	63
Winter Blend	3.5 oz	26
Green Giant		
American Mixtures Broccoli Carrots Cauliflower	¾ cup (2.6 oz)	25
American Mixtures Broccoli Carrots Waterchestnuts	¾ cup (3 oz)	30
American Mixtures Carrots Green Bean Cauliflower	¾ cup (2.7 oz)	25
American Mixtures Cauliflower Broccoli Sugar Snap & Sweet Pea	¾ cup (2.8 oz)	35
American Mixtures Corn Broccoli Red Pepper	¾ cup (3.1 oz)	60
American Mixtures Green Beans Potatoes Onions Red Peppers	¾ cup (2.8 oz)	45
American Mixtures Sweet Peas Potatoes Carrots	⅔ cup (3 oz)	70
Butter Sauce Broccoli Cauliflower Carrots Corn Sweet Peas	¾ cup (3.6 oz)	60
Butter Sauce Broccoli Pasta Sweet Peas Corn Red Peppers	¾ cup (3.5 oz)	70
Butter Sauce Mixed	¾ cup (3.6 oz)	70
Cheese Sauce Broccoli Cauliflower Carrots	⅔ cup (4.3 oz)	80
Harvest Fresh Broccoli Cauliflower Carrots	1 cup (3.4 oz)	30
Harvest Fresh Mixed Vegetables	⅔ cup (3.1 oz)	50
Harvest Fresh Sweet Peas & Pearl Onions	½ cup (2.7 oz)	55
Mixed	¾ cup (2.9 oz)	50
Select Sweet Peas & Pearl Onions	⅔ cup (3.1 oz)	60

FOOD	PORTION	CALS.
Ore Ida		
Stew Vegetables	⅔ cup (3 oz)	50
Soglowek		
Golden Vegetarian Nuggets	4 pieces (2.5 oz)	190
Tree Of Life		
Mixed	½ cup (3 oz)	65
Veg-All		
Country Wisconsin Blend	3.5 oz	52
Scandinavian Blend	3.5 oz	48
Vegetables For Soup (Eight)	3.5 oz	34
Vegetables For Soup (Potatoes)	3.5 oz	53
Vegetables For Stew 4-Way	3.5 oz	51
Vegetables For Stew 5-Way	3.5 oz	54
TAKE-OUT		
caponata	¼ cup	28
gyoza potstickers vegetable	8 (4.9 oz)	210
ratatouille	1 serv (3.5 oz)	96
succotash	½ cup	111

VENISON

FOOD	PORTION	CALS.
roasted	3 oz	134
Broken Arrow Ranch		
Antelope Chili Meat	3.5 oz	115
Antelope Ground Venison	3.5 oz	110
Antelope Stew Meat	3.5 oz	110
Nilgai Chili Meat	3.5 oz	115
Nilgai Leg	3.5 oz	100
Nilgai Stew Meat	3.5 oz	110
Venison & Beef Smoked Sausage	6 oz	432
Venison Meat Chunks	6 oz	175
Venison Salami	6 oz	252

VINEGAR

FOOD	PORTION	CALS.
balsamic	1 tbsp (0.5 oz)	5
Hain		
Cider	1 tbsp	2
Nakano		
Rice	1 tbsp	0
Regina		
Red Wine	1 oz	4
Tree Of Life		
Apple Cider Organic	1 tbsp (0.5 oz)	0
Brown Rice	1 tbsp (0.5 oz)	2

FOOD	PORTION	CALS.
Victoria		
Balsamic	1 tbsp (0.5 oz)	5
WAFFLES		
FROZEN		
buttermilk	1 4 in sq (1.2 oz)	88
plain	1 4 in sq (1.2 oz)	88
Aunt Jemima		
Blueberry	2 (2.5 oz)	190
Buttermilk	2 (2.5 oz)	170
Cinnamon	2 (2.5 oz)	180
Oatmeal	2 (2.5 oz)	170
Whole Grain	2 (2.5 oz)	170
Belgian Chef		
Belgian	2 (2.5 oz)	140
Downyflake		
Blueberry	2	180
Buttermilk	2	190
Multi-Grain	2	250
Oat Bran	2	260
Regular	2	120
Regular Jumbo	2	170
Rice Bran	2	210
Roman Meal	2	280
Waffles	2	180
Eggo		
Apple Cinnamon	2 (2.7 oz)	220
Banana Bread	2 (2.7 oz)	200
Blueberry	2 (2.7 oz)	220
Buttermilk	2 (2.7 oz)	220
Golden Oat	2 (2.7 oz)	150
Homestyle	2 (2.7 oz)	220
Minis Cinnamon Toast	12 (3.2 oz)	290
Minis Cinnamon Toast	12 (3.2 oz)	280
Minis Homestyle	12 (3.3 oz)	260
Nut & Honey	2 (2.7 oz)	240
Nutri-Grain	2 (2.7 oz)	190
Nutri-Grain Multi-Bran	2 (2.7 oz)	180
Nutri-Grain Raisin & Bran	2 (2.9 oz)	210
Special K	2 (2 oz)	120
Strawberry	2 (2.7 oz)	220
Kellogg's		
Homestyle Low Fat	2 (2.7 oz)	180
Nutri-Grain Low Fat	2 (2.7 oz)	160

FOOD	PORTION	CALS.
Kellogg's (CONT.)		
Nutri-Grain Low Fat Blueberry	2 (2.7 oz)	160
Van's		
7 Grain Belgain	2	152
Belgian Original	2	145
Belgian Original Toaster	2	145
Blueberry Toaster	2	157
Blueberry Wheat Free Toaster	2	225
Fat Free	2	155
Mini	4	107
Multigrain Toaster	2	160
Organic Whole Wheat	2	190
Organic Whole Wheat Blueberry	2	190
Wheat Free Cinnamon Apple Toaster	2	220
Wheat Free Toaster	2	220
HOME RECIPE		
plain	1 (7 in diam)	218
MIX		
plain as prep	1 7 in diam (2.6 oz)	218

WALNUTS
FOOD	PORTION	CALS.
Planters		
Black	1 pkg (2 oz)	340
Gold Measure Halves	1 pkg (2 oz)	380
Halves	⅓ cup (1.2 oz)	220
Pieces	¼ cup (1 oz)	190

WASABI
FOOD	PORTION	CALS.
root raw	1 (5.9 oz)	184
root raw sliced	1 cup (4.6 oz)	142

WATER
FOOD	PORTION	CALS.
Canada Dry		
Sparkling Water	8 fl oz	0
Crystal Geyser		
Sparking Natural Wild Cherry	1 bottle 12 fl oz	0
Sparkling Lemon	1 bottle (12 fl oz)	0
Sparkling Mineral	1 bottle (12 fl oz)	0
Sparkling Natural Cola Berry	1 bottle (12 fl oz)	0
Sparkling Orange	1 bottle (12 fl oz)	0
Evian		
Water	1 liter	0
Glacier Springs		
Drinking Water	8 fl oz	0
Glennpatrick		
Irish Spring Pure	8 oz	0

FOOD	PORTION	CALS.
LaCroix		
Sparking Berry	12 fl oz	0
Sparkling Lemon	12 fl oz	0
Sparkling Lime	12 fl oz	0
Sparkling Orange	12 fl oz	0
Sparkling Regular	12 fl oz	0
Spring	1 bottle (12 oz)	0
Mountain Valley		
Mineral Water	1 qt	0
Mt Shasta		
Natural Spring	1 bottle (20 oz)	0
San Pellegrino		
Acqua Panna	8 fl oz	0
Mineral Water	1 liter (33.8 oz)	0
Saratoga		
Sparkling	1 liter	0
Snapple		
Natural Spring	8 fl oz	0
Water Joe		
Caffeine Enhanced	8 fl oz	0

WATERCRESS
(*see also* CRESS)

raw chopped	½ cup	2

WATERMELON
FRESH

cut up	1 cup	50
wedge	1/16	152
SEEDS		
dried	1 oz	158

WATERMELON JUICE
Kool-Aid

Splash Drink	1 serv (8 oz)	110

WAX BEANS
CANNED
Del Monte

Cut Golden	½ cup (4.3 oz)	20
Seneca		
Cuts Natural Pack	½ cup	25
Wax Beans	½ cup	25

WHALE

raw	3.5 oz	134

FOOD	PORTION	CALS.

WHEAT
(*see also* BULGUR, BRAN, CEREAL, COUSCOUS, FLOUR, WHEAT GERM)

sprouted	1 cup (3.8 oz)	214
Arrowhead		
Kamut Grain	¼ cup (1.7 oz)	140
Seitan Quick Mix	⅓ cup (1.4 oz)	150
Hodgson Mill		
Vital Wheat Gluten Plus Ascorbic Acid	1 tbsp (0.3 oz)	30
Near East		
Taboule Salad Mix as prep	⅔ cup	120
Wheat Pilaf as prep	1 cup	220
Sonoma		
Wheat Nuts Salted	2 tbsp (0.5 oz)	60
White Wave		
Seitan	½ pkg (4 oz)	140
Seitan Fajita Strips	⅓ cup (1.8 oz)	60
Seitan Marinated Slices	3 slices (1.8 oz)	60

WHEAT GERM

plain toasted	¼ cup (1 oz)	108
Arrowhead		
Wheat Germ	3 tbsp (0.5 oz)	50
Hodgson Mill		
Wheat Germ	2 tbsp (0.5 oz)	55
Stone-Buhr		
Untoasted	2 tbsp (0.5 oz)	58

WHEY

acid dry	1 tbsp (3 g)	10
acid fluid	1 cup (8 fl oz)	59
sweet dry	1 tbsp (8 g)	26
sweet fluid	1 cup (8 fl oz)	66
whey cheese	3.5 oz	440

WHIPPED TOPPINGS
(*see also* CREAM)

Cool Whip		
Extra Creamy	2 tbsp (0.3 oz)	25
Free	2 tbsp (0.3 oz)	15
Lite	2 tbsp (0.3 oz)	20
Original	2 tbsp (0.3 oz)	25
Dream Whip		
Mix as prep	2 tbsp (0.3 oz)	20
Estee		
Whipped Topping	1 serv	10

FOOD	PORTION	CALS.
Hood		
Instant	2 tbsp	20
Light Instant	2 tbsp	15
Kraft		
Dairy Whip Light Cream	2 tbsp (0.2 oz)	10
Fat Free	1 tbsp (0.3 oz)	15
La Creme		
Topping	1 tbsp	16
Pet		
Whip	1 tbsp	14
Reddiwip		
Lite	2 tbsp (8 g)	15
Non-Dairy	2 tbsp (8 g)	20
Real Whipped Heavy Cream	2 tbsp (8 g)	30
Real Whipped Light Cream	2 tbsp (8 g)	20

WHITE BEANS
CANNED
Goya		
Spanish Style	7.5 oz	130
Progresso		
Cannellini	½ cup (4.6 oz)	100

WHITEFISH
baked	3 oz	146
smoked	1 oz	39

WHITING
cooked	3 oz	98

WILD RICE
cooked	1 cup (5.7 oz)	166
Haddon House		
Extra Fancy	¼ cup (1.6 oz)	170

WINE
(*see also* CHAMPAGNE, WINE COOLERS)

madeira	3.5 oz	169
port	3.5 oz	156
red	3.5 oz	74
rose	3.5 oz	73
sweet dessert	2 oz	90
white	3.5 oz	70
Boone's		
Country Kwencher	1 fl oz	24
Delicious Apple	1 fl oz	21

FOOD	PORTION	CALS.
Boone's (CONT.)		
Sangria	1 fl oz	22
Snow Creek Berry	1 fl oz	18
Strawberry Hill	1 fl oz	22
Sun Peak Peach	1 fl oz	18
Wild Island	1 fl oz	18
Carlo Rossi		
Blush	1 fl oz	21
Burgundy	1 fl oz	22
Chablis	1 fl oz	21
Paisano	1 fl oz	23
Red Sangria	1 fl oz	24
Rhine	1 fl oz	21
Vin Rose'	1 fl oz	21
White Grenache	1 fl oz	20
Fairbanks		
Cream Sherry	1 fl oz	42
Port	1 fl oz	44
Sherry	1 fl oz	34
White Port	1 fl oz	44
Gallo		
Blush Chablis	1 fl oz	22
Burgundy	1 fl oz	22
Cabernet Sauvignon	1 fl oz	22
Chablis Blanc	1 fl oz	20
Chardonnay	1 fl oz	23
Classic Burgundy	1 fl oz	21
French Colombard	1 fl oz	21
Hearty Burgundy	1 fl oz	22
Johannisbery Riesling '88	1 fl oz	20
Pink Chablis	1 fl oz	20
Red Rose'	1 fl oz	23
Rhine	1 fl oz	22
Sauvignon Blanc '90	1 fl oz	20
White Grenache '92	1 fl oz	20
White Grenache New Vintage	1 fl oz	20
White Zinfandel '91	1 fl oz	18
White Zinfandel New Vintage	1 fl oz	18
Zinfandel '87	1 fl oz	23
Sheffield Cellars		
Sherry	1 fl oz	44
Tawny Port	1 fl oz	45
Vermouth Extra Dry	1 fl oz	28
Vermouth Sweet	1 fl oz	43

FOOD	PORTION	CALS.
Sheffield Cellars (CONT.)		
Very Dry Sherry	1 fl oz	32
WINE COOLERS		
Bartles & Jaymes		
Berry	12 fl oz	210
Margarita	12 fl oz	260
Original	12 fl oz	190
Peach	12 fl oz	210
Pina Colada	12 fl oz	280
Planter's Punch	12 fl oz	230
Strawberry	12 fl oz	210
Strawberry Daquiri	12 fl oz	230
Tropical	12 fl oz	230
WINGED BEANS		
drled cooked	1 cup	252
WOLFFISH		
atlantic baked	3 oz	105
YAM		
(*see also* SWEET POTATO)		
CANNED		
Allen		
Cut	⅔ cup (5.8 oz)	160
Princella		
Cut	⅔ cup (5.8 oz)	160
Royal Prince		
Whole	4 pieces (5.9 oz)	200
Sugary Sam		
Cut	⅔ cup (5.8 oz)	160
Trappey		
Whole	4 pieces (5.9 oz)	200
YAMBEAN		
cooked	¾ cup	38
YAUTIA (TANNIER)		
raw sliced	1 cup (4.7 oz)	132
root raw	1 (10.7 oz)	299
YEAST		
baker's compressed	1 cake (0.6 oz)	18
baker's dry	1 pkg (¼ oz)	21
baker's dry	1 tbsp	35
brewer's dry	1 tbsp	25

FOOD	PORTION	CALS.
Fleischmann's		
Active Dry	1 pkg (¼ oz)	20
Fresh Active	1 pkg (0.6 oz)	15
Household Yeast	0.5 oz	15
RapidRise	1 pkg (¼ oz)	20
Red Star		
Yeast	4 tbsp (0.5 oz)	47
Yeast Flakes	3 tbsp (0.5 oz)	47

YELLOW BEANS

canned	½ cup	13

YELLOWEYE BEANS
CANNED

B&M		
Baked	½ cup (4.6 oz)	170

DRIED

Bean Cuisine		
Dried	½ cup	115

YELLOWTAIL

baked	3 oz	159

YOGURT
(*see also* YOGURT FROZEN)

Breyers		
Blended Blueberry	4.4 oz	130
Blended Peach	4.4 oz	130
Blended Strawberry	4.4 oz	130
Light Nonfat Apple Pie A La Mode	8 oz	120
Light Nonfat Berry Banana Split	8 oz	120
Light Nonfat Black Cherry Jubilee	8 oz	120
Light Nonfat Blueberries N' Cream	8 oz	120
Light Nonfat Cherry Bon-Bon	8 oz	120
Light Nonfat Cherry Vanilla Cream	8 oz	120
Light Nonfat Classic Strawberry	8 oz	120
Light Nonfat Key Lime Pie	8 oz	120
Light Nonfat Lemon Chiffon	8 oz	120
Light Nonfat Peaches N' Cream	8 oz	120
Light Nonfat Raspberries N' Cream	8 oz	120
Light Nonfat Strawberry Cheesecake	8 oz	120
Lowfat Black Cherry	8 oz	240
Lowfat Blueberry	8 oz	230
Lowfat Mixed Berry	8 oz	320
Lowfat Peach	8 oz	240
Lowfat Pineapple	8 oz	240

FOOD	PORTION	CALS.
Breyers (CONT.)		
Lowfat Red Raspberry	8 oz	230
Lowfat Strawberry	8 oz	230
Lowfat Strawberry Banana	8 oz	240
Lowfat Vanilla	8 oz	220
Smooth & Creamy Apple Cobbler	8 oz	230
Smooth & Creamy Black Cherry Parfait	8 oz	240
Smooth & Creamy Black Cherry Parfait	4.4 oz	130
Smooth & Creamy Blueberries 'N Cream	8 oz	240
Smooth & Creamy Blueberries 'N Cream	4.4 oz	130
Smooth & Creamy Classic Strawberry	8 oz	230
Smooth & Creamy Classic Strawberry	4.4 oz	130
Smooth & Creamy Orange Vanilla Cream	8 oz	230
Smooth & Creamy Peaches 'N Cream	4.4 oz	130
Smooth & Creamy Peaches 'N Cream	8 oz	230
Smooth & Creamy Raspberries 'N Cream	8 oz	230
Smooth & Creamy Strawberry Banana Split	8 oz	240
Smooth & Creamy Strawberry Cheesecake	8 oz	240
Colombo		
Banana Strawberry	8 oz	210
Black Cherry	8 oz	200
Blueberry	8 oz	200
Fat Free Apples 'n Spice	8 oz	190
Fat Free Apricot	8 oz	190
Fat Free Banana Strawberry	8 oz	200
Fat Free Blueberry	8 oz	190
Fat Free Cappuccino	8 oz	180
Fat Free Cherry	8 oz	190
Fat Free Cranberry Strawberry	8 oz	200
Fat Free French Roast	8 oz	180
Fat Free Fruit Cocktail	8 oz	190
Fat Free Lemon	8 oz	170
Fat Free Peach	8 oz	190
Fat Free Plain	8 oz	110
Fat Free Raspberry	8 oz	190
Fat Free Strawberry	8 oz	190
Fat Free Strawberry Pineapple Orange	8 oz	190
Fat Free Vanilla	8 oz	170
French Vanilla	8 oz	180
Light 100 Blueberry	8 oz	100
Light 100 Cherry Vanilla	8 oz	100
Light 100 Coffee & Cream	8 oz	100
Light 100 Creamy Vanilla	8 oz	100

FOOD	PORTION	CALS.
Colombo (CONT.)		
Light 100 Fruit Medley	8 oz	100
Light 100 Juicy Peach	8 oz	100
Light 100 Lemon Creme	8 oz	100
Light 100 Mandarin Orange	8 oz	100
Light 100 Mixed Berries	8 oz	100
Light 100 Raspberry	8 oz	100
Light 100 Strawberry	8 oz	100
Peach Melba	8 oz	200
Plain	8 oz	120
Raspberry	8 oz	200
Strawberry	8 oz	200
Dannon		
Chunky Fruit Nonfat Apple Cinnamon	6 oz	160
Chunky Fruit Nonfat Blueberry	6 oz	160
Chunky Fruit Nonfat Cherry Vanilla	6 oz	160
Chunky Fruit Nonfat Peach	6 oz	160
Chunky Fruit Nonfat Strawberry	6 oz	160
Chunky Fruit Nonfat Strawberry Banana	6 oz	160
Daniamls Lowfat Tropical Punch	4.4 oz	130
Danimals Lowfat Blueberry	4.4 oz	130
Danimals Lowfat Grape Lemonade	4.4 oz	120
Danimals Lowfat Lemon Ice	4.4 oz	120
Danimals Lowfat Orange Banana	4.4 oz	130
Danimals Lowfat Strawberry	4.4 oz	130
Danimals Lowfat Vanilla	4.4 oz	120
Danimals Lowfat Wild Raspberry	4.4 oz	120
Double Delights Banana Creme Strawberry	6 oz	160
Double Delights Bavarian Creme Raspberry	6 oz	170
Double Delights Cheesecake Cherry	6 oz	170
Double Delights Cheesecake Strawberry	6 oz	170
Double Delights Chocolate Cheesecake	6 oz	220
Double Delights Chocolate Dipped Strawberry	6 oz	210
Double Delights Chocolate Eclair	6 oz	220
Double Delights Vanilla Strawberry	6 oz	170
Double Delights Vanilla Peach & Apricot	6 oz	170
Fruit On The Bottom Lowfat Apple Cinnamon	8 oz	240
Fruit On The Bottom Lowfat Blueberry	8 oz	240
Fruit On The Bottom Lowfat Boysenberry	8 oz	240
Fruit On The Bottom Lowfat Cherry	8 oz	240
Fruit On The Bottom Lowfat Minipack Mixed Berry	4.4 oz	130

FOOD	PORTION	CALS.
Dannon (CONT.)		
Fruit On The Bottom Lowfat Minipack Strawberry	4.4 oz	130
Fruit On The Bottom Lowfat Mixed Berries	8 oz	240
Fruit On The Bottom Lowfat Orange	8 oz	240
Fruit On The Bottom Lowfat Peach	8 oz	240
Fruit On The Bottom Lowfat Raspberry	8 oz	240
Fruit On The Bottom Lowfat Strawberry	8 oz	240
Fruit On The Bottom Lowfat Strawberry Banana	8 oz	240
Light 'N Crunchy Mint Chocolate Chip	8 oz	140
Light 'N Crunchy Nonfat Caramel Apple Crunch	8 oz	140
Light 'N Crunchy Nonfat Lemon Blueberry Cobbler	8 oz	140
Light 'N Crunchy Nonfat Mocha Cappuccino	8 oz	140
Light 'N Crunchy Nonfat Raspberry w/ Granola	8 oz	140
Light 'N Crunchy Nonfat Vanilla Chocolate Crunch	8 oz	130
Light Duets Cherry Cheesecake	6 oz	90
Light Duets Peaches N' Cream	6 oz	90
Light Duets Raspberry Royale	6 oz	90
Light Duets Strawberry Cheesecake	6 oz	90
Light Nonfat Banana Cream Pie	8 oz	100
Light Nonfat Blueberry	8 oz	100
Light Nonfat Cappuccino	8 oz	100
Light Nonfat Cherry Vanilla	8 oz	100
Light Nonfat Coconut Cream Pie	8 oz	100
Light Nonfat Creme Caramel	8 oz	100
Light Nonfat Lemon Chiffon	8 oz	100
Light Nonfat Mint Chocolate Cream Pie	8 oz	100
Light Nonfat Peach	8 oz	100
Light Nonfat Raspberry	8 oz	100
Light Nonfat Strawberry	8 oz	100
Light Nonfat Strawberry Banana	8 oz	100
Light Nonfat Strawberry Kiwi	8 oz	100
Light Nonfat Tangerine Chiffon	8 oz	100
Light Nonfat Vanilla	8 oz	100
Lowfat Coffee	8 oz	210
Lowfat Cranberry Raspberry	8 oz	210
Lowfat Lemon	8 oz	210
Lowfat Vanilla	8 oz	210

FOOD	PORTION	CALS.
Dannon (CONT.)		
Minipack Blended Nonfat Blueberry	4.4 oz	120
Minipack Blended Nonfat Cherry	4.4 oz	110
Minipack Blended Nonfat Peach	4.4 oz	120
Minipack Blended Nonfat Raspberry	4.4 oz	120
Minipack Blended Nonfat Strawberry	4.4 oz	120
Minipack Blended Nonfat Strawberry Banana	4.4 oz	120
Sprinkl'ins Cherry Vanilla	1 (4.1 oz)	130
Sprinkl'ins Strawberry	1 (4.1 oz)	130
Sprinkl'ins Strawberry Banana	1 (4.1 oz)	130
Sprinkl'ins Vanilla w/ Cherry Crystals	1 (4.1 oz)	110
Sprinkl'ins Vanilla w/ Orange Crystals	1 (4.1 oz)	110
Friendship		
Coffee	8 oz	210
Fruit Crunch Peach	6 oz	190
Fruit Crunch Strawberry	6 oz	190
Fruit Crunch Strawberry Banana	6 oz	190
Plain	8 oz	150
Hood		
Fat Free Blueberry	1 (8 oz)	190
Fat Free Cherry	1 (8 oz)	190
Fat Free Peach	1 (8 oz)	190
Fat Free Plain	1 (8 oz)	130
Fat Free Raspberry	1 (8 oz)	190
Fat Free Strawberry	1 (8 oz)	190
Fat Free Strawberry Banana	1 (8 oz)	190
Fat Free Vanilla	1 (8 oz)	190
Fat Free Swiss Blueberry	1 (8 oz)	210
Fat Free Swiss Lemon	1 (8 oz)	210
Fat Free Swiss Raspberry	1 (8 oz)	210
Fat Free Swiss Strawberry	1 (8 oz)	210
Fat Free Swiss Strawberry Banana	1 (8 oz)	210
Fat Free Swiss Vanilla	1 (8 oz)	210
Jell-O		
Lowfat Cherry	4.4 oz	130
Lowfat Grape	4.4 oz	130
Lowfat Raspberry	4.4 oz	130
Lowfat Tropical Berry Twist	4.4 oz	130
Lowfat Tropical Punch	4.4 oz	130
Lowfat Watermelon	4.4 oz	130
Lowfat Wild Berry	4.4 oz	130
Lowfat Wild Strawberry	4.4 oz	130

FOOD	PORTION	CALS.
La Yogurt		
French Style Banana	6 oz	180
French Style Blueberry	6 oz	180
French Style Cherry	6 oz	180
French Style Cherry Vanilla	6 oz	190
French Style Guava	6 oz	180
French Style Key Lime	6 oz	180
French Style Mango	6 oz	180
French Style Mixed Berry	6 oz	180
French Style Nonfat Blueberry	6 oz	70
French Style Nonfat Cherry	6 oz	75
French Style Nonfat Raspberry	6 oz	70
French Style Nonfat Strawberry	6 oz	70
French Style Nonfat Strawberry Banana	6 oz	70
French Style Peach	6 oz	180
French Style Pina Colada	6 oz	180
French Style Raspberry	6 oz	180
French Style Strawberry	6 oz	180
French Style Strawberry Banana	6 oz	180
French Style Strawberry Fruit Cup	6 oz	180
French Style Tropical Orange	6 oz	180
French Style Vanilla	6 oz	170
Latin Style Banana	6 oz	190
Latin Style Guava	6 oz	190
Latin Style Mango	6 oz	190
Latin Style Papaya	6 oz	190
Latin Style Passion Fruit	6 oz	190
Latin Style Strawberry Kiwi	6 oz	180
Light N'Lively		
Free Blueberry	4.4 oz	70
Free Peach	4.4 oz	70
Free Strawberry	4.4 oz	70
Free Strawberry Banana Cream	4.4 oz	70
Free Strawberry Fruit Cup	4.4 oz	70
Lowfat Blueberry	4.4 oz	130
Lowfat Peach	4.4 oz	130
Lowfat Pineapple	4.4 oz	130
Lowfat Red Raspberry	4.4 oz	120
Lowfat Strawberry	4.4 oz	130
Lowfat Strawberry Banana Cream	4.4 oz	130
Lowfat Strawberry Fruit Cup	4.4 oz	130
Lite Line		
Swiss Style Cherry Vanilla	1 cup	240
Swiss Style Peach	1 cup	230

FOOD	PORTION	CALS.
Lite Line (CONT.)		
Swiss Style Plain	1 cup	140
Swiss Style Strawberry	1 cup	240
Meadow Gold		
Plain	1 cup	160
Sundae Style Raspberry	1 cup	250
Mountain High		
Blueberry	1 cup	220
Plain	1 cup	200
Yoplait		
99% Fat Free Blueberry	6 oz	180
99% Fat Free Boysenberry	6 oz	180
99% Fat Free Cherry	6 oz	180
99% Fat Free Harvest Peach	6 oz	180
99% Fat Free Harvest Peach	6 oz	120
99% Fat Free Key Lime Pie	6 oz	180
99% Fat Free Lemon	6 oz	180
99% Fat Free Mixed Berry	6 oz	180
99% Fat Free Mixed Berry	6 oz	120
99% Fat Free Orange	6 oz	180
99% Fat Free Pina Colada	6 oz	180
99% Fat Free Pineapple	6 oz	180
99% Fat Free Raspberry	6 oz	180
99% Fat Free Strawberry	6 oz	180
99% Fat Free Strawberry	6 oz	120
99% Fat Free Strawberry Banana	6 oz	120
99% Fat Free Strawberry Banana	6 oz	180
99% Fat Free Strawberry Cheesecake	6 oz	180
Custard Style Banana	6 oz	190
Custard Style Banana	6 oz	190
Custard Style Blueberry	6 oz	190
Custard Style Cherry Vanilla	6 oz	190
Custard Style Key Lime Pie	6 oz	190
Custard Style Lemon	6 oz	190
Custard Style Peaches'n Cream	6 oz	190
Custard Style Raspberry	6 oz	190
Custard Style Raspberry Cheesecake	6 oz	190
Custard Style Strawberry	6 oz	190
Custard Style Strawberry Banana	6 oz	190
Custard Style Strawberry Vanilla	4 oz	120
Custard Style Vanilla	6 oz	190
Go-Gurt Strawberry Banana Burst	1 pkg (2.25 oz)	80
Go-Gurt Watermelon Meltdown	1 pkg (2.25 oz)	80
Light Amaretto Cheesecake	6 oz	90

FOOD	PORTION	CALS.
Yoplait (CONT.)		
Light Apricot Mango	6 oz	90
Light Banana Cream	6 oz	90
Light Blueberry	6 oz	90
Light Boston Cream Pie	6 oz	90
Light Caramel Apple	6 oz	90
Light Cherry	6 oz	90
Light Key Lime Pie	6 oz	90
Light Lemon Cream Pie	6 oz	90
Light Peach	6 oz	90
Light Peach Melba	6 oz	90
Light Raspberry	6 oz	90
Light Raspberry	6 oz	90
Light Strawberry	6 oz	90
Light Strawberry Banana	6 oz	90
Light White Chocolate Strawberry	6 oz	90
Original Cafe Au Lait	6 oz	170
Original Coconut Cream Pie	6 oz	200
Original French Vanilla	6 oz	180
Trix Raspberry Rainbow	6 oz	190
Trix Strawberry Banana Bash	6 oz	190
Trix Strawberry Punch	4 oz	130
Trix Triple Cherry	6 oz	190
Trix Watermelon Burst	4 oz	130
Trix Wild Berry Blue	4 oz	130

YOGURT FROZEN

FOOD	PORTION	CALS.
chocolate soft serve	½ cup (4 fl oz)	115
vanilla soft serve	½ cup (4 fl oz)	114
Ben & Jerry's		
Cherry Garcia	½ cup (3.7 oz)	170
Chocolate Fudge Brownie	½ cup (3.7 oz)	190
Coffee Almond Fudge	½ cup (3.7 oz)	200
English Toffee Crunch	½ cup (3.7 oz)	190
No Fat Cappuccino	½ cup (3.3 oz)	140
Pop Cherry Garcia	1 (3.8 oz)	290
Breyers		
Chocolate	½ cup (2.6 oz)	130
Fat Free Chocolate	½ cup (2.6 oz)	100
Fat Free Cookies N Cream	½ cup (2.6 oz)	110
Fat Free Peach	½ cup (2.6 oz)	90
Fat Free Strawberry	½ cup (2.6 oz)	100
Fat Free Take Two Vanilla Chocolate	½ cup (2.6 oz)	100
Fat Free Vanilla	½ cup (2.6 oz)	100

FOOD	PORTION	CALS.
Breyers (CONT.)		
Fat Free Vanilla Fudge Twirl	½ cup (2.6 oz)	110
Vanilla	½ cup (2.6 oz)	120
Vanilla Chocolate Strawberry	½ cup (2.6 oz)	120
Dannon		
Light Cappuccino	½ cup (2.8 oz)	80
Light Cherry Vanilla Swirl	½ cup (2.8 oz)	90
Light Chocolate	½ cup (2.7 oz)	80
Light Mint Chocolate Fudge	½ cup (2.8 oz)	90
Light Peach Raspberry Melba	½ cup (2.8 oz)	90
Light Strawberry Cheesecake	½ cup (2.8 oz)	90
Light Vanilla	½ cup (2.8 oz)	80
Light 'N Crunchy Carmel Toffee Crunch	½ cup (2.8 oz)	110
Light 'N Crunchy Rocky Road	½ cup (2.8 oz)	110
Light 'N Crunchy Vanilla Streusel	½ cup (2.8 oz)	110
Light Duets Strawberry Sundae	6 oz	90
Light Nonfat Cappuccino	8 oz	100
Light'N Crunchy Banana Cream Pie	½ cup (2.8 oz)	110
Light'N Crunchy Mocha Chocolate Chunk	½ cup (2.8 oz)	110
Light'N Crunchy Peanut Chocolate Crunch	½ cup (2.8 oz)	110
Light'N Crunchy Triple Chocolate	½ cup (2.8 oz)	110
Edy's		
Banana Strawberry	3 oz	80
Blueberry	3 oz	80
Cherry	3 oz	80
Chocolate	3 oz	80
Chocolate Chip	3 oz	100
Citrus Heights	3 oz	80
Cookies'N'Cream	3 oz	100
Marble Fudge	3 oz	100
Perfectly Peach	3 oz	80
Raspberry	3 oz	80
Raspberry Vanilla Swirl	3 oz	80
Strawberry	3 oz	80
Vanilla	3 oz	80
Elan		
Blueberry	4 oz	130
Caramel Almond Praline	4 oz	150
Chocolate	4 oz	130
Chocolate Almond	4 oz	160
Coffee	4 oz	130
Coffee Decaffeinated	4 oz	130
Peach	4 oz	130
Rum Raisin	4 oz	135

FOOD	PORTION	CALS.
Elan (CONT.)		
Strawberry	4 oz	125
Vanilla	4 oz	130
Fi-Bar		
Chocolate	1	190
Strawberry	1	190
Vanilla	1	190
Friendly's		
Apple Bettie	½ cup (2.6 oz)	140
Fabulous Fudge Swirl	½ cup (2.6 oz)	140
Fudge Berry Swirl	½ cup (2.6 oz)	150
Lowfat Perfectly Peach	½ cup (2.6 oz)	110
Lowfat Purely Chocolate	½ cup (2.6 oz)	120
Lowfat Raspberry Delight	½ cup (2.6 oz)	120
Lowfat Simply Vanilla	½ cup (2.6 oz)	120
Lowfat Strawberry Patch	½ cup (2.6 oz)	110
Mint Chocolate Chip	½ cup (2.6 oz)	130
Strawberry Cheesecake Blast	½ cup (2.6 oz)	140
Toffee Almond Crunch	½ cup (2.6 oz)	160
Good Humor		
Creamsicle Raspberry	1 (2.8 oz)	100
Frista Cup	1 (6.2 oz)	220
Haagen-Dazs		
Banana Nut Blast	½ cup (3.5 oz)	220
Bars Cherry Chocolate Fudge	1 (2.6 oz)	240
Bars Peach	1 (2.5 oz)	90
Bars Pina Colada	1 (2.5 oz)	100
Bars Raspberry & Vanilla	1 (2.5 oz)	90
Bars Strawberry Daiquiri	1 (2.5 oz)	90
Chocolate	½ cup (3.4 oz)	160
Coffee	½ cup (3.4 oz)	160
Fat Free Bar Raspberry & Vanilla	1 (2.5 oz)	90
Fat Free Cherry Vanilla	½ cup (3.3 oz)	140
Fat Free Chocolate	½ cup (3.3 oz)	140
Fat Free Coffee	½ cup (3.3 oz)	140
Fat Free Vanilla	½ cup (3.3 oz)	140
Fat Free Vanilla Fudge	½ cup (3.3 oz)	160
Orange Tango	½ cup (3.5 oz)	130
Pina Colada	½ cup (3.4 oz)	130
Raspberry Randevous	½ cup (3.5 oz)	130
Strawberry Cheesecake Craze	½ cup (3.6 oz)	220
Strawberry Duet	½ cup (3.4 oz)	130
Vanilla	½ cup (3.4 oz)	160

FOOD	PORTION	CALS.
Hood		
Bavarian Truffle & Twist	½ cup (2.6 oz)	150
Coffee Toffee Chunk Sundae	½ cup (2.6 oz)	150
Combo Bars	1 (2.2 oz)	90
Cookies & Cream	½ cup (2.6 oz)	140
Grandma's Raisin Oatmeal Cookie Dough	½ cup (2.6 oz)	140
Mixed Berry Swirl	½ cup (2.6 oz)	120
Natural Strawberry	½ cup (2.6 oz)	110
Natural Strawberry Banana	½ cup (2.6 oz)	110
Natural Vanilla	½ cup (2.6 oz)	120
Nonfat Caramel & Brownie Sundae	½ cup (2.6 oz)	120
Nonfat Chocolate Marshmallow	½ cup (2.6 oz)	110
Nonfat Double Raspberry	½ cup (2.6 oz)	120
Nonfat Mocha Fudge	½ cup (2.6 oz)	120
Nonfat Olde Fashioned Vanilla	½ cup (2.6 oz)	110
Nonfat Peach Cobbler A La Mode	½ cup (2.6 oz)	110
Nonfat Strawberry	½ cup (2.6 oz)	100
Nonfat Vanilla Fudge	½ cup (2.6 oz)	120
Raspberry Swirl	½ cup (2.6 oz)	130
Sundae Cups Chocolate & Strawberry	1 (2.2 oz)	110
Vanilla Chocolate Strawberry	½ cup (2.6 oz)	120
Vanilla Swiss Almond Sundae	½ cup (2.6 oz)	150
Sealtest		
Chocolate	½ cup (2.7 oz)	120
Mocha Fudge	½ cup (2.6 oz)	130
Vanilla	½ cup (2.6 oz)	120
Tofutti		
Better Than Yogurt Chocolate Fudge	4 fl oz	120
Better Than Yogurt Coffee Mashmallow Swirl	4 fl oz	100
Better Than Yogurt Passion Island Fruit	4 fl oz	100
Better Than Yogurt Peach Mango	4 fl oz	100
Better Than Yogurt Strawberry Banana	4 fl oz	100
Better Than Yogurt Vanilla Fudge	4 fl oz	120
Turkey Hill		
Chocolate Cherry Cordial	½ cup (2.6 oz)	130
Chocolate Chip Cookie Dough	½ cup (2.6 oz)	140
Death By Chocolate	½ cup (2.6 oz)	150
Nonfat Chocolate Cherry Cordial	½ cup (2.4 oz)	100
Nonfat Chocolate Marshmallow	½ cup (2.4 oz)	130
Nonfat Coffee Cappuccino	½ cup (2.4 oz)	110
Nonfat Mint Cookie 'N Cream	½ cup (2.4 oz)	110
Nonfat Neapolitan	½ cup (2.4 oz)	100
Nonfat Raspberry Chocolate Bliss	½ cup (2.4 oz)	110

FOOD	PORTION	CALS.
Turkey Hill (CONT.)		
Nonfat Southern Lemon Pie	½ cup (2.4 oz)	110
Nonfat Vanilla Fudge	½ cup (2.4 oz)	110
Peach Raspberry	½ cup (2.6 oz)	110
Strawberry	½ cup (2.6 oz)	110
Tin Roof Sundae	½ cup (2.6 oz)	140
Vanilla & Chocolate	½ cup (2.6 oz)	110
Vanilla Bean	½ cup (2.6 oz)	110

ZUCCHINI
CANNED
Del Monte

With Italian Tomato Sauce	½ cup (4.2 oz)	30

Progresso

Italian Style	½ cup (4.2 oz)	40

FRESH

baby raw	1 (0.5 oz)	3
raw sliced	½ cup	9
sliced cooked	½ cup	14

FROZEN
Big Valley

Zucchini	¾ cup (3 oz)	10

Empire

Breaded	1 (2.9 oz)	100

TAKE-OUT

indian paalkora	1 serv	46

PART • TWO

RESTAURANT

FOODS

FOOD	PORTION	CALS.

ARBY'S
BEVERAGES

2 % Milk	0.5 oz	5
Chocolate Shake	1 (12 oz)	451
Coca Cola Classic	1 serv (12 oz)	140
Coffee	1 serv (8 oz)	3
Diet Coke	1 serv (12 oz)	0
Diet Pepsi	1 serv (12 oz)	0
Diet Seven Up	1 serv (12 oz)	0
Dr. Pepper	1 serv (12 oz)	160
Hot Chocolate	1 serv (8 oz)	110
Iced Tea	1 serv (16 oz)	6
Jamocha Shake	1 (12 oz)	384
Nehi Orange	1 serv (12 oz)	195
Orange Juice	1 serv (6 oz)	82
Pepsi Cola	1 serv (12 oz)	150
RC Cola	1 serv (12 oz)	165
RC Diet Rite	1 serv (12 oz)	1
Seven Up	1 serv (12 oz)	144
Upper Ten	1 serv (12 oz)	169
Vanilla Shake	1 (12 oz)	360

BREAKFAST SELECTIONS

Bacon	2 strips (0.53 oz)	90
Biscuit Plain	1 (2.9 oz)	280
Blueberry Muffin	1 (2.3 oz)	230
Cinnamon Nut Danish	1 (3.5 oz)	360
Croissant Plain	1 (2 oz)	220
Egg Portion	1 serv (1.6 oz)	95
Ham	1 serv (1.5 oz)	45
Sausage	1 (1.3 oz)	163
Swiss	1 serv (0.5 oz)	45
Table Syrup	1 serv (1 oz)	100
Toastix	6 pieces (4.4 oz)	430

DESSERTS

Apple Turnover	1 (3.2 oz)	330
Cheesecake Plain	1 serv (3 oz)	320
Cherry Turnover	1 (3.2 oz)	320
Chocolate Chip Cookie	1 (1 oz)	125
Polar Swirl Butterfinger	1 (11.6 oz)	457
Polar Swirl Heath	1 (11.6 oz)	543
Polar Swirl Oreo	1 (11.6 oz)	329
Polar Swirl Peanut Butter Cup	1 (11.6 oz)	517
Polar Swirl Snickers	1 (11.6 oz)	511

FOOD	PORTION	CALS.
MAIN MENU SELECTIONS		
Arby's Sauce	1 serv (0.5 oz)	15
Baked Potato Broccoli'n Cheddar	1 (15.7 oz)	571
Baked Potato Deluxe	1 (15.3 oz)	736
Baked Potato Plain	1 (11.5 oz)	355
Baked Potato w/ Margarine & Sour Cream	1 (14 oz)	578
Barbeque Sauce	1 serv (0.5 oz)	30
Beef Stock Au Jus	1 serv (2 oz)	10
Breaded Chicken Fillet	1 (7.2 oz)	536
Cheddar Cheese Sauce	1 serv (0.75 oz)	35
Cheddar Curly Fried	1 serv (4.25 oz)	333
Chicken Cordon Bleu	1 (8.5 oz)	623
Chicken Finger	2 (3.6 oz)	290
Curly Fries	1 serv (3.5 oz)	300
Fish Fillet Sandwich	1 (7.7 oz)	529
French Fries	1 serv (2.5 oz)	246
Garden Salad	1 (11.9 oz)	61
Grilled Chicken BBQ	1 (7.1 oz)	388
Grilled Chicken Deluxe	1 (8.1 oz)	430
Ham 'n Cheese Sandwich	1 (5.9 oz)	359
Ham'n Cheese Melt	1 (4.9 oz)	329
Honey Mayonnaise Reduced Calorie	1 serv (0.5 oz)	70
Horsey Sauce	1 serv (0.5 oz)	60
Italian Sub	1 (10.1 oz)	675
Italian Sub Sauce	1 serv (0.5 oz)	70
Ketchup	1 serv (0.5 oz)	16
Light Roast Beef Deluxe	1 (6.4 oz)	296
Light Roast Chicken Deluxe	1 (6.8 oz)	276
Light Roast Chicken Salad	1 serv (14.4 oz)	149
Light Roast Turkey Deluxe	1 (6.8 oz)	260
Mayonnaise	1 serv (0.5 oz)	110
Mayonnaise Light Cholesterol Free	1 serv (0.25 oz)	12
Mustard German Style	1 serv (0.16 oz)	5
Parmesan Cheese Sauce	1 serv (0.5 oz)	70
Potato Cakes	2 (3 oz)	204
Roast Beef Arby's Melt w/ Cheddar	1 (5.2 oz)	368
Roast Beef Arby-Q	1 (6.4 oz)	431
Roast Beef Bac'n Cheddar Deluxe	1 (8.1 oz)	539
Roast Beef Beef'n Cheddar	1 (6.7 oz)	487
Roast Beef Gaint	1 (8.1 oz)	555
Roast Beef Junior	1 (4.4 oz)	324
Roast Beef Regular	1 (5.4 oz)	388
Roast Beef Sub	1 (10.8 oz)	700
Roast Beef Super	1 (8.7 oz)	523

FOOD	PORTION	CALS.
Roast Chicken Club	1 (8.5 oz)	546
Roast Chicken Deluxe	1 (7.6 oz)	433
Roast Chicken Santa Fe	1 (6.4 oz)	436
Side Salad	1 (5 oz)	23
Sub Roll French Dip	1 (6.8 oz)	475
Sub Roll Hot Ham 'n Swiss	1 (9.3 oz)	500
Sub Roll Pilly Beef'n Swiss	1 (10.4 oz)	755
Sub Roll Triple Cheese Melt	1 (8.4 oz)	720
Tartar Sauce	1 serv (1 oz)	140
Turkey Sub	1 (9.8 oz)	550
SALAD DRESSINGS		
Buttermilk Ranch Reduced Calorie	1 serv (2 oz)	50
Honey French	1 serv (2 oz)	280
Italian Reduced Calorie	1 serv (2 oz)	20
Red Ranch	1 serv (0.5 oz)	75
Thousand Island	1 serv (2 oz)	260
SOUPS		
Boston Clam Chowder	1 serv (8 oz)	190
Cream of Broccoli	1 serv (8 oz)	160
Lumberjack Mixed Vegetable	1 serv (8 oz)	90
Old Fashioned Chicken Noodle	1 serv (8 oz)	80
Potato w/ Bacon	1 serv (8 oz)	170
Timberline Chili	1 serv (8 oz)	220
Wisconsin Cheese	1 serv (8 oz)	280

AU BON PAIN
BAKED SELECTIONS

FOOD	PORTION	CALS.
Apple Coffee Cake	1 piece (4.6 oz)	480
Bagel Chocolate Chip	1 (5 oz)	380
Bagel Dutch Apple w/ Walnut Streussel	1 (5 oz)	360
Baguette Loaf	1 slice (1.8 oz)	140
Biscotti	1 (1.5 oz)	200
Biscotti Chocolate	1 (1.7 oz)	240
Braided Roll	1 (1.8 oz)	170
Cinnamon Roll	1 (7 oz)	710
Cookie Chocolate Chip	1 (2.1 oz)	280
Cookie Oatmeal Raisin	1 (2.1 oz)	250
Cookie Peanut Butter	1 (2.1 oz)	280
Cookie Shortbread	1 (2.4 oz)	390
Croissant Almond	1 (4.3 oz)	560
Croissant Apple	1 (3.4 oz)	280
Croissant Chocolate	1 (3.4 oz)	440
Croissant Cinnamon Raisin	1 (3.7 oz)	380
Croissant Plain	1 (2.1 oz)	270

FOOD	PORTION	CALS.
Croissant Raspberry Cheese	1 (3.5 oz)	380
Croissant Sweet Cheese	1 (3.6 oz)	390
Danish Cheese Swirl	1 (3.8 oz)	450
Danish Lemon Swirl	1 (4 oz)	450
Danish Raspberry	1 (3.6 oz)	370
Danish Sweet Cheese	1 (3.6 oz)	420
Four Grain Loaf	1 slice (1.8 oz)	130
French Sandwich Roll	1 (1.8 oz)	120
Hazelnut Fudge Brownie	1 (4 oz)	380
Holiday Cookie Cranberry Almond Macaroon	1 (1.5 oz)	160
Holiday Cookie Cranberry Almond Macaroon w/ Chocolate	1 (1.9 oz)	210
Holiday Cookie English Toffee	1 (1.8 oz)	220
Holiday Cookie Ginger Pecan	1 (2 oz)	260
Mochaccino Bar	1 (4 oz)	404
Muffin Blueberry	1 (4.5 oz)	410
Muffin Carrot	1 (5 oz)	480
Muffin Chocolate Chip	1 (4.5 oz)	490
Muffin Corn	1 (4.6 oz)	470
Muffin Pumpkin w/ Streusel Topping	1 (5.5 oz)	470
Muffin Low Fat Chocolate Cake	1 (4 oz)	290
Muffin Low Fat Triple Berry	1 (4.2 oz)	270
Multigrain Loaf	1 slice (1.8 oz)	130
Parisienne Loaf	1 slice (1.8 oz)	120
Pear Ginger Tea Cake	1 piece (4 oz)	380
Pecan Roll	1 (6.8 oz)	900
Roll 3 Seed Pecan Raisin	1 (2.7 oz)	250
Roll Hearth Sandwich	1 (2.8 oz)	220
Rolls Petit Pan	1 (2.5 oz)	200
Rye Loaf	1 slice (1.8 oz)	110
Scone Cinnamon	1 (4.1 oz)	520
Scone Current	1 (3.7 oz)	430
Scone Orange	1 (4.1 oz)	440
Sourdough Bagel Asiago Cheese	1 (4.2 oz)	380
Sourdough Bagel Cinnamon Raisin	1 (4.5 oz)	390
Sourdough Bagel Cranberry Walnut	1 (5 oz)	460
Sourdough Bagel Everything	1 (4.2 oz)	360
Sourdough Bagel Honey 8 Grain	1 (4.2 oz)	360
Sourdough Bagel Mocha Chip Swirl	1 (5 oz)	370
Sourdough Bagel Plain	1 (4 oz)	350
Sourdough Bagel Sesame	1 (4.2 oz)	380
Sourdough Bagel Wild Blueberry	1 (4.5 oz)	380
Valentine Cookie Chocolate Dipped Shortbread	1 (2.8 oz)	410

FOOD	PORTION	CALS.
Valentine Cookie Red Sugar Shortbread Heart	1 (2.4 oz)	350
Valentine Cookie Shortbread	1 (2.4 oz)	340
BEVERAGES		
Frozen Java Blast	1 serv (16 oz)	220
Frozen Mocha Blast	1 serv (16 oz)	320
Hot Apple Cider	1 med (16 oz)	310
Hot Apple Cider	1 sm (10 oz)	190
Hot Apple Cider	1 lg (20 oz)	350
Hot Hazelnut Blast	1 serv (16 oz)	310
Hot Mocha Blast	1 lg (17 oz)	310
Hot Mocha Blast	1 med (13 oz)	260
Hot Mocha Blast	1 sm (9 oz)	160
Hot Raspberry Mocha Blast	1 serv (16 oz)	300
Hot Raspberry Mocha Blast	1 serv (10 oz)	180
Hot Raspberry Mocha Blast	1 serv (20 oz)	350
Hot Strawberry Chocolate Blast	1 serv (16 oz)	330
Hot Vanilla Chocolate Blast	1 serv (16 oz)	310
Iced Caffee Latte	1 lg (20.5 oz)	270
Iced Caffee Latte	1 sm (9 oz)	130
Iced Caffee Latte	1 med (12 oz)	150
Iced Cappuccino	1 sm (9 oz)	110
Iced Cappuccino	1 lg (20.5 oz)	270
Iced Cappuccino	1 med (12 oz)	150
Iced Cocoa	1 lg (20.5 oz)	440
Iced Cocoa	1 sm (9 oz)	200
Iced Cocoa	1 med (12 oz)	280
Iced Hazelnut Blast	1 serv (16 oz)	310
Iced Mocha Blast	1 med (12 oz)	260
Iced Mocha Blast	1 lg (20.5 oz)	360
Iced Mocha Blast	1 sm (9 oz)	180
Iced Raspberry Mocha Blast	1 serv (24 oz)	330
Iced Raspberry Mocha Blast	1 serv (16 oz)	310
Iced Raspberry Mocha Blast	1 serv (12 oz)	160
Iced Strawberry Chocolate Blast	1 serv (16 oz)	310
Iced Vanilla Chocolate Blast	1 serv (16 oz)	310
Iced Tea Peach	1 med (12 oz)	130
Iced Tea Peach	1 sm (12 oz)	90
Iced Tea Peach	1 lg (16 oz)	170
Iced Tea Raspberry	1 lg (16 oz)	150
Iced Tea Raspberry	1 med (12 oz)	110
Iced Tea Raspberry	1 sm (8 oz)	80
Whipped Cream	1 serv (1.2 oz)	160

FOOD	PORTION	CALS.
SALAD DRESSINGS		
Bleu Cheese	1 serv (3 oz)	370
Buttermilk Ranch	1 serv (3 oz)	310
Ceasar	1 serv (3 oz)	380
Fat Free Tomato Basil	1 serv (3 oz)	70
Greek	1 serv (3 oz)	440
Lemon Basil Vinaigrette	1 serv (3 oz)	330
Lite Honey Mustard	1 serv (3 oz)	280
Lite Italian	1 serv (3 oz)	230
Sesame French	1 serv (3 oz)	370
SALADS AND SALAD BARS		
Caesar	1 serv (8.9 oz)	270
Chicken Caesar	1 serv (11.4 oz)	360
Garden	1 sm (7.5 oz)	100
Garden	1 lg (10.6 oz)	160
Mozzarella & Roasted Pepper Salad	1 serv (13.7 oz)	340
Pesto Chicken Salad	1 serv (10.7 oz)	230
Tuna	1 serv (15 oz)	490
SANDWICHES AND FILLINGS		
Bagel Spreads Lite Strawberry	1 serv (2 oz)	150
Bagel Spreads Lite Vanilla Hazelnut	1 serv (2 oz)	150
Cheddar	½ serv (1.5 oz)	170
Chicken Tarragon	1 serv (4 oz)	240
Club Sandwich Hot Roasted Turkey	1 (14.9 oz)	950
Country Ham	1 serv (3.7 oz)	150
Cracked Pepper Chicken	1 serv (3.9 oz)	140
Cream Cheese Lite	1 serv (2 oz)	130
Cream Cheese Lite Honey Walnut	1 serv (2 oz)	260
Cream Cheese Lite Raspberry	1 serv (2 oz)	200
Cream Cheese Lite Sun-Dried Tomato	1 serv (2 oz)	130
Cream Cheese Plain	1 serv (2 oz)	190
Cream Cheese Veggie Lite	1 serv (2 oz)	100
Grilled Chicken	1 serv (3.9 oz)	140
Hot Croissant Ham & Cheese	1 (4.2 oz)	380
Hot Croissants Spinach & Cheese	1 (3.6 oz)	270
Provolone	½ serv (1.5 oz)	150
Roast Beef	1 serv (3.7 oz)	140
Sandwich Arizona Chicken	1 (12.7 oz)	720
Sandwich Buffalo Chicken	1 (13.7 oz)	640
Sandwich California Chicken	1 (13.2 oz)	820
Sandwich Fresh Mozzarella Tomato & Pesto	1 (10.5 oz)	650
Sandwich Honey Dijon Chicken	1 (15.3 oz)	730
Sandwich Parmesan Chicken	1 (11.1 oz)	740
Sandwich Steak & Cheese Melt	1 (11.7 oz)	750

FOOD	PORTION	CALS.
Sandwich Thai Chicken	1 (8.3 oz)	420
Swiss	½ serv (1.5 oz)	160
Tuna Salad	1 serv (4.5 oz)	360
Turkey Breast	1 serv (3.7 oz)	120
Wraps Chicken Caesar	1 (9.9 oz)	630
Wraps Southwestern Tuna	1 (14.4 oz)	950
Wraps Summer Turkey	1 (11.7 oz)	340
SOUPS		
Beef Barley	1 serv (12 oz)	112
Beef Barley	1 serv (16 oz)	150
Beef Barley	1 serv (8 oz)	75
Beef Stew	1 serv (8 oz)	140
Bohemian Cabbage	1 serv (8 oz)	70
Bohemian Cabbage	1 serv (12 oz)	110
Bohemian Cabbage	1 serv (16 oz)	140
Bread Bowl	1 (9 oz)	640
Broccoli & Cheddar	1 serv (8 oz)	260
Broccoli & Cheddar	1 serv (16 oz)	520
Broccoli & Cheddar	1 serv (12 oz)	390
Caribbean Black Bean	1 serv (16 oz)	250
Caribbean Black Bean	1 serv (12 oz)	180
Caribbean Black Bean	1 serv (8 oz)	120
Chicken Chili	1 serv (12 oz)	350
Chicken Chili	1 serv (8 oz)	240
Chicken Chili	1 serv (16 oz)	470
Chicken Noodle	1 serv (16 oz)	170
Chicken Noodle	1 serv (12 oz)	120
Chicken Noodle	1 serv (8 oz)	80
Chili	1 serv (12 oz)	340
Chili	1 serv (16 oz)	460
Chili	1 serv (8 oz)	230
Clam Chowder	1 serv (8 oz)	270
Clam Chowder	1 serv (16 oz)	540
Clam Chowder	1 serv (12 oz)	400
Corn Chowder	1 serv (16 oz)	530
Corn Chowder	1 serv (12 oz)	390
Corn Chowder	1 serv (8 oz)	260
Cream Of Broccoli	1 serv (16 oz)	440
Cream Of Broccoli	1 serv (12 oz)	330
Cream Of Broccoli	1 serv (8 oz)	220
Cream Of Chicken With Wild Rice	1 serv (16 oz)	330
French Onion	1 serv (12 oz)	120
French Onion	1 serv (16 oz)	170
French Onion	1 serv (8 oz)	80

FOOD	PORTION	CALS.
In A Bread Bowl Beef Barley	1 serv (21 oz)	760
In A Bread Bowl Carribean Black Bean	1 serv (21 oz)	830
In A Bread Bowl Chicken Chili	1 serv (21 oz)	990
In A Bread Bowl Chicken Noodle	1 serv (21 oz)	760
In A Bread Bowl Clam Chowder	1 serv (21 oz)	1050
In A Bread Bowl Cream of Broccoli	1 serv (21 oz)	970
In A Bread Bowl French Onion	1 serv (21 oz)	760
In A Bread Bowl New England Potato & Cheese w/ Ham	1 serv (21 oz)	860
In A Bread Bowl Tomato Florentine	1 serv (21 oz)	760
In A Bread Bowl Vegetarian Chili	1 serv (21 oz)	870
Louisiana Beans & Rice	1 serv (16 oz)	360
Louisiana Beans & Rice	1 serv (8 oz)	180
Louisiana Beans & Rice	1 serv (12 oz)	280
New England Potato & Cheese w/ Ham	1 serv (8 oz)	150
New England Potato & Cheese w/ Ham	1 serv (12 oz)	220
New England Potato & Cheese w/ Ham	1 serv (16 oz)	290
Potato Leek	1 serv (12 oz)	320
Potato Leek	1 serv (8 oz)	200
Potato Leek	1 serv (16 oz)	400
Sante Fe Chicken Tortilla	1 serv (16 oz)	300
Sante Fe Chicken Tortilla	1 serv (8 oz)	150
Sante Fe Chicken Tortilla	1 serv (12 oz)	230
Seafood Gumbo	1 serv (8 oz)	130
Seafood Gumbo	1 serv (12 oz)	190
Seafood Gumbo	1 serv (16 oz)	260
Tomato Florentine	1 serv (8 oz)	61
Tomato Florentine	1 serv (16 oz)	122
Tomato Florentine	1 serv (12 oz)	90
Tomato Tortellini	1 serv (12 oz)	90
Tomato Tortellini	1 serv (8 oz)	60
Tomato Tortellini	1 serv (16 oz)	110
Vegetable Stew	1 serv (8 oz)	60
Vegetable Stew	1 serv (12 oz)	100
Vegetable Stew	1 serv (16 oz)	130
Vegetarian Lentil	1 serv (16 oz)	270
Vegetarian Lentil	1 serv (8 oz)	130
Vegetarian Lentil	1 serv (12 oz)	200
Vegetarian Chili	1 serv (16 oz)	278
Vegetarian Chili	1 serv (12 oz)	210
Vegetarian Chili	1 serv (8 oz)	139
Vegetarian Corn & Green Chili Bisque	1 serv (8 oz)	190
Vegetarian Corn & Green Chili Bisque	1 serv (16 oz)	380
Vegetarian Corn & Green Chili Bisque	1 serv (12 oz)	300

FOOD	PORTION	CALS.
AUNTIE ANNE'S		
Caramel Dip	1 serv (1.5 oz)	135
Cheese Sauce	1 serv (1 oz)	70
Chocolate Dip	1 serv (1.25 oz)	130
Cream Cheese Light	1 serv (.75 oz)	45
Cream Cheese Pineapple	1 serv (.75 oz)	70
Cream Cheese Strawberry	1 serv (.75 oz)	70
Dutch Ice Kiwi Banana	1 (12 oz)	160
Dutch Ice Kiwi Banana	1 (18 oz)	250
Dutch Ice Lemonade	1 (12 oz)	270
Dutch Ice Lemonade	1 (18 oz)	405
Dutch Ice Mocha	1 (18 oz)	340
Dutch Ice Mocha	1 (18 oz)	500
Dutch Ice Orange Creme	1 (18 oz)	360
Dutch Ice Orange Creme	1 (12 oz)	240
Dutch Ice Raspberry	1 (18 oz)	220
Dutch Ice Raspberry	1 (12 oz)	150
Dutch Ice Strawberry	1 (18 oz)	280
Dutch Ice Strawberry	1 (12 oz)	190
Marinara Sauce	1 serv (1 oz)	10
Pretzel Almond w/ Butter	1	400
Pretzel Almond w/o Butter	1	350
Pretzel Cinnamon Raisin w/o Butter	1	350
Pretzel Cinnamon Sugar w/ Butter	1	450
Pretzel Garlic w/ Butter	1	350
Pretzel Garlic w/o Butter	1	320
Pretzel Glazein' Raisin w/ Butter	1	510
Pretzel Glazin' Raisin w/o Butter	1	470
Pretzel Jalapeno w/ Butter	1	310
Pretzel Jalapeno w/o Butter	1	270
Pretzel Original w/ Butter	1	370
Pretzel Original w/o Butter	1	340
Pretzel Sesame w/ Butter	1	410
Pretzel Sesame w/o Butter	1	350
Pretzel Sour Cream & Onion w/ Butter	1	340
Pretzel Sour Cream & Onion w/o Butter	1	310
Pretzel Whole Wheat w/ Butter	1	370
Pretzel Whole Wheat w/o Butter	1	350
Sweet Mustard	1 serv (1 oz)	60
BASKIN-ROBBINS		
FROZEN YOGURT		
Maui Brownie Madness	½ cup	140
Perils Of Pauline	½ cup	140

FOOD	PORTION	CALS.
ICE CREAM		
Banana Strawberry	½ cup	130
Baseball Nut	½ cup	160
Black Walnut	½ cup	160
Cherries Jubilee	½ cup	140
Chocolate	½ cup	150
Chocolate Almond	½ cup	180
Chocolate Chip	½ cup	150
Chocolate Chip Cookie Dough	½ cup	170
Chocolate Fudge	½ cup	160
Chocolate Mousse Royale	½ cup	170
Chocolate Raspberry Truffle	½ cup	180
Chunky Heath Bar	½ cup	170
Cookies N Cream	½ cup	170
Dirt'N Worms	½ cup	160
Egg Nog	½ cup	150
Everybody's Favorite Candy Bar	½ cup	170
French Vanilla	½ cup	160
French Vanilla	½ cup	170
Fudge Brownie	½ cup	170
Fudge Brownie	½ cup	180
German Chocolate Cake	½ cup	180
Gold Medal Ribbon	½ cup	150
Gold Medal Ribbon	½ cup	150
Jamoca	½ cup	140
Jamoca Almond Fudge	½ cup	150
Lemon Custard	½ cup	150
Lowfat Carmel Apple AlaMod	½ cup	100
Lowfat Espresso'N Cream	½ cup	100
Mint Chocolate Chip	½ cup	150
No Sugar Added Call Me Nuts	½ cup	110
No Sugar Added Cherry Cordial	½ cup	100
No Sugar Added Mad About Chocolate	½ cup	100
No Sugar Added Pineapple Coconut	½ cup	90
No Sugar Added Thin Mint	½ cup	100
Nonfat Berry Innocent Cheese	½ cup	110
Nonfat Check-It-Out Cherry	½ cup	100
Nonfat Jamoca Swirl	½ cup	110
Ocean Commotion	½ cup	150
Old Fashion Butter Pecan	½ cup	160
Oregon Blueberry	½ cup	140
Peanut Butter N Chocolate	½ cup	180
Pink Bubblegum	½ cup	150

FOOD	PORTION	CALS.
Pistachio Almond	½ cup	170
Pralines N Cream	½ cup	160
Pumpkin Pie	½ cup	130
Quarterback Crunch	½ cup	160
Reeses Peanut Butter	½ cup	180
Rocky Road	½ cup	170
Rum Raisin	½ cup	140
Strawberry Cheesecake	½ cup	150
Triple Chocolate Passion	½ cup	180
Vanilla	½ cup	140
Very Berry Strawberry	½ cup	130
Winter White Chocolate	½ cup	150
World Class Chocolate	½ cup	160
ICES AND ICE POPS		
Daiquiri Ice	½ cup	110
Sherbet Blue Raspberry	½ cup	120
Sherbet Orange	½ cup	120
Sherbet Rainbow	½ cup	120
Sorbet Pink Raspberry Lemon	½ cup	120
The Mask Ice	½ cup	120
Watermelon Ice	½ cup	110
Watermelon Ice	½ cup	110

BEN & JERRY'S

Sugar Cone	1	48
FROZEN YOGURT		
Cherry Garcia	½ cup (3.3 oz)	150
Chocolate Chip Cookie Dough	½ cup (3.3 oz)	190
Chocolate Fudge Brownie	½ cup (3.3 oz)	180
No Fat Black Raspberry	½ cup (3.4 oz)	140
No Fat Vanilla	½ cup (3.4 oz)	140
No Fat Vanilla Swirl	½ cup (3.4 oz)	130
Peach Raspberry Trifle	½ cup (3.3 oz)	150
Vanilla w/ Heath Toffee Crunch	½ cup (3.3 oz)	190
ICE CREAM		
Butter Pecan	½ cup (3.1 oz)	270
Cherry Garcia	½ cup (3.1 oz)	210
Chocolate Chip Cookie Dough	½ cup (3.1 oz)	180
Chocolate Fudge Brownie	½ cup (3.1 oz)	230
Chubby Hubby	½ cup (3.1 oz)	280
Chunky Monkey	½ cup (3.1 oz)	220
Coffee Coffee Buzz Buzz	½ cup (3.1 oz)	240
Coffee Ole	½ cup (3.1 oz)	200
Coffee w/ Heath Toffee Crunch	½ cup (3.1 oz)	250

FOOD	PORTION	CALS.
Cool Britannia	½ cup (3.1 oz)	210
Deep Deep Chocolate	½ cup (3.1 oz)	210
Holy Cannoli	½ cup (3.1 oz)	240
Low Fat Blond Brownie Sundae	½ cup (3.1 oz)	160
Low Fat Coffee & Biscotti	½ cup (3.1 oz)	160
Low Fat Sweet Cream & Cookies	½ cup (3.1 oz)	160
Low Fat Vanilla & Chocolate Mint Patty	½ cup (3.1 oz)	170
Maple Walnut	½ cup (3.1 oz)	240
Mint Chocolate Chunk	½ cup (3.1 oz)	240
Mint Chocolate Cookie	½ cup (3.1 oz)	230
New York Super Fudge Chunk	½ cup (3.1 oz)	250
Peanut Butter Cup	½ cup (3.1 oz)	270
Peanut Butter & Jelly	½ cup (3.1 oz)	230
Phish Food	½ cup (3.1 oz)	230
Pistachio Pistachio	½ cup (3.1 oz)	230
Rainforest Crunch	½ cup (3.1 oz)	250
Southern Peach	½ cup (3.1 oz)	180
Strawberry	½ cup (3.1 oz)	180
Sweet Cream Cookie	½ cup (3.1 oz)	230
Vanilla Caramel Fudge	½ cup (3.1 oz)	230
Vanilla Chocolate Chunk	½ cup (3.1 oz)	240
Vanilla Fudge Brownie	½ cup (3.1 oz)	210
Vanilla World's Best	½ cup (3.1 oz)	200
Vanilla w/ Heath Toffee Crunch	½ cup (3.1 oz)	250
Wavy Gravy	½ cup (3.1 oz)	260
White Russian	½ cup (3.1 oz)	200
SORBETS		
Cranberry Orange	½ cup (3.2 oz)	110
Doonesberry	½ cup (3.2 oz)	100
Mango Lime	½ cup (3.2 oz)	110
Pina Colada	½ cup (3.2 oz)	110
Purple Passion Fruit	½ cup (3.2 oz)	100
Strawberry Kiwi	½ cup (3.2 oz)	110

BIG BOY
DESSERTS

FOOD	PORTION	CALS.
Frozen Yogurt Fat Free	1 serv	118
Frozen Yogurt Shake	1	156
MAIN MENU SELECTIONS		
Baked Cod w/ Salad Baked Potato Roll & Margarine	1 meal	744
Baked Potato	1	163
Breast of Chicken Pita w/ Mozzarella & Ranch Dressing	1	361

FOOD	PORTION	CALS.
Breast of Chicken w/ Mozzarella Salad Baked Potato Roll & Margarine	1 meal	697
Cabbage Soup	1 bowl	40
Cabbage Soup	1 cup	34
Cajun Cod w/ Salad Baked Potato Roll & Margarine	1 meal	736
Chicken & Pasta Primavera w/ Salad Roll & Margarine	1 meal	676
Chicken 'n Vegetable Stir Fry w/ Salad Baked Potato Roll & Margarine	1 meal	795
Dinner Roll	1	210
Plain Egg Beaters Omelette w/ Whole Wheat Bread & Margarine	1 meal	305
Promise Margarine	1 pat	25
Rice Pilaf	1 serv	153
Scrambled Egg Beaters w/ Whole Wheat Bread & Margarine	1 meal	305
Southwest Chicken w/ Salad Baked Potato Roll & Margarine	1 meal	702
Spaghetti Marinara w/ Salad Roll & Margarin	1 meal	754
Turkey Pita w/ Ranch Dressing	1	245
Vegetable Stir Fry w/ Salad Baked Potato Roll & Margarine	1 meal	616
Vegetarian Egg Beaters Omelette w/ Whole Wheat Bread & Margarine	1 meal	330
SALAD DRESSINGS		
Italian Fat Free	1 oz	11
Lo Cal Oriental	1 oz	20
Lo Cal Ranch	1 oz	41
SALADS AND SALAD BARS		
Chicken Breast Salad w/ Roll & Margarine	1 serv	523
Oriental Chicken Breast Salad w/ Dinner Roll & Margarine	1 serv	660
Tossed Salad	1	35

BLIMPIE
6 INCH SUB

FOOD	PORTION	CALS.
5 Meatball	1 (7.8 oz)	500
Blimpie Best	1 (8.5 oz)	410
Cheese Trio	1 (8.2 oz)	510
Club	1 (9.8 oz)	450
Grilled Chicken	1 (9.1 oz)	400
Ham & Swiss	1 (8.2 oz)	400
Ham Salami Provolone	1 (9.8 oz)	590

FOOD	PORTION	CALS.
Roast Beef	1 (8.5 oz)	340
Steak & Cheese	1 (7.1 oz)	550
Tuna	1 (10.2 oz)	570
Turkey	1 (8.2 oz)	320
SALADS AND SALAD BARS		
Grilled Chicken Salad	1 serv (16.2 oz)	350

BOJANGLES
BAKED SELECTIONS

FOOD	PORTION	CALS.
Biscuit	1	243
Multi-Grain Roll	1	150
Sweet Biscuit Apple Cinnamon	1	330
Sweet Biscuit Bo*Berry	1	220
Sweet Biscuit Cinnamon	1	320
MAIN MENU SELECTIONS		
Biscuit Sandwich Bacon	1	290
Biscuit Sandwich Bacon Egg & Cheese	1	550
Biscuit Sandwich Cajun Filet	1	454
Biscuit Sandwich Country Ham	1	270
Biscuit Sandwich Egg	1	400
Biscuit Sandwich Sausage	1	350
Biscuit Sandwich Smoked Sausage	1	380
Biscuit Sandwich Steak	1	649
Bo Rounds	1 serv	235
Buffalo Bites	1 serv	180
Cajun Pintos	1 serv	110
Cajun Roast Skinfree Breast	1 serv	143
Cajun Roast Skinfree Leg	1 serv	161
Cajun Roast Skinfree Thigh	1 serv	215
Cajun Roast Wing	1 serv	231
Cajun Spiced Breast	1 serv	278
Cajun Spiced Leg	1 serv	310
Cajun Spiced Thigh	1 serv	264
Cajun Spiced Wing	1 serv	355
Chicken Supremes	1 serv	337
Corn On The Cob	1 serv	140
Dirty Rice	1 serv	166
Green Beans	1 serv	25
Macaroni & Cheese	1 serv	198
Marinated Cole Slaw	1 serv	136
Potatoes w/o Gravy	1 serv	80
Sandwich Cajun Filet w/ Mayonnaise	1	437
Sandwich Cajun Steak w/ Horseradish Sauce & Pickles	1	434

FOOD	PORTION	CALS.
Sandwich Cjun Filet w/o Mayonnaise	1	337
Sandwich Grilled Filet w/ Mayonnaise	1	335
Sandwich Grilled Filet w/o Mayonnaise	1 serv (5.2 oz)	329
Seasoned Fries	1 serv	344
Southern Style Breast	1 serv	261
Southern Style Leg	1 serv	254
Southern Style Thigh	1 serv	308
Southern Style Wing	1 serv	337

BOSTON MARKET
BAKED SELECTIONS

Brownie	1 (3.3 oz)	450
Cookie Chocolate Chip	1 (2.8 oz)	340
Cookie Oatmeal Raisin	1 (2.8 oz)	320
Honey Wheat Roll	½ roll (2 oz)	150

MAIN MENU SELECTIONS

½ Chicken w/ Skin	1 serv (10 oz)	630
¼ Dark Meat Chicken No Skin	1 serv (3.6 oz)	210
¼ Dark Meat Chicken w/ Skin	1 serv (4.6 oz)	330
¼ White Meat Chicken No Skin Or Wing	1 serv (3.6 oz)	160
¼ White Meat Chicken w/ Skin	1 serv (5.4 oz)	330
BBQ Baked Beans	¾ cup (7.1 oz)	330
Butternut Squash Low Fat	¾ cup (6.8 oz)	160
Caesar Salad Entree	1 serv (10 oz)	520
Caesar Salad w/o Dressing	1 serv (8 oz)	240
Caesar Side Salad	1 (4 oz)	210
Chicken Caesar Salad	1 serv (13 oz)	670
Chicken Gravy	1 serv (1 oz)	15
Chicken Salad Sandwich	1 (10.7 oz)	680
Chicken Sandwich w/ Cheese & Sauce	1 (12.4 oz)	750
Chicken Sandwich w/o Cheese & Sauce Low Fat	1 (10 oz)	430
Chunky Chicken Salad	¾ cup (5.5 oz)	370
Cole Slaw	¾ cup (6.5 oz)	280
Corn Bread	1 (2.4 oz)	200
Cranberry Relish Low Fat	¾ cup (7.9 oz)	370
Creamed Spinach	¾ cup (6.4 oz)	280
Fruit Salad Low Fat	¾ cup (5.5 oz)	70
Green Bean Casserole	¾ cup (6 oz)	170
Ham & Turkey Club w/ Cheese & Sauce	1 (13.3 oz)	890
Ham & Turkey Club w/o Cheese & Sauce	1 (9.3 oz)	430
Ham Sandwich w/ Cheese & Sauce	1 (11.8 oz)	760
Ham Sandwich w/o Cheese & Sauce	1 (9.3 oz)	450
Ham w/ Cinnamon Apples	1 serv (8 oz)	350

FOOD	PORTION	CALS.
Homestyle Mashed Potatoes & Gravy	¾ cup (6.6 oz)	200
Hot Cinnamon Apples	¾ cup (6.4 oz)	250
Macaroni & Cheese	¾ cup (6.7 oz)	280
Mashed Potatoes	⅔ cup (5.6 oz)	180
Meat Loaf & Brown Gravy	1 serv (7 oz)	390
Meat Loaf & Chunky Tomato Sauce	1 serv (8 oz)	370
Meat Loaf Sandwich w/ Cheese	1 (13.8 oz)	860
Meat Loaf Sandwich w/o Cheese	1 (12.3 oz)	690
Mediterranean Pasta Salad	¾ cup (4.5 oz)	170
New Potatoes Low Fat	¾ cup (4.6 oz)	130
Original Chicken Pot Pie	1 serv (14.9 oz)	750
Rice Pilaf	⅔ cup (5.1 oz)	180
Rotisserie Turkey Breast Skinless Low Fat	1 serv (5 oz)	170
Steamed Vegetables Low Fat	⅔ cup (3.7 oz)	35
Stuffing	¾ cup (6.1 oz)	310
Tortellini Salad	¾ cup (5.6 oz)	380
Turkey Sandwich w/ Cheese & Sauce	1 (11.8 oz)	710
Turkey Sandwich w/o Cheese & Sauce	1 (9.3 oz)	400
Whole Kernel Corn Low Fat	¾ cup (5.8 oz)	180
Zucchini Marinara	¾ cup (6.6 oz)	80
SOUPS		
Chicken Low Fat	¾ cup (6.8 oz)	80
Chicken Tortilla	1 cup (8.4 oz)	220

BROWN'S CHICKEN

Breadsticks w/ Garlic Butter	1	199
Breast	3.5 oz	284
Coleslaw	3.5 oz	131
Corn Fritters	3.5 oz	415
Corn On Cob	1 ear (3 inch)	126
Fettucini Alfredo	1 serv (12 oz)	1507
French Fries	3.5 oz	503
Gizzard	3.5 oz	387
Leg	3.5 oz	287
Liver	3.5 oz	341
Mostaccioli w/ Meat	1 serv (12 oz)	835
Mostaccioli w/o Meat	1 serv (12 oz)	792
Mushrooms	3.5 oz	289
Potato Salad	3.5 oz	94
Ravioli w/ Meat	1 serv (12 oz)	865
Ravioli w/o Meat	1 serv (12 oz)	822
Shrimp	3.5 oz	277
Thigh	3.5 oz	355
Wing	3.5 oz	385

FOOD	PORTION	CALS.
BRUEGGER'S BAGELS		
Blueberry	1 (3.5 oz)	300
Cinnamon Raisin	1 (3.5 oz)	290
Egg	1 (3.5 oz)	280
Everything	1 (3.6 oz)	290
Garlic	1 (3.6 oz)	280
Honey Grain	1 (3.6 oz)	300
Onion	1 (3.6 oz)	280
Orange Cranberry	1 (3.5 oz)	290
Pesto	1 (3.5 oz)	280
Plain	1 (3.5 oz)	280
Poppy Seed	1 (3.6 oz)	280
Pumpernickel	1 (3.5 oz)	280
Salt	1 (3.6 oz)	270
Sesame	1 (3.6 oz)	290
Spinach	1 (3.5 oz)	280
Sun Dried Tomato	1 (3.5 oz)	280
Wheat Bran	1 (3.5 oz)	280
BURGER KING		
BEVERAGES		
Cocoa Cola Classic	1 med (22 fl oz)	260
Coffee	1 serv (12 oz)	5
Diet Coke	1 med (22 fl oz)	1
Milk 2%	1 (8 oz)	130
Shake Chocolate	1 med (10 oz)	320
Shake Chocolate Syrup Added	1 med (12 oz)	440
Shake Strawberry Syrup Added	1 med (12 oz)	420
Shake Vanilla	1 med (10 oz)	300
Sprite	1 med (22 fl oz)	260
Tropicana Orange Juice	1 serv (11 oz)	140
BREAKFAST SELECTIONS		
AM Express Grape Jam	1 serv (0.4 oz)	30
AM Express Strawberry Jam	1 serv (0.4 oz)	30
AM Express Dip	1 serv (1 oz)	80
Biscuit	1 (3.3 oz)	330
Biscuit w/ Bacon Egg & Cheese	1 (6 oz)	510
Biscuit w/ Egg	1 (5.3 oz)	420
Biscuit w/ Sausage	1 (4.8 oz)	530
Cini-minis	4	550
Croissan'wich Sausage Egg & Cheese	1 (5.7 oz)	550
Croissan'wich w/ Sausage & Cheese	1 (3.7 oz)	450
French Toast Sticks	1 serv (4.9 oz)	500
Hash Browns	1 sm (2.6 oz)	240
Land O'Lakes Whipped Classic Blend	1 serv (0.4 oz)	65

FOOD	PORTION	CALS.
MAIN MENU SELECTIONS		
American Cheese	2 slices (0.9 oz)	90
BK Big Fish Sandwich	1 (8.8 oz)	720
BK Broiler Chicken Sandwich	1 (8.7 oz)	530
Bacon Bits	1 serv (3 g)	15
Big King Sandwich	1 (7.9 oz)	660
Broiled Chicken Salad w/o Dressing	1 serv (10.6 oz)	190
Bull's Eye Barbecue Sauce	1 serv (0.5 oz)	20
Cheeseburger	1 (5 oz)	380
Chicken Sandwich	1 (8 oz)	710
Chicken Tenders	8 pieces (4.3 oz)	350
Coated French Fries Salted	1 med (4.1 oz)	400
Croutons	1 serv (0.2 oz)	30
Dipping Sauce Barbecue	1 serv (1 oz)	35
Dipping Sauce Honey	1 serv (1 oz)	90
Dipping Sauce Ranch	1 serv (1 oz)	170
Dipping Sauce Sweet & Sour	1 serv (1 oz)	45
Double Cheeseburger	1 (7.5 oz)	600
Double Cheeseburger w/ Bacon	1 (7.6 oz)	640
Double Whopper	1 (12.3 oz)	870
Double Whopper w/ Cheese	1 (13.2 oz)	960
Dutch Apple Pie	1 serv (4 oz)	300
French Fries Salted	1 med (4.1 oz)	370
Garden Salad w/o Dressing	1 (7.5 oz)	100
Hamburger	1 (4.5 oz)	330
Ketchup	1 serv (0.5 oz)	15
King Sauce	1 serv (0.5 oz)	70
Lettuce	1 leaf (0.7 oz)	0
Mayonnaise	1 serv (1 oz)	210
Mustard	1 serv (3 g)	0
Onion	1 serv (0.5 oz)	5
Onion Rings	1 serv (4.4 oz)	310
Pickles	4 slices (0.5 oz)	0
Side Salad w/o Dressing	1 (4.7 oz)	60
Tartar Sauce	1 serv (1 oz)	180
Tomato	2 slices (1 oz)	5
Whopper	1 (9.5 oz)	640
Whopper Jr.	1 (5.9 oz)	420
Whopper Jr. w/ Cheese	1 (6.3 oz)	460
Whopper w/ Cheese	1 (10.3 oz)	730
SALAD DRESSINGS		
Bleu Cheese	1 serv (1 oz)	160
French	1 serv (1 oz)	140
Ranch	1 serv (1 oz)	180

FOOD	PORTION	CALS.
Reduced Calorie Light Italian	1 serv (1 oz)	15
Thousand Island	1 serv (1 oz)	140

CAPTAIN D'S
DESSERTS

Carrot Cake	1 piece (4 oz)	434
Cheesecake	1 piece (4 oz)	420
Chocolate Cake	1 piece (4 oz)	303
Lemon Pie	1 piece (4 oz)	351
Pecan Pie	1 piece (4 oz)	458

MAIN MENU SELECTIONS

Baked Potato	1	278
Breadstick	1	113
Broiled Chicken Lunch	1 serv	503
Broiled Chicken Platter	1 serv	802
Broiled Chicken Sandwich	1 (8.2 oz)	451
Broiled Fish & Chicken Platter	1 serv	777
Broiled Fish & Chicken Lunch	1 serv	478
Broiled Fish Lunch	1 serv	435
Broiled Fish Platter	1 serv	734
Broiled Shrimp Lunch	1 serv	421
Broiled Shrimp Platter	1 serv	720
Cheese	1 slice (1 oz)	54
Cob Corn	1 serv (9.5 oz)	251
Cocktail Sauce	1 lg serv (1 fl oz)	34
Cocktail Sauce	1 serv (1 fl oz)	137
Cole Slaw	1 pt (16 oz)	633
Cole Slaw	1 serv (4 oz)	158
Crackers	4 (0.5 oz)	50
Cracklins	1 serv (1 oz)	218
Dinner Salad w/o Dressing	1 (2.5 oz)	27
French Fried Potatoes	1 serv (3.5 oz)	302
Fried Okra	1 serv (4 oz)	300
Green Beans Seasoned	1 serv (4 oz)	46
Hushpuppies	6 (6.7 oz)	756
Hushpuppy	1 (1.1 oz)	126
Imitation Sour Cream	1 serv	29
Margarine	1 serv	102
Non-Dairy Creamer	1 serv	14
Rice	1 serv (4 oz)	124
Stuffed Crab	1 serv	91
Sugar	1 pkg	18
Sweet & Sour Sauce	1 serv (1.8 fl oz)	52
Sweet & Sour Sauce	1 lg serv (4 fl oz)	206

FOOD	PORTION	CALS.
Tartar Sauce	1 lg serv (4 fl oz)	298
Tartar Sauce	1 serv (1 fl oz)	75
Vegetable Medley	1 serv	36
White Beans	1 serv (4 oz)	126
SALAD DRESSINGS		
Blue Cheese	1 pkg (1 fl oz)	105
French	1 pkg (1 fl oz)	111
Light Italian	1 serv	16
Ranch	1 pkg (1 fl oz)	92

CARL'S JR.
BAKED SELECTIONS

FOOD	PORTION	CALS.
Cheese Danish	1 (4.1 oz)	400
Cheesecake Strawberry Swirl	1 serv (3.5 oz)	300
Chocolate Cake	1 serv (3 oz)	300
Chocolate Chip Cookie	1 (2.5 oz)	370
Cinnamon Roll	1 (4.2 oz)	420
Muffin Blueberry	1 (4.2 oz)	340
Muffin Bran	1 (4.7 oz)	370
BEVERAGES		
Coco-Cola Classic	1 reg (16 fl oz)	190
Coffee	1 reg (12 oz)	10
Diet 7UP	1 reg (16 oz)	0
Diet Coke	1 reg (16 oz)	0
Dr. Pepper	1 reg (16 oz)	200
Hot Chocolate	1 reg (12 oz)	110
Iced Tea	1 reg (14 fl oz)	5
Milk 1%	1 (10 fl oz)	150
Minute Maid Orange Soda	1 reg (16 oz)	230
Orange Juice	1 (6 fl oz)	90
Ramblin' Root Beer	1 reg (16 oz)	230
Shake Chocolate	1 sm (13.5 oz)	390
Shake Strawberry	1 sm (13.5 oz)	400
Shake Vanilla	1 sm (13.5 fl oz)	330
Sprite	1 reg (16 fl oz)	190
BREAKFAST SELECTIONS		
Bacon	2 strips (0.3 oz)	40
Breakfast Burrito	1 (5.3 oz)	430
Breakfast Quesadilla Cheese	1 (5.2 oz)	300
English Muffin w/ Margarine	1 (2.6 oz)	230
French Toast Dips w/o Syrup	1 serv (3.7 oz)	410
Grape Jelly	1 serv (0.5 oz)	35
Hash Brown Nuggets	1 serv (3.3 oz)	270
Sausage	1 patty (1.8 oz)	200

FOOD	PORTION	CALS.
Scrambed Eggs	1 serv (3.5 oz)	160
Strawberry Jam	1 serv (0.5 oz)	35
Sunrise Sandwich	1 (4.6 oz)	370
Table Syrup	1 serv (1 oz)	90
MAIN MENU SELECTIONS		
American Cheese	1 slice (0.5 oz)	60
BBQ Chicken Sandwich	1 (6.7 oz)	310
BBQ Sauce	1 serv (1.1 oz)	50
Big Burger	1 (6.8 oz)	470
Breadstick	1 (0.3 oz)	35
Carl's Catch Fish Sandwich	1 (7.5 oz)	560
Chicken Club Sandwich	1 (8.8 oz)	550
Chicken Stars	6 pieces (3 oz)	230
CrissCut Fries	1 lg (5.7 oz)	550
Croutons	1 serv (7 g)	35
Double Western Bacon Cheeseburger	1 (11.5 oz)	970
Famous Big Star Hamburger	1 (8.6 oz)	610
French Fries	1 reg (4.4 oz)	370
Great Stuff Potato Bacon & Cheese	1 (14.2 oz)	630
Great Stuff Potato Broccoli & Cheese	1 (14.2 oz)	530
Great Stuff Potato Plain	1 (9.4 oz)	290
Great Stuff Potato Sour Cream & Chive	1 (10.9 oz)	430
Hamburger	1 (3.1 oz)	200
Honey Sauce	1 serv (1 oz)	90
Hot & Crispy Sandwich	1 (5 oz)	400
Mustard Sauce	1 serv (1 oz)	45
Onion Rings	1 serv (5.3 oz)	520
Salsa	1 serv (0.9 oz)	10
Sante Fe Chicken Sandwich	1 (7.9 oz)	530
Super Star Hamburger	1 (11.2 oz)	820
Sweet N'Sour Sauce	1 serv (1 oz)	50
Swiss Cheese	1 slice (0.5 oz)	45
Western Bacon Cheeseburger	1 (8.1 oz)	870
Zucchini	1 serv (5.9 oz)	380
SALAD DRESSINGS		
1000 Island	2 fl oz	250
Blue Cheese	2 fl oz	310
French Fat Free	2 fl oz	70
House	2 fl oz	220
Italian Fat Free	2 fl oz	15
SALADS AND SALAD BARS		
Salad-To-Go Charbroiled Chicken	1 serv (12 oz)	260
Salad-To-Go Garden	1 (4.8 oz)	50

FOOD	PORTION	CALS.

CARVEL
FROZEN YOGURT
Vanilla Low Fat No Sugar Added	4 fl oz	110

ICE CREAM
Brown Bonnet Cone	1 (4.7 oz)	380
Brown Bonnet Cone No Fat Vanilla	1 (4.7 oz)	300
Cake	1 pkg (7 oz)	450
Cake	1 pkg (4 oz)	270
Cake Cheesecake	1 serv (4 oz)	280
Cake Chocolate Vanilla Chocolate Crunchies	1/15 cake (3.4 oz)	230
Cake Cookies & Cream	1 serv (4 oz)	270
Cake Fudge Drizzle	1/8 cake (4 oz)	310
Cake Fudgie The Whale	1/14 cake (3.6 oz)	290
Cake Holiday	1/15 cake (3.4 oz)	240
Cake S'mores	1 serv (4 oz)	270
Cake Sinfully Chocolate	1 serv (4 oz)	280
Cake Strawberries & Cream	1/8 cake (3.8 oz)	240
Chocolate	4 fl oz	190
Chocolate No Fat	4 fl oz	120
Flying Saucer Chocolate	1 (4 oz)	230
Flying Saucer Chocolate w/ Sprinkles	1 (4 oz)	330
Flying Saucer Low Fat Chocolate	1 (4 oz)	190
Flying Saucer Low Fat Vanilla	1 (4 oz)	180
Flying Saucer Vanilla	1 (4 oz)	240
Flying Saucer Vanilla w/ Sprinkles	1 (4 oz)	340
Nature's Crunch	1 (4.2 g)	450
Olde Fashion Sundae Butterscotch	1 (8 oz)	500
Olde Fashion Sundae Chocolate	1 (8 oz)	470
Olde Fashion Sundae Strawberry	1 (8 oz)	420
Sheet Cake Chocolate Vanilla Chocolate Crunchies	1/26 cake (3.3 oz)	230
Sinful Love Bar	1 (4.2 oz)	460
Thick Shake Chocolate	1 (16 oz)	719
Thick Shake Low Fat Chocolate	1 (16 oz)	490
Thick Shake Low Fat Strawberry	1 (16 oz)	460
Thick Shake Low Fat Vanilla	1 (16 oz)	460
Thick Shake No Fat Chocolate	1 (16 oz)	524
Thick Shake No Fat Strawberry	1 (16 oz)	453
Thick Shake No Fat Vanilla	1 (16 oz)	462
Thick Shake Strawberry	1 (16 oz)	648
Thick Shake Vanilla	1 (16 oz)	657
Vanilla	4 fl oz	200
Vanilla No Fat	4 fl oz	120

FOOD	PORTION	CALS.
SHERBET		
Black Raspberry	½ cup (3.4 oz)	150
Blueberry	½ cup (3.4 oz)	150
Lemon	½ cup (3.5 oz)	150
Lime	½ cup (3.5 oz)	150
Mango	½ cup (3.5 oz)	140
Orange	½ cup (3.5 oz)	150
Peach	½ cup (3.4 oz)	150
Pineapple	½ cup (3.5 oz)	150
Strawberry	½ cup (3.5 oz)	150
CHICK-FIL-A		
BEVERAGES		
Coca-Cola Classic	1 serv (9 oz)	110
Diet Coke	1 serv (9 oz)	0
Diet Lemonade	1 serv (9 oz)	5
Ice Tea Sweetened	1 serv (9 oz)	150
Iced Tea Unsweetened	1 serv (9 fl oz)	0
Lemonade	1 serv (9 oz)	90
DESSERTS		
Cheesecake	1 slice (3.1 oz)	270
Cheesecake w/ Blueberry Topping	1 slice (4.1 oz)	290
Cheesecake w/ Strawberry Topping	1 slice (4.1 oz)	290
Fudge Nut Brownie	1 (2.6 oz)	350
Icedream Cone	1 sm (4.5 oz)	140
Icedream Cup	1 sm (7.5 oz)	350
Lemon Pie	1 slice (4 oz)	320
MAIN MENU SELECTIONS		
Carrot & Raisin Salad	1 sm (2.7 oz)	150
Chargrilled Chicken Club Sandwich w/o Dressing	1 (8.2 oz)	390
Chargrilled Chicken Deluxe Sandwich	1 (7.4 oz)	290
Chargrilled Chicken Garden Salad	1 serv (14 oz)	170
Chargrilled Chicken Sandwich	1 (5.3 oz)	280
Chargrilled Chicken w/o Bun Or Pickles	1 piece (2.8 oz)	130
Chick-n-Strips	4 (4.2 oz)	230
Chick-n-Strips Salad	1 serv (15.9 oz)	290
Chicken Sandwich	1 (5.9 oz)	290
Chicken Deluxe Sandich	1 (8 oz)	300
Chicken Salad Plate	1 serv (16.5 oz)	290
Chicken Salad Sandwich On Whole Wheat	1 (5.9 oz)	320
Chicken w/o Bun Or Pickles	1 piece (3.7 oz)	160
Cole Slaw	1 sm (2.8 oz)	130
Hearty Breast of Chicken Soup	1 cup (7.6 oz)	110

FOOD	PORTION	CALS.
Nuggets	8 (3.9 oz)	290
Tossed Salad	1 serv (4.6 oz)	70
Waffle Potato Fries	1 sm (3 oz)	290
Waffle Potato Fries w/o Salt	1 sm (3 oz)	290

CHILI'S
DESSERTS

Diet By Chocolate Cake	1 serv	370
Diet By Chocolate Cake w/ Yogurt	1 serv	465
Diet By Chocolate Cake w/ Yogurt & Fudge Topping	1 serv	534

MAIN MENU SELECTIONS

Guiltless Grill Chicken Fijitas	1 serv	726
Guiltless Grill Chicken Platter	1 serv	563
Guiltless Grill Chicken Salad w/ Dressing	1 serv	254
Guiltless Grill Chicken Sandwich	1	527
Guiltless Grill Veggie Pasta	1 serv	590
Guiltless Grill Veggie Pasta w/ Chicken	1 serv	696

CHURCH'S CHICKEN

Apple Pie	1 serv (3.1 oz)	280
Biscuit	1 (2.1 oz)	250
Breast	1 serv (2.8 oz)	200
Cajun Rice	1 serv (3.1 oz)	130
Cole Slaw	1 serv (3 oz)	92
Corn On The Cob	1 serv (5.7 oz)	139
French Fries	1 serv (2.7 oz)	210
Leg	1 serv (2 oz)	140
Okra	1 serv (2.8 oz)	210
Potatoes & Gravy	1 serv (3.7 oz)	90
Tender Strip	1 (1.1 oz)	80
Thigh	1 serv (2.8 oz)	230
Wing	1 serv (3.1 oz)	250

COLOMBO FROZEN YOGURT

Alpine Strawberry Nonfat	4 fl oz	100
Banana Strawberry Nonfat	4 fl oz	50
Brazlian Banana Nonfat	4 fl oz	100
Butter Pecan Nonfat	4 fl oz	100
Cappuccino Nonfat	4 fl oz	100
Cherry Amaretto Nonfat	4 fl oz	50
Cherry Vanilla Nonfat	4 fl oz	100
Chocolate Nonfat	4 fl oz	50

FOOD	PORTION	CALS.
Coconut Cooler Nonfat	4 fl oz	100
Cool Berry Blue Nonfat	4 fl oz	100
Country Pumpkin Nonfat	4 fl oz	100
Double Dutch Chocolate Nonfat	4 fl oz	100
Egg Nog Nonfat	4 fl oz	100
French Vanilla Lowfat	4 fl oz	110
French Vanilla Nonfat	4 fl oz	100
Georgia Peach Nonfat	4 fl oz	100
German Fudge Chocolate Nonfat	4 fl oz	100
Hawaiian Pineapple Nonfat	4 fl oz	100
Hazelnut Amaretto Nonfat	4 fl oz	100
Honey Almond Nonfat	4 fl oz	100
Irish Cream Nonfat	4 fl oz	100
New York Cheesecake Nonfat	4 fl oz	100
Old World Chocolate Lowfat	4 fl oz	110
Orange Bavarian Creme Nonfat	4 fl oz	100
Peanut Butter Lowfat	4 fl oz	110
Pecan Praline Nonfat	4 fl oz	100
Pina Colada Nonfat	4 fl oz	100
Raspberry Nonfat	4 fl oz	50
Rockin' Raspberry Nonfat	4 fl oz	100
Simply Vanilla Lowfat	4 fl oz	110
Simply Vanilla Nonfat	4 fl oz	100
Strawberry Nonfat	4 fl oz	50
Tropical Tango Nonfat	4 fl oz	100
Vanilla Nonfat	4 fl oz	50
White Chocolate Almond Nonfat	4 fl oz	100
Wild Strawberry Lowfat	4 fl oz	110

DAIRY QUEEN
FOOD SELECTIONS

FOOD	PORTION	CALS.
Chicken Breast Fillet Sandwich	1 (6.7 oz)	430
Chicken Strip Basket	1 serv (14.5 oz)	1000
Chili 'n' Cheese Dog	1 (5 oz)	330
DQ Homestyle Bacon Double Cheeseburger	1 (8.9 oz)	610
DQ Homestyle Cheeseburger	1 (5.3 oz)	340
DQ Homestyle Double Cheeseburger	1 (7.7 oz)	540
DQ Homestyle Hamburger	1 (4.8 oz)	290
DQ Ultimate Burger	1 (9.4 oz)	670
French Fries	1 med (3.9 oz)	350
French Fries	1 lg (4.9 oz)	440
Grilled Chicken Sandwich	1 (6.5 oz)	310
Hot Dog	1 (3.5 oz)	240

FOOD	PORTION	CALS.
Onion Rings	1 serv (4 oz)	320
ICE CREAM		
Banana Split	1 (12.9 oz)	510
Blizzard Chocolate Sandwich Cookie	1 med (11.4 oz)	640
Blizzard Chocolate Sandwich Cookie	1 sm (12 oz)	520
Blizzard Chocolate Chip Cookie Dough	1 med (15.4 oz)	950
Blizzard Chocolate Chip Cookie Dough	1 sm (12 oz)	660
Breeze Heath	1 med (14.2 oz)	710
Breeze Heath	1 sm (10.2 oz)	470
Breeze Strawberry	1 sm (12 oz)	320
Breeze Strawberry	1 med (13.4 oz)	460
Buster Bar	1 (5.2 oz)	450
Chocolate Malt	1 med (19.9 oz)	880
Chocolate Malt	1 sm (14.7 oz)	650
Cone Chocolate	1 med (6.9 oz)	340
Cone Chocolate	1 sm (5 oz)	240
Cone Vanilla	1 sm (5 oz)	230
Cone Vanilla	1 med (6.9 oz)	330
Cone Vanilla	1 lg (8.9 oz)	410
Cone Yogurt	1 med (6.9 oz)	260
Cone Dipped	1 med (7.7 oz)	490
Cone Dipped	1 sm (5.5 oz)	340
Cup Of Yogurt	1 med (6.7 oz)	230
DQ 8 Inch Round Cake Undecorated	⅛ of cake (6.2 oz)	340
DQ Fudge Bar No Sugar Added	1 (2.3 oz)	50
DQ Lemon Freez'r	½ cup (3.2 oz)	80
DQ Nonfat Frozen Yogurt	½ cup (3 oz)	100
DQ Sandwich	1 (2.1 oz)	150
DQ Soft Serve Chocolate	½ cup (3.3 oz)	150
DQ Soft Serve Vanilla	½ cup (3.3 oz)	140
DQ Treatzza Pizza Heath	⅛ of pie (2.3 oz)	180
DQ Treatzza Pizza M&M	⅛ of pie (2.4 oz)	190
DQ Vanilla Orange Bar No Sugar Added	1 (2.3 oz)	60
Dilly Bar Chocolate	1 (3 oz)	210
Fudge Cake Supreme	1 serv (11.2 oz)	890
Misty Slush	1 med (20.9 oz)	290
Misty Slush	1 sm (15.9 oz)	220
Peanut Buster Parfait	1 (10.7 oz)	730
Shake Chocolate	1 med (18.9 oz)	770
Shake Chocolate	1 sm (13.9 oz)	560
Starkiss	1 (3 oz)	80
Strawberry Shortcake	1 (8.5 oz)	430
Sundae Chocolate	1 med (8.2 oz)	400,
Sundae Chocolate	1 sm (5.7 oz)	280
Yogurt Sundae Strawberry	1 med (8.2 oz)	280

FOOD	PORTION	CALS.

D'ANGELO SANDWICH SHOPS
SALADS AND SALAD BARS

FOOD	PORTION	CALS.
Antipasto Salad w/o Dressing	1	420
Caesar Salad w/ Dressing	1	740
Caesar Salad w/o Dressing	1	490
Chicken Caesar Salad w/ Dressing	1	860
Chicken Caesar Salad w/o Dressing	1	600
Chicken Salad w/o Dressing	1	390
Chicken Salad D'Lite	1	325
D'Lite Turkey	1 serv	355
Greek Salad w/ Dressing	1	940
Greek Salad w/ Tuna & Dressing	1	1010
Greek Salad w/ Tuna w/o Dressing	1	490
Greek Salad w/o Dressing	1	420
Roast Beef Salad w/o Dressing	1	400
Roast Beef Salad D'Lite	1	350
Tossed Garden Salad w/o Dressing	1	270
Tuna Salad w/o Dressing	1	330
Tuna Salad D'Lite	1	305
Turkey Salad w/o Dressing	1	400

SANDWICHES

FOOD	PORTION	CALS.
BLT w/ Cheese	1	1170
BLT w/ Cheese Medium Sub	1	870
BLT w/ Cheese Pokket	1	570
BLT w/ Cheese Small Sub	1	600
Barbecue Curls	1	480
Buffalo Chicken Wrap w/ Blue Cheese Dressing	1	621
Buffalo Chicken Wrap w/o Dressing	1	417
Caesar Salad w/ Dressing Pokket	1	590
Caesar Salad w/o Dressing Pokket	1	460
Caesar Salad w/ Chicken w/ Dressing Pokket	1	700
Caesar Salad w/ Chicken w/ Dressing Pokket	1	570
Caesar Wrap w/ Dressing	1	484
Caesar Wrap w/ Fat Free Dressing	1	484
Capicola Ham & Cheese Large Sub	1	740
Capicola Ham & Cheese Medium Sub	1	550
Capicola Ham & Cheese Pokket	1	350
Capicola Ham & Cheese Small Sub	1	390
Cheeseburger Large Sub	1	1060
Cheeseburger Medium Sub	1	780
Cheeseburger Pokket	1	490
Cheeseburger Small Sub	1	530

FOOD	PORTION	CALS.
Chicken Salad Large Sub	1	1370
Chicken Salad Medium Sub	1	970
Chicken Salad Pokket	1	650
Chicken Salad Small Sub	1	690
Chicken Stir Fry D'Lite Pokket	1	360
Chicken Stir Fry D'Lite Sub	1	280
Chicken Stir Fry Large Sub	1	800
Chicken Stir Fry Medium Sub	1	560
Chicken Stir Fry Pokket	1	360
Chicken Stir Fry Small Sub	1	380
Classic Vegetable D'Lite Pokket	1	340
Classic Vegetable Large Sub	1	860
Classic Vegetable Medium Sub	1	610
Classic Vegetable Pokket	1	400
Classic Vegetable Small Sub	1	430
Crunchy Vegetable D'Lite Pokket	1	350
Crunchy Vegetable D'Lite Small Sub	1	385
Crunchy Vegetable Large Sub	1	880
Crunchy Vegetable Pokket	1	410
Crunchy Vegetables Medium Sub	1	620
Crunchy Vegetables Small Sub	1	440
Ginger Chicken Stir Fry D'Lite Pokket	1	400
Greek Pokket	1	910
Grilled Spicy Steak D'Lite Pokket	1	425
Grilled Steak Cheese Large Sub	1	1160
Grilled Steak Cheese Medium Sub	1	820
Grilled Steak Cheese Pokket	1	550
Grilled Steak Cheese Small Sub	1	580
Grilled Steak Combo Large Sub	1	1170
Grilled Steak Combo Medium Sub	1	830
Grilled Steak Combo Pokket	1	550
Grilled Steak Combo Small Sub	1	590
Grilled Steak D'Lite Pokket	1	390
Grilled Steak Large Sub	1	990
Grilled Steak Medium Sub	1	680
Grilled Steak Mushrooms Large Sub	1	1000
Grilled Steak Mushrooms Medium Sub	1	690
Grilled Steak Mushrooms Pokket	1	450
Grilled Steak Mushrooms Small Sub	1	480
Grilled Steak Onion Large Sub	1	1000
Grilled Steak Onion Medium Sub	1	700
Grilled Steak Onion Small Sub	1	480
Grilled Steak Onions Pokket	1	450

FOOD	PORTION	CALS.
Grilled Steak Peppers	1	690
Grilled Steak Peppers Large Sub	1	1000
Grilled Steak Peppers Pokket	1	540
Grilled Steak Pokket	1	440
Grilled Steak Small Sub	1	470
Ham & Cheese Large Sub	1	760
Ham & Cheese Medium Sub	1	550
Ham & Cheese Pokket	1	370
Ham & Cheese Small Sub	1	400
Ham Salami & Cheese Large Sub	1	870
Ham Salami & Cheese Medium Sub	1	630
Ham Salami & Cheese Pokket	1	420
Ham Salami & Cheese Smalle Sub	1	450
Hamburger Large Sub	1	920
Hamburger Medium Sub	1	680
Hamburger Pokket	1	430
Hamburger Small Sub	1	460
Italian Cold Cut Large Sub	1	1130
Italian Cold Cut Medium Sub	1	820
Italian Cold Cut Pokket	1	550
Italian Cold Cut Small Sub	1	580
Meatball Large Sub	1	1010
Meatball Medium Sub	1	750
Meatball Pokket	1	480
Meatball Small Sub	1	520
Meatball w/ Cheese Large Sub	1	1170
Meatball w/ Cheese Medium Sub	1	880
Meatball w/ Cheese Pokket	1	580
Meatball w/ Cheese Small Sub	1	620
Pastrami Large Sub	1	1250
Pastrami Medium Sub	1	860
Pastrami Pokket	1	550
Pastrami Small Sub	1	580
Pastrami w/ Cheese Large Sub	1	1640
Pastrami w/ Cheese Medium Sub	1	1170
Pastrami w/ Cheese Pokket	1	780
Pastrami w/ Cheese Small Sub	1	820
Roast Beef D'Lite Pokket	1	330
Roast Beef D'Lite Small Sub	1	365
Roast Beef Large Sub	1	710
Roast Beef Medium Sub	1	520
Seafood Salad Large Sub	1	1210

FOOD	PORTION	CALS.
Seafood Salad Medium Sub	1	860
Seafood Salad Pokket	1	570
Seafood Salad Small Sub	1	610
Stuffed Turkey D'Lite Pokket	1	510
Stuffed Turkey D'Lite Small Sub	1	545
Stuffed Turkey Large Sub	1	1070
Stuffed Turkey Medium Sub	1	790
Tuna Salad Large Sub	1	1510
Tuna Salad Medium Sub	1	1070
Tuna Salad Pokket	1	720
Tuna Salad Small Sub	1	760
Turkey D'Lite Pokket	1	330
Turkey D'Lite Small Sub	1	365
Turkey Large Sub	1	710
Turkey Medium Sub	1	520
Turkey Club Large Sub	1	860
Turkey Club Medium Sub	1	630
Turkey Club Pokket	1	400
Turkey Club Small Sub	1	430

DELTACO
BEVERAGES

FOOD	PORTION	CALS.
Coffee	1 serv	6
Coke Classic	1 lg	287
Coke Classic	1 med	198
Coke Classic	1 sm	144
Coke Classic Best Value	1 serv	395
Diet Coke	1 lg	2
Diet Coke	1 sm	1
Diet Coke	1 med	1
Diet Coke Best Value	1 serv	2
Iced Tea	1 sm	3
Iced Tea	1 med	4
Iced Tea	1 lg	6
Iced Tea Best Value	1 serv	8
M&M's Toppers	1 serv	256
Milk	1 serv	126
Mr Pibb	1 sm	142
Mr Pibb	1 med	195
Mr Pibb	1 lg	283
Mr Pibb Best Value	1 serv	390
Orange Juice	1 serv	83
Oreos Toppers	1 serv	257
Shake Chocolate	1 sm	549

FOOD	PORTION	CALS.
Shake Chocolate	1 med	755
Shake Orange	1 sm	609
Shake Orange	1 med	837
Shake Strawberry	1 sm	486
Shake Strawberry	1 med	668
Shake Vanilla	1 med	707
Shake Vanilla	1 sm	514
Snickers Toppers	1 serv	254
Sprite	1 sm	144
Sprite	1 lg	287
Sprite	1 med	198
Sprite Best Value	1 serv	395
BREAKFAST SELECTIONS		
Burrito Beef And Egg	1	529
Burrito Breakfast	1	256
Burrito Egg And Cheese	1	443
Burrito Egg and Bean	1	470
Burrito Steak And Egg	1	500
CHILDREN'S MENU SELECTIONS		
Kid's Meal Hamburger	1 meal	617
Kid's Meal Taco	1 meal	532
MAIN MENU SELECTIONS		
American Cheese	1 slice	53
Beans And Cheese	1	122
Burrito Chicken	1	264
Burrito Combination	1	413
Burrito Del Beef	1	440
Burrito Deluxe Chicken	1	549
Burrito Deluxe Combo	1	453
Burrito Deluxe Del Beef	1	479
Burrito Green	1	229
Burrito Green Regular	1	330
Burrito Macho Beef	1	893
Burrito Macho Combo	1	774
Burrito Red	1	235
Burrito Red Regular	1	342
Burrito Spicy Chicken	1	392
Burrito The Works	1	448
Cheeseburger	1	284
Chicken Salad	1	254
Chicken Salad Deluxe	1	716
Del Burger	1	385
Del Cheeseburger	1	439
Double Del Cheeseburger	1	618
French Fries	1 sm	242

FOOD	PORTION	CALS.
French Fries	1 reg	404
French Fries	1 lg	566
Fries Chili Cheese	1 serv	562
Fries Deluxe Chili Cheese	1 serv	600
Fries Nacho	1 serv	669
Guacamole	1 oz	60
Hamburger	1	231
Hot Sauce	1 pkg	2
Nacho Cheese Sauce	1 side order	100
Nachos	1 serv	390
Nachos Macho	1	1089
Quesadilla	1	257
Quesadilla Chicken	1	544
Quesadilla Regular	1	483
Quesadilla Spicy Jack	1	254
Quesadilla Spicy Jack Chicken	1	537
Quesadilla Spicy Jack Regular	1	476
Salsa	2 oz	14
Salsa Dressing	1 oz	33
Soft Taco	1	146
Soft Taco Chicken	1	197
Soft Taco Deluxe Double Beef	1	211
Soft Taco Double Beef	1	178
Sour Cream	1 oz	60
Taco	1	140
Taco Chicken	1	186
Taco Deluxe Double Beef	1	205
Taco Double Beef	1	172
Taco Salad	1	235
Taco Salad Deluxe	1	741
Tostada	1	140

DENNY'S
BEVERAGES

FOOD	PORTION	CALS.
2% Milk	1 serv (10 oz)	151
Chocolate Milk	1 serv (10 oz)	235
Coffee French Vanilla	1 serv (8 oz)	76
Coffee Hazelnut	1 serv (8 oz)	66
Coffee Irish Cream	1 serv (8 oz)	73
Grapefruit Juice	1 serv (10 oz)	115
Hot Chocolate	1 serv (8 oz)	90
Lemonade	1 serv (16 oz)	150
Orange Juice	1 serv (10 oz)	126
Raspberry Ice Tea	1 serv (16 oz)	78
Tomato Juice	1 serv (10 oz)	56

FOOD	PORTION	CALS.
BREAKFAST SELECTIONS		
All American Slam	1 serv (15 oz)	1028
Applesauce	1 serv (3 oz)	60
Bacon	4 strips (1 oz)	162
Bagel Dry	1 (3 oz)	235
Banana	1 (4 oz)	110
Banana Strawberry Medley	1 serv (4 oz)	108
Biscuit Plain	1 (3 oz)	375
Biscuit w/ Sausage Gravy	1 serv (7 oz)	570
Blueberry Topping	1 serv (3 oz)	106
Canadian Bacon	1 serv (3 oz)	110
Cantaloup	1 serv (3 oz)	32
Cheddar Cheese Omelette	1 serv (13 oz)	770
Cherry Topping	1 serv (3 oz)	86
Chicken Fried Steak & Eggs	1 serv (14 oz)	723
Country Scramble	1 serv (16 oz)	795
Cream Cheese	1 oz	100
Egg	1 (2 oz)	134
Egg Beaters	1 serv (2.3 oz)	71
Eggs Benedict	1 serv (19 oz)	860
English Muffin Dry	1 (4 oz)	125
Farmer's Omelette	1 serv (18 oz)	912
French Slam	1 serv (14 oz)	1029
French Toast	2 pieces (8 oz)	510
Fresh Fruit Mix	1 serv (3 oz)	36
Grapefruit	½ (5 oz)	60
Grapes	1 serv (3 oz)	55
Grits	1 serv (4 oz)	80
Ham	1 serv (3 oz)	94
Ham'n'Cheddar Omelette	1 serv (14 oz)	743
Hashed Browns	1 serv (4 oz)	218
Hashed Browns Covered	1 serv (6 oz)	318
Hashed Browns Covered & Smothered	1 serv (8 oz)	359
Honeydew	1 serv (3 oz)	31
Junior Meals Basic Breakfast	1 serv (9 oz)	558
Junior Meals Junior French Slam	1 serv (7 oz)	461
Junior Meals Junior Grand Slam	1 serv (5 oz)	397
Junior Meals Junior Waffle Supreme	1 serv (4 oz)	190
Meat Lover's Sampler	1 serv (14 oz)	806
Moon Over My Hammy	1 serv (12 oz)	807
Muffin Blueberry	1 (3 oz)	309
Oatmeal	1 serv (4 oz)	100
Original Grand Slam	1 serv (10 oz)	795
Pancakes	3 (5 oz)	491

FOOD	PORTION	CALS.
Pork Chop & Eggs	1 serv (12 oz)	555
Porterhouse Steak & Eggs	1 serv (18 oz)	1223
Ready To Eat Cereal	1 serv (1 oz)	100
Sausage	4 links (3 oz)	354
Sausage Cheddar Omelette	1 serv (16 oz)	1036
Scram Slam	1 serv (18 oz)	974
Senior Belgian Waffle Slam	1 serv (6 oz)	399
Senior Omelette	1 serv (12 oz)	623
Senior Starter	1 serv (7 oz)	336
Senior Triple Play	1 serv (8 oz)	537
Sirloin Steak & Eggs	1 serv (13 oz)	808
Slim Slam	1 serv (14 oz)	638
Southern Slam	1 serv (13 oz)	1065
Strawberries w/ Sugar	1 serv (3 oz)	115
Strawberry Topping	1 serv (3 oz)	115
Sunshine Slam	1 serv (8 oz)	537
Super Play It Again Slam	1 serv (15 oz)	1192
Syrup	3 tbsp (1.5 oz)	143
Syrup Reduced Calorie	1 serv (1.5 oz)	25
T-Bone Steak & Eggs	1 serv (16 oz)	1045
Toast Dry	1 slice (1 oz)	92
Ultimate Omelette	1 serv (17 oz)	780
Vegggie Cheese Omelette	1 serv (16 oz)	714
Waffle	1 (6 oz)	304
Whipped Margarine	1 serv (0.5 oz)	87
Whipped Cream	1 serv (2 oz)	23
DESSERTS		
Apple Pie	1 serv (7 oz)	430
Apple Pie w/ Equal	1 serv (7 oz)	370
Banana Split	1 serv (19 oz)	894
Blueberry Topping	1 serv (3 oz)	106
Cheesecake Pie	1 serv (4 oz)	470
Cherry Topping	1 serv (3 oz)	86
Cherry Pie	1 serv (7 oz)	540
Chocolate Topping	1 serv (2 oz)	317
Chocolate Cake	1 serv (4 oz)	370
Chocolate Pecan Pie	1 serv (6 oz)	790
Chocolate Shake	1 serv (10 oz)	579
Coconut Cream Pie	1 serv (7 oz)	480
Double Scoop Sundae	1 serv (6 oz)	375
Dutch Apple Pie	1 serv (7 oz)	440
French Silk Pie	1 serv (6 oz)	650
Fudge Topping	1 serv (2 oz)	201
German Chocolate Pie	1 serv (7 oz)	580

FOOD	PORTION	CALS.
Hot Fudge Cake Sundae	1 serv (8 oz)	687
Ice Cream Float	1 serv (12 oz)	280
Key Lime Pie	1 serv (6 oz)	600
Lemon Meringue Pie	1 serv (7 oz)	460
Pecan Pie	1 serv (6 oz)	600
Single Scoop Sundae	1 serv (3 oz)	188
Strawberry Topping	1 serv (3 oz)	115
Vanilla Shake	1 serv (11 oz)	581
MAIN MENU SELECTIONS		
BBQ Sauce	1 serv (1.5 oz)	47
Bacon Cheddar Burger	1 (14 oz)	935
Bacon Lettuce & Tomato Sandwich	1 (6 oz)	634
Baked Potato Plain	1 (6 oz)	186
Battered Cod Dinner w/ Tartar Sauce	1 serv (9 oz)	732
Broccoli In Butter Sauce	2 serv (4 oz)	50
Brown Gravy	1 serv (1 oz)	13
Buffalo Chicken Strips	1 serv (10 oz)	734
Buffalo Wings	12 pieces (15 oz)	856
Carrots In Honey Glaze	2 serv (4 oz)	80
Charleston Chicken Sandwich	1 (11 oz)	632
Chicken Quesadilla	1 serv (16 oz)	827
Chicken Fried Chicken	1 serv (6 oz)	327
Chicken Fried Steak w/ Gravy	1 serv (4 oz)	265
Chicken Gravy	1 serv (1 oz)	14
Chicken Melt Sandwich	1 (7 oz)	520
Chicken Strip w/ Dressing	1 serv (10 oz)	635
Chicken Strips	5 pieces (10 oz)	720
Classic Burger	1 (11 oz)	673
Classic Burger w/ Cheese	1 (13 oz)	836
Club Sandwich	1	485
Corn In Butter Sauce	2 serv (4 oz)	120
Cornbread Stuffing Plain	1 serv (2 oz)	182
Cottage Cheese	1 serv (3 oz)	72
Country Gravy	1 serv (1 oz)	17
Delidinger Sandwich	1 (14 oz)	852
Deluxe Grilled Cheese Sandwich	1 (7 oz)	482
Dinner Roll	1 (1.5 oz)	132
French Fries Unsalted	1 serv (4 oz)	323
Fried Fish Sandwich	1 (11 oz)	905
Gardenburger Patty	1 patty (3.4 oz)	160
Gardenburger Patty w/ Bun & Fat Free Honey Mustard Dressing	1 serv (11.1 oz)	653
Green Beans w/ Bacon	2 serv (4 oz)	60
Green Peas In Butter Sauce	2 serv (4 oz)	100

FOOD	PORTION	CALS.
Grilled Mushrooms	1 serv (2 oz)	14
Grilled Alaskan Salmon	1 serv (7 oz)	296
Grilled Chicken Breast	1 serv (4 oz)	130
Grilled Chicken Dinner	1 serv (4 oz)	130
Grilled Chicken Sandwich	1 (11 oz)	509
Grilled Chopped Steak w/ Gravy	1 serv (10 oz)	400
Ham & Swiss On Rye	1 (9 oz)	533
Hashed Browns	1 serv (4 oz)	218
Herb Toast	1 serv (2 oz)	200
Horseradish Sauce	1 serv (1.5 oz)	170
Junior Meals Junior Burger	1 serv (3 oz)	261
Junior Meals Junior Chicken Strips	1 serv (5 oz)	318
Junior Meals Junior Fried Fish	1 serv (5 oz)	465
Junior Meals Junior Grilled Cheese	1 serv (4 oz)	375
Junior Meals Junior Shrimp Basket	1 serv (4 oz)	291
Lunch Basket Charleston Chicken Ranch Melt	1 serv (14 oz)	975
Lunch Basket Chicken Strips	1 serv (8 oz)	568
Lunch Basket Classic Burger	1 serv (12 oz)	674
Lunch Basket Delidinger	1 serv (14 oz)	852
Lunch Basket Five Star Philly	1 serv (10 oz)	657
Lunch Basket Patty Melt	1 serv (8 oz)	696
Mashed Potatoes Plain	1 serv (6 oz)	105
Mayonnaise	2 tbsp (1 oz)	200
Mozzarella Sticks w/ Sauce	8 pieces (10 oz)	756
Onion Ring Basket	1 serv (5 oz)	439
Onion Rings	1 serv (3 oz)	264
Patty Melt Sandwich	1 (8 oz)	695
Pork Chop Dinner w/ Gravy	1 serv (8 oz)	386
Porterhouse Steak	1 (14 oz)	708
Pot Roast Dinner w/ Gravy	1 serv (7 oz)	260
Rice Pilaf	1 serv (3 oz)	112
Roast Turkey & Stuffing	1 serv (12 oz)	701
Sampler	1 serv (15 oz)	1120
Seasoned Fries	1 serv (4 oz)	261
Senior Battered Cod	1 serv (5 oz)	465
Senior Chicken Fried Steak	1 serv (8 oz)	341
Senior Grilled Cheese Sandwich	1 serv	360
Senior Grilled Chicken Breast	1 serv (6 oz)	219
Senior Liver w/ Bacon & Onions	1 serv (8 oz)	322
Senior Pork Chop	1 serv (4 oz)	193
Senior Pot Roast	1 serv (5 oz)	149
Senior Roast Turkey & Stuffing	1 serv (8 oz)	596
Senior Turkey Sandwich	1	340

FOOD	PORTION	CALS.
Senior Sandwich Ham & Swiss	1 serv (9 oz)	497
Shrimp Dinner	1 serv (8 oz)	558
Sirloin Steak Dinner	1 serv (5.5 oz)	271
Sliced Tomatoes	3 slices (2 oz)	13
Sour Cream	1 serv (1.5 oz)	91
Steak & Shrimp Dinner w/ Gravy	1 serv (9 oz)	645
Super Bird Sandwich	1 (9 oz)	620
T-Bone Steak Dinner	1 serv (10 oz)	530
Turkey Breast On Multigrain	1 (9 oz)	476
SALAD DRESSINGS		
Bleu Cheese	1 oz	124
Caesar	1 oz	142
Creamy Italian	1 oz	106
Fat Free Honey Mustard	1 oz	38
French	1 oz	106
Oriental Peanut Dressing	1 serv (1 oz)	106
Ranch	1 oz	101
Reduced Calorie French	1 oz	76
Reduced Calorie Italian	1 oz	32
Thousand Island	1 oz	104
SALADS AND SALAD BARS		
Buffalo Chicken Salad	1 serv (17 oz)	615
Fried Chicken Salad	1 serv (13 oz)	506
Garden Chicken Delight Salad	1 serv (16 oz)	277
Grilled Chicken Caesar Salad w/ Dressing	1 serv (13 oz)	655
Oriental Chicken Salad w/ Dressing	1 serv (20 oz)	568
Side Caesar w/ Dressing	1 serv (6 oz)	338
Side Garden Salad w/ Dressing	1 serv (7 oz)	113
SOUPS		
Cheese	1 serv (8 oz)	293
Chicken Noodle	1 serv (8 oz)	60
Clam Chowder	1 serv (8 oz)	214
Cream Of Broccoli	1 serv (8 oz)	193
Cream of Potato	1 serv (8 oz)	222
Split Pea	1 serv (8 oz)	146
Vegetable Beef	1 serv (8 oz)	79

DOMINO'S PIZZA
12 INCH MEDIUM PIZZAS

Add A Topping Anchovies	1 topping serv	23
Add A Topping Bacon	1 topping serv	81
Add A Topping Banana Peppers	1 topping serv	3
Add A Topping Canned Mushrooms	1 topping serv	4
Add A Topping Cheddar Cheese	1 topping serv	57

FOOD	PORTION	CALS.
Add A Topping Cooked Beef	1 topping serv	56
Add A Topping Extra Cheese	1 topping serv	48
Add A Topping Fresh Mushrooms	1 topping serv	4
Add A Topping Green Olives	1 topping serv	12
Add A Topping Green Peppers	1 topping serv	3
Add A Topping Ham	1 topping serv	18
Add A Topping Italian Sausage	1 topping serv	55
Add A Topping Onion	1 topping serv	4
Add A Topping Pepperoni	1 topping serv	62
Add A Topping Pineapple Tidbits	1 topping serv	10
Add A Topping Ripe Olives	1 topping serv	14
Deep Dish Cheese	2 slices (6.3 oz)	477
Hand Tossed Cheese	2 slices (5.2 oz)	347
Thin Crust Cheese	¼ pie (3.7 oz)	271
14 INCH LARGE PIZZAS		
Add A Topping Anchovies	1 topping serv	23
Add A Topping Anchovies	1 topping serv	23
Add A Topping Bacon	1 topping serv	75
Add A Topping Banana Peppers	1 topping serv	3
Add A Topping Canned Mushrooms	1 topping serv	3
Add A Topping Cheddar Cheese	1 topping serv	48
Add A Topping Cheddar Cheese	1 topping serv	48
Add A Topping Cooked Beef	1 topping serv	44
Add A Topping Extra Cheese	1 topping serv	45
Add A Topping Extra Cheese	1 topping serv	45
Add A Topping Fresh Mushrooms	1 topping serv	3
Add A Topping Green Olives	1 topping serv	11
Add A Topping Green Peppers	1 topping serv	2
Add A Topping Ham	1 topping serv	17
Add A Topping Italian Sausage	1 topping serv	44
Add A Topping Onion	1 topping serv	3
Add A Topping Pepperoni	1 topping serv	55
Add A Topping Pineapple Tidbits	1 topping serv	8
Add A Topping Ripe Olives	1 topping serv	12
Deep Dish Cheese	2 slices (6.1 oz)	455
Hand-Tossed Cheese	2 slices (4.8 oz)	317
Thin Crust Cheese	⅙ pie (3.5 oz)	253
6 INCH DEEP DISH PIZZAS		
Add A Topping Anchovies	1 topping serv	45
Add A Topping Bacon	1 topping serv	82
Add A Topping Banana Peppers	1 topping serv	3
Add A Topping Canned Mushrooms	1 topping serv	2
Add A Topping Cheddar Cheese	1 topping serv	86
Add A Topping Cooked Beef	1 topping serv	44

FOOD	PORTION	CALS.
Add A Topping Extra Cheese	1 topping serv	57
Add A Topping Fresh Mushrooms	1 topping serv	2
Add A Topping Green Olives	1 topping serv	10
Add A Topping Green Peppers	1 topping serv	2
Add A Topping Ham	1 topping serv	17
Add A Topping Italian Sausage	1 topping serv	44
Add A Topping Onion	1 topping serv	3
Add A Topping Pepperoni	1 topping serv	50
Add A Topping Pineapple Tidbits	1 topping serv	5
Add A Topping Ripe Olives	1 topping serv	11
Cheese	1 pie (7.6 oz)	595
MAIN MENU SELECTIONS		
Breadstick	1 (0.8 oz)	78
Buffalo Wings Barbeque	1 piece (0.9 oz)	50
Buffalo Wings Hot	1 piece (0.9 oz)	45
Cheesy Bread	1 piece (1 oz)	103
Garden Salad	1 sm (4.3 oz)	22
Garden Salad	1 lg (7.7 oz)	39
SALAD DRESSINGS		
Marzetti Blue Cheese	1 serv (1.5 oz)	220
Marzetti Creamy Caesar	1 serv (1.5 oz)	200
Marzetti Fat Free Ranch	1 serv (1.5 oz)	40
Marzetti Honey French	1 serv (1.5 oz)	210
Marzetti House Italian	1 serv (1.5 oz)	220
Marzetti Light Italian	1 serv (1.5 oz)	20
Marzetti Ranch	1 serv (1.5 oz)	260
Marzetti Thousand Island	1 serv (1.5 oz)	200

DUNKIN' DONUTS
BAGELS AND CREAM CHEESE

FOOD	PORTION	CALS.
Bagel Blueberry	1 (4.4 oz)	330
Bagel Cinnamon Raisin	1 (4.4 oz)	340
Bagel Egg	1 (4.4 oz)	340
Bagel Everything	1 (4.4 oz)	340
Bagel Garlic	1 (4.4 oz)	330
Bagel Onion	1 (4.4 oz)	320
Bagel Plain	1 (4.4 oz)	330
Bagel Plain	1 (3 oz)	200
Bagel Poppy	1 (4.4 oz)	340
Bagel Pumpernickel	1 (4.4 oz)	340
Bagel Salt	1 (4.4 oz)	320
Bagel Sesame	1 (4.4 oz)	350
Bagel Whole Wheat	1 (4.4 oz)	320
Bagel Sticks Cinnamon Sugar	1 (2.9 oz)	210

FOOD	PORTION	CALS.
Bagel Sticks Jalapeno Cheddar	1 (2.9 oz)	210
Bagel Sticks Santa Fe Ranch	1 (2.9 oz)	210
Bagel Sticks Spinach Romano	1 (2.9 oz)	210
Cream Cheese Classic Lite	2 tbsp (1 oz)	60
Cream Cheese Classic Plain	2 tbsp (1 oz)	100
Cream Cheese Garden Veggie	2 tbsp (1 oz)	90
Cream Cheese Honey Walnut	2 tbsp (1 oz)	100
Cream Cheese Savory Chive	2 tbsp (1 oz)	100
Cream Cheese Smoked Salmon	2 tbsp (1 oz)	100
Cream Cheese Strawberry	2 tbsp (1 oz)	100
Super Bagel Glazed Apple Cinnamon	1 (4.6 oz)	350
BAKED SELECTIONS		
Bismark	1 (2.8 oz)	310
Bow Tie	1 (2.5 oz)	250
Brownie Blondie w/ Chocolate Chips	1 (2.4 oz)	300
Brownie Fudge	1 (2.4 oz)	290
Brownie Peanut Butter Blondie	1 (2.4 oz)	330
Cake Donut Blueberry	1 (2.4 oz)	230
Cake Donut Blueberry Crumb	1 (2.6 oz)	260
Cake Donut Butternut	1 (2.6 oz)	340
Cake Donut Chocolate	1 (2.1 oz)	210
Cake Donut Chocolate Coconut	1 (2.4 oz)	250
Cake Donut Chocolate Glazed	1 (2.5 oz)	250
Cake Donut Cinnamon	1 (2.3 oz)	300
Cake Donut Coconut	1 (2.5 oz)	320
Cake Donut Double Chocolate	1 (2.6 oz)	260
Cake Donut Old Fashioned	1 (2.1 oz)	280
Cake Donut Peanut	1 (2.6 oz)	340
Cake Donut Powdered	1 (2.4 oz)	310
Cake Donut Sugared	1 (2.4 oz)	310
Cake Donut Toasted Coconut	1 (2.5 oz)	320
Cake Donut Whole Wheat Glazed	1 (2.7 oz)	230
Coffee Roll	1 (2.6 oz)	280
Coffee Roll Chocolate Frosted	1 (2.7 oz)	290
Coffee Roll Cinnamon Raisin	1 (3.1 oz)	330
Coffee Roll Maple Frosted	1 (2.7 oz)	300
Coffee Roll Vanilla Frosted	1 (2.7 oz)	300
Cookie Chocolate Chocolate Chunk	1 (1.5 oz)	200
Cookie Chocolate Chunk	1 (1.5 oz)	200
Cookie Chocolate Chunk w/ Nut	1 (1.5 oz)	200
Cookie Chocolate White Chocolate Chunk	1 (1.5 oz)	200
Cookie Oatmeal Raisin Pecan	1 (1.5 oz)	190
Cookie Peanut Butter Chocolate Chunk w/ Nuts	1 (1.5 oz)	210

FOOD	PORTION	CALS.
Cookie Peanut Butter Chocolate Chunk w/ Peanuts	1 (1.5 oz)	210
Croissant Almond	1 (2.7 oz)	360
Croissant Cheese	1 (2.5 oz)	240
Croissant Chocolate	1 (2.5 oz)	370
Croissant Plain	1 (2.1 oz)	270
Crullers/Sticks Dunkin' Donut	1 (2.1 oz)	240
Crullers/Sticks Glazed	1 (3 oz)	340
Crullers/Sticks Glazed Chocolate	1 (3.2 oz)	410
Crullers/Sticks Jelly	1 (3.2 oz)	330
Crullers/Sticks Plain	1 (2.1 oz)	260
Crullers/Sticks Powdered	1 (2.3 oz)	290
Crullers/Sticks Sugar	1 (2.2 oz)	270
Eclair	1 (3.2 oz)	290
English Muffin	1 (2 oz)	130
French Roll	1 (2.1 oz)	140
Fritter Apple	1 (3.3 oz)	300
Fritter Glazed	1 (2.7 oz)	290
Muffin Banana Nut	1 (3.3 oz)	340
Muffin Blueberry	1 (3.3 oz)	310
Muffin Cherry	1 (3.3 oz)	330
Muffin Chocolate Chip	1 (3.3 oz)	400
Muffin Corn	1 (3.3 oz)	350
Muffin Cranberry Orange Nut	1 (3.5 oz)	310
Muffin Honey Raisin Bran	1 (3.3 oz)	330
Muffin Lemon Poppy Seed	1 (3.3 oz)	360
Muffin Oat Bran	1 (3.2 oz)	290
Muffin Lowfat Apple n' Spice	1 (3.3 oz)	220
Muffin Lowfat Banana	1 (3.3 oz)	240
Muffin Lowfat Blueberry	1 (3.3 oz)	230
Muffin Lowfat Bran	1 (3.3 oz)	260
Muffin Lowfat Cherry	1 (3.3 oz)	230
Muffin Lowfat Corn	1 (3.3 oz)	250
Muffin Lowfat Cranberry Orange	1 (3.3 oz)	230
Munchkins Butternut	3 (2 oz)	230
Munchkins Chocolate Glazed	3 (2 oz)	180
Munchkins Cinnamon	4 (2 oz)	240
Munchkins Coconut	3 (1.7 oz)	200
Munchkins Glazed Cake	3 (2.1 oz)	220
Munchkins Glazed Raised	4 (2.1 oz)	210
Munchkins Jelly	3 (1.9 oz)	170
Munchkins Lemon	3 (2 oz)	160
Munchkins Plain	4 (1.8 oz)	200
Munchkins Powdered Sugar	4 (2 oz)	240

FOOD	PORTION	CALS.
Munchkins Sugar Raised	6 (1.9 oz)	210
Munchkins Toasted Coconut	3 (1.8 oz)	210
Tart Apple	1 (3.4 oz)	310
Tart Blueberry	1 (3.4 oz)	300
Tart Lemon	1 (3.4 oz)	280
Tart Raspberry	1 (3.4 oz)	310
Tart Strawberry	1 (3.4 oz)	310
Turnover Apple	1 (3.8 oz)	350
Turnover Blueberry	1 (3.8 oz)	370
Turnover Lemon	1 (3.8 oz)	350
Turnover Raspberry	1 (3.8 oz)	380
Turnover Strawberry	1 (3.8 oz)	380
Yeast Donut Apple Crumb	1 (2.6 oz)	250
Yeast Donut Apple n' Spice	1 (2.5 oz)	230
Yeast Donut Bavarian Kreme	1 (2.5 oz)	250
Yeast Donut Black Raspberry	1 (2.4 oz)	240
Yeast Donut Boston Kreme	1 (2.8 oz)	270
Yeast Donut Chocolale Kreme Filled	1 (2.6 oz)	320
Yeast Donut Chocolate Frosted	1 (2.1 oz)	210
Yeast Donut Glazed	1 (1.6 oz)	160
Yeast Donut Jelly Filled	1 (2.4 oz)	240
Yeast Donut Lemon	1 (2.5 oz)	240
Yeast Donut Maple Frosted	1 (2.1 oz)	210
Yeast Donut Marble Frosted	1 (2.1 oz)	210
Yeast Donut Strawberry	1 (2.4 oz)	240
Yeast Donut Strawberry Frosted	1 (2.1 oz)	220
Yeast Donut Sugar Raised	1 (1.6 oz)	170
Yeast Donut Vanilla Frosted	1 (2.1 oz)	220
BEVERAGES		
Coffee Coolatta w/ 2% Milk	1 (15.7 oz)	210
Coffee Coolatta w/ Cream	1 (15.7 oz)	370
Coffee Coolatta w/ Skim Milk	1 (15.7 oz)	190
Coffee Coolatta w/ Whole Milk	1 (15.7 oz)	230
Cream	1 serv (1 oz)	60
Dark Roast	1 serv (10 oz)	5
Decaf	1 serv (10 oz)	0
French Vanilla	1 serv (10 oz)	5
Hazelnut	1 serv (10 oz)	5
Hazelnut Coolatta w/ 2% Milk	1 (15.7 oz)	210
Hazelnut Coolatta w/ Cream	1 (15.7 oz)	370
Hazelnut Coolatta w/ Skim Milk	1 (15.7 oz)	200
Hazelnut Coolatta w/ Whole Milk	1 (15.7 oz)	230
Mocha Coolatta w/ 2% Milk	1 (15.7 oz)	220
Mocha Coolatta w/ Cream	1 (15.7 oz)	380

FOOD	PORTION	CALS.
Mocha Coolatta w/ Skim Milk	1 (15.7 oz)	200
Mocha Coolatta w/ Whole Milk	1 (15.7 oz)	230
Regular	1 serv (10 oz)	5
Vanilla Coolatta w/ 2% Milk	1 (15.7 oz)	220
Vanilla Coolatta w/ Cream	1 (15.7 oz)	380
Vanilla Coolatta w/ Skim Milk	1 (15.7 oz)	200
Vanilla Coolatta w/ Whole Milk	1 (15.7 oz)	230
SANDWICHES		
Croissant Sandwich Broccoli & Cheese	1 (6.1 oz)	370
Croissant Sandwich Chicken Salad	1 (7.6 oz)	540
Croissant Sandwich Egg & Cheese	1 (5 oz)	430
Croissant Sandwich Egg, Bacon & Cheese	1 (5.4 oz)	500
Croissant Sandwich Egg, Ham & Cheese	1 (6 oz)	530
Croissant Sandwich Egg, Sausage & Cheese	1 (6.9 oz)	630
Croissant Sandwich Ham & Cheese	1 (6.7 oz)	710
Croissant Sandwich Roast Beef & Cheese	1 (6 oz)	490
Croissant Sandwich Seafood Salad	1 (7.6 oz)	480
Croissant Sandwich Tuna Salad	1 (7.5 oz)	540
SOUPS		
Beef Barley	1 serv (8 oz)	90
Beef Noodle	1 serv (8 oz)	90
Chicken Noodle	1 serv (8 oz)	80
Chili	1 serv (8 oz)	170
Chili Con Carne w/ Beans	1 serv (8 oz)	300
Cream Of Broccoli	1 serv (8 oz)	200
Cream Of Potato	1 serv (8 oz)	190
Harvest Vegetable	1 serv (8 oz)	80
Manhattan Clam Chowder	1 serv (8 oz)	70
Minestrone	1 serv (8 oz)	100
New England Clam Chowder	1 serv (8 oz)	200
Split Pea w/ Ham	1 serv (8 oz)	190

EINSTEIN BROS BAGELS
BAGELS

Bagel Chips Cinnamon Raisin Swirl	1 serv (1 oz)	90
Bagel Chips Plain	1 serv (1 oz)	90
Bagel Chips Sourdough Dill	1 serv (1 oz)	90
Bagel Chips Sun Dried Tomato	1 serv (1 oz)	90
Bagel Chips Sunflower	1 serv (1 oz)	100
Bagel Chips Wild Blueberry	1 serv (1 oz)	90
Chocolate Chip	1 (4 oz)	380
Chopped Garlic	1 (4.2 oz)	377
Chopped Onion	1 (4 oz)	340
Cinnamon Raisin Swirl	1 (4 oz)	360

FOOD	PORTION	CALS.
Cinnamon Sugar	1	330
Dark Pumpernickel	1 (3.8 oz)	330
Everything	1 (4 oz)	342
Honey 8 Grain	1 (4 oz)	320
Nutty Banana	1 (4 oz)	370
Plain	1 (3.7 oz)	330
Poppy Dip'd	1 (3.9 oz)	348
Salt	1 (3.9 oz)	330
Sesame Dip'd	1 (4.1 oz)	381
Spinach Herb	1 (3.8 oz)	320
Sun Dried Tomato	1 (3.8 oz)	320
Veggie Confetti	1 (3.8 oz)	330
Wild Blueberry	1 (4 oz)	360
SANDWICHES AND FILLINGS		
Butter & Margarine Blend	1 serv (0.4 oz)	60
Capers	1 tbsp	0
Cheddar Cheese	1 serv (0.75 oz)	110
Classic New York Lox & Bagel	1 (11.4 oz)	560
Cream Cheese Cheddarpeno	1 serv (1 oz)	90
Cream Cheese Chive	1 serv (1 oz)	90
Cream Cheese Maple Walnut Raisin	1 serv (1 oz)	100
Cream Cheese Plain	1 serv (1 oz)	100
Cream Cheese Smoked Salmon	1 serv (1 oz)	90
Cream Cheese Strawberry	1 serv (1 oz)	90
Cream Cheese Sun Dried Tomato	1 serv (1 oz)	90
Cucumbers	1 serv (1 oz)	0
Fruit Spreads	1 tbsp	40
Ham	1 serv (2.5 oz)	75
Ham & Cheese Sandwich	1 (9.9 oz)	520
Honey	1 tbsp	64
Hummus	2 tbsp	60
Hummus Sandwich	1 (6 oz)	440
Lettuce	1 leaf	0
Lite Cream Cheese Plain	1 serv (1 oz)	60
Lite Cream Cheese Spinach Dill	1 serv (1 oz)	60
Lite Cream Cheese Veggie	1 serv (1 oz)	60
Lite Cream Cheese Wildberry	1 serv (1 oz)	70
Lowfat Chicken Salad Sandwich	1 (11.6 oz)	440
Lowfat Tuna Salad Sandwich	1 (11.6 oz)	440
Marshall's Loz	1 serv (2 oz)	90
Mayonnaise Lite Reduced Calorie	1 serv (0.5 oz)	50
Peanut Butter	1 serv (1.1 oz)	190
Peanut Butter & Jelly Sandwich	1 (6 oz)	595
Scrambled Egg Sandwich	1 (7.7 oz)	480

FOOD	PORTION	CALS.
Scrambled Egg Sandwich w/ Meat & Cheese	1 (8.9 oz)	520
Smoked Turkey	1 serv (2.5 oz)	75
Smoked Turkey Sandwich	1 (9.9 oz)	480
Spouts Alfalfa	1 serv (0.5 oz)	0
Sweet Onions	1 serv (1 oz)	0
Swiss Cheese	1 serv (0.75 oz)	100
Tasty Turkey Sandwich	1 (10 oz)	530
Tomato	1 serv (1.5 oz)	0
Turkey Pastrami 99% Fat Free	1 serv (2.5 oz)	75
Turkey Pastrami Sandwich	1 (9.7 oz)	460
Veg Out Sandwich	1 (8.9 oz)	350
Whitefish Salad Sandwich	1 (9.2 oz)	630

EL POLLO LOCO
MAIN MENU SELECTIONS

FOOD	PORTION	CALS.
Broccoli Slaw	1 serv (5 oz)	203
Burrito BRC	1 (9.3 oz)	482
Burrito Classic Chicken	1 (9.3 oz)	556
Burrito Grilled Steak	1 (11.3 oz)	705
Burrito Loco Grande	1 (13.1 oz)	632
Burrito Smokey Black Bean	1 (9.3 oz)	566
Burrito Spicy Hot Chicken	1 (9.8 oz)	559
Burrito Whole Wheat Chicken	1 (10.8 oz)	592
Chicken Breast	1 piece (3 oz)	160
Chicken Leg	1 piece (1.75 oz)	90
Chicken Soft Taco	1 (4 oz)	224
Chicken Thigh	1 piece (2 oz)	180
Chicken Wing	1 (1.5 oz)	110
Chicken Tamale	1 (3.5 oz)	190
Cole Slaw	1 serv (5 oz)	206
Corn-On-Cob	1 ear (5.5 oz)	146
Cornbread Stuffing	1 serv (6 oz)	281
Crispy Green Beans	1 serv (5 oz)	41
Cucumber Salad	1 serv (4.2 oz)	34
Fiesta Corn	1 serv (5 oz)	152
Flame Broiled Chicken Salad	1 serv (14.9 oz)	167
French Fries	1 serv (4.4 oz)	323
Garden Salad	1 serv (6.4 oz)	29
Gravy	1 serv (1 oz)	14
Honey Glazed Carrots	1 serv (5 oz)	104
Lime Parfait	1 serv (5 oz)	125
Macaroni & Cheese	1 serv (6 oz)	238
Mashed Potatoes	1 serv (5 oz)	97
Pinto Beans	1 serv (6 oz)	185

FOOD	PORTION	CALS.
Polo Bowl	1 serv (19 oz)	504
Potato Salad	1 serv (6 oz)	256
Rainbow Pasta Salad	1 serv (5 oz)	157
Salad Shell	1 (5.6 oz)	440
Smokey Black Beans	1 serv (5 oz)	255
Southwest Cole Slaw	1 serv (5 oz)	178
Spanish Rice	1 serv (4 oz)	130
Spiced Apples	1 serv (5 oz)	146
Steak Bowl	1 serv (15.2 oz)	616
Taco Al Carbon Chicken	1 serv (4.4 oz)	265
Taco Al Carbon Steak	1 (4.4 oz)	394
Taquito	1 serv (5 oz)	370
Tortilla Corn	1 (1.1 oz)	70
Tortilla Flour	1 (1 oz)	90
Tortilla Wrap Chicken Caesar	1 (10.47 oz)	518
Tortilla Wrap Southwest	1 (11.97 oz)	632
Tostada Salad Chicken	1 serv (14.7 oz)	332
Tostado Salad Steak	1 serv (13.2 oz)	525
SALAD DRESSINGS		
Blue Cheese	1 serv (2 oz)	300
Light Italian	1 serv (2 oz)	25
Ranch	1 serv (2 oz)	350
Thousand Island	1 serv (2 oz)	270

FOSTERS FREEZE
Soft Serve Vanilla	1 serv (4 oz)	152

FRIENDLY'S
FROZEN YOGURT

Apple Bettie	½ cup (2.6 oz)	140
Chocolate Fudge Brownie	½ cup (2.6 oz)	160
Fabulous Fudge Swirl	½ cup (2.6 oz)	140
Fudge Berry Swirl	½ cup (2.6 oz)	150
Lowfat Perfectly Peach	½ cup (2.6 oz)	110
Lowfat Purely Chocolate	½ cup (2.6 oz)	120
Lowfat Raspberry Delight	½ cup (2.6 oz)	120
Lowfat Simply Vanilla	½ cup (2.6 oz)	120
Lowfat Strawberry Patch	½ cup (2.6 oz)	110
Mint Chocolate Chip	½ cup (2.6 oz)	130
Strawberry Cheesecake Blast	½ cup (2.6 oz)	140
Toffee Almond Crunch	½ cup (2.6 oz)	160
ICE CREAM		
Black Raspberry	½ cup	150
Chocolate Almond Chip	½ cup	170
Forbidden Chocolate	½ cup	150

FOOD	PORTION	CALS.
Fudge Nut Brownie	½ cup	200
Heath English Toffee	½ cup (2.7 oz)	190
Purely Pictachio	½ cup	160
Vanilla	½ cup	150
Vienna Mocha Chunk	½ cup	180

FRULLATI CAFE
BAKED SELECTIONS

FOOD	PORTION	CALS.
Muffin Banana Nut	1 (4 oz)	394
Muffin Cranberry Orange	1 (4 oz)	357
Muffin Fat Free Apple Streusel	1 (4 oz)	260
Muffin Fat Free Chocolate	1 (4 oz)	260
Muffin Fat Free Very Berry	1 (4 oz)	260
Muffin Sugar Free Blueberry	1 (4 oz)	308
Muffin Wild Blueberry	1 (4 oz)	344

BEVERAGES

FOOD	PORTION	CALS.
Apple Juice	1 serv (12 oz)	131
Carrot Juice	1 serv (12 oz)	111
Celery Juice	1 serv (12 oz)	22
Lemondae	1 serv	209
Lemondae Apple	1 serv	245
Lemondae Cherry	1 serv	237
Lemondae Orange	1 serv	270
Lemondae Strawberry	1 serv	234
Orange Banana Juice	1 serv (12 oz)	150
Orange Juice	1 serv (12 oz)	126
Smoothie A La Frullati	1 sm	275
Smoothie A La Frullati	1 lg	426
Smoothie Affinity	1 lg	378
Smoothie Affinity	1 sm	226
Smoothie Fiesta	1 lg	257
Smoothie Fiesta	1 sm	234
Smoothie Peach Banana	1 sm	266
Smoothie Peach Banana	1 lg	289
Smoothie Pina Colada	1 sm	236
Smoothie Pina Colada	1 lg	387
Smoothie Strawberry Banana	1 sm	165
Smoothie Strawberry Banana	1 lg	188
Smoothie Strawberry Blueberry	1 sm	90
Smoothie Strawberry Blueberry	1 lg	113
Smoothie Strawberry Fruit	1 lg	101
Smoothie Strawberry Fruit	1 sm	79
Smoothie Strawberry Watermelon	1 lg	123
Smoothie Strawberry Watermelon	1 sm	100

FOOD	PORTION	CALS.
DESSERTS		
Frozen Yogurt	1 reg	205
Frozen Yogurt	1 lg	263
Frozen Yogurt	1 sm	146
Yogurt Smoothie Cappuccino	1 serv	472
Yogurt Smoothie Chocolate Fudge	1 serv	555
Yogurt Smoothie Fiesta	1 serv	432
Yogurt Smoothie Oreo Cookie	1 serv	566
Yogurt Smoothie Peach	1 serv	486
Yogurt Smoothie Peach Banana	1 serv	519
Yogurt Smoothie Peanut Butter	1 serv	630
Yogurt Smoothie Pina Colada	1 serv	519
Yogurt Smoothie Strawberry Banana	1 serv	514
Yogurt Smoothie Strawberry Fruit	1 serv	487
Yogurt Smoothie Strawberry Vanilla	1 serv	462
Yogurt Smoothie Strawberry Watermelon	1 serv	503
SALADS AND SALAD BARS		
Fruit Salad	1 lg	148
Fruit Salad	1 sm	99
Garden Salad	1 sm	56
Garden Salad w/ Italian Fat Free Dressing	1 lg	72
Pasta Salad	1 lg	256
Pasta Salad	1 sm	179
SANDWICHES		
Chicken On Croissant	1	481
Chicken On Honey Wheat	1	297
Chicken On Jewish Rye	1	261
Chicken On Pita	1	281
Chicken On White	1	291
Ham & Cheese On Croissant	1	797
Ham & Cheese On Honey Wheat	1	613
Ham & Cheese On Jewish Rye	1	577
Ham & Cheese On Pita	1	597
Ham & Cheese On White	1	607
Roast Beef On Croissant	1	631
Roast Beef On Honey Wheat	1	348
Roast Beef On Jewish Rye	1	312
Roast Beef On Pita	1	332
Roast Beef On White	1	342
Tuna On Croissant	1	480
Tuna On Honey Wheat	1	295
Tuna On Jewish Rye	1	259
Tuna On Pita	1	280
Tuna On White	1	289

FOOD	PORTION	CALS.
Turkey On Croissant	1	566
Turkey On Honey Wheat	1	342
Turkey On Jewish Rye	1	306
Turkey On Pita	1	326
Turkey On White	1	338
Veggie On Croissant	1	510
Veggie On Honey Wheat	1	227
Veggie On Jewish Rye	1	191
Veggie On Pita	1	211
Veggie On White	1	221

GODFATHER'S PIZZA

FOOD	PORTION	CALS.
Golden Crust Cheese	⅛ med (3.1 oz)	212
Golden Crust Cheese	⅒ lg (3.5 oz)	242
Golden Crust Combo	⅛ med (4.4 oz)	271
Golden Crust Combo	⅒ lg (4.9 oz)	305
Original Crust Cheese	⅒ jumbo (5.8 oz)	382
Original Crust Cheese	¼ mini (1.9 oz)	131
Original Crust Cheese	⅛ med (3.5 oz)	231
Original Crust Cheese	⅒ lg (4 oz)	258
Original Crust Combo	⅒ lg (5.6 oz)	338
Original Crust Combo	⅛ med (5.1 oz)	306
Original Crust Combo	⅒ jumbo (8.3 oz)	503
Original Crust Combo	¼ mini (2.9 oz)	176

GODIVA

FOOD	PORTION	CALS.
Almond Butter Dome	3 pieces (1.5 oz)	240
Bouchee Au Chocolat	1 piece (1.5 oz)	210
Bouchee Ivory Raspberry	1 pieces (1 oz)	160
Gold Ballotin	3 pieces (1.5 oz)	210
Truffle Amaretto Di Saronno	2 pieces (1.5 oz)	210
Truffle Deluxe Liqueur	2 pieces (1.5 oz)	210

HAAGEN-DAZS
FROZEN YOGURT

FOOD	PORTION	CALS.
Brownie Nut Blast	½ cup (3.5 oz)	215
Chocolate	½ cup (3.4 oz)	160
Coffee	½ cup (3.4 oz)	161
Orange Tango	½ cup (3.5 oz)	132
Pina Colada	½ cup (3.4 oz)	139
Raspberry Randezvous	½ cup (3.5 oz)	132
Soft Serve Coffee	½ cup (3.3 oz)	145
Soft Serve Nonfat Chocolate	½ cup (3.3 oz)	116
Soft Serve Nonfat Chocolate Mousse	½ cup (3.3 oz)	86
Soft Serve Nonfat Vanilla	½ cup (3.3 oz)	114

FOOD	PORTION	CALS.
Soft Serve Nonfat Vanilla Mousse	½ cup (3.3 oz)	78
Strawberry Cheesecake Craze	½ cup (3.6 oz)	213
Strawberry Duet	½ cup (3.4 oz)	135
Vanilla	½ cup (3.4 oz)	162
Vanilla Almond Crunch	½ cup (3.4 oz)	198
ICE CREAM		
Bar Chocolate	1 (2.7 oz)	247
Bar Coffee	1 (2.7 oz)	249
Bar Vanilla	1 (2.7 oz)	251
Belgian Chocolate Chocolate	½ cup (3.6 oz)	315
Brownies A La Mode	½ cup (3.5 oz)	284
Butter Pecan	½ cup (3.7 oz)	304
Cappuccino Commotion	½ cup (3.6 oz)	305
Caramel Cone Explosion	½ cup (3.6 oz)	298
Chocolate	½ cup (3.7 oz)	249
Chocolate Chocolate Chip	½ cup (3.7 oz)	282
Chocolate Chocolate Mint	½ cup (3.6 oz)	285
Coffee	½ cup (3.7 oz)	251
Coffee Chip	½ cup (3.6 oz)	285
Cookie Dough Dynamo	½ cup (3.6 oz)	298
Cookies & Cream	½ cup (3.6 oz)	264
Deep Chocolate Peanut Butter	½ cup (3.7 oz)	339
Macadamia Brittle	½ cup (3.7 oz)	282
Macadamia Nut	½ cup (3.6 oz)	309
Midnight Cookies & Cream	½ cup (3.6 oz)	285
Peanut Butter Burst	½ cup (2.6 oz)	314
Pralines & Cream	½ cup (3.6 oz)	278
Rum Raisin	½ cup (3.7 oz)	256
Strawberry	½ cup (3.7 oz)	242
Strawberry Cheesecake Craze	½ cup (3.7 oz)	273
Swiss Chocolate Almond	½ cup (3.6 oz)	288
Triple Brownie Overload	½ cup (3.5 oz)	298
Vanilla	½ cup (3.7 oz)	252
Vanilla Chip	½ cup (3.6 oz)	286
Vanilla Fudge	½ cup (3.7 oz)	268
Vanilla Swiss Almond	½ cup (3.7 oz)	288
SORBET		
Mango	½ cup (4 oz)	107
Raspberry	½ cup (4 oz)	110
Soft Serve Lemonade	½ cup (3.3 oz)	113
Soft Serve Mango	½ cup (3.3 oz)	107
Soft Serve Raspberry	½ cup (3.3 oz)	108
Strawberry	½ cup (4 oz)	118
Zesty Lemon	½ cup (4 oz)	111

FOOD	PORTION	CALS.
HARDEE'S		
BEVERAGES		
Orange Juice	1 serv (11 oz)	140
Shake Chocolate	1 (12.2 oz)	370
Shake Peach	1 (12.1 oz)	390
Shake Strawberry	1 (12.7 oz)	420
Shake Vanilla	1 (12.2 oz)	350
BREAKFAST SELECTIONS		
Apple Cinnamon 'N' Raisin Biscuit	1 (2.18 oz)	200
Bacon & Egg Biscuit	1 (5.5 oz)	570
Bacon Egg & Cheese Biscuit	1 (5.9 oz)	610
Big Country Breakfast Bacon	1 serv (9.4 oz)	820
Big Country Breakfast Sausage	1 serv (11.4 oz)	1000
Biscuit 'N' Gravy	1 (7.8 oz)	510
Country Ham Biscuit	1 (3.8 oz)	430
Frisco Breakfast Sandwich Ham	1 (7.4 oz)	500
Ham Biscuit	1 (4 oz)	400
Ham Egg & Cheese Biscuit	1 (6.5 oz)	540
Hash Rounds	1 serv (2.8 oz)	230
Jelly Biscuit	1 (3.5 oz)	440
Rise 'N' Shine Biscuit	1 (2.9 oz)	390
Sausage Biscuit	1 (4.1 oz)	510
Sausage & Egg Biscuit	1 (6.3 oz)	630
Three Pancakes	1 serv (4.8 oz)	280
Ultimate Omelet Biscuit	1 (5.8 oz)	570
DESSERTS		
Big Cookie	1 (2.0 oz)	280
Cone Chocolate	1 (4.1 oz)	180
Cone Vanilla	1 (4.1 oz)	170
Cool Twist Cone Vanilla/ Chocolate	1 (4.1 oz)	180
Peach Cobbler	1 serv (6 oz)	310
Sundae Hot Fudge	1 (5.5 oz)	290
Sundae Strawberry	1 (5.8 oz)	210
MAIN MENU SELECTIONS		
Baked Beans	1 serv (5 oz)	170
Big Roast Beef Sandwich	1 (6.5 oz)	460
Cheeseburger	1 (4.3 oz)	310
Chicken Fillet Sandwich	1 (7.5 oz)	480
Cole Slaw	1 serv (4 oz)	240
Cravin' Bacon Cheeseburger	1 (8.1 oz)	690
Fisherman's Fillet	1 (8.3 oz)	560
French Fries	1 med (5 oz)	350
French Fries	1 lg (6 oz)	430

FOOD	PORTION	CALS.
French Fries	1 sm (3.4 oz)	240
Fried Chicken Breast	1 piece (5.2 oz)	370
Fried Chicken Leg	1 piece (2.4 oz)	170
Fried Chicken Thigh	1 piece (4.2 oz)	330
Fried Chicken Wing	1 piece (2.3 oz)	200
Frisco Burger	1 (8.1 oz)	720
Gravy	1 serv (1.5 oz)	20
Grilled Chicken Sandwich	1 (7.1 oz)	350
Hamburger	1 (3.9 oz)	270
Hot Ham 'N' Cheese	1 (5.1 oz)	310
Mashed Potatoes	1 serv (4 oz)	70
Mesquite Bacon Cheeseburger	1 (4.5 oz)	370
Mushroom 'N' Swiss Burger	1 (6.8 oz)	490
Quarter Pound Double Cheeseburger	1 (6 oz)	470
Regular Roast Beef	1 (4.3 oz)	320
The Boss	1 (7 oz)	570
The Works Burger	1 (8.1 oz)	530
SALAD DRESSINGS		
Fat Free French	1 serv (2 oz)	70
Ranch	1 serv (2 oz)	290
Thousand Island	1 serv (2 oz)	250
SALADS AND SALAD BARS		
Garden Salad	1 (10.2 oz)	220
Grilled Chicken Salad	1 (11.5 oz)	150
Side Salad	1 (4.6 oz)	25

H.SALT SEAFOOD

Chicken	3 oz	108
Cod	3 oz	62
Hamburger	3 oz	228
Pork Loin	3 oz	254
Sirloin Steak	3 oz	239

IHOP

Pancake Buckwheat	1 (2.5 oz)	134
Pancake Buttermilk	1 (2 oz)	108
Pancake Country Griddle	1 (2.25 oz)	134
Pancake Egg	1 (2 oz)	102
Pancake Harvest Grain 'N Nut	1 (2.25 oz)	160
Waffle	1 (4 oz)	305
Waffle Belgian	1 (6 oz)	408
Waffle Belgian Harvest Grain 'N Nut	1 (6 oz)	445

JACK IN THE BOX
BEVERAGES

2% Milk	1 serv (8 fl oz)	130

FOOD	PORTION	CALS.
Barq's Root Beer	1 reg (20 fl oz)	180
Classic Ice Cream Shake Chocolate	1 reg (11 fl oz)	630
Classic Ice Cream Shake Oreo Cookie	1 reg (12 oz)	740
Classic Ice Cream Shake Strawberry	1 reg (10 fl oz)	640
Classic Ice Cream Shake Vanilla	1 reg (11 oz)	610
Classice Ice Cream Shake Cappuccino	1 reg (11 oz)	630
Coca-Cola Classic	1 reg (20 fl oz)	170
Coffee	1 reg (12 fl oz)	5
Diet Coke	1 reg (20 fl oz)	0
Dr Pepper	1 reg (20 fl oz)	190
Iced Tea	1 reg (20 fl oz)	0
Minute Maid Lemonade	1 reg (20 fl oz)	190
Orange Juice	1 serv (10 oz)	150
Sprite	1 reg (20 fl oz)	160
BREAKFAST SELECTIONS		
Breakfast Jack	1 (4.2 oz)	300
Country Crock Spread	1 pat (5 g)	25
Grape Jelly	1 serv (0.5 oz)	40
Hash Browns	1 serv (2 oz)	160
Pancake Syrup	1 serv (1.5 oz)	120
Pancakes w/ Bacon	1 serv (5.6 oz)	400
Sausage Croissant	1 (6.4 oz)	670
Sourdough Breakfast Sandwich	1 (5.2 oz)	380
Supreme Croissant	1 (6 oz)	570
Ultimate Breakfast Sandwich	1 (8.5 oz)	620
DESSERTS		
Carrot Cake	1 serv (3.5 oz)	370
Cheesecake	1 serv (3.5 oz)	310
Double Fudge Cake	1 serv (3 oz)	300
Hot Apple Turnover	1 (3.8 oz)	340
MAIN MENU SELECTIONS		
¼ lb Burger	1 (6 oz)	510
American Cheese	1 slice (0.4 oz)	45
Bacon & Cheddar Potato Wedges	1 serv (9.3 oz)	800
Bacon Ultimate Cheeseburger	1 (10.4 oz)	1150
Barbeque Dipping Sauce	1 serv (1 fl oz)	45
Cheeseburger	1 (4 oz)	330
Chicken & Fries	1 serv (9.3 oz)	730
Chicken Caesar Sandwich	1 (8.3 oz)	520
Chicken Fajita Pita	1 (6.6 oz)	280
Chicken Sandwich	1 (5.9 oz)	450
Chicken Strips Breaded	5 pieces (5.3 oz)	360
Chicken Supreme Sandwich	1 (8.2 oz)	680
Chili Cheese Curly Fries	1 serv (8.1 oz)	650

FOOD	PORTION	CALS.
Double Cheeseburger	1 (5.3 oz)	450
Egg Rolls	3 pieces (6 oz)	440
Egg Rolls	5 pieces (10 oz)	730
Fish & Chips	1 serv (9 oz)	720
French Fries	1 reg (4.1 oz)	360
Grilled Chicken Fillet Sandwich	1 (8.1 oz)	520
Hamburger	1 (3.6 oz)	280
Jumbo Fries	1 serv (5 oz)	430
Jumbo Jack	1 (7.8 oz)	560
Jumbo Jack w/ Cheese	1 (8.6 oz)	650
Ketchup	1 pkg (0.3 oz)	10
Monster Taco	1 (4 oz)	290
Onion Rings	1 serv (4.2 oz)	460
Pilly Cheesesteak Sandwich	1 (7.6 oz)	520
Salsa	1 serv (1 oz)	10
Seasoned Curly Fries	1 serv (4.5 oz)	420
Sour Cream	1 serv (1 oz)	60
Sourdough Jack	1 (7.8 oz)	670
Soy Sauce	1 serv (0.3 oz)	5
Spicy Crispy Chicken Sandwich	1 (7.9 oz)	560
Stuffed Jalapenos	10 pieces (7.6 oz)	680
Stuffed Jalapenos	7 pieces (5.3 oz)	470
Super Scoop French Fries	1 serv (7 oz)	610
Sweet & Sour Dipping Sauce	1 serv (1 oz)	40
Swiss-Style Cheese	1 slice (0.4 oz)	40
Taco	1 (2.7 oz)	190
Tartar Dipping Sauce	1 pkg (1.5 oz)	220
Teriyaki Bowl Chicken	1 serv (17.6 oz)	670
Ultimate Cheeseburger	1 (9.8 oz)	1030
SALAD DRESSINGS		
Blue Cheese	1 serv (2 fl oz)	210
Buttermilk House	1 serv (2 fl oz)	290
Buttermilk House Dipping Sauce	1 serv (0.9 oz)	130
Low Calorie Italian	1 serv (2 fl oz)	25
Thousand Island	1 serv (2 fl oz)	250
SALADS AND SALAD BARS		
Croutons	1 serv (0.4 oz)	50
Garden Chicken Salad	1 serv (8.9 oz)	200
Side Salad	1 (3 oz)	50

KENNY ROGERS ROASTERS
MAIN MENU SELECTIONS

½ Chicken w/ Skin	1 serv (9 oz)	515
½ Chicken w/o Skin & Wing	1 serv (7 oz)	313

FOOD	PORTION	CALS.
¼ Chicken Dark Meat w/ Skin	1 serv (4.35 oz)	271
¼ Chicken Dark Meat w/o Skin & Wing	1 serv (3.3 oz)	169
¼ Chicken White Meat w/ Skin	1 serv (4.7 oz)	244
¼ Chicken White Meat w/o Skin & Wing	1 serv (3.75 oz)	144
Baked Sweet Potato	1 (9 oz)	263
Chicken Caesar Salad	1 serv (9.4 oz)	285
Cinnamon Apples	1 serv (5.3 oz)	199
Cole Slaw	1 serv (5 oz)	225
Corn Muffin	1 (2 oz)	175
Corn On The Cob	1 (2.25 oz)	68
Corn Stuffing	1 serv (7.1 oz)	326
Creamy Parmesan Spinach	1 serv (5.3 oz)	119
Garlic Parsley Potatoes	1 serv (6.5 oz)	259
Honey Baked Beans	1 serv (5 oz)	148
Italian Green Beans	1 serv (6.1 oz)	116
Macaroni & Cheese	1 serv (5.5 oz)	197
Pasta Salad	1 serv (5 oz)	236
Pita BBQ Chicken	1 (7.3 oz)	401
Pita Chicken Caesar	1 (9.2 oz)	606
Pita Roasted Chicken	1 (10.8 oz)	685
Pot Pie Chicken	1 (12 oz)	708
Potato Salad	1 serv (7 oz)	390
Real Mashed Potatoes	1 serv (8 oz)	295
Rice Pilaf	1 serv (5 oz)	173
Roasted Chicken Salad	1 serv (16.9 oz)	292
Sandwich Turkey	1 (9.2 oz)	385
Side Salad	1 serv (4.7 oz)	23
Sour Cream & Dill Pasta Salad	1 serv (5 oz)	233
Steamed Vegetables	1 serv (4.25 oz)	48
Sweet Corn Niblets	1 serv (5 oz)	112
Tomato Cucumber Salad	1 serv (6 oz)	123
Turkey Sliced Breast	1 serv (4.5 oz)	158
Zucchini & Squash Santa Fe	1 serv (5 oz)	70
SALAD DRESSINGS		
Blue Cheese	1 serv (2.5 oz)	370
Buttermilk Ranch	1 serv (2.5 oz)	430
Caesar	1 serv (2.5 oz)	340
Honey French	1 serv (2.5 oz)	350
Honey Mustard	1 serv (2.5 oz)	320
Italian Fat Free	1 serv (2.5 oz)	35
Thousand Island	1 serv (2.5 oz)	330
SOUPS		
Chicken Noodle	1 bowl (10 oz)	91
Chicken Noodle	1 cup (6 oz)	55

FOOD	PORTION	CALS.
KFC		
BBQ Baked Beans	1 serv (5.5 oz)	190
Biscuit	1 (2 oz)	180
Chicken Pot Pie	1 (13 oz)	770
Chicken Twister	1 (8.7 oz)	550
Cole Slaw	1 serv (5 oz)	180
Corn On The Cob	1 ear (5.7 oz)	150
Cornbread	1 (2 oz)	228
Crispy Strips Colonel's	3 (3.25 oz)	261
Crispy Strips Spicy Buffalo	3 (4.2 oz)	350
Extra Tasty Crispy Breast	1 (5.9 oz)	470
Extra Tasty Crispy Drumstick	1 (2.4 oz)	190
Extra Tasty Crispy Thigh	1 (4.2 oz)	370
Extra Tasty Crispy Whole Wing	1 (1.9 oz)	200
Green Beans	1 serv (4.7 oz)	45
Hot & Spicy Breast	1 (6.5 oz)	530
Hot & Spicy Drumstick	1 (2.3 oz)	190
Hot & Spicy Thigh	1 (3.8 oz)	370
Hot & Spicy Whole Wing	1 (1.9 oz)	210
Hot Wings	6 (4.8 oz)	471
Macaroni & Cheese	1 serv (5.4 oz)	180
Mashed Potatoes With Gravy	1 serv (4.8 oz)	120
Mean Greens	1 serv (5.4 oz)	70
Original Recipe Breast	1 (5.4 oz)	400
Original Recipe Chicken Sandwich	1 (7.3 oz)	497
Original Recipe Drumstick	1 (2.2 oz)	140
Original Recipe Thigh	1 (3.2 oz)	250
Original Recipe Whole Wing	1 (1.6 oz)	140
Potato Salad	1 serv (5.6 oz)	230
Potato Wedges	1 serv (4.8 oz)	280
Tender Roast Breast w/ Skin	1 (4.9 oz)	251
Tender Roast Breast w/o Skin	1 (4.2 oz)	169
Tender Roast Drumstick w/ Skin	1 (1.9 oz)	97
Tender Roast Drumstick w/o Skin	1 (1.2 oz)	67
Tender Roast Thigh w/ Skin	1 (3.2 oz)	207
Tender Roast Thigh w/o Skin	1 (2.1 oz)	106
Tender Roast Wing w/ Skin	1 (1.8 oz)	121
Value BBQ Chicken Sandwich	1 (5.3 oz)	256
KRISPY KREME		
Chocolate Iced Cake	1 (2 oz)	230
Chocolate Iced Creme Filled	1 (2.3 oz)	270
Chocolate Iced Cruller	1 (1.7 oz)	240
Chocolate Iced Custard Filled	1 (2.7 oz)	250

FOOD	PORTION	CALS.
Cinnamon Apple Filled	1 (2.3 oz)	210
Cinnamon Bun	1 (2.1 oz)	220
Glazed Blueberry	1 (2.4 oz)	300
Glazed Creme Filled	1 (2.3 oz)	270
Glazed Cruller	1 (1.5 oz)	220
Glazed Devil's Food	1 (1.9 oz)	240
Lemon Filled	1 (2.2 oz)	210
Maple Iced	1 (1.8 oz)	200
Original Glazed	1 (1.3 oz)	180
Powdered Cake	1 (1.8 oz)	220
Raspberry Filled	1 (2 oz)	210

KRYSTAL
BEVERAGES
Chocolate Shake	1 (16 fl oz)	275

BREAKFAST SELECTIONS
Biscuit	1 (2.5 oz)	244
Biscuit Bacon	1 (2.9 oz)	306
Biscuit Bacon, Egg & Cheese	1 (4.7 oz)	421
Biscuit Country Ham	1 (3.7 oz)	334
Biscuit Egg	1 (4 oz)	327
Biscuit Gravy	1 (7.5 oz)	419
Biscuit Sausage	1 (4.1 oz)	437
Sunriser	1 (3.8 oz)	259

DESSERTS
Apple Pie	1 serv (4.5 oz)	300
Donut Plain	1 (1.3 oz)	150
Donut w/ Chocolate Icing	1 (1.8 oz)	212
Donut w/ Vanilla Icing	1 (1.8 oz)	198
Lemon Meringue Pie	1 serv (4 oz)	340
Pecan Pie	1 serv (4 oz)	450

MAIN MENU SELECTIONS
Bacon Cheeseburger	1 (7.4 oz)	521
Big K	1 (8 oz)	540
Burger Plus	1 (6.5 oz)	415
Burger Plus w/ Cheese	1 (7.1 oz)	473
Cheese Krystal	1 (2.5 oz)	187
Chili	1 lg (12 oz)	327
Chili	1 reg (8 oz)	218
Chili Cheese Pup	1 (2.7 oz)	211
Chili Pup	1 (2.5 oz)	182
Corn Pup	1 (2.3 oz)	214
Crispy Crunchy Chicken Sandwich	1 (5.75 oz)	467
Double Cheese Krystal	1 (4.5 oz)	337

FOOD	PORTION	CALS.
Double Krystal	1 (4 oz)	277
Fries	1 reg (4.1 oz)	358
Fries	1 sm (3 oz)	262
Fries	1 lg (5.3 oz)	463
Krys Kross Fries	1 serv (4.3 oz)	486
Krys Kross Fries Chili Cheese	1 serv (6.8 oz)	625
Krys Kross Fries w/ Cheese	1 serv (5.3 oz)	515
Krystal	1 (2.2 oz)	158
Plain Pup	1 (1.9 oz)	160

LITTLE CAESARS
MAIN MENU SELECTIONS

FOOD	PORTION	CALS.
Crazy Bread	1 piece (1.4 oz)	106
Crazy Sauce	1 serv (6 oz)	170
Deli-Style Sandwich Ham & Cheese	1 (11.6 oz)	728
Deli-Style Sandwich Italian	1 (11.9 oz)	740
Deli-Style Sandwich Veggie	1 (11.9 oz)	647
Hot Oven-Baked Sandwich Cheeser	1 (12.1 oz)	822
Hot Oven-Baked Sandwich Meatsa	1 (15 oz)	1036
Hot Oven-Baked Sandwich Pepperoni	1 (11.2 oz)	899
Hot Oven-Baked Sandwich Supreme	1 (13.1 oz)	894
Hot Oven-Baked Sandwich Veggie	1 (13.7 oz)	669

PIZZA

FOOD	PORTION	CALS.
Baby Pan!Pan!	1 serv (8.4 oz)	616
Pan!Pan! Cheese	1 med slice (2.9 oz)	181
Pan!Pan! Pepperoni	1 med slice (3 oz)	199
Pizza!Pizza! Cheese	1 med slice (3.2 oz)	201
Pizza!Pizza! Pepperoni	1 med slice (3.3 oz)	220

SALAD DRESSINGS

FOOD	PORTION	CALS.
1000 Island	1 serv (1.5 oz)	183
Blue Cheese	1 serv (1.5 oz)	160
Caesar	1 serv (1.5 oz)	255
French	1 serv (1.5 oz)	166
Greek	1 serv (1.5 oz)	268
Italian	1 serv (1.5 oz)	200
Italian Fat Free	1 serv (1.5 oz)	15
Ranch	1 serv (1.5 oz)	221

SALADS AND SALAD BARS

FOOD	PORTION	CALS.
Antipasto Salad	1 serv (8.4 oz)	176
Caesar Salad	1 serv (5 oz)	140
Greek Salad	1 serv (10.3 oz)	168
Tossed Salad	1 serv (8.5 oz)	116

LONG JOHN SILVER'S
MAIN MENU SELECTIONS

FOOD	PORTION	CALS.
Batter-Dipped Chicken	1 piece (2 oz)	120

FOOD	PORTION	CALS.
Batter-Dipped Fish	1 piece (3 oz)	170
Batter-Dipped Shrimp	1 piece (0.4 oz)	35
Breaded Chicken Strips	1 piece (1.15 oz)	100
Breaded Clams	1 serv (3 oz)	300
Breaded Fish	1 piece (1.6 oz)	110
Cheese Sticks	1 serv (1.6 oz)	160
Chicken Salsa	1 reg (11 oz)	690
Corn Cobbette w/ Butter	1 piece (3.3 oz)	140
Corn Cobbette w/o Butter	1 (3.1 oz)	80
Fish Cajun	1 lg (23 oz)	1450
Flavorbaked Chicken	1 piece (2.6 oz)	110
Flavorbaked Fish	1 piece (2.3 oz)	90
Fries	1 reg (3 oz)	250
Fries	1 lg (5 oz)	420
Honey Mustard Sauce	1 serv (0.4 oz)	20
Hushpuppy	1 (0.8 oz)	60
Ketchup	1 serv (.32 oz)	10
Popcorn Chicken Munchers	1 serv (4 oz)	380
Popcorn Fish Munchers	1 serv (4 oz)	300
Popcorn Shrimp Munchers	1 serv (4 oz)	320
Rice	1 serv (3 oz)	140
Sandwich Batter Dipped Fish No Sauce	1 (5.4 oz)	320
Sandwich Flavorbaked Chicken	1 (5.8 oz)	290
Sandwich Flavorbaked Fish	1 (6 oz)	320
Sandwich Ultimate Fish	1 (6.4 oz)	430
Shrimp Sauce	1 serv (0.4 oz)	15
Side Salad	1 (4.3 oz)	25
Slaw	1 serv (3.4 oz)	140
Sweet'N'Sour Sauce	1 serv (0.4 oz)	20
Tartar Sauce	1 serv (0.4 oz)	35
Wraps Chicken Cajun	1 reg (11 oz)	720
Wraps Chicken Cajun	1 lg (22 oz)	1440
Wraps Chicken Ranch	1 reg (11 oz)	730
Wraps Chicken Ranch	1 lg (22 oz)	1450
Wraps Chicken Salsa	1 lg (22 oz)	1370
Wraps Chicken Tartar	1 lg (22 oz)	1450
Wraps Chicken Tartar	1 reg (11 oz)	730
Wraps Fish Cajun	1 reg (11.5 oz)	730
Wraps Fish Ranch	1 reg (11.5 oz)	730
Wraps Fish Ranch	1 lg (23 oz)	1460
Wraps Fish Salsa	1 reg (11.5 oz)	690
Wraps Fish Salsa	1 lg (23 oz)	1380
Wraps Fish Tartar	1 reg (11.5 oz)	730
Wraps Fish Tartar	1 lg (23 oz)	1470

FOOD	PORTION	CALS.
Wraps Popcorn Shrimp Cajun	1 lg (22 oz)	1450
Wraps Popcorn Shrimp Cajun	1 reg (11 oz)	720
Wraps Popcorn Shrimp Ranch	1 lg (22 oz)	1460
Wraps Popcorn Shrimp Ranch	1 reg (11 oz)	720
Wraps Popcorn Shrimp Salsa	1 lg (22 oz)	1380
Wraps Popcorn Shrimp Salsa	1 reg (11 oz)	690
Wraps Popcorn Shrimp Tartar	1 reg (11 oz)	730
Wraps Popcorn Shrimp Tartar	1 lg (22 oz)	1460
SALAD DRESSINGS		
Fat-Free French	1 serv (1.5 oz)	50
Fat-Free Ranch	1 serv (1.5 oz)	50
Italian	1 serv (1 oz)	130
Malt Vinegar	1 serv (0.3 oz)	0
Ranch Dressing	1 serv (1 oz)	170
Thousand Island	1 serv (1 oz)	110

LYONS RESTAURANTS
MAIN MENU SELECTIONS

Light & Healthy Halibut Brochette	1 serv	502
Light & Healthy Lime & Cilantro Chicken	1 serv	511

MACHEEZMO MOUSE
CHILDREN'S MENU SELECTIONS

El Bento Kid	1 serv (7 oz)	235
Quesadilla Kid Cheese	1 serv (5 oz)	360
Quesadilla Kid Chicken	1 serv (7 oz)	430
Taco Kid Cheese	1 serv (6 oz)	285
Taco Kid Chicken	1 (8 oz)	355
MAIN MENU SELECTIONS		
Beans	1 oz	35
Bento Stick	1 oz	30
Boss Sauce	1 oz	30
Broccoli	1 oz	4
Burrito Chicken	1 (13 oz)	580
Burrito Combo	1 (14 oz)	630
Burrito Vegetarian	1 (14 oz)	655
Cheese	1 oz	81
Chicken	1 oz	35
Chili	1 oz	43
Chips	1 oz	140
Cilantro	1 oz	8
Dinner Rice, Beans, Broccoli	1 serv (10 oz)	328
Dinner Rice, Beans, Salad	1 serv (12 oz)	344
El Bento	1 serv (16 oz)	600
El Bento Deluxe	1 serv (20 oz)	740

FOOD	PORTION	CALS.
Enchilada Chicken	1 (12 oz)	533
Enchilada Chili	1 (12 oz)	549
Enchilada Veggie	1 (14 oz)	623
Enchilada Sauce	1 oz	6
Fresh Greens	1 oz	2
Green Sauce	1 oz	5
Guacamole	1 oz	100
Marinated Veggies	1 oz	10
Mexican Cheese	1 oz	100
Mustard Dressing	1 oz	25
Power Salad Chicken	1 serv (16 oz)	275
Power Salad Veggie	1 serv (13 oz)	200
Rice	1 oz	45
Salad Chicken	1 serv (15 oz)	430
Salad Veggie Taco	1 serv (16 oz)	655
Salsa	1 oz	4
Snack Famouse #5	1 serv (14 oz)	585
Snack Nacho Grande	1 serv (9 oz)	841
Snack Quesadilla Cheese	1 serv (6 oz)	377
Snack Quesadilla Chicken	1 serv (10 oz)	450
Snack Tacos Chicken	1 serv (6 oz)	290
Snack Tacos Chili	1 serv (6 oz)	314
Snack Tacos Veggie	1 serv (6 oz)	290
Sour Cream	1 oz	23
Tortilla Corn	3 (1 oz)	60
Tortilla Flour	1 oz	80
Tortilla Wheat	1 oz	80
Veggie Deluxe	1 serv (18 oz)	665
Yogurt Nonfat	1 oz	20

MANHATTAN BAGEL

FOOD	PORTION	CALS.
Blueberry	1 (4 oz)	260
Cheddar Cheese	1 (4 oz)	270
Chocolate Chip	1 (4 oz)	290
Cinnamon Raisin	1 (4 oz)	280
Egg	1 (4 oz)	270
Everything	1 (4 oz)	290
Garlic	1 (4 oz)	270
Jalapeno Cheddar	1 (4 oz)	260
Marble	1 (4 oz)	260
Oat Bran	1 (4 oz)	260
Oat Bran Raisin Walnut	1 (4 oz)	270
Onion	1 (4 oz)	270
Plain	1 (4 oz)	260

FOOD	PORTION	CALS.
Poppy	1 (4 oz)	300
Pumpernickel	1 (4 oz)	250
Rye	1 (4 oz)	260
Salt	1 (4 oz)	260
Sesame	1 (4 oz)	310
Spinach	1 (4 oz)	270
Sun-Dried Tomato	1 (4 oz)	260
Whole Wheat	1 (4 oz)	260

MAX & IRMA'S

Black Bean Roll Up	1 serv	401
Fat Free French	2 tbsp	126
Fat Free Honey Mustard	2 tbsp	60
Fruit Smoothie	1 serv	114
Garden Grill	1 serv	467
Garlic Breadstick	1	156
Gourmet Garden Grill	1 serv	484
Grilled Zucchini & Mushroom Pasta	1 serv	448
Grilled Zucchini & Mushroom Pasta w/ Chicken	1 serv	621
Hula Bowl w/ Fat Free Honey Mustard Dressing	1 serv	526
Lo-Cal Ranch	2 tbsp	54
Tijuana Tortilla Wrap	1	692

MCDONALD'S
BAKED SELECTIONS

Apple Pie Baked	1 (2.7 oz)	260
Chocolate Chip Cookie	1 (1.2 oz)	170
Cinnamon Roll	1 (3.3 oz)	400
Danish Apple	1 (3.7 oz)	360
Danish Cheese	1 (3.7 oz)	410
Lowfat Muffin Apple Bran	1 (4 oz)	300
McDonaldland Cookies	1 pkg (1.5 oz)	180

BEVERAGES

Coca-Cola Classic	1 sm (16 oz)	150
Cocoa-Cola Classic	1 lg (32 oz)	310
Cocoa-Cola Classic	1 child serv (12 oz)	110
Cocoa-Cola Classic	1 med (21 oz)	210
Diet Coke	1 sm (16 oz)	1
Diet Coke	1 med (21 oz)	0
Diet Coke	1 child serv (12 oz)	0
Diet Coke	1 lg (32 oz)	0
Hi-C Orange	1 sm (16 oz)	160
Hi-C Orange	1 lg (32 oz)	350

FOOD	PORTION	CALS.
Hi-C Orange	1 med (21 oz)	240
Hi-C Orange	1 child serv (12 oz)	120
Milk 1%	1 serv (8 oz)	100
Orange Juice	1 serv (6 oz)	80
Shake Chocolate	1 sm (14.5 oz)	360
Shake Strawberry	1 sm (14.5 oz)	360
Shake Vanilla	1 sm (14.5 oz)	360
Sprite	1 sm (16 fl oz)	150
Sprite	1 med (21 oz)	210
Sprite	1 child serv (12 oz)	110
Sprite	1 lg (32 oz)	310
BREAKFAST SELECTIONS		
Bacon Egg & Cheese Biscuit	1 (5.5 oz)	470
Biscuit	1 (2.9 oz)	290
Breakfast Burrito	1 (4.1 oz)	320
Egg McMuffin	1 (4.8 oz)	290
English Muffin	1 (1.9 oz)	140
Hash Browns	1 serv (1.9 oz)	130
Hotcakes Margarine & Syrup	2 serv (7.8 oz)	570
Hotcakes Plain	1 serv (5.3 oz)	310
Sausage	1 (1.5 oz)	170
Sausage Biscuit	1 (4.5 oz)	470
Sausage Biscuit With Egg	1 (6.2 oz)	550
Sausage McMuffin	1 (3.9 oz)	360
Sausage McMuffin With Egg	1 (5.7 oz)	440
Scrambled Eggs	2 (3.6 oz)	160
DESSERTS		
Nuts For Sundaes	1 serv (7 g)	40
Reduced Fat Ice Cream Cone Vanilla	1 (3.2 oz)	150
Sundae Hot Caramel	1 (6.4 oz)	360
Sundae Hot Fudge	1 (6.3 oz)	340
Sundae Strawberry	1 (6.2 oz)	290
MAIN MENU SELECTIONS		
Arch Deluxe	1 (8.4 oz)	550
Arch Deluxe With Bacon	1 (8.7 oz)	590
Barbeque Sauce	1 pkg (1 oz)	45
Big Mac	1 (7.5 oz)	560
Cheeseburger	1 (4.2 oz)	320
Chicken McNuggets	6 pieces (3.7 oz)	290
Chicken McNuggets	4 pieces (2.5 oz)	190
Chicken McNuggets	9 pieces (5.6 oz)	430
Crispy Chicken Deluxe	1 (7.8 oz)	500
Fish Filet Deluxe	1 (8 oz)	560
French Fries	1 sm (2.4 oz)	210

FOOD	PORTION	CALS.
French Fries	1 lg (5.2 oz)	450
French Fries	1 super (6.2 oz)	540
Grilled Chicken Deluxe	1 (7.8 oz)	440
Grilled Chicken Deluxe Plain w/o Mayonnaise	1 (7.2 oz)	300
Grilled Chicken Salad Deluxe	1 serv (9 oz)	120
Hamburger	1 (3.7 oz)	260
Honey	1 pkg (0.5 oz)	45
Honey Mustard	1 pkg (0.5 oz)	40
Hot Mustard	1 pkg (1 oz)	60
Light Mayonnaise	1 pkg (0.4 oz)	40
Quarter Pounder	1 (6 oz)	420
Quarter Pounder With Cheese	1 (7 oz)	530
Sweet 'N Sour Sauce	1 pkg (1 oz)	50
SALAD DRESSINGS		
Caesar	1 pkg (2.1 oz)	160
Fat Free Herb Vinaigrette	1 pkg (2.1 oz)	50
Ranch	1 pkg (2.1 oz)	230
Reduced Calorie Red French	1 pkg (2.1 oz)	160
SALADS AND SALAD BARS		
Croutons	1 pkg (0.4 oz)	50
Garden Salad	1 serv (6.2 oz)	35

MORRISON'S
DESSERTS

Boston Cream Cake	1 slice	218
MAIN MENU SELECTIONS		
Baked Potato	1	220
Broccoli	1 serv (4 oz)	37
Cabbage	1 serv (4 oz)	36
Cantaloupe Compote	1 serv (4 oz)	130
Cauliflower	1 serv (4 oz)	68
Chicken Stew & Dumplings	1 serv (7 oz)	362
Chicken Teriyaki	1 serv (5.5 oz)	232
French Bread	1 slice	207
Grilled Chicken Pecan Salad	1 serv (6 oz)	298
Lima Beans	1 serv (4 oz)	170
Okra & Tomatoes	1 serv (5 oz)	40
Pinto Beans	1 serv (4 oz)	105
Plain Jello	1 serv (3 oz)	131
Rutabagas	1 serv (4 oz)	33
Sliced Tomato	4 slices	40
Soft Roll	1 (2 oz)	170
Strawberries & Banana Bowl	1 serv (6 oz)	203
Strawberries Peaches & Bananas	1 serv (6 oz)	203

FOOD	PORTION	CALS.
Turnip Greens	1 serv (4 oz)	30
Watermelon	1 serv (6 oz)	102
Yellow Squash	1 serv (4 oz)	22
SALADS AND SALAD BARS		
Garden Salad	1 serv (2.5 oz)	75
Tossed Salad	1 serv (3 oz)	30

MRS. FIELDS

FOOD	PORTION	CALS.
Brownie Double Fudge	1 (3.1 oz)	420
Brownie Fudge Walnut	1 (3.4 oz)	500
Brownie Pecan Fudge	1 (2.8 oz)	390
Brownie Pecan Pie	1 (3 oz)	400
Cookie Chewy Fudge	1 (1.7 oz)	230
Cookie Coconut Macadamia	1 (1.7 oz)	250
Cookie Milk Chocolate Chip	1 (1.7 oz)	240
Cookie Milk Chocolate Macadamia	1 (1.7 oz)	250
Cookie Milk Chocolate w/ Walnuts	1 (1.7 oz)	250
Cookie Oatmeal Raisin	1 (1.7 oz)	220
Cookie Peanut Butter	1 (1.7 oz)	240
Cookie Semi-Sweet Chocolate	1 (1.7 oz)	230
Cookie Semi-Sweet Chocolate w/ Walnuts	1 (1.8 oz)	240
Cookie Triple Chocolate	1 (1.7 oz)	230
Cookie White Chunk Macadamia	1 (1.7 oz)	260
Muffin Banana Walnut	1 (3.9 oz)	460
Muffin Blueberry	1 (4 oz)	390
Muffin Chocolate Chip	1 (4 oz)	450
Muffin Mandarin Orange	1 (4 oz)	420
Peanut Butter Dream Bar	1 (5 oz)	750
PRETZELS		
Hot Sam Bavarian	1 reg (2.5 oz)	200
Hot Sam Bavarian	1 lg (5.1 oz)	390
Hot Sam Bavarian Stix	10 (5 oz)	390
Hot Sam Sweet Dough	1 (4.5 oz)	360
Hot Sam Sweet Dough Blueberry	1 (4.5 oz)	400

MY FAVORITE MUFFIN

FOOD	PORTION	CALS.
Basic Muffin	⅓ muffin	220
Double Chocolate	⅓ muffin	190
Fat Free Bavarian	⅓ muffin	100
Fat Free Bavarian Chocolate	⅓ muffin	130

NATHAN'S

FOOD	PORTION	CALS.
BEVERAGES		
Lemonade	22 fl oz	260
Lemonade	32 fl oz	378
Lemonade	16 fl oz	189

FOOD	PORTION	CALS.
MAIN MENU SELECTIONS		
Breaded Chicken Sandwich	1 (7.2 oz)	510
Charbroiled Chicken Sandwich	1 (4.5 oz)	288
Cheese Steak Sandwich	1 (6.1 oz)	485
Chicken 2 Pieces	1 serv (7.1 oz)	693
Chicken 4 Pieces	1 serv (14.2 oz)	1382
Chicken Platter 2 Pieces	1 serv (14.8 oz)	1096
Chicken Platter 4 Pieces	1 serv (21.9 oz)	1788
Chicken Salad	1 serv (12.7 oz)	154
Double Burger	1 (7.3 oz)	671
Filet of Fish Platter	1 serv (22 oz)	1455
Filet of Fish Sandwich	1 (5.2 oz)	403
Frank Nuggets	11 pieces (5.1 oz)	563
Frank Nuggets	15 pieces (6.9 oz)	764
Frank Nuggets	7 pieces (3.2 oz)	357
Frankfurter	1 (3.2 oz)	310
French Fries	1 serv (8.6 oz)	514
Fried Clam Platter	1 serv (13.1 oz)	1024
Fried Clam Sandwich	1 (5.4 oz)	620
Fried Shrimp	1 serv (4.4 oz)	348
Fried Shrimp Platter	1 serv (12.6 oz)	796
Hamburger	1 (4.7 oz)	434
Knish	1 (5.9 oz)	318
Pastrami Sandwich	1 (4.1 oz)	325
Sauteed Onions	1 serv (3.5 oz)	39
Super Burger	1 (7.6 oz)	533
Turkey Sandwich	1 (4.9 oz)	270
SALADS AND SALAD BARS		
Garden Salad	1 serv (10.9 oz)	193

NEWPORT CREAMERY

BEVERAGES		
Skim Milk	1 serv (16 oz)	206
ICE CREAM		
Reduced Fat No Sugar Added Chocolate	½ cup (2.6 oz)	110
Reduced Fat No Sugar Added Coffee	½ cup (2.6 oz)	100
Soft Serve Nonfat Frozen Yogurt Cone or Dish	1 reg (5 oz)	125
SALAD DRESSINGS		
Corn Oil & Vinegar	1 tbsp	45
Fat Free Ranch	1½ oz	48
Low-Cal French	1½ oz	48
SALADS AND SALAD BARS		
Chef's Salad	1 serv	215

FOOD	PORTION	CALS.
Chicken Fajita	1 serv	295
Grilled Chicken	1 serv	247
SANDWICHES		
Lite Chicken Salad	1	379
Lite Grilled Cheese	1	274
Lite Grilled Chicken Breast Pocket	1	327
Lite Sliced Turkey	1	288
Lite Tuna Salad	1	358
Lite Vegetarian Pocket Broccoli Mushrooms Onions Peppers Cheese	1	211
Lite Vegetarian Pocket Broccoli Cheese	1	214
Lite Vegetarian Pocket Peppers Onions Mushrooms Cheese	1	230
Low Fat Cheese	1 slice	73
Mayonnaise	2 tsp	71
Smart Sides Broccoli	1 serv	23
Smart Sides Cottage Cheese	1 serv	90
Smart Sides Side Salad	1 serv	30

OLIVE GARDEN

FOOD	PORTION	CALS.
Garden Fare Apple Carmellina	1 serv (12.2 oz)	560
Garden Fare Dinner Capellini Pomodoro	1 serv (21.1 oz)	610
Garden Fare Dinner Capellini Primavera	1 serv (20.1 oz)	400
Garden Fare Dinner Capellini Primavera w/ Chicken	1 serv (23.8 oz)	560
Garden Fare Dinner Chicken Giardino	1 serv (20.6 oz)	550
Garden Fare Dinner Linguine Alla Marinara	1 serv (16.3 oz)	500
Garden Fare Dinner Penne Fra Diavolo	1 serv (14.3 oz)	420
Garden Fare Dinner Shrimp Primavera	1 serv (28.4 oz)	740
Garden Fare Lunch Capellini Pamodoro	1 serv (11.7 oz)	360
Garden Fare Lunch Capellini Primavera	1 serv (11.2 oz)	260
Garden Fare Lunch Capellini Primavera w/ Chicken	1 serv (14.9 oz)	420
Garden Fare Lunch Chicken Giardino	1 serv (12.8 oz)	360
Garden Fare Lunch Linguine Alla Marinara	1 serv (10.2 oz)	310
Garden Fare Lunch Penne Fra Diavolo	1 serv (10.2 oz)	300
Garden Fare Lunch Shrimp Primavera	1 serv (15.2 oz)	410
Minestrone Soup	1 serv (6 oz)	80

PERKINS

FOOD	PORTION	CALS.
Low Fat Brownie	1 (5.4 oz)	260
Low Fat Muffin Banana	1 (5.8 oz)	330
Low Fat Muffin Blueberry	1 (5.8 oz)	270
Low Fat Muffin Honey Bran	1 (5.8 oz)	270
Low Fat Muffin Plain	1 (5.8 oz)	300

FOOD	PORTION	CALS.
PICCADILLY CAFETERIA		
BAKED SELECTIONS		
Corn Sticks	1 (2 oz)	165
French Bread	1 slice	132
Garlic Bread	1 serv (15.8 oz)	1154
Mexican Corn Bread	1 piece	220
Roll	1 (2 oz)	130
Roll Whole Wheat	1 (1.7 oz)	117
Texas Toast	1 serv (15.5 oz)	1088
BEVERAGES		
Iced Tea	1 serv (6.5 oz)	2
Punch	1 serv (9 oz)	133
DESSERTS		
Apple Pie	1 slice (7.2 oz)	439
Cantaloupe	1 serv (9 oz)	89
Cantaloupe	1 serv (5.5 oz)	55
Chocolate Cream Pie	1 slice (7.5 oz)	512
Custard	1 cup (5.4 oz)	183
Custard Pie	1 slice (6.2 oz)	412
Dole Whip Topping	1 serv (3 oz)	68
Fresh Fruit Plate	1 serv (21.1 oz)	389
Gelatin	1 serv (4.75 oz)	128
Honeydew Melon	1 serv (5.5 oz)	55
Honeydew Melon	1 serv (9 oz)	89
Lemon Chiffon Pie	1 slice (6.3 oz)	481
Pound Cake	1 slice (3.8 oz)	371
Watermelon	1 serv (11 oz)	100
MAIN MENU SELECTIONS		
Au Jus	1 serv (3 oz)	5
Baby Lima Beans	1 serv (4.5 oz)	151
Baked Potato	1	218
Baked Potato w/ Topping	1	350
Beef Chopped Steak Fried	1 serv (4 oz)	311
Beef Leg Roast	1 serv (4 oz)	311
Beef Liver Fried	1 serv (4.5 oz)	430
Beef Tips Braised	1 serv (10 oz)	470
Black-eyed Peas w/ Pork Jowls	1 serv (4 oz)	108
Broccoli Buttered	1 serv (4 oz)	77
Broccoli & Rice Au Gratin	½ cup	184
Carrots Young Buttered	½ cup	90
Cauliflower Buttered	1 serv	80
Chicken Baked w/o Skin	¼ chicken	352
Chicken Teriyaki	1 serv (4 oz)	445

FOOD	PORTION	CALS.
Chicken Teriyaki Polynesian	1 serv (4 oz)	537
Corn	1 serv (4.5 oz)	128
Cornbread Stuffing	1 serv (4.5 oz)	164
Crackers	4 (0.4 oz)	51
Cranberry Sauce	1 serv (1.5 oz)	64
Eggplant Escalloped	½ cup	180
Fish Baked	1 serv (7 oz)	195
Green Beans	1 serv (4.5 oz)	77
Ham Baked	1 serv (4 oz)	224
Macaroni & Cheese	½ cup	317
Mashed Potatoes	1 serv (4.8 oz)	120
Meatballs Baked & Spaghetti	1 serv (11.5 oz)	108
New Potatoes Boiled	½ cup	148
Okra Smothered	1 serv (4 oz)	121
Onion Sauce	1 serv (4 oz)	152
Rice	½ cup	99
Rice Polynesian	1 serv (4 oz)	140
Spaghetti Baked	1 serv (9.5 oz)	256
Squash Baked Italian	1 serv (4.75 oz)	73
Squash Mixed Yellow & Zucchini	1 serv (4 oz)	72
Squash Yellow Baked French Style	⅓ cup	86
Turkey Breast	1 serv (3 oz)	99
Vegetables Unseasoned	1 serv (5 oz)	29
SALADS AND SALAD BARS		
Broccoli Salad	1 serv (4 oz)	202
Cabbage Combination Salad	1 serv (4.5 oz)	50
Carrot & Raisin Salad	1 serv (4.5 oz)	321
Cole Slaw w/ Cream	1 serv (4 oz)	182
Cucumber & Celery Salad	1 serv (4 oz)	82
Fruit Salad	1 serv (6 oz)	59
Neptune Salad	1 serv	361
Spinach Tossed Salad	1 serv (4 oz)	88
Spring Salad Bowl	1 serv (4 oz)	22
SOUPS		
Gumbo Chicken	1 serv (8 oz)	92
Gumbo Seafood	1 serv (8 oz)	98
Vegetable	1 serv (8 oz)	49

PIZZA HUT
MAIN MENU SELECTIONS

Bread Stick	1 (1.3 oz)	130
Bread Stick Dipping Sauce	1 serv (1.2 oz)	30
Cavatini Pasta	1 serv (12.5 oz)	480
Cavatini Supreme Pasta	1 serv (13.9 oz)	560

FOOD	PORTION	CALS.
Garlic Bread	1 slice (1.3 oz)	150
Ham & Cheese Sandwich	1 (9.7 oz)	550
Hot Buffalo Wings	4 pieces (2.1 oz)	210
Spaghetti Marinara	1 serv (16.6 oz)	490
Spaghetti Meat Sauce	1 serv (16.4 oz)	600
Spaghetti Meatballs	1 serv (18.8 oz)	850
Supreme Sandwich	1 (10.2 oz)	640
Wild Buffalo Wings	5 pieces (2.9 oz)	200
PIZZA		
Beef Topping Hand Tossed	1 slice (3.9 oz)	280
Beef Topping Pan	1 slice (3.9 oz)	310
Beef Topping Stuffed Crust	1 slice (5.6 oz)	410
Beef Topping Thin 'N Crispy	1 slice (3.1 oz)	240
Cheese Hand Tossed	1 slice (3.9 oz)	280
Cheese Pan	1 slice (3.9 oz)	300
Cheese Stuffed Crust	1 slice (5.4 oz)	380
Cheese Thin'N Crispy	1 slice (2.6oz)	210
Chicken Supreme Pan	1 slice (4.1 oz)	280
Chicken Supreme Stuffed Crust	1 slice (6.4 oz)	390
Chicken Supreme Thin 'N Crispy	1 slice (4.2 oz)	240
Dessert Apple	1 slice (2.8 oz)	250
Dessert Cherry	1 slice (2.8 oz)	250
Ham Hand Tossed	1 slice (3.4 oz)	230
Ham Pan	1 slice (3.4 oz)	250
Ham Stuffed Crust	1 slice (5.4 oz)	380
Ham Thin 'N Crispy	1 slice (2.4 oz)	190
Italian Sausage Hand Tossed	1 slice (4 oz)	300
Italian Sausage Pan	1 slice (4.3 oz)	350
Italian Sausage Stuffed Crust	1 slice (5.7 oz)	430
Italian Sausage Thin 'N Crispy	1 slice (3.4 oz)	300
Meat Lover's Hand Tossed	1 slice (3.9 oz)	290
Meat Lover's Pan	1 slice (4.4 oz)	360
Meat Lover's Stuffed Crust	1 slice (6.6 oz)	500
Meat Lover's Thin 'N Crispy	1 slice (3.7 oz)	310
Pepperoni Hand Tossed	1 slice (3.4 oz)	260
Pepperoni Lover's Hand Tossed	1 slice (4 oz)	320
Pepperoni Lover's Pan	1 slice (4.1 oz)	350
Pepperoni Lover's Stuffed Crust	1 slice (6.1 oz)	480
Pepperoni Lover's Thin 'N Crispy	1 slice (3.1 oz)	270
Pepperoni Pan	1 slice (3.4 oz)	280
Pepperoni Stuffed Crust	1 slice (5.3 oz)	410
Pepperoni Thin 'N Crispy	1 slice (2.3 oz)	220
Personal Pan Cheese	1 pie (8.1 oz)	630
Personal Pan Pepperoni	1 pie (8.1 oz)	670

FOOD	PORTION	CALS.
Personal Pan Supreme	1 pie (9.5 oz)	710
Pork Topping Hand Tossed	1 slice (3.9 oz)	290
Pork Topping Pan	1 slice (3.6 oz)	300
Pork Topping Stuffed Crust	1 slice (5.6 oz)	420
Pork Topping Thin 'N Crispy	1 slice (3.2 oz)	270
Super Supreme Hand Tossed	1 slice (4.7 oz)	290
Super Supreme Pan	1 slice (4.6 oz)	340
Super Supreme Stuffed Crust	1 slice (7.2 oz)	470
Super Supreme Thin 'N Crispy	1 slice (4 oz)	280
Supreme Hand Tossed	1 slice (3.9 oz)	270
Supreme Pan	1 slice (4 oz)	300
Supreme Stuffed Crust	1 slice (6.4 oz)	440
Supreme Thin 'N Crispy	1 slice (3.4 oz)	250
Veggie Lover's Hand Tossed	1 slice (4 oz)	240
Veggie Lover's Pan	1 slice (3.9 oz)	240
Veggie Lover's Stuffed Crust	1 slice (5.9 oz)	390
Veggie Lover's Thin 'N Crispy	1 slice (2.6 oz)	170

POLLO TROPICAL
(see TropiGrill)

POPEYE'S

Apple Pie	1 serv (3.1 oz)	290
Biscuit	1 serv (2.3 oz)	250
Breast Mild	1 (3.7 oz)	270
Breast Spicy	1 (3.7 oz)	270
Cajun Rice	1 serv (3.9 oz)	150
Cole Slaw	1 serv (4 oz)	149
Corn On The Cob	1 serv (5.2 oz)	127
French Fries	1 serv (3 oz)	240
Leg Mild	1 (1.7 oz)	120
Leg Spicy	1 (1.7 oz)	120
Nuggets	1 serv (4.2 oz)	410
Nuggets Mild Tender	1 (1.2 oz)	110
Nuggets Spicy Tender	1 (1.2 oz)	110
Onion Rings	1 serv (3.1 oz)	310
Potatoes & Gravy	1 serv (3.8 oz)	100
Red Beans & Rice	1 serv (5.9 oz)	270
Shrimp	1 serv (2.8 oz)	250
Thigh Mild	1 (3.1 oz)	300
Thigh Spicy	1 (3.1 oz)	300
Wing Mild	1 (1.6 oz)	160
Wing Spicy	1 (1.6 oz)	160

PUDGIE'S FAMOUS CHICKEN

Fried Chicken	3.5 oz	233

FOOD	PORTION	CALS.
QUINCY'S		
BAKED SELECTIONS		
Banana Nut Bread	1 serv (2 oz)	165
Biscuit	1 (2.5 oz)	270
Cornbread	1 serv (2 oz)	140
Yeast Roll	1 (2 oz)	160
BREAKFAST SELECTIONS		
Bacon	1 serv (0.25 oz)	35
Corned Beef Hash	1 serv (4.5 oz)	210
Country Ham	1 serv (1.5 oz)	90
Escalloped Apples	1 serv (3.5 oz)	120
Oatmeal	1 serv (1 oz)	175
Pancakes	1 (1.5 oz)	95
Sausage Gravy	1 serv (4 oz)	70
Sausage Links	1 (2 oz)	225
Sausage Patties	1 (2 oz)	230
Scrambled Eggs	1 serv (2 oz)	95
Steak Fingers	1 serv (3.5 oz)	360
Syrup	1 oz	75
DESSERTS		
Banana Pudding	1 serv (5 oz)	240
Brownie Pudding Cake	1 serv (4 oz)	310
Caramel Topping	1 serv (1 oz)	105
Chocolate Chip Cookies	1 (0.5 oz)	60
Cobbler Apple	1 serv (6 oz)	255
Cobbler Cherry	1 serv (6 oz)	410
Cobbler Peach	1 serv (6 oz)	305
Frozen Yogurt	1 serv (4 oz)	135
Fudge Topping	1 serv (1 oz)	105
Sugar Cookie	1 (0.5 oz)	60
MAIN MENU SELECTIONS		
1/3 Pound Hamburger	1 serv (8 oz)	565
BBQ Beans	1 serv (4 oz)	114
Bacon Cheese Burger	1 (9 oz)	663
Baked Potato	1 (6 oz)	115
Broccoli	1 serv (4 oz)	34
Cheese Sauce	1 serv (1 oz)	58
Chopped Steak Steak	1 serv (8 oz)	499
Cinnamon Apples	1 serv (4 oz)	172
Corn	1 serv (4 oz)	96
Country Steak w/ Gravy	1 serv (8 oz)	530
Cowboy Steak	1 serv (14 oz)	580
Filet w/ Bacon	1 serv (8 oz)	340

FOOD	PORTION	CALS.
Green Beans	1 serv (4 oz)	61
Grilled Chicken	1 reg serv (5 oz)	120
Grilled Chicken Sandwich	1 (9 oz)	324
Grilled Salmon	1 serv (7 oz)	228
Homestyle Chicken Fillet	1 serv (3 oz)	217
Junior Sirloin Steak	1 serv (5.5 oz)	194
Large Sirloin Steak	1 serv (10 oz)	368
Mashed Potatoes	1 serv (4 oz)	54
NY Strip Steak	1 serv (10 oz)	450
Philly Cheese Steak	1 serv (11 oz)	588
Porterhouse Steak	1 serv (17 oz)	683
Regular Sirloin Steak	1 serv (8 oz)	285
Ribeye Steak	1 serv (10 oz)	452
Rice Pilaf	1 serv (4 oz)	119
Roasted BBQ Chicken	1 serv (14 oz)	941
Roasted Herb Chicken	1 serv (14 oz)	875
Sirloin Tips w/ Mushroom Gravy	1 serv (6 oz)	196
Sirloin Tips w/ Peppers & Onions	1 serv (5 oz)	203
Smothered Steak Sandwich	1 (9 oz)	429
Smothered Strip Steak	1 serv (10 oz)	622
Southern Breaded Shrimp	1 serv (7 oz)	546
Spicy BBQ Chicken Sandwich	1 (10 oz)	368
Steak & Shrimp	1 serv (9 oz)	677
Steak Fries	1 serv (4 oz)	358
T-Bone Steak	1 serv (13 oz)	521
SALAD DRESSINGS		
Blue Cheese	1 serv (1 oz)	155
French	1 serv (1 oz)	125
Honey Mustard	1 serv (1 oz)	100
Italian	1 serv (1 oz)	135
Light Creamy Italian	1 serv (1 oz)	65
Light French	1 serv (1 oz)	85
Light Italian	1 serv (1 oz)	20
Light Thousand Island	1 serv (1 oz)	65
Parmesan Peppercorn	1 serv (1 oz)	150
Ranch	1 serv (1 oz)	110
SOUPS		
Chili With Beans	1 serv (6 oz)	235
Clam Chowder	1 serv (6 oz)	180
Cream Of Broccoli	1 serv (6 oz)	170
Vegetable Beef	1 serv (6 oz)	90

RALLY'S
BEVERAGES

Coke	1 serv (20 oz)	177

FOOD	PORTION	CALS.
Coke	1 serv (32 oz)	264
Coke	1 serv (42 oz)	372
Coke	1 serv (16 oz)	132
Diet Coke	1 serv (32 oz)	1
Diet Coke	1 serv (42 oz)	2
Diet Coke	1 serv (20 oz)	1
Fanta Orange	1 serv (42 oz)	424
Fanta Orange	1 serv (20 oz)	202
Fanta Orange	1 serv (32 oz)	301
Fanta Orange	1 serv (16 oz)	150
Mr. Pibb	1 serv (42 oz)	334
Mr. Pibb	1 serv (32 oz)	237
Mr. Pibb	1 serv (16 oz)	113
Mr. Pibb	1 serv (20 oz)	159
Root Beer	1 serv (32 oz)	294
Root Beer	1 serv (20 oz)	197
Root Beer	1 serv (42 oz)	414
Root Beer	1 serv (16 oz)	146
Shake Banana	1 serv	399
Shake Chocolate	1 serv	411
Shake Strawberry	1 serv	399
Shake Vanilla	1 serv	320
Sprite	1 serv (16 oz)	132
Sprite	1 serv (20 oz)	161
Sprite	1 serv (32 oz)	264
Sprite	1 serv (42 oz)	338
MAIN MENU SELECTIONS		
Big Buford	1	743
Chicken Fillet Sandwich	1	399
Chili w/ Cheese & Onion	1 serv (13 oz)	669
Chili w/ Cheese & Onion	1 serv (7 oz)	360
French Fries	1 reg (4 oz)	211
French Fries	1 lg (6 oz)	317
French Fries	1 extra lg (8 oz)	423
Onion Rings	1 serv	210
Rallyburger	1	433
Rallyburger w/ Cheese	1	488
Spicy Chicken Sandwich	1	437
Super Barbecue Bacon	1	593
Super Double Cheeseburger	1	762

RAX
BEVERAGES

Chocolate Shake	1 (11 fl oz)	445

FOOD	PORTION	CALS.
Coke	16 fl oz	205
Diet Coke	16 fl oz	1
DESSERTS		
Chocolate Chip Cookie	1 (2 oz)	262
MAIN MENU SELECTIONS		
Bacon	1 slice (0.1 oz)	14
Baked Potato	1 (10 oz)	264
Baked Potato w/ 1 Tbsp Margarine	1 (10.5 oz)	364
Barbecue Sauce	1 pkg (0.4 oz)	11
Beef Bacon 'N Cheddar	1 (6.7 oz)	523
Cheddar Cheese Sauce	1 fl oz	29
Country Fried Chicken Breast Sandwich	1 (7.4 oz)	618
Deluxe Roast Beef	1 (7.9 oz)	498
French Fries	1 serv (3.25 oz)	282
Grilled Chicken Breast Sandwich	1 (6.9 oz)	402
Grilled Chicken Garden Salad w/ French Dressing	1 serv (12.7 oz)	477
Grilled Chicken Garden Salad w/ Lite Italian Dressing	1 serv (12.7 oz)	264
Mushroom Sauce	1 fl oz	16
Philly Melt	1 (8.2 oz)	396
Regular Rax	1 (4.7 oz)	262
Swiss Slice	1 slice (0.4 oz)	42
SALAD DRESSINGS		
French	2 fl oz	275
Lite Italian	2 fl oz	63
SALADS AND SALAD BARS		
Gourmet Garden Salad w/ French Dressing	1 serv (10.7 oz)	409
Gourmet Garden Salad w/ Lite Italian Dressing	1 serv (10.7 oz)	305
Gourmet Garden Salad w/o Dressing	1 serv (8.7 oz)	134
Grilled Chicken Garden Salad w/o Dressing	1 serv (10.7 oz)	202

RED LOBSTER
CHILDREN'S MENU SELECTIONS

FOOD	PORTION	CALS.
Cheeseburger	1 serv	1040
Fried Chicken Fingers	1 serv	680
Fried Shrimp	1 serv	650
Grilled Chicken Teneders	1 serv	580
Hamburger	1 serv	920
Popcorn Shrimp	1 serv	650
Popcorn Shrimp & Cheesesticks	1 serv	750
Spaghetti & Cheesesticks	1 serv	830
DESSERTS		
Carrot Cake	1 serv (6.5 oz)	730

FOOD	PORTION	CALS.
Cheesecake	1 serv (5.5 oz)	530
Fudge Overboard	1 serv	620
Ice Cream	1 serv (4.5 oz)	140
Key Lime Pie	1 serv (5 oz)	450
Raspberry Cobbler	1 serv (3 oz)	530
Sensational 7	1 serv	790
MAIN MENU SELECTIONS		
Admiral's Feast	1 serv	1060
Appetizer Calamari	1 serv	350
Appetizer Chicken Fingers	1 serv	390
Appetizer Chilled Shrimp In The Shell	1 serv (6 oz)	110
Appetizer Crab & Shrimp Cakes	1 serv	480
Appetizer Crab Add-On	1 serv	60
Appetizer Fresh Fried Mushrooms	1 serv	790
Appetizer Lobster Quesadilla	1 serv	760
Appetizer Lobster Stuffed Mushroom	1 serv	400
Appetizer Mozzarella Cheesesticks	1 serv	730
Appetizer Parmesan Zucchini	1 serv	620
Appetizer Shrimp Cocktail	1 serv	50
Appetizer Stuffed Mushrooms	1 serv	420
Applesauce	1 serv (4 oz)	90
Atlantic Cod	1 serv (8 oz)	200
Atlantic Cod	1 lunch serv (5 oz)	110
Atlantic Salmon	1 lunch serv (5 oz)	200
Atlantic Salmon	1 serv (8 oz)	340
Baked Atlantic Cod	1 serv	220
Baked Atlantic Haddock	1 serv	220
Baked Flounder	1 lunch serv	190
Baked Potato	1 (8 oz)	130
Broccoli	1 serv (3 oz)	25
Broiled Fisherman's Platter	1 serv	600
Broiled Rock Lobster Tail	1 tail	190
Broiled Seafarer's Platter	1 serv	450
Caesar Salad w/ Dressing	1 serv	240
Catfish	1 serv (8 oz)	220
Catfish	1 lunch serv (5 oz)	130
Catfish Santa Fe	1 serv	340
Catfish Sante Fe	1 lunch serv	180
Chicken Fingers	1 lunch serv	390
Chicken Fresco	1 serv	1320
Chicken Fresco	1 lunch serv	660
Clam Strips	1 serv	720
Clam Strips	1 lunch serv	360
Cocktail Sauce	1 oz	30

FOOD	PORTION	CALS.
Cole Slaw	1 serv (4 oz)	190
Crab Alfredo	1 serv	1170
Crab Alfredo	1 lunch serv	590
Fish & Shrimp Combo	1 serv	730
Fish Nuggets	1 lunch serv	320
Fish Seasoning Add On For Blackened Dinner	1 serv	70
Fish Seasoning Add On For Blackened Lunch	1 serv	50
Fish Seasoning Add On For Broiled Dinner	1 serv	45
Fish Seasoning Add On For Broiled Lunch	1 serv	35
Fish Seasoning Add On For Grilled Dinner	1 serv	35
Fish Seasoning Add On For Grilled Lunch	1 serv	25
Fish Seasoning Add On For Lemon Pepper Dinner	1 serv	35
Fish Seasoning Add On For Lemon Pepper Lunch	1 serv	30
Fish Seasoning Add On For Sante Fe Style Dinner	1 serv	60
Fish Seasoning Add On For Sante Fe Style Lunch	1 serv	40
Flounder	1 lunch serv (5 oz)	130
Flounder	1 serv (8 oz)	220
French Fries	1 serv (4 oz)	350
Fried Flounder	1 lunch serv	230
Fried Shrimp	1 lunch serv	270
Fried Shrimp	12 lg	500
Garden Salad w/o Dressing	1 serv	50
Garlic Cheese Biscuit	1	140
Grilled Cheeseburger	1	580
Grilled Chicken Breasts	1 serv	230
Grilled Chicken Salad w/o Dressing	1 serv	320
Grouper	1 lunch serv (5 oz)	130
Grouper	1 serv (8 oz)	220
Haddock	1 serv (8 oz)	210
Haddock	1 lunch serv (5 oz)	120
Halibut	1 lunch serv (5 oz)	150
Halibut	1 serv (8 oz)	260
King Salmon	1 lunch serv (5 oz)	250
King Salmon	1 serv (8 oz)	420
Lake Trout	1 lunch serv (5 oz)	200
Lake Trout	1 serv (8 oz)	340
Lemon Pepper Grilled Maki Mahi	1 serv	240
Lobster Shrimp & Scallop Scampi	1 lunch serv	430
Lobster Shrimp & Scallop Scampi	1 serv	870
Mahi Mahi	1 lunch serv (5 oz)	130

FOOD	PORTION	CALS.
Mahi Mahi	1 serv (8 oz)	220
Maine Lobster Steamed	1 serv (1.25 lb)	160
Maine Lobster Stuffed	1 serv (2 lb)	430
Marinara Sauce	1 serv	50
Melted Butter	1 oz	200
Neptune's Feast	1 serv	1210
New York Strip Steak	1 serv	560
Perch	1 serv (8 oz)	220
Perch	1 lunch serv (5 oz)	130
Pollack	1 lunch serv (5 oz)	120
Pollock	1 serv (8 oz)	120
Popcorn Shrimp	1 lunch serv	380
Popcorn Shrimp	1 serv	580
Red Rockfish	1 lunch serv (5 oz)	130
Red Rockfish	1 serv (8 oz)	230
Red Snapper	1 lunch serv (5 oz)	140
Red Snapper	1 serv (8 oz)	240
Rice Pilaf	1 serv (4 oz)	180
Roasted Vegetables	1 serv (6 oz)	120
Roasted Vegetables	1 lunch serv (4 oz)	80
Sailor's Platter	1 lunch serv	250
Sandwich Blackened Catfish	1	340
Sandwich Broiled Fish	1	300
Sandwich Cajun Grilled Chicken	1	370
Sandwich Classic Fish	1	520
Sandwich Grilled Chicken	1	290
Sassy Sauce	1 oz	80
Seafood Broil	1 lunch serv	310
Shrimp & Chicken	1 serv	340
Shrimp Caesar Salad w/o Dressing	1 serv	240
Shrimp Carbonara	1 serv	1290
Shrimp Carbonara	1 lunch serv	650
Shrimp Combo	1 serv	380
Shrimp Feast	1 serv	470
Shrimp Milano	1 serv	1190
Shrimp Milano	1 lunch serv	590
Shrimp Scampi	1 lunch serv	110
Smothered Chicken	1 serv	530
Snow Crab Legs	1 serv	110
Sockeye Salmon	1 lunch serv (5 oz)	240
Sockeye Salmon	1 serv (8 oz)	410
Sole	1 serv (8 oz)	220
Sole	1 lunch serv (5 oz)	130
Soup Bread Salad w/o Dressing	1 lunch serv	430

FOOD	PORTION	CALS.
Steak & Fried Shrimp	1 serv	780
Steak & Rock Lobster Tail	1 serv	570
Swordfish	1 serv (8 oz)	290
Swordfish	1 lunch serv (5 oz)	170
Tartar Sauce	1 oz	160
Teriyaki Grilled Chicken Breast	1 serv	240
Twice Baked Potato	1	430
Walleye	1 serv (8 oz)	210
Walleye	1 lunch serv (5 oz)	120
Yellow Lake Perch	1 serv (8 oz)	220
Yellow Lake Perch	1 lunch serv (5 oz)	130
SALAD DRESSINGS		
Blue Cheese	1 serv	170
Buttermilk Ranch	1 serv	110
Caesar	1 serv	170
Dijon Honey Mustard	1 serv	140
Fat Free Ranch	1 serv	50
Lite Red Wine Vinaigrette	1 serv	50
SOUPS		
Bayou Style Gumbo	1 serv (6 oz)	120
Broccoli Cheese	1 serv	160
Clam Chowder	1 serv (6 oz)	130

ROY ROGERS
BEVERAGES

FOOD	PORTION	CALS.
Orange Juice	11 fl oz	140
BREAKFAST SELECTIONS		
3 Pancakes	1 serv (4.8 oz)	280
3 Pancakes w/ 1 Sausage	1 serv (6.2 oz)	430
3 Pancakes w/ 2 Bacon	1 serv (5.3 oz)	350
Bagel Cinnamon Raisin	1 (4 oz)	300
Bagel Plain	1 (4 oz)	300
Big Country Platters w/ Bacon	1 serv (7.6 oz)	740
Big Country Platters w/ Ham	1 serv (9.4 oz)	710
Big Country Platters w/ Sausage	1 serv (9.6 oz)	920
Biscuit	1 (2.9 oz)	390
Biscuit Bacon	1 (3.1 oz)	420
Biscuit Bacon & Egg	1 (4.2 oz)	470
Biscuit Cinnamon 'N' Raisin	1 (2.8 oz)	370
Biscuit Ham & Cheese	1 (4.5 oz)	450
Biscuit Ham & Egg	1 (5.1 oz)	460
Biscuit Ham, Egg & Cheese	1 (5.6 oz)	500
Biscuit Sausage	1 (4.1 oz)	510
Biscuit Sausage & Egg	1 (5.2 oz)	560

FOOD	PORTION	CALS.
Hashrounds	1 serv (2.8 oz)	230
Sourdough Ham, Egg & Cheese	1 (6.8 oz)	480
DESSERTS		
Strawberry Shortcake	1 serv (6.6 oz)	480
ICE CREAM		
Ice Cream Cone	1 (4.1 oz)	180
Sundae Hot Fudge	1 (6 oz)	320
Sundae Strawberry	1 (5.5 oz)	260
MAIN MENU SELECTIONS		
¼ Cheeseburger	1 (6 oz)	510
¼ Hamburger	1 (5.5 oz)	460
¼ Roaster Dark Meat	7.4 oz	490
¼ Roaster Dark Meat w/ Skin Off	4 oz	190
¼ Roaster White Meat	8.6 oz	500
¼ Roaster White Meat w/ Skin Off	4.7 oz	190
Bacon Cheeseburger	1 (5.9 oz)	520
Baked Beans	1 serv (5 oz)	160
Baked Potato	1 (3.9 oz)	130
Baked Potato w/ Margarine	1 (4.4 oz)	240
Baked Potato w/ Margarine & Sour Cream	1 (5.4 oz)	300
Cheeseburger	1 (4.2 oz)	300
Chicken Fillet Sandwich	1 (8.3 oz)	500
Cole Slaw	1 serv (5 oz)	295
Cornbread	1 serv (2.7 oz)	310
Fisherman's Fillet	1 (6.5 oz)	490
Fried Chicken Breast	1 (5.2 oz)	370
Fried Chicken Leg	1 (2.4 oz)	170
Fried Chicken Thigh	1 (4.2 oz)	330
Fried Chicken Wing	1 (2.3 oz)	200
Fry	1 lg (6.1 oz)	430
Fry	1 reg (5 oz)	350
Gravy	1 serv (1.5 fl oz)	20
Grilled Chicken Sandwich	1 (8.3 oz)	340
Hamburger	1 (3.8 oz)	260
Mashed Potatoes	1 serv (5 oz)	92
Nuggets	6 (4 oz)	290
Nuggets	9 (6.2 oz)	460
Pizza	1 serv (4.75 oz)	282
Roast Beef Sandwich	1 (5.7 oz)	260
Sourdough Bacon Cheeseburger	1 (9.1 oz)	770
Sourdough Grilled Chicken	1 (10.1 oz)	500
SALADS AND SALAD BARS		
Garden Salad	1 (9.3 oz)	190
Grilled Chicken Salad	1 serv (9.8 oz)	120
Side Salad	1 (4.9 oz)	20

FOOD	PORTION	CALS.
SCHLOTZSKY'S DELI		
PIZZA		
Chicken & Pesto	1	634
Onion & Mushroom	1	577
Smoked Turkey & Jalapeno	1	589
Vegetarian	1	555
SALAD AND SALAD BARS		
Chicken Chef	1 serv	192
Turkey Club	1 serv	233
SANDWICHES		
Chicken Breast	1 sm	514
Dijon Chicken Breast	1 sm	469
Smoked Turkey	1 sm	510
The Original	1 sm	598
SOUPS		
Creole Vegetable	1 serv (8 fl oz)	120
Red Bean	1 serv (8 fl oz)	110
Shrimp & Okra	1 serv (8 fl oz)	100
Spicy Chicken	1 serv (8 fl oz)	120
SHAKEY'S		
MAIN MENU SELECTIONS		
3 Piece Fried Chicken And Potatoes	1 serv	947
5 Piece Fried Chicken And Potatoes	1 serv	1700
Hot Ham And Cheese	1	550
Potatoes	15 pieces	950
Spaghetti With Meat Sauce And Garlic Bread	1 serv	940
PIZZA		
Thick Crust Cheese	1 slice	170
Thick Crust Green Pepper, Black Olives, Mushrooms	1 slice	162
Thick Crust Pepperoni	1 slice	185
Thick Crust Sausage, Mushrooms	1 slice	179
Thick Crust Sausage, Pepperoni	1 slice	177
Thick Crust Shakey's Special	1 slice	208
Thin Crust Cheese	1 slice	133
Thin Crust Onion, Green Pepper, Black Olives, Mushrooms	1 slice	125
Thin Crust Pepperoni	1 slice	148
Thin Crust Sausage, Mushroom	1 slice	141
Thin Crust Sausage, Pepperoni	1 slice	166
Thin Crust Shakey's Special	1 slice	171
SHONEY'S		
BEVERAGES		
Clear Soda	1 sm	52

FOOD	PORTION	CALS.
Clear Soda	1 lg	105
Coffee Regular & Decaf	1 cup	8
Cola	1 sm	69
Cola	1 lg	139
Creamer	3/8 oz	14
Hot Chocolate	1 cup	110
Hot Tea	1 cup	0
Milk 2%	1 cup	121
Orange Juice	4 oz	54
Sugar	1 pkg	13
BREAKFAST SELECTIONS		
100% Natural	1/2 cup	244
Ambrosia Salad	1/4 cup	75
Apple	1	81
Apple Butter	1 tbsp	37
Apple Grape Surprise	1/4 cup	19
Apple Ring	1	15
Apple sliced	1 slice	13
Bacon	1 strip	36
Beef Stick	1	43
Biscuit	1	170
Blueberries	1/4 cup	21
Blueberry Muffin	1	107
Bread Pudding	1 sq	305
Breakfast Ham	1 slice	26
Brunch Cake Apple	1 sq	160
Brunch Cake Banana	1 sq	152
Brunch Cake Carrot	1 sq	150
Brunch Cake Pineapple	1 sq	147
Brunch Cake Sour Cream	1 sq	160
Buttered Toast	2 slices	163
Cantaloupe Sliced	1 slice	8
Cantaloupe diced	1/2 cup	28
Captain Crunch Berry	1/2 cup	73
Cheese Sauce	1 ladle	26
Chicken Pieces	1 piece	40
Chocolate Pudding	1/4 cup	81
Cinnamon Honey Bun	1	344
Cottage Cheese	1 tbsp	12
Cottage Fries	1/4 cup	62
Country Gravy	1/4 cup	82
Croissant	1	260
Donut Mini Cinnamon	1 (14 g)	56
DoughNugget	1	157

FOOD	PORTION	CALS.
Egg Fried	1	159
Egg Scrambled	¼ cup	95
English Muffin w/ margarine	1	140
Fluff	¼ cup	16
French Toast	1 slice	69
Fruit Delight	¼ cup	54
Fruit Topping All Flavors	1 tbsp	24
Glaced Fruit	¼ cup	51
Golden Pound Cake	1 slice	134
Grape Jelly	1 tbsp	60
Grapefruit Canned	¼ cup	24
Grapes	25	57
Grits	¼ cup	57
Hashbrowns	¼ cup	43
Home Fries	¼ cup	53
Honey Bun	1	265
Honeydew Sliced	1 slice	13
Jelly Packet	1	40
Jr. Bun Chocolate	1	141
Jr. Bun Honey	1	141
Jr. Bun Maple	1	141
Kiwi Sliced	1 slice	11
Marble Cake w/ Icing	1 slice	136
Mixed Fruit	¼ cup	37
Mushroom Topping	1 oz	25
Oleo Whipped	1 tbsp	70
Omelette Topping	1 spoonful	23
Orange	1 med	65
Orange Sections	1 section	7
Oriental Salad	¼ cup	79
Pancake	1	41
Pear	1	98
Pineapple Bits	1 tbsp	9
Pineapple Fresh Sliced	1 slice	10
Pistachio Pineapple Salad	¼ cup	98
Prunes	1 tbsp	19
Raisin Bran	½ cup	87
Raisin English Muffin w/ Margarine	1	158
Sausage Link	1	91
Sausage Patty	1	136
Sausage Rice	¼ cup	110
Shortcake	1	60
Sirloin Steak Charbroiled	6 oz	357
Smoked Sausage	1	103

FOOD	PORTION	CALS.
Snow Salad	1/4 cup	72
Strawberries	5	23
Syrup Light	1 ladle	60
Syrup Low-Cal	2.2 oz	98
Tangerine	1	37
Trix	1/2 cup	54
Waldorf Salad	1/4 cup	81
Watermelon Diced	1/2 cup	50
Watermelon Sliced	1 slice	9
Whipped Topping	1 scoop	10
CHILDREN'S MENU SELECTIONS		
Jr. Burger All-American	1 serv	234
Kid's Chicken Dinner (fried)	1 serv	244
Kid's Fish N' Chips (includes fries)	1 serv	337
Kid's Fried Shrimp	1 serv	194
Kid's Spaghetti	1 serv	247
DESSERTS		
Apple Pie A La Mode	1 slice	492
Carrot Cake	1 slice	500
Strawberry Pie	1 slice	332
Walnut Brownie A La Mode	1	576
ICE CREAM		
Hot Fudge Cake	1 slice	522
Hot Fudge Sundae	1	451
Strawberry Sundae	1	380
MAIN MENU SELECTIONS		
All-American Burger	1	501
BBQ Sauce	1 souffle cup	41
Bacon Burger	1	591
Baked Fish	1 serv	170
Baked Fish Light	1 serv	170
Baked Ham Sandwich	1	290
Baked Potato	10 oz	264
Beef Patty Light	1 serv	289
Charbroiled Chicken	1 serv	239
Charbroiled Chicken Sandwich	1	451
Chicken Fillet Sandwich	1	464
Chicken Tenders	1 serv	388
Cocktail Sauce	1 souffle cup	36
Country Fried Sandwich	1	588
Country Fried Steak	1 serv	449
Fish N' Chips (includes fries)	1 serv	639
Fish N' Shrimp	1 serv	487
Fish Sandwich	1	323

FOOD	PORTION	CALS.
French Fries	4 oz	252
French Fries	3 oz	189
Fried Fish Light	1 serv	297
Grecian Bread	1 slice	80
Grilled Bacon & Cheese Sandwich	1	440
Grilled Cheese Sandwich	1	302
Half O'Pound	1 serv	435
Ham Club On Whole Wheat	1	642
Hawaiian Chicken	1 serv	262
Italian Feast	1 serv	500
Lasagna	1 serv	297
Liver N' Onions	1 serv	411
Mushroom Swiss Burger	1	616
Old-Fashioned Burger	1	470
Onion Rings	1	52
Patty Melt	1	640
Philly Steak Sandwich	1	673
Reuben Sandwich	1	596
Ribeye	6 oz	605
Rice	3.5 oz	137
Sauteed Mushrooms	3 oz	75
Sauteed Onions	2.5 oz	37
Seafood Platter	1 serv	566
Shoney Burger	1	498
Shrimp Bite-Size	1 serv	387
Shrimp Broiled	1 serv	93
Shrimp Charbroiled	1 serv	138
Shrimp Sampler	1 serv	412
Shrimper's Feast	1 serv	383
Shrimper's Feast Large	1 serv	575
Sirloin	6 oz	357
Slim Jim Sandwich	1	484
Spaghetti	1 serv	496
Steak N' Shrimp (charbroiled shrimp)	1 serv	361
Steak N' Shrimp (fried shrimp)	1 serv	507
Sweet N' Sour Sauce	1 souffle cup	58
Tartar Sauce	1 souffle cup	84
Turkey Club On Whole Wheat	1	635
SALAD DRESSINGS		
Biscayne Lo-Cal	2 tbsp	62
Blue Cheese	2 tbsp	113
Creamy Italian	2 tbsp	135
French	2 tbsp	124
Golden Italian	2 tbsp	141

FOOD	PORTION	CALS.
Honey Mustard	2 tbsp	165
Ranch	2 tbsp	95
Rue French	2 tbsp	122
Thousand Island	2 tbsp	130
W.W. Italian	2 tbsp	10
SALADS AND SALAD BARS		
Ambrosia Salad	¼ cup	75
Apple Grape Surprise	¼ cup	19
Apple Ring	1	15
Bacon Bits	1 spoonful	15
Beet Onion Salad	¼ cup	25
Broccoli	¼ cup	4
Broccoli Cauliflower Carrot Salad	¼ cup	53
Broccoli Cauliflower Ranch	¼ cup	65
Broccoli & Cauliflower	¼ cup	98
Carrot	¼ cup	10
Carrot Apple Salad	¼ cup	99
Cauliflower	¼ cup	8
Celery	1 tbsp	5
Cheese Shredded	1 tbsp	21
Chocolate Pudding	¼ cup	81
Chow Mein Noodles	1 spoonful	13
Cole Slaw	¼ cup	69
Cottage Cheese	1 tbsp	12
Croutons	1 spoonful	13
Cucumber	1 tbsp	1
Cucumber Lite	¼ cup	12
Don's Pasta	¼ cup	82
Egg Diced	1 tbsp	15
Fruit Delight	¼ cup	54
Fruit Topping All Flavors	¼ cup	64
Glaced Fruit	¼ cup	51
Granola	1 spoonful	25
Grapefruit	¼ cup	24
Green Pepper	1 tbsp	1
Italian Vegetable	¼ cup	11
Jello	¼ cup	40
Jello Fluff	¼ cup	16
Kidney Bean Salad	¼ cup	55
Lettuce	1.8 oz	7
Macaroni Salad	¼ cup	207
Margarine Whipped	1 tsp	23
Melba Toast	2	20
Mixed Fruit Salad	¼ cup	37

FOOD	PORTION	CALS.
Mixed Squash	¼ cup	49
Mushrooms	1 tbsp	1
Oil	1 tsp	45
Olives Black	2	10
Olives Green	2	8
Onion Sliced	1 tbsp	1
Oriental Salad	¼ cup	79
Pea Salad	¼ cup	73
Pepperoni	1 tbsp	30
Pickle Chips	1 slice	5
Pickle Spear	1 spear	2
Pineapple Bits	1 tbsp	9
Pistachio Pineapple Salad	¼ cup	98
Prunes	1 tbsp	19
Radish	1 tbsp	1
Raisins	1 spoonful	26
Rotelli Pasta	¼ cup	78
Seign Salad	¼ cup	72
Snow Delight	¼ cup	72
Spaghetti Salad	¼ cup	81
Spinach	¼ cup	1
Spring Pasta	¼ cup	38
Summer Salad	¼ cup	114
Sunflower Seeds	1 spoonful	40
Three Bean Salad	¼ cup	96
Trail Mix	1 spoonful	30
Turkey Ham	1 tbsp	12
Waldorf	¼ cup	81
Wheat Bread	1 slice	71
SOUPS		
Bean	6 fl oz	63
Beef Cabbage	6 fl oz	86
Broccoli Cauliflower	6 fl oz	124
Cheddar Chowder	6 fl oz	91
Cheese Florentine Ham	6 fl oz	110
Chicken Gumbo	6 fl oz	60
Chicken Noodle	6 fl oz	62
Chicken Rice	6 fl oz	72
Clam Chowder	6 fl oz	94
Corn Chowder	6 fl oz	148
Cream Of Broccoli	6 fl oz	75
Cream Of Chicken	6 fl oz	136
Cream Of Chicken Vegetable	6 fl oz	79
Onion	6 fl oz	29

FOOD	PORTION	CALS.
Potato	6 fl oz	102
Tomato Florentine	6 fl oz	63
Tomato Vegetable	6 fl oz	46
Vegetable Beef	6 fl oz	82

SIZZLER
DESSERTS

Chocolate & Vanilla Soft Serve	4 oz	136
Chocolate Syrup	1 oz	90
Strawberry Topping	1 oz	70
Whipped Topping	1 tbsp	12

HOT BUFFET

Broccoli Cheese Soup	1 serv (4 oz)	139
Chicken Noodle Soup	1 serv (4 oz)	31
Chicken Wings	1 oz	73
Clam Chowder	1 serv (4 oz)	118
Fettucine	2 oz	80
Focaccia Bread	2 pieces	108
Marinara Sauce	1 oz	13
Meatballs	4	157
Minestrone Soup	1 serv (4 oz)	36
Nacho Cheese Soup	1 serv (4 oz)	120
Potato Skins	2 oz	160
Refried Beans	¼ cup	62
Saltine Crackers	2	25
Spaghetti	2 oz	80
Taco Filling	2 oz	103
Taco Shells	1	50
Vegetable Sirloin Soup	1 serv (4 oz)	60

MAIN MENU SELECTIONS

Buttery Dipping Sauce	1 serv (1.5 oz)	330
Cheese Toast	1 piece	273
Cocktail Sauce	1 serv (1.5 oz)	40
Dakota Ranch Steak	1 (6 oz)	316
Dakota Ranch Steak	1 (8 oz)	421
Dakota Ranch Steak	1 (9.5 oz)	500
French Fries	1 serv (4 oz)	358
Hamburger	1	626
Hibachi Chicken Breast w/ Pineapple	5 oz	193
Hibachi Sauce	1 serv (1.5 oz)	57
Lemon Herb Chicken Breast	5 oz	140
Malibu Chicken Patty	1	310
Malibu Sauce	1 serv (1.5 oz)	283
Margarine Whipped	1½ tbsp	105

FOOD	PORTION	CALS.
Potato Baked Plain	1 (4 oz)	105
Rice Pilaf	1 serv (6 oz)	256
Salmon	8 oz	110
Sante Fe Chicken Breast	5 oz	150
Shrimp Broiled	5 oz	150
Shrimp Fried	4 pieces	223
Shrimp Mini	4 oz	152
Shrimp Scampi	5 oz	143
Sour Dressing	2 tbsp	60
Swordfish	8 oz	315
Tartar Sauce	1 serv (1.5 oz)	170
SALAD DRESSINGS		
Blue Cheese	1 oz	111
Honey Mustard	1 oz	160
Italian Lite	1 oz	14
Japanese Rice Vinegar Fat Free	1 oz	10
Parmesan Italian	1 oz	100
Ranch	1 oz	120
Ranch Reduced Calorie	1 oz	90
Thousand Island	1 oz	143
SALADS AND SALAD BARS		
Alfafa Sprouts	¼ cup	2
Avocado	½	153
Bean Sprouts	¼ cup	8
Beets	¼ cup	13
Bell Peppers	2 oz	8
Broccoli	½ cup	12
Cabbage Red	¼ cup	5
Cantoupe	½ cup	28
Carrot & Raisin Salad	2 oz	130
Carrots	¼ cup	12
Chinese Chicken Salad	2 oz	54
Chives	1 oz	62
Cottage Cheese	2 oz	51
Cucumber	2 oz	7
Eggs	1 oz	44
Garbanzo Beans	¼ cup	63
Grapes	½ cup	29
Guacamole	1 oz	42
Honeydew Melon	½ cup	30
Iceberg Lettuce	1 cup	7
Jicama	2 oz	13
Kidney Beans	¼ cup	52
Kiwifruit	2 oz	35

FOOD	PORTION	CALS.
Mediterranean Minted Fruit Salad	2 oz	29
Mexican Fiesta Salad	2 oz	54
Mushrooms	¼ cup	4
Old Fashioned Potato Salad	2 oz	84
Onions Red	2 tbsp	8
Peaches	¼ cup	34
Peas	¼ cup	31
Pineapple	½ cup	38
Real Bacon Bits	1 tbsp	27
Red Herb Potato Salad	2 oz	121
Romaine Lettuce	1 cup	9
Salsa	1 oz	7
Seafood Louis Pasta Salad	2 oz	64
Seafood Salad	2 oz	56
Spicy Jicama Salad	2 oz	16
Spinach	½ cup	6
Strawberries	½ cup	22
Teriyaki Beef Salad	2 oz	49
Tomatoes Cherry	¼ cup	12
Tuna Pasta Salad	2 oz	133
Turkey Ham	1 oz	62
Watermelon	½ cup	26
Zucchini	¼ cup	5

SKIPPER'S
BEVERAGES

Coke Classic	1 (12 fl oz)	144
Coke Diet	1 (12 fl oz)	2
Milk Lowfat	1 (12 fl oz)	181
Root Beer	1 (12 fl oz)	154
Root Beer Float	1 (12 oz)	302
Sprite	1 (12 fl oz)	142

DESSERTS

Jell-O	1 serv (2.75 oz)	55

MAIN MENU SELECTIONS

Baked Fish With Margarine & Seas	1 serv (4.4 oz)	147
Baked Potato	1 (6 oz)	145
Captain's Cut	1 piece (2.6 oz)	160
Cocktail Sauce	1 tbsp	20
Coleslaw	1 serv (5 oz)	289
Corn Muffin	1 (2 oz)	91
English Style Fish	1 piece (2.4 oz)	187
French Fries	1 serv (3.5 oz)	239
Green Salad (no dressing)	1 serv (4 oz)	24

FOOD	PORTION	CALS.
Ketchup	1 tbsp	17
Margarine	1 serv (0.5 oz)	50
Shrimp Fried Cajun	1 serv (4 oz)	342
Shrimp Fried Jumbo	1 piece (.65 oz)	51
Shrimp Fried Original	1 serv (4 oz)	266
Tartar Original	1 tbsp	65
SOUPS		
Clam Chowder	1 cup (6 fl oz)	100
Clam Chowder	1 pint (12 fl oz)	200

SMOOTHIE KING

FOOD	PORTION	CALS.
Activator Banana	1 (20 oz)	429
Activator Chocolate	1 (20 oz)	429
Activator Strawberry	1 (20 oz)	559
Activator Vanilla	1 (20 oz)	429
Angel Food	1 (20 oz)	330
Blackberry Dream	1 (20 oz)	343
Caribbean Way	1 (20 oz)	392
Celestial Cherry High	1 (20 oz)	285
Coconut Surprise	1 (20 oz)	457
Cranberry Supreme	1 (20 oz)	577
Cranberry Cooler	1 (20 oz)	538
GoGuava	1 (20 oz)	300
Grape Expectations	1 (20 oz)	399
Grape Expectations II	1 (20 oz)	529
Hawaiian Cafe Au Lei	1 (20 oz)	286
High Protein Almond Mocha	1 (20 oz)	402
High Protein Banana	1 (20 oz)	412
High Protein Chocolate	1 (20 oz)	401
High Protein Lemon	1 (20 oz)	390
High Protein Pineapple	1 (20 oz)	380
Hulk Chocolate	1 (20 oz)	846
Hulk Strawberry	1 (20 oz)	953
Hulk Vanilla	1 (20 oz)	846
Immune Builder	1 (20 oz)	333
Instant Vigor	1 (20 oz)	359
Island Treat	1 (20 oz)	334
Lemon Twist Banana	1 (20 oz)	339
Lemon Twist Strawberry	1 (20 oz)	399
Light & Fluffy	1 (20 oz)	389
Malt	1 (20 oz)	887
Mo'cuccino	1 (20 oz)	440
Muscle Punch	1 (20 oz)	339
Muscle Punch Plus	1 (20 oz)	340

FOOD	PORTION	CALS.
Peach Slice	1 (20 oz)	341
Peach Slice Plus	1 (20 oz)	471
Peanut Power	1 (20 oz)	502
Peanut Power Plus Grape	1 (20 oz)	703
Peanut Power Plus Strawberry	1 (20 oz)	632
Pep Upper	1 (20 oz)	334
Pineapple Pleasure	1 (20 oz)	313
Power Punch	1 (20 oz)	430
Power Punch Plus	1 (20 oz)	499
Raspberry Sunrise	1 (20 oz)	335
Shake	1 (20 oz)	875
Slim & Trim Chocolate	1 (20 oz)	270
Slim & Trim Strawberry	1 (20 oz)	357
Slim & Trim Vanilla	1 (20 oz)	227
Super Punch	1 (20 oz)	425
Super Punch Plus	1 (20 oz)	516
Yogurt D'Lite	1 (20 oz)	341
Youth Fountain	1 (20 oz)	267

SONIC DRIVE-IN

FOOD	PORTION	CALS.
#1 Hamburger	1 (6.6 oz)	409
#2 Hamburger	1 (6.6 oz)	323
B-L-T Sandwich	1 (6.1 oz)	327
Bacon Cheeseburger	1 (7.2 oz)	548
Chicken Sandwich Breaded	1 (7.4 oz)	455
Chili Pie	1 (3.7 oz)	327
Corn Dog	1 (3 oz)	280
Extra Long Cheese Coney	1 (8.9 oz)	635
Extra Long Cheese Coney w/ Onions	1 (9.4 oz)	640
Fish Sandwich	1 (6.1 oz)	277
French Fries	1 lg (6.7 oz)	315
French Fries	1 reg (5 oz)	233
French Fries w/ Cheese	1 lg (7.7 oz)	219
Grilled Cheese Sandwich	1 (2.8 oz)	288
Grilled Chicken Sandwich w/o Dressing	1 (6.4 oz)	215
Hickory Burger	1 (5.1 oz)	314
Jalapeno Burger Double Meat & Cheese	1 (9.1 oz)	638
Mini Burger	1 (3.5 oz)	246
Mini Cheeseburger	1 (3.9 oz)	281
Onion Rings	1 reg (3.5 oz)	404
Onion Rings	1 lg (5 oz)	577
Regular Cheese Coney	1 (5 oz)	358
Regular Cheese Coney w/ Onions	1 (5.3 oz)	361
Regular Hot Dog	1 (3.5 oz)	258

FOOD	PORTION	CALS.
Steak Sandwich Breaded	1 (3.9 oz)	631
Super Sonic Burger w/ Mustard Double Meat & Cheese	1 (10.1 oz)	644
Super Sonic Burger w/ Mayo Double Meat & Cheese	1 (10.1 oz)	730
Tater Tots	1 serv (3 oz)	150
Tater Tots w/ Cheese	1 serv (3.6 oz)	220

STARBUCKS

FOOD	PORTION	CALS.
Americano Grande	1 serv	10
Americano Short	1 serv	5
Americano Tall	1 serv	5
Cappuccino Grande Lowfat Milk	1 serv	110
Cappuccino Grande Nonfat Milk	1 serv	80
Cappuccino Grande Whole Milk	1 serv	140
Cappuccino Short Lowfat Milk	1 serv	60
Cappuccino Short Nonfat Milk	1 serv	40
Cappuccino Short Whole Milk	1 serv	70
Cappuccino Tall Lowfat Milk	1 serv	80
Cappuccino Tall Nonfat Milk	1 serv	60
Cappuccino Tall Whole Milk	1 serv	110
Cocoa w/ Whipping Cream Grande Lowfat Milk	1 serv	350
Cocoa w/ Whipping Cream Grande Nonfat Milk	1 serv	310
Cocoa w/ Whipping Cream Grande Whole Milk	1 serv	400
Cocoa w/ Whipping Cream Short Lowfat Milk	1 serv	180
Cocoa w/ Whipping Cream Short Nonfat Milk	1 serv	160
Cocoa w/ Whipping Cream Short Whole Milk	1 serv	210
Cocoa w/ Whipping Cream Tall Lowfat Milk	1 serv	270
Cocoa w/ Whipping Cream Tall Nonfat Milk	1 serv	230
Cocoa w/ Whipping Cream Tall Whole Milk	1 serv	300
Drip Coffee Grande	1 serv	10
Drip Coffee Short	1 serv	5
Drip Coffee Tall	1 serv	10
Espresso Doppio	1 serv	5
Espresso Macchiato Doppio Lowfat Milk	1 serv	15
Espresso Macchiato Doppio Nonfat Milk	1 serv	15
Espresso Macchiato Doppio Whole Milk	1 serv	15
Espresso Macchiato Solo Lowfat Milk	1 serv	10
Espresso Macchiato Solo Nonfat Milk	1 serv	10
Espresso Macchiato Solo Whole Milk	1 serv	15
Espresso Solo	1 serv	5

FOOD	PORTION	CALS.
Espresso Con Panna Doppio	1 serv	45
Espresso Con Panna Solo	1 serv	40
Latte Grande Lowfat Milk	1 serv	170
Latte Grande Nonfat Milk	1 serv	130
Latte Grande Whole Milk	1 serv	220
Latte Short Lowfat Milk	1 serv	80
Latte Short Nonfat Milk	1 serv	60
Latte Short Whole Milk	1 serv	100
Latte Tall Lowfat Milk	1 serv	140
Latte Tall Nonfat Milk	1 serv	110
Latte Tall Whole Milk	1 serv	180
Latte Iced Grande Lowfat Milk	1 serv	170
Latte Iced Grande Nonfat Milk	1 serv	130
Latte Iced Grande Whole Milk	1 serv	210
Latte Iced Short Lowfat Milk	1 serv	90
Latte Iced Short Nonfat Milk	1 serv	70
Latte Iced Short Whole Milk	1 serv	120
Latte Iced Tall Lowfat Milk	1 serv	120
Latte Iced Tall Nonfat Milk	1 serv	90
Latte Iced Tall Whole Milk	1 serv	150
Mocha w/ Whipping Cream Grande Lowfat Milk	1 serv	350
Mocha w/ Whipping Cream Grande Nonfat Milk	1 serv	310
Mocha w/ Whipping Cream Grande Whole Milk	1 serv	390
Mocha w/ Whipping Cream Short Lowfat Milk	1 serv	170
Mocha w/ Whipping Cream Short Nonfat Milk	1 serv	150
Mocha w/ Whipping Cream Short Whole Milk	1 serv	180
Mocha w/ Whipping Cream Tall Lowfat Milk	1 serv	260
Mocha w/ Whipping Cream Tall Nonfat Milk	1 serv	230
Mocha w/ Whipping Cream Tall Whole Milk	1 serv	290
Mocha w/o Whipping Cream Grande Lowfat Milk	1 serv	230
Mocha w/o Whipping Cream Grande Nonfat Milk	1 serv	190
Mocha w/o Whipping Cream Grande Whole Milk	1 serv	260
Mocha w/o Whipping Cream Short Lowfat Milk	1 serv	120
Mocha w/o Whipping Cream Short Nonfat Milk	1 serv	100

FOOD	PORTION	CALS.
Mocha w/o Whipping Cream Short Whole Milk	1 serv	150
Mocha w/o Whipping Cream Tall Lowfat Milk	1 serv	170
Mocha w/o Whipping Cream Tall Nonfat Milk	1 serv	140
Mocha w/o Whipping Cream Tall Whole Milk	1 serv	190
Mocha Syrup Grande	1 serv (2 oz)	80
Mocha Syrup Short	1 serv (1 oz)	40
Mocha Syrup Tall	1 serv (1.5 oz)	60
Steamed Lowfat Milk Grande	1 serv	180
Steamed Lowfat Milk Short	1 serv	90
Steamed Lowfat Milk Tall	1 serv	140
Steamed Nonfat Milk Grande	1 serv	130
Steamed Nonfat Milk Short	1 serv	60
Steamed Nonfat Milk Tall	1 serv	100
Steamed Whole Milk Grande	1 serv	230
Steamed Whole Milk Short	1 serv	110
Steamed Whole Milk Tall	1 serv	180
Whipping Cream Grande	1 serv (1.1 oz)	110
Whipping Cream Short	1 serv (0.7 oz)	70
Whipping Cream Tall	1 serv (0.8 oz)	80
ICE CREAM		
Biscotte Bliss	½ cup	240
Caffe Almond Fudge	½ cup	260
Caffe Almond Roast	1 bar	280
Dark Roast Expresso Swirl	½ cup	220
Frappuccino Coffee	1 bar	110
Italian Roast Coffee	½ cup	230
Javachip	½ cup	250
Low Fat Latte	½ cup	170
Low Fat Mocha Mambo	½ cup	170
Vanilla Mochachip	½ cup	270

STUFF'N TURKEY

FOOD	PORTION	CALS.
Chef's Salad	1 serv	288
Grilled Turkey Breast	1 serv	244
Homemade Turkey Salad	1 serv	651
Real Fresh Roasted Turkey Breast	1 serv	384
Rotisserie Turkey Breast	1 serv	251
Thanksgiving Dinner On A Sandwich	1 serv	605
Turkey Barbecue	1 serv	478
Turkey Powerhouse	1 serv	482

SUBWAY
COOKIES

FOOD	PORTION	CALS.
Chocolate Chip	1	210

FOOD	PORTION	CALS.
Chocolate Chip M&M	1	210
Chocolate Chunk	1	210
Double Chocolate Brazil Nut	1	230
Oatmeal Raisin	1	200
Peanut Butter	1	220
Sugar	1	230
White Chocolate Macadamia Nut	1	230
SALAD DRESSINGS		
Creamy Italian	1 tbsp	65
Fat Free French	1 tbsp	15
Fat Free Italian	1 tbsp	5
Fat Free Ranch	1 tbsp	12
French	1 tbsp	65
Ranch	1 tbsp	87
Thousand Island	1 tbsp	65
SALADS AND SALAD BARS		
B.L.T.	1 serv	140
Bread Bowl	1 serv	330
Chicken Taco	1 serv	250
Classic Italian B.M.T.	1 serv	274
Cold Cut Trio	1 serv	191
Ham	1 serv	116
Meatball	1 serv	233
Pizza	1 serv	277
Roast Beef	1 serv	117
Roasted Chicken Breast	1 serv	162
Steak & Cheese	1 serv	212
Subway Club	1 serv	126
Subway Melt	1 serv	195
Subway Seafood & Crab	1 serv	244
Subway Seafood & Crab w/ Light Mayonnaise	1 serv	161
Tuna	1 serv	356
Tuna w/ Light Mayonnaise	1 serv	205
Turkey Breast	1 serv	102
Turkey Breast & Ham	1 serv	109
Veggie Delight	1 serv	51
SANDWICHES		
6 Inch Cold Ham	1	302
6 Inch Cold Tuna w/ Light Mayonnaise	1	391
6 Inch Cold Sub B.L.T.	1	327
6 Inch Cold Sub Classic Italian B.M.T.	1	460
6 Inch Cold Sub Cold Cut Trio	1	378
6 Inch Cold Sub Roast Beef	1	303

FOOD	PORTION	CALS.
6 Inch Cold Sub Subway Club	1	312
6 Inch Cold Sub Subway Seafood & Crab	1	430
6 Inch Cold Sub Subway Seafood & Crab w/ Light Mayonniase	1	347
6 Inch Cold Sub Tuna	1	542
6 Inch Cold Sub Turkey Breast	1	289
6 Inch Cold Sub Turkey Breast & Ham	1	295
6 Inch Cold Sub Veggie Delight	1	237
6 Inch Hot Subway Melt	1	382
6 Inch Hot Sub Chicken Taco Sub	1	436
6 Inch Hot Sub Meatball	1	419
6 Inch Hot Sub Pizza Sub	1	464
6 Inch Hot Sub Roasted Chicken Breast	1	348
6 Inch Hot Sub Steak & Cheese	1	398
Bacon	2 strips	45
Cheese	2 triangles	41
Deli Sandwich Bologna	1	292
Deli Sandwich Ham	1	234
Deli Sandwich Roast Beef	1	245
Deli Sandwich Tuna	1	354
Deli Sandwich Tuna w/ Light Mayonnaise	1	279
Deli Sandwich Turkey Breast	1	235
Light Mayonnaise	1 tsp	18
Mayonnaise	1 tsp	37
Mustard	2 tsp	8
Olive Oil Blend	1 tsp	45
Vinegar	1 tsp	1

TACO BELL
BEVERAGES

FOOD	PORTION	CALS.
2% Lowfat Milk	1 serv (8 oz)	110
Coffee Black	1 serv (12 oz)	5
Diet Pepsi	1 serv (16 oz)	0
Dr. Pepper	1 serv (16 oz)	208
Lipton Iced Tea Sweetened	1 serv (16 oz)	140
Lipton Iced Tea Unsweetened	1 serv (16 oz)	0
Mountain Dew	1 serv (16 oz)	227
Orange Juice	1 serv (6 oz)	80
Pepsi Cola	1 serv (16 oz)	200
Slice	1 serv (16 oz)	200

BREAKFAST MENU SELECTIONS

FOOD	PORTION	CALS.
Breakfast Quesadilla Cheese	1 (5.5 oz)	380
Breakfast Quesadilla w/ Bacon	1 (6 oz)	450
Breakfast Quesadilla w/ Sausage	1 (6 oz)	430

FOOD	PORTION	CALS.
Country Breakfast Burrito	1 (4 oz)	270
Double Bacon & Egg Burrito	1 (6.25 oz)	480
Fiesta Breakfast Burrito	1 (3.5 oz)	280
Grande Breakfast Burrito	1 (6.25 oz)	420
Hash Brown Nuggets	1 serv (3.5 oz)	280
MAIN MENU SELECTIONS		
7-Layer Burrito	1 (10 oz)	530
BLT Soft Taco	1 (4.5 oz)	340
Bacon Cheeseburger Burrito	1 (8.5 oz)	570
Bean Burrito	1 (7 oz)	380
Big Beef Burrito Supreme	1 (10.5 oz)	520
Big Beef MexiMelt	1 (4.75 oz)	290
Big Chicken Burrito Supreme	1 (9 oz)	510
Border Sauce Fire	1 serv (0.3 oz)	0
Border Sauce Hot	1 serv (0.3 oz)	0
Border Sauce Mild	1 serv (0.3 oz)	0
Burger Sauce	1 serv (0.5 oz)	60
Burrito Supreme	1 (9 oz)	440
Cheddar Cheese	1 serv (0.25 oz)	30
Cheese Quesadilla	1 (4.25 oz)	350
Chicken Fajita Wrap	1 (8 oz)	470
Chicken Fajita Wrap Supreme	1 (9 oz)	520
Chicken Quesadilla	1 (6 oz)	410
Chicken Club Burrito	1 (8 oz)	540
Chili Cheese Burrito	1 (5 oz)	330
Choco Taco Ice Cream Dessert	1 serv (4 oz)	310
Cinnamon Twists	1 serv (1 oz)	140
Club Sauce	1 serv (0.5 oz)	80
Double Decker Taco	1 (5.75 oz)	340
Double Decker Taco Supreme	1 (7 oz)	390
Fajita Sauce	1 serv (0.5 oz)	70
Green Sauce	1 serv (1 oz)	5
Grilled Chicken Burrito	1 (7 oz)	410
Grilled Chicken Soft Taco	1 (4.5 oz)	240
Grilled Steak Soft Taco	1 (4.5 oz)	230
Grilled Steak Soft Taco Supreme	1 (5.75 oz)	290
Guacamole	1 serv (0.75 oz)	35
Mexican Pizza	1 serv (7.75 oz)	570
Mexican Rice	1 serv (4.75 oz)	190
Nacho Cheese Sauce	2 serv (2 oz)	120
Nachos	1 serv (3.5 oz)	320
Nachos Beef Beef Supreme	1 serv (7 oz)	450
Nachos Bellgrande	1 serv (11 oz)	770
Picante Sauce	1 serv (0.3 oz)	0

FOOD	PORTION	CALS.
Pico De Gallo	1 serv (0.75 oz)	5
Pintos 'n Cheese	1 serv (4.5 oz)	190
Red Sauce	1 serv (1 oz)	10
Soft Taco	1 (3.5 oz)	220
Soft Taco Supreme	1 (5 oz)	260
Sour Cream	1 serv (0.75 oz)	40
Steak Fajita Wrap	1 (8 oz)	470
Steak Fajita Wrap Supreme	1 (9 oz)	510
Taco	1 (2.75 oz)	180
Taco Supreme	1 (4 oz)	220
Taco Salad w/ Salsa	1 (19 oz)	850
Taco Salad w/ Salsa w/o Shell	1 (16.5 oz)	420
Three Cheese Blend	1 serv (0.25 oz)	25
Tostada	1 (6.25 oz)	300
Veggie Fajita Wrap	1 (8 oz)	420
Veggie Fajita Wrap Supreme	1 (9 oz)	470

TACO JOHN'S
CHILDREN'S MENU SELECTIONS

Kid's Meal Softshell Taco	1 serv (8.5 oz)	617
Kids's Meal Crispy Taco	1 serv (8 oz)	579

DESSERTS

Choco Taco	1 serv (3.5 oz)	320
Churro	1 serv (1.5 oz)	147
Flauta Apple	1 serv (2 oz)	84
Flauta Cherry	1 serv (2 oz)	143
Flauta Cream Cheese	1 serv (2 oz)	181
Italian Ice	1 serv (4 oz)	80

MAIN MENU SELECTIONS

Bean Burrito	1 (6.5 oz)	387
Beans Refried	1 serv (9.5 oz)	357
Beef Burrito	1 (6.5 oz)	449
Chicken Fajita Burrito	1 (6.25)	370
Chicken Fajita Salad w/o Dressing	1 serv (12.25 oz)	557
Chicken Fajita Softshell	1 (4.5 oz)	200
Chili	1 serv (9.25 oz)	350
Chimichanga Platter	1 serv (18 oz)	979
Combination Burrito	1 (6.5 oz)	418
Crispy Tacos	1 serv (3.25 oz)	182
Double Enchilada Platter	1 serv (18.25 oz)	967
Meat & Potato Burrito	1 (7.75 oz)	503
Mexi Rolls w/ Nacho Cheese	1 serv (9.75 oz)	863
Mexican Rice	1 serv (8 oz)	567
Nacho Cheese	1 serv (2 oz)	300

FOOD	PORTION	CALS.
Nachos	1 serv (3.5 oz)	333
Potato Oles	1 serv (4.6 oz)	363
Potato Oles	1 lg serv (6.1 oz)	484
Potato Oles Bravo	1 serv (8.9 oz)	579
Potato Oles w/ Nacho Cheese	1 serv (6.6 oz)	483
Ranch Burrito	1 (7 oz)	447
Sampler Platter	1 serv (25.5 oz)	1406
Sierra Chicken Fillet Sandwich	1 (8.5 oz)	534
Smothered Burrito Platter	1 serv (19.5 oz)	1031
Softshell Tacos	1 serv (4.25 oz)	230
Sour Cream	1 oz	60
Super Burrito	1 (8.5 oz)	465
Super Nachos	1 serv (13 oz)	919
Taco Bravo	1 serv (6.25 oz)	346
Taco Burger	1 (5 oz)	280
Taco Salad w/o Dressing	1 (12.4 oz)	584

TACOTIME

FOOD	PORTION	CALS.
Casita Burrito Meat	1 serv (12 oz)	647
Cheddar Cheese	1 serv (0.75 oz)	86
Chicken	1 serv (2.5 oz)	109
Chips	1 serv (2 oz)	266
Crisp Burriot Chicken	1 (4.75 oz)	422
Crisp Burrito Bean	1 (5.25 oz)	427
Crisp Burrito Meat	1 (5.25 oz)	552
Crisp Taco	1 (4 oz)	295
Crustos	1 serv (3.5 oz)	373
Double Soft Bean Burrito	1 (9.5 oz)	506
Double Soft Combination Burrito	1 (9.5 oz)	617
Double Soft Meat Burrito	1 serv (6.5 oz)	726
Empanada Cherry	1 (4 oz)	250
Enchilada Sauce	1 serv (1 oz)	12
Flour Tortilla 10 in	1 (2.75 oz)	213
Flour Tortilla 7 in	1 (1.75 oz)	88
Flour Tortilla 8 in	1 (1.25 oz)	107
Fried Flour Tortilla 10 in	1 (2.75 oz)	318
Fried Flour Tortilla 8 in	1 (1.4 oz)	205
Guacamole	1 serv (1 oz)	29
Hot Sauce	1 serv (1 oz)	10
Lettuce	1 serv (0.5 oz)	2
Mexi Fries	1 lg (8 oz)	532
Mexi Fries	1 reg (4 oz)	266
Mexican Dressing No Fat	1 serv (2 oz)	20
Mexican Rice	1 serv (4 oz)	159

FOOD	PORTION	CALS.
Nachos	1 serv (10.5 oz)	680
Nachos Deluxe	1 serv (15.25 oz)	1048
Natural Super Taco Meat	1 (11.25 oz)	627
Olives	1 serv (0.50 oz)	16
Quesadilla Cheese	1 serv (3.25 oz)	205
Ranchero Salsa	1 serv (2 oz)	21
Refritos	1 serv (2.5 oz)	97
Refritos	1 serv (7 oz)	326
Rolled Soft Flour Taco	1 (7 oz)	512
Shredded Beef	1 serv (2.5 oz)	70
Soft Taco Chicken	1 (7 oz)	387
Sour Cream	1 serv (1 oz)	55
Sour Cream Dressing	1 serv (1.5 oz)	137
Super Shredded Beef Soft Taco	1 (8 oz)	368
Taco Cheeseburger	1 (7.5 oz)	633
Taco Meat	1 serv (2.5 oz)	208
Taco Salad Chicken w/o Dressing	1 serv (9 oz)	370
Taco Salad w/o Dressing	1 serv (7.75 oz)	479
Taco Shell 6 in	1 (1.25 oz)	110
Thousand Island Dressing	1 serv (1 oz)	160
Tomato	1 serv (0.5 oz)	3
Tostada Delight Salad Meat	1 (9.75 oz)	628
Value Soft Bean Burrito	1 (6.75 oz)	380
Value Soft Meat Burrito	1 (6.75 oz)	491
Value Soft Taco	1 (5.25 oz)	316
Veggie Burrito	1 (11 oz)	491
Wheat Tortilla 11 in	1 (3.5 oz)	175

TCBY

FOOD	PORTION	CALS.
Hand Dipped All Flavors 96% Fat Free	½ cup (3 oz)	140
Hand Dipped All Flavors Nonfat	½ cup (2.9 oz)	120
Lowfat Ice Cream All Flavors No Sugar Added	½ cup (2.6 oz)	110
Nonfat Ice Cream All Flavors	½ cup (2.9 oz)	120
Soft Serve All Flavors 96% Fat Free	½ cup (3.4 fl oz)	140
Soft Serve All Flavors No Sugar Added Nonfat	½ cup (2.8 oz)	80
Soft Serve All Flavors Nonfat	½ cup (3.4 oz)	110
Sorbet All Flavors Nonfat & Nondairy	½ cup (3.4 oz)	100

TGI FRIDAY'S

FOOD	PORTION	CALS.
Chili Yogurt	1 serv	30
Corn Salsa	1 serv	175
Fresh Vegetable Medley w/ Potato	1 serv	470
Fresh Vegetable Medley w/ Rice	1 serv	407

FOOD	PORTION	CALS.
Friday's Gardenburger	1	445
Garden Dagwood Sandwich	1 serv	375
Pacific Coast Chicken	1 serv	415
Pacific Coast Tuna	1 serv	410
Pea Salsa	1 serv (6.4 oz)	175
Plum Sauce	1 serv	105
Salad & Baked Potato	1 serv	250
Turkey Burger	1 (9.8 oz)	410

TJ CINNAMONS

FOOD	PORTION	CALS.
Doughnuts Cake	2	454
Doughnuts Raised	2	352
Mini-Cinn Plain	1	75
Mini-Cinn With Icing	1	80
Original Gourmet Cinnamon Roll Plain	1	630
Original Gourmet Cinnamon Roll With Icing	1	686
Petite Cinnamon Roll Plain	1	185
Petite Cinnamon Roll With Icing	1	202
Sticky Bun Cinnamon Pecan	1	607
Sticky Bun Petite Cinnamon Pecan	1	255
Triple Chocolate Classic Roll Plain	1	412
Triple Chocolate Classic Roll With Icing	1	462

TROPIGRILL

(Restaurants in this chain may also be called Pollo Tropical. Menu items are the same for both.)

FOOD	PORTION	CALS.
Banana Tropical	1 serv (7.6 oz)	498
Black Beans (combo meal portion)	1 serv (4.8 oz)	153
Black Beans (side)	1 serv (8.4 oz)	269
Boiled Yuca	1 serv (12 oz)	334
Boneless Breast	1 serv (3.1 oz)	140
Cheese Potatoes	1 serv (7.4 oz)	177
Chicken ¼ Dark Meat	1 serv (4.5 oz)	298
Chicken ¼ Dark Meat w/o Skin	1 serv (3.4 oz)	170
Chicken ¼ White Meat	1 serv (5 oz)	295
Chicken ¼ White Meat w/o Skin	1 serv (3.8 oz)	167
Chicken Caesar Sandwich	1 (6.4 oz)	457
Chicken Sandwich	1 (7.9 oz)	442
Congri	1 serv (7.1 oz)	439
Vegetable Kabob	1 (3.1 oz)	106
White Rice	1 serv (6.8 oz)	341
Yellow Rice	1 serv (7 oz)	294
Yucatan Fries	1 serv (5.3 oz)	440

UNO RESTAURANT

FOOD	PORTION	CALS.
DeepDish Pizza	1 serv	770

FOOD	PORTION	CALS.
VILLAGE INN		
French Toast Cinnamon Raisin	1 serv	809
Fruit & Nut Pancakes Low Cholesterol	1 serv	936
Omelette Chcken & Cheese	1 serv	721
Omelette Fresh Veggie	1 serv	704
Omelette Mushroom & Cheese	1 serv	680
Turkey & Vegetable Scrambled Sensation	1 serv	726
WENDY'S		
BEVERAGES		
Coffee Decaffeinated Black	1 cup (6 fl oz)	0
Coffee Black	1 cup (6 fl oz)	0
Cola	11 oz	130
Diet Cola	11 oz	0
Hot Chocolate	1 cup (6 fl oz)	80
Lemon-Lime Soda	11 oz	130
Lemonade	1l oz	130
Milk 2%	1 (8 fl oz)	110
Tea Hot	1 cup (6 fl oz)	0
Tea Iced	1 cup (6 fl oz)	0
CHILDREN'S MENU SELECTIONS		
Kid's Meal Cheeseburger	1 (4.3 oz)	320
Kid's Meal Hamburger	1 (3.9 oz)	270
Kids'Meal Chicken Nuggets	4 pieces (2.1 oz)	190
DESSERTS		
Chocolate Chip Cookie	1 (2 oz)	270
Frosty Dairy Dessert	1 sm (12 oz)	330
Frosty Dairy Dessert	1 lg (20 fl oz)	540
Frosty Dairy Dessert	1 med (16 fl oz)	440
MAIN MENU SELECTIONS		
¼ lb Hamburger Patty	1 (2.6 oz)	200
2 Oz Hamburger Patty	1 (1.3 oz)	100
American Cheese	1 slice (0.6 oz)	70
American Cheese Jr.	1 slice (0.4 oz)	45
Bacon	1 strip (4 g)	20
Baked Potato Bacon & Cheese	1 (13.3 oz)	530
Baked Potato Broccoli & Cheese	1 (14.4 oz)	470
Baked Potato Cheese	1 (13.4 oz)	570
Baked Potato Chili & Cheese	1 (15.4 oz)	630
Baked Potato Plain	1 (10 oz)	310
Baked Potato Sour Cream & Chives	1 (11 oz)	380
Big Bacon Classic	1 (9.9 oz)	580
Breaded Chicken Fillet	1 (3.5 oz)	230
Breaded Chicken Sandwich	1 (7.3 oz)	440

FOOD	PORTION	CALS.
Cheddar Cheese Shredded	2 tbsp (0.6 oz)	70
Chicken Club Sandwich	1 (7.6 oz)	470
Chicken Nuggets	5 pieces (2.6 oz)	230
Chili	1 lg (12 oz)	310
Chili	1 sm (8 oz)	210
French Fries	1 Great Biggie (6.7 oz)	570
French Fries	1 sm (3.2 oz)	270
French Fries	1 Biggie (5.6 oz)	470
French Fries	1 med (4.6 oz)	390
Grilled Chicken Fillet	1 (2.9 oz)	110
Grilled Chicken Sandwich	1 (6.6 oz)	310
Honey Mustard Reduced Calorie	1 tsp (7 g)	25
Jr. Bacon Cheeseburger	1 (5.8 oz)	380
Jr. Cheeseburger	1 (4.6 oz)	320
Jr. Cheeseburger Deluxe	1 (6.3 oz)	360
Jr. Hamburger	1 (4.1 oz)	270
Kaiser Bun	1 (2.4 oz)	190
Ketchup	1 tsp (7 g)	10
Lettuce	1 leaf (0.5 oz)	0
Mayonnaise	1½ tsp (9 g)	30
Mustard	½ tsp (5 g)	5
Nuggets Sauce Barbeque	1 pkg (1 oz)	45
Nuggets Sauce Honey Mustard	1 pkg (1 oz)	130
Nuggets Sauce Sweet & Sour	1 pkg (1 oz)	50
Onion	4 rings (0.5 oz)	5
Pickles	4 slices (0.4 oz)	0
Pita Dressing Caesar Vinaigrette Reduced Fat Reduced Calorie	1 tbsp (0.6 oz)	70
Pita Dressing Garden Ranch Sauce Reduced Fat Reduced Calorie	1 tbsp (0.6 oz)	50
Plain Single	1 (4.7 oz)	360
Saltines	2 (0.2 oz)	25
Sandwich Bun	1 (2 oz)	160
Single With Everything	1 (7.7 oz)	420
Sour Cream	1 pkt (1 oz)	60
Spicy Buffalo Wing Sauce	1 pkg (1 oz)	25
Spicy Chicken Fillet	1 (3.6 oz)	210
Spicy Chicken Sandwich	1 (7.5 oz)	410
Stuffed Pita Chicken Caesar w/Dressing	1 (8.3 oz)	490
Stuffed Pita Classic Greek w/Dressing	1 (8.2 oz)	440
Stuffed Pita Garden Ranch Chicken w/ Dressing	1 (9.9 oz)	480
Stuffed Pita Garden Veggie w/ Dressing	1 (9 oz)	400
Tomatoes	1 slice (0.9 oz)	5
Whipped Margarine	1 pkg (0.5 oz)	60

FOOD	PORTION	CALS.
SALAD DRESSINGS		
Blue Cheese	2 tbsp (1 oz)	180
French	2 tbsp (1 oz)	120
French Fat Free	2 tbsp (1 oz)	35
Hidden Valley Ranch	2 tbsp (1 oz)	90
Hidden Valley Ranch Reduced Fat Reduced Calorie	2 tbsp (1 oz)	60
Italian Reduced Fat Reduced Calorie	2 tbsp (1 oz)	40
Italian Caesar	2 tbsp (1 oz)	150
Salad Oil	1 tbsp (0.5 oz)	120
Thousand Island	2 tbsp (1 oz)	90
Wine Vinegar	1 tbsp (0.5 oz)	0
SALADS AND SALAD BARS		
Applesauce	2 tbsp (1.4 oz)	30
Bacon Bits	2 tbsp (0.5 oz)	45
Bananas & Strawberry Glaze	¼ cup (1.6 oz)	30
Broccoli	¼ cup (0.5 oz)	0
Cantaloupe Sliced	1 piece (1.6 oz)	15
Carrots	¼ cup (0.6 oz)	5
Cauliflower	¼ cup (0.6 g)	0
Ceasar Side Salad w/o Dressing	1 (3.1 oz)	100
Cheese Shredded Imitation	2 tbsp (0.6 oz)	50
Chicken Salad	2 tbsp (1.2 oz)	70
Cottage Cheese	2 tbsp (1.1 oz)	30
Croutons	2 tbsp (0.2 oz)	25
Cucumbers	2 slices (0.5 oz)	0
Deluxe Garden Salad w/o Dressing	1 (9.5 oz)	110
Eggs Hard Cooked	2 tbsp (0.9 oz)	40
Green Peas	2 tbsp (0.7 oz)	15
Green Peppers	2 pieces (0.3 oz)	0
Grilled Chicken Caesar Salad w/o Dressing	1 (9.2 oz)	260
Grilled Chicken Salad w/o Dressing	1 (11.9 oz)	200
Lettuce Iceberg/Romaine	1 cup (2.6 oz)	10
Mushrooms	¼ cup (0.5 oz)	0
Orange Sliced	2 slices (1.1 oz)	15
Parmesan Blend Grated	2 tbsp (0.5 oz)	70
Pasta Salad	2 tbsp (1.2 oz)	35
Peaches Sliced	1 piece (1 oz)	15
Pepperoni Sliced	6 slices (0.2 oz)	30
Potato Salad	2 tbsp (1.3 oz)	80
Pudding Chocolate	¼ cup (1.8 oz)	70
Red Onions	3 rings (0.5 oz)	0
Side Salad w/o Dressing	1 (5.4 oz)	60
Soft Breadstick	1 (1.5 oz)	130

FOOD	PORTION	CALS.
Sunflower Seeds & Raisins	2 tbsp (0.5 oz)	80
Taco Chips	15 (1.5 oz)	210
Taco Salad w/o Dressing	1 (16.4 oz)	380
Tomatoes Wedged	1 piece (0.9 oz)	5
Turkey Ham Diced	2 tbsp (0.8 oz)	50
Watermelon Wedged	1 piece (2.2 oz)	20

WHATABURGER

BAKED SELECTIONS

Biscuit	1	280
Blueberry Muffin	1	239
Cinnamon Roll	1	320
Cookie Chocolate Chunk	1	247
Cookie White Chocolate Macadamia Nut	1	269
Fried Apple Turnover	1	215

BEVERAGES

Cherry Coke	1 reg	227
Coffee	1 sm	5
Coke Classic	1 reg	211
Creamer	1 pkg	10
Diet Coke	1 reg	2
Dr. Pepper	1 reg	207
Iced Tea	1 reg	5
Lemon Juice	1 pkg	1
Milk 2%	1 serv	113
Orange Juice	1 serv (10 oz)	140
Root Beer	1 reg	237
Shake Chocolate	1 junior	364
Shake Strawberry	1 junior	352
Shake Vanilla	1 junior	325
Sprite	1 reg	211
Sugar	1 pkg	15
Sweet And Low	1 pkg	4

BREAKFAST SELECTIONS

Biscuit w/ Bacon	1	359
Biscuit w/ Bacon Egg & Cheese	1	511
Biscuit w/ Egg & Cheese	1	434
Biscuit w/ Sausage	1	446
Biscuit w/ Sausage Egg & Cheese	1	601
Biscuit w/ Sausage Gravy	1	479
Breakfast Platter w/ Bacon	1 serv	695
Breakfast Platter w/ Sausage	1 serv	785
Breakfast On A Bun w/ Bacon	1	365
Breakfast On A Bun w/ Sausage	1	455

FOOD	PORTION	CALS.
Butter	1 pkg	36
Egg Omelette Sandwich	1	288
Grape Jelly	1 pkg	45
Hashbrown	1 serv	150
Honey	1 pkg	25
Margarine	1 pkg	25
Pancake Syrup	1 pkg	180
Pancakes	3	259
Pancakes w/ Bacon	1 serv	335
Pancakes w/ Sausage	1 serv	426
Srambled Eggs	2	189
Strawberry Jam	1 pkg	40
Taquito Bacon & Egg	1	335
MAIN MENU SELECTIONS		
Bacon	1 slice	38
Cheese Slice	1 lg	89
Cheese Slice	1 sm	46
Chicken Strips	2	120
Club Crackers	1 pkg	30
Croutons	1 pkg	30
Fajita Beef	1	326
Fajita Grilled Chicken	1	272
French Fries	1 junior	221
French Fries	1 reg	332
French Fries	1 lg	442
Garden Salad	1	56
Grilled Chicken Salad	1 serv	150
Grilled Chicken Sandwich	1	442
Grilled Chicken Sandwich w/o Bun Oil w/ Mustard	1	300
Grilled Chicken Sandwich w/o Bun Oil & Dressing	1	358
Grilled Chicken Sandwich w/o Dressing	1	385
Jalapeno Pepper	1	3
Justaburger	1	276
Ketchup	1 pkg	30
Onion Rings	1 lg	493
Onion Rings	1 reg	329
Peppered Gravy	1 serv (3 oz)	75
Picante Sauce	1 pkg	5
Taquito Potato & Egg	1	446
Taquito Sausage & Egg	1	443
Texas Toast	1 slice	147
Whataburger	1	598

FOOD	PORTION	CALS.
Whataburger Double Meat	1	823
Whataburger Jr.	1	300
Whataburger w/o bun oil	1	407
Whatacatch Sandwich	1	467
Whatachick'n Sandwich	1	501
SALAD DRESSINGS		
Low Fat Ranch	1 pkg	66
Low Fat Vinaigrette	1 pkg	37
Ranch	1 pkg	320
Thousand Island	1 pkg	160

WHITE CASTLE

Bun Only	1	74
Cheese Only	0.3 oz	31
Cheeseburger	2 (3.6 oz)	310
Fish w/o Tarter Sandwich	1	155
French Fries	1 reg	301
Grilled Chicken Sandwich	2 (4 oz)	250
Grilled Chicken Sandwich w/ Sauce	2 (4.8 oz)	290
Hamburger	2 (3.2 oz)	270
Onion Rings	1 reg	245
Sausage Sandwich	1	196
Sausage & Egg Sandwich	1	322

WINCHELL'S DONUTS

Apple Fritter	1 (4.25 oz)	580
Cinnamon Crumb	1 (2 oz)	240
Cinnamon Roll	1 (3 oz)	360
Glazed Jelly	1 (3 oz)	300
Glazed Round	1 (1.75 oz)	210
Glazed Twist	1 (1.75 oz)	210
Iced Chocolate Bar	1 (2 oz)	220
Iced Chocolate Cake	1 (2 oz)	230
Iced Chocolate Devil's Food	1 (2 oz)	240
Iced Chocolate French	1 (1.9 oz)	220
Iced Chocolate Raised	1 (1.75 oz)	210
Plain	1 (1.6 oz)	200
Plain Donut Hole	1 (0.4 oz)	50

ZUZU

Bean & Cheese Burrito Platter	1 serv	475
Beans	1 cup	210
Cheese Enchilada Platter	1 serv	395
Chicken Burrito Platter	1 serv	580
Chicken Taco Platter	1 serv	440

FOOD	PORTION	CALS.
Chicken Taco w/o Mexican Cream	1	125
Frozen Yogurt	1 serv	200
Green Salad w/o Dressing or Avocado	1	20
Grilled Chicken Salad w/o Dressing	1 serv	305
Rice	1 cup	150
Salsa Roja Epazote	¼ cup	8
Tortilla Corn	1	35
Tortilla Flour	1	60